# Management of Venous and Arterial Thrombosis

# Management of Venous and Arterial Thrombosis

Editors

**Lucia Stančiaková**
**Maha Othman**
**Peter Kubisz**

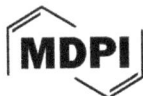

Basel • Beijing • Wuhan • Barcelona • Belgrade • Novi Sad • Cluj • Manchester

*Editors*
Lucia Stančiaková
Comenius University
in Bratislava
Martin
Slovakia

Maha Othman
Queen´s University
Kingston, ON
Canada

Peter Kubisz
Comenius University
in Bratislava
Martin
Slovakia

*Editorial Office*
MDPI
St. Alban-Anlage 66
4052 Basel, Switzerland

This is a reprint of articles from the Special Issue published online in the open access journal *Journal of Clinical Medicine* (ISSN 2077-0383) (available at: https://www.mdpi.com/journal/jcm/special_issues/venos_arterial_throm).

For citation purposes, cite each article independently as indicated on the article page online and as indicated below:

Lastname, A.A.; Lastname, B.B. Article Title. *Journal Name* **Year**, *Volume Number*, Page Range.

ISBN 978-3-7258-1179-3 (Hbk)
ISBN 978-3-7258-1180-9 (PDF)
doi.org/10.3390/books978-3-7258-1180-9

Cover image courtesy of Lucia Stančiaková

© 2024 by the authors. Articles in this book are Open Access and distributed under the Creative Commons Attribution (CC BY) license. The book as a whole is distributed by MDPI under the terms and conditions of the Creative Commons Attribution-NonCommercial-NoDerivs (CC BY-NC-ND) license.

# Contents

**Lucia Stančiaková, Maha Othman and Peter Kubisz**
Management of Venous and Arterial Thrombosis
Reprinted from: *J. Clin. Med.* **2024**, *13*, 2744, doi:10.3390/jcm13102744 . . . . . . . . . . . . . . . . . 1

**Marianna Vachalcová, Monika Jankajová, Marta Jakubová, Karolina Angela Sieradzka, Tibor Porubän, Gabriel Valočik, et al.**
Rare Source of Embolism in a Young Patient: Case Report and Literature Review
Reprinted from: *J. Clin. Med.* **2022**, *11*, 2038, doi:10.3390/jcm11072038 . . . . . . . . . . . . . . . . . 5

**Francesco Nappi, Francesca Bellomo and Sanjeet Singh Avtaar Singh**
Insights into the Role of Neutrophils and Neutrophil Extracellular Traps in Causing Cardiovascular Complications in Patients with COVID-19: A Systematic Review
Reprinted from: *J. Clin. Med.* **2022**, *11*, 2460, doi:10.3390/jcm11092460 . . . . . . . . . . . . . . . . . 11

**Antonio Leidi, Stijn Bex, Marc Righini, Amandine Berner, Olivier Grosgurin and Christophe Marti**
Risk Stratification in Patients with Acute Pulmonary Embolism: Current Evidence and Perspectives
Reprinted from: *J. Clin. Med.* **2022**, *11*, 2533, doi:10.3390/jcm11092533 . . . . . . . . . . . . . . . . . 41

**Carlos Constantin Otto, Zoltan Czigany, Daniel Heise, Philipp Bruners, Drosos Kotelis, Sven Arke Lang, et al.**
Prognostic Factors for Mortality in Acute Mesenteric Ischemia
Reprinted from: *J. Clin. Med.* **2022**, *11*, 3619, doi:10.3390/jcm11133619 . . . . . . . . . . . . . . . . . 56

**Sabina Ugovšek and Miran Šebeštjen**
Non-Lipid Effects of PCSK9 Monoclonal Antibodies on Vessel Wall
Reprinted from: *J. Clin. Med.* **2022**, *11*, 3625, doi:10.3390/jcm11133625 . . . . . . . . . . . . . . . . . 69

**Corinne Frere, Benjamin Crichi, Clémentine Wahl, Elodie Lesteven, Jérôme Connault, Cécile Durant, et al.**
The Ottawa Score Performs Poorly to Identify Cancer Patients at High Risk of Recurrent Venous Thromboembolism: Insights from the TROPIQUE Study and Updated Meta-Analysis
Reprinted from: *J. Clin. Med.* **2022**, *11*, 3729, doi:10.3390/jcm11133729 . . . . . . . . . . . . . . . . . 85

**Arkadiusz Pietrasik, Aleksandra Gąsecka, Paweł Kurzyna, Katarzyna Wrona, Szymon Darocha, Marta Banaszkiewicz, et al.**
Characteristics and Outcomes of Patients Consulted by a Multidisciplinary Pulmonary Embolism Response Team: 5-Year Experience
Reprinted from: *J. Clin. Med.* **2022**, *11*, 3812, doi:10.3390/jcm11133812 . . . . . . . . . . . . . . . . . 96

**Haixu Yu, Wei Rong, Jie Yang, Jie Lu, Ke Ma, Zhuohui Liu, et al.**
Tumor Necrosis Factor-Related Apoptosis-Inducing Ligand (TRAIL): A Novel Biomarker for Prognostic Assessment and Risk Stratification of Acute Pulmonary Embolism
Reprinted from: *J. Clin. Med.* **2022**, *11*, 3908, doi:10.3390/jcm11133908 . . . . . . . . . . . . . . . . . 110

**Claudia Minutti-Zanella, Laura Villarreal-Martínez and Guillermo J. Ruiz-Argüelles**
Primary Thrombophilia XVII: A Narrative Review of Sticky Platelet Syndrome in México
Reprinted from: *J. Clin. Med.* **2022**, *11*, 4100, doi:10.3390/jcm11144100 . . . . . . . . . . . . . . . . . 122

**Philipp Bücke, Victoria Hellstern, Alexandru Cimpoca, José E. Cohen, Thomas Horvath, Oliver Ganslandt, et al.**
Endovascular Treatment of Intracranial Vein and Venous Sinus Thrombosis—A Systematic Review
Reprinted from: *J. Clin. Med.* **2022**, *11*, 4215, doi:10.3390/jcm11144215 . . . . . . . . . . . . . . . . . . **130**

**Radhika Kiritsinh Jadav, Reza Mortazavi and Kwang Choon Yee**
Blood Biomarkers for Triaging Patients for Suspected Stroke: Every Minute Counts
Reprinted from: *J. Clin. Med.* **2022**, *11*, 4243, doi:10.3390/jcm11144243 . . . . . . . . . . . . . . . . . . **144**

**Qian Gao, Kaiyuan Zhen, Lei Xia, Wei Wang, Yaping Xu, Chaozeng Si, et al.**
Assessment of the Effect on Thromboprophylaxis with Multifaceted Quality Improvement Intervention based on Clinical Decision Support System in Hospitalized Patients: A Pilot Study
Reprinted from: *J. Clin. Med.* **2022**, *11*, 4997, doi:10.3390/jcm11174997 . . . . . . . . . . . . . . . . . . **156**

**Sarah Mubeen, Daniel Domingo-Fernández, Sara Díaz del Ser, Dhwani M. Solanki, Alpha T. Kodamullil, Martin Hofmann-Apitius, et al.**
Exploring the Complex Network of Heme-Triggered Effects on the Blood Coagulation System
Reprinted from: *J. Clin. Med.* **2022**, *11*, 5975, doi:10.3390/jcm11195975 . . . . . . . . . . . . . . . . . . **167**

**Francesco Nappi, Omar Giacinto, Mario Lusini, Marialuisa Garo, Claudio Caponio, Antonio Nenna, et al.**
Patients with Bicuspid Aortopathy and Aortic Dilatation
Reprinted from: *J. Clin. Med.* **2022**, *11*, 6002, doi:10.3390/jcm11206002 . . . . . . . . . . . . . . . . . . **183**

**Matej Samoš, Tomáš Bolek, Lucia Stančiaková, Martin Jozef Péč, Kristína Brisudová, Ingrid Škorňová, et al.**
Tailored Direct Oral Anticoagulation in Patients with Atrial Fibrillation: The Future of Oral Anticoagulation?
Reprinted from: *J. Clin. Med.* **2022**, *11*, 6369, doi:10.3390/jcm11216369 . . . . . . . . . . . . . . . . . . **211**

**Lucia Stančiaková, Jana Žolková, Ľubica Vadelová, Andrea Hornáková, Zuzana Kolková, Martin Vážan, et al.**
DNA Polymorphisms in Pregnant Women with Sticky Platelet Syndrome
Reprinted from: *J. Clin. Med.* **2022**, *11*, 6532, doi:10.3390/jcm11216532 . . . . . . . . . . . . . . . . . . **220**

**Peter Blaško, Matej Samoš, Tomáš Bolek, Lucia Stančiaková, Ingrid Škorňová, Martin Jozef Péč, et al.**
Resistance on the Latest Oral and Intravenous P2Y12 ADP Receptor Blockers in Patients with Acute Coronary Syndromes: Fact or Myth?
Reprinted from: *J. Clin. Med.* **2022**, *11*, 7211, doi:10.3390/jcm11237211 . . . . . . . . . . . . . . . . . . **239**

**Tomáš Bolek, Matej Samoš, Jakub Jurica, Lucia Stančiaková, Martin Jozef Péč, Ingrid Škorňová, et al.**
COVID-19 and the Response to Antiplatelet Therapy
Reprinted from: *J. Clin. Med.* **2023**, *12*, 2038, doi:10.3390/jcm12052038 . . . . . . . . . . . . . . . . . . **254**

**Nebojsa Antonijevic, Dragan Matic, Biljana Beleslin, Danijela Mikovic, Zaklina Lekovic, Marija Marjanovic, et al.**
The Influence of Hyperthyroidism on the Coagulation and on the Risk of Thrombosis
Reprinted from: *J. Clin. Med.* **2024**, *13*, 1756, doi:10.3390/jcm13061756 . . . . . . . . . . . . . . . . . . **264**

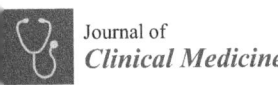

Editorial

# Management of Venous and Arterial Thrombosis

Lucia Stančiaková [1,*], Maha Othman [2] and Peter Kubisz [1,†]

1. National Centre of Haemostasis and Thrombosis, Department of Haematology and Transfusion Medicine, Jessenius Faculty of Medicine in Martin, Comenius University in Bratislava, Martin University Hospital, 036 59 Martin, Slovakia; peter.kubisz@uniba.sk
2. Department of Biomedical and Molecular Sciences, School of Medicine, Queen's University, Kingston, ON K7L 3N6, Canada; othman@queensu.ca
* Correspondence: stanciakova2@uniba.sk
† This author has passed away.

A thrombus is a hemostatic plug localized in a blood vessel. This blockage might lead to partial or complete obstruction of blood flow in arteries, veins, or microcirculation [1].

Acute myocardial infarction (MI) is mainly a consequence of coronary atherosclerosis, and it is caused by thrombotic occlusion of an arterial lumen [2]. The pathology of myocardial infarction (MI) is divided into ST-elevation MI (STE-MI) and non-ST-elevation MI (NSTE-MI). MI is a major cause of human death, and more than 3 million people develop STE-MI every year. Although the worldwide rate of MI-related mortality has decreased, the incidence of heart failure is still high [3]. Moreover, one of the complications is a thromboembolism precipitated by left-ventricular thrombosis based on chronic dysfunction in this area [4]. One of the ways of reducing the prevalence of MI-related disorders is to identify high on-treatment platelet reactivity, which is still challenging and often inaccurately identified [5].

Stroke is also a prevalent vascular disorder that leads to significant morbidity and mortality of affected individuals. Biomarkers including C-reactive protein, interleukins 6 and 10, low-density lipoprotein cholesterol, total cholesterol, and homocysteine can serve as predictors of cognitive decline after this ischemic complication [6]. Congenital heart abnormalities might contribute to microthrombi formation and valvular incompetence, potentially eventuating in embolization as well [7].

Deep venous thrombosis (DVT) is a blood clot developed in non-superficial veins. Thus, venous thromboembolism (VTE) refers to an in situ thrombus and a dislodged thrombus—an embolus occurring predominantly in the lungs and serving as a life-threatening pulmonary embolism (PE) [1]. VTE is the third-most-frequent underlying cause of death. Its incidence is estimated at 1.43 per 1000 people a year; for DVT, it is 0.93 per 1000 people a year, and for PE, it is 0.50 per 1000 people a year. Due to improvements in the diagnostics for and treatment of VTE in the last few decades, there has also been a decrease in VTE-associated deaths, plummeting from 12.8 to 6.5 deaths per 100,000 people [8]. However, VTE can lead to further clinical conditions with significant morbidity and mortality, including the extension of thrombi, recurrence, chronic thromboembolic pulmonary hypertension, and post-thrombotic syndrome [9].

One of the clinical manifestations of thrombosis at the level of microcirculation is the pregnancy loss caused by impaired placental blood flow. Such complication might be caused by various prothrombotic conditions including enhanced platelet activation playing the role in the pathogenesis of the sticky platelet syndrome [10].

A strategy consisting of D-dimer testing with a borderline increasing with age has been developed for diagnosing VTE [11]. Assessment of D-dimer levels has a high negative predictive value, with a negative test indicating an absence of thrombosis in an organism [12]. Unfortunately, an elevated concentration of D-dimers is nonspecific, especially in cancer patients. The high prevalence of VTE in this population decreases its negative

**Citation:** Stančiaková, L.; Othman, M.; Kubisz, P. Management of Venous and Arterial Thrombosis. *J. Clin. Med.* **2024**, *13*, 2744. https://doi.org/10.3390/jcm13102744

Received: 31 March 2024
Accepted: 11 April 2024
Published: 7 May 2024

**Copyright:** © 2024 by the authors. Licensee MDPI, Basel, Switzerland. This article is an open access article distributed under the terms and conditions of the Creative Commons Attribution (CC BY) license (https://creativecommons.org/licenses/by/4.0/).

predictive value and undermines pretest probability assessed via the Geneva or Wells scores otherwise used to guide evaluation for a PE [13].

The Pulmonary Embolism Severity Index (PESI) and its simplified version are designed to distill clinical information, including vital functions and comorbidities, into a risk score. The PESI score indicates increased all-cause mortality at 30 days after a diagnosis of PE. Its simplified form (sPESI) has limited specificity in predicting mortality among high-risk patients. Risk indicators for PE include serologic markers of right-ventricular dysfunction and myocardial injury, echocardiography, computed tomography pulmonary angiography (CTPA), and the evaluation of hemodynamic status via right-heart catheterization [14].

Anticoagulant drugs are used in the acute (the first week), long-term (7 days up to 3 months), and extended (3 months and longer) treatment of VTE. Anticoagulation can be managed with low-molecular-weight heparin (LMWH), fondaparinux, unfractionated heparin (UFH), direct oral anticoagulants (DOACs), and/or vitamin K antagonists (VKAs). Deciding which type of anticoagulant to use depends on the indication, the underlying condition, the preference of the patient, and bleeding risk [15], as assessed using various strategies of VTE prophylaxis. For most of these drugs, under specific occasions, we can test their effectiveness that might be associated with a lower rate of thromboembolic episodes [16]. Moreover, there are novel treatment options for both arterial and venous thromboembolic episodes, such as proprotein convertase subtilisin/kexin type 9 (PCSK9) inhibitors that decrease the levels of lipoprotein (a) [17,18].

Systemic thrombolytic therapy reduces pulmonary arterial pressure and length of hospitalization [14]. In severe cases of iliofemoral DVT, catheter-directed thrombolytic systems and mechanical thrombectomy show promising results not only in terms of decreasing the risk of PE development and death but also in terms of ameliorating its later consequences [19]. Such endovascular treatment might be a rescue option for patients with a deteriorating clinical state or those for whom standard forms of therapy failed or was associated with contraindications [20].

Along with activated epithelium, neutrophils produce pro-inflammatory cytokines and chemokines to promote local inflammation. Under the conditions of sustained activation, aside from the potential effect of circulating free hemoglobin, heme, and iron, they contribute to the release of neutrophile extracellular traps (NETs) [21,22]. Such NETs are associated with hypofibrinolysis and correlate with elevated lactate levels that indicate increased mortality in patients with acute PE [23]. Increased serum lactate levels are also a promising biomarker of the prognosis of patients with acute mesenteric ischemia [24].

One of the infections associated with inflammation and an increased risk of thromboembolic episodes is coronavirus disease 2019 (COVID-19) caused by SARS-CoV-2 infection [25]. However, the optimal dose of anticoagulants and the need for additional antiplatelet treatment for critically ill patients with COVID-19 require further investigation [26].

We, the Editors, are honored to have received so many high-quality articles addressing these and other topics written by recognized experts in the field of thrombosis and hemostasis. The excellence of these articles was verified by positive reactions and their increased number of citations to date. Predominantly, we sincerely hope that the information included in the articles of this Special Issue will help to improve the management of patients with thromboembolisms, thus increasing their quality of life. We hope that the readers will enjoy it as well.

**Author Contributions:** Conceptualization, L.S., M.O. and P.K.; resources, L.S. and P.K.; writing—original draft preparation, L.S.; supervision, M.O. and P.K.; funding acquisition, L.S. and P.K. All authors have read and agreed to the published version of the manuscript.

**Funding:** This study was supported by donations from the project of the Scientific Grant Agency (Vega) 1/0549/19, Vega 1/0168/16, Vega 1/0479/21, and the Agency for the Support of Research and Development (APVV) APVV-16-0020 given to our faculty.

**Conflicts of Interest:** The authors declare no conflict of interest. Funding came in the form of the abovementioned projects in the above section. The funders had no role in the design, execution, interpretation, or writing of this study.

## References

1. Gollamudi, J.; Sartain, S.E.; Navaei, A.H.; Aneja, S.; Dhawan, P.K.; Tran, D.; Joshi, J.; Gidudu, J.; Gollamudi, J.; Chiappini, E.; et al. Thrombosis and thromboembolism: Brighton collaboration case definition and guidelines for data collection, analysis, and presentation of immunization safety data. *Vaccine* **2022**, *40*, 6431–6444. [CrossRef] [PubMed]
2. Jeon, W.; Lee, S.-J.; Park, S.-H.; Lee, S.-W.; Shin, W.-Y.; Jin, D.-K. Acute myocardial infarction caused by a floating thrombus in the proximal ascending aorta. *Korean J. Int. Med.* **2015**, *30*, 921–924. [CrossRef] [PubMed]
3. Salari, N.; Morddarvanjoghi, F.; Abdolmaleki, A.; Rasoulpoor, S.; Khaleghi, A.A.; Hezarkhani, L.A.; Shohaimi, S.; Mohammadi, M. The global prevalence of myocardial infarction: A systematic review and meta-analysis. *BMC Cardiovasc. Disord.* **2023**, *23*, 206. [CrossRef] [PubMed]
4. Delewi, R.; Zijlstra, F.; Piek, J.J. Left ventricular thrombus formation after acute myocardial infarction. *Heart* **2012**, *98*, 1743–1749. [CrossRef] [PubMed]
5. Birocchi, S.; Rocchetti, M.; Minardi, A.; Podda, G.M.; Squizzato, A.; Cattaneo, M. Guided Anti-P2Y12 Therapy in Patients Undergoing PCI: Three Systematic Reviews with Meta-analyses of Randomized Controlled Trials with Homogeneous Design. *Thromb. Haemost.* **2023**. online ahead of print. [CrossRef] [PubMed]
6. Guo, X.; Phan, C.; Batarseh, S.; Wei, M.; Dye, J. Risk factors and predictive markers of post-stroke cognitive decline-A mini review. *Front. Aging Neurosci.* **2024**, *16*, 1359792. [CrossRef] [PubMed]
7. Pleet, A.B.; Massey, E.W.; Vengrow, M.E. TIA, stroke, and the bicuspid aortic valve. *Neurology* **1981**, *31*, 1540–1542. [CrossRef] [PubMed]
8. Pastori, D.; Cormaci, V.M.; Marucci, S.; Franchino, G.; Del Sole, F.; Capozza, A.; Fallarino, A.; Corso, C.; Valeriani, E.; Menichelli, D.; et al. A Comprehensive Review of Risk Factors for Venous Thromboembolism: From Epidemiology to Pathophysiology. *Int. J. Mol. Sci.* **2023**, *24*, 3169. [CrossRef] [PubMed]
9. Patel, K.; Fasanya, A.; Yadam, S.; Joshi, A.A.; Singh, A.C.; DuMont, T. Pathogenesis and Epidemiology of Venous Thromboembolic Disease. *Crit. Care Nurs. Q.* **2017**, *40*, 191–200. [CrossRef]
10. Yagmur, E.; Bast, E.; Mühlfeld, A.S.; Koch, A.; Weiskirchen, R.; Tacke, F.; Neulen, J. High Prevalence of Sticky Platelet Syndrome in Patients with Infertility and Pregnancy Loss. *J. Clin. Med.* **2019**, *8*, 1328. [CrossRef]
11. Cosmi, B.; Legnani, C.; Libra, A.; Palareti, G. D-Dimers in diagnosis and prevention of venous thrombosis: Recent advances and their practical implications. *Pol. Arch. Intern. Med.* **2023**, *133*, 16604. [CrossRef] [PubMed]
12. Parakh, R.S.; Sabath, D.E. Venous Thromboembolism: Role of the Clinical Laboratory in Diagnosis and Management. *J. Appl. Lab. Med.* **2019**, *3*, 870–882. [CrossRef] [PubMed]
13. Dave, H.M.; Khorana, A.A. Management of venous thromboembolism in patients with active cancer. *Cleve Clin. J. Med.* **2024**, *91*, 109–117. [CrossRef] [PubMed]
14. Brunton, N.; McBane, R.; Casanegra, A.I.; Houghton, D.E.; Balanescu, D.V.; Ahmad, S.; Caples, S.; Motiei, A.; Henkin, S. Risk Stratification and Management of Intermediate-Risk Acute Pulmonary Embolism. *J. Clin. Med.* **2024**, *13*, 257. [CrossRef] [PubMed]
15. Bartholomew, J.R. Update on the management of venous thromboembolism. *Cleve Clin. J. Med.* **2017**, *84*, 39–46. [CrossRef] [PubMed]
16. Ferreira, L.B.; Lanna de Almeida, R.; Arantes, A.; Abdulazeem, H.; Weerasekara, I.; Ferreira, L.S.D.N.; Fonseca de Almeida Messias, L.; Siuves Ferreira Couto, L.; Parreiras Martins, M.A.; Suelen Antunes, N.; et al. Telemedicine-Based Management of Oral Anticoagulation Therapy: Systematic Review and Meta-analysis. *J. Med. Internet Res.* **2023**, *25*, e45922. [CrossRef] [PubMed]
17. Marston, N.A.; Gurmu, Y.; Melloni, G.E.M.; Bonaca, M.; Gencer, B.; Sever, P.S.; Pedersen, T.R.; Keech, A.C.; Roselli, C.; Lubitz, S.A.; et al. The Effect of PCSK9 (Proprotein Convertase Subtilisin/Kexin Type 9) Inhibition on the Risk of Venous Thromboembolism. *Circulation* **2020**, *141*, 1600–1607. [CrossRef] [PubMed]
18. Schwartz, G.G.; Steg, P.G.; Szarek, M.; Bittner, V.A.; Diaz, R.; Goodman, S.G.; Kim, Y.-U.; Jukema, J.W.; Pordy, R.; Roe, M.T.; et al. Peripheral Artery Disease and Venous Thromboembolic Events After Acute Coronary Syndrome: Role of Lipoprotein(a) and Modification by Alirocumab: Prespecified Analysis of the Odyssey Outcomes Randomized Clinical Trial. *Circulation* **2020**, *141*, 1608–1617. [CrossRef] [PubMed]
19. Rossi, F.H.; Osse, F.J.; Thorpe, P.E. The paradigm shift in treatment of severe venous thromboembolism. *J. Vasc. Bras.* **2024**, *24*, e20230095. [CrossRef]
20. Saposnik, G.; Bushnell, C.; Coutinho, J.M.; Field, T.S.; Furie, K.L.; Galadanci, N.; Kam, W.; Kirkham, F.C.; McNair, N.D.; Singhal, A.B.; et al. Diagnosis and Management of Cerebral Venous Thrombosis: A Scientific Statement from the American Heart Association. *Stroke* **2024**, *55*, e77–e90. [CrossRef]
21. Caillon, A.; Trimaille, A.; Favre, J.; Jesel, L.; Morel, O.; Kauffenstein, G. Role of neutrophils, platelets, and extracellular vesicles and their interactions in COVID-19-associated thrombopathy. *J. Thromb. Haemost.* **2022**, *20*, 17–31. [CrossRef] [PubMed]
22. L'Acqua, C.; Hod, E. New perspectives on the thrombotic complications of haemolysis. *Br. J. Haematol.* **2015**, *168*, 175–185. [CrossRef] [PubMed]

23. Ząbczyk, M.; Natorska, J.; Janion-Sadowska, A.; Malinowski, K.P.; Janion, M.; Undas, A. Elevated Lactate Levels in Acute Pulmonary Embolism Are Associated with Prothrombotic Fibrin Clot Properties: Contribution of NETs Formation. *J. Clin. Med.* **2020**, *9*, 953. [CrossRef] [PubMed]
24. Memet, O.; Zhang, L.; Shen, J. Serological biomarkers for acute mesenteric ischemia. *Ann. Transl. Med.* **2019**, *7*, 394. [CrossRef] [PubMed]
25. Ansari, S.A.; Merza, N.; Salman, M.; Raja, A.; Zafar Sayeed, B.; Ur Rahman, H.A.; Bhimani, S.; Saeed Shaikh, A.; Naqi, U.; Farooqui, A.; et al. Safety and efficacy of antithrombotics in outpatients with symptomatic COVID-19: A systematic review and meta-analysis. *Curr. Probl. Cardiol.* **2024**, *49*, 102451. [CrossRef]
26. Meng, J.; Tang, H.; Xiao, Y.; Liu, W.; Wu, Y.; Xiong, Y.; Gao, S. Appropriate thromboprophylaxis strategy for COVID-19 patients on dosage, antiplatelet therapy, outpatient and post-discharge prophylaxis: A meta-analysis of randomized controlled trials. *Int. J. Surg.* **2024**. *online ahead of print.* [CrossRef]

**Disclaimer/Publisher's Note:** The statements, opinions and data contained in all publications are solely those of the individual author(s) and contributor(s) and not of MDPI and/or the editor(s). MDPI and/or the editor(s) disclaim responsibility for any injury to people or property resulting from any ideas, methods, instructions or products referred to in the content.

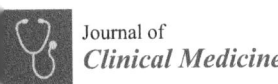 

*Case Report*

# Rare Source of Embolism in a Young Patient: Case Report and Literature Review

Marianna Vachalcová [1,2], Monika Jankajová [1,*], Marta Jakubová [2], Karolina Angela Sieradzka [1,2], Tibor Porubän [1], Gabriel Valočik [1,2], Peter Šafár [3], Daniela Ondušová [2], Ján Petruš [1] and Ingrid Schusterová [2]

[1] 1st Department of Cardiology, East-Slovak Institute of Cardiovascular Diseases, 04011 Kosice, Slovakia; marianna.vachalcova@gmail.com (M.V.); sieradzka.ina@gmail.com (K.A.S.); porubantibor@gmail.com (T.P.); gvalocik@vusch.sk (G.V.); jpetrus@vusch.sk (J.P.)

[2] Department of Functional Diagnostic, East-Slovak Institute of Cardiovascular Diseases, 04011 Kosice, Slovakia; mjakubova@vusch.sk (M.J.); dondusova@vusch.sk (D.O.); ischusterova@vusch.sk (I.S.)

[3] Department of Cardiothoracic Surgery, East-Slovak Institute of Cardiovascular Diseases, 04011 Kosice, Slovakia; psafar@vusch.sk

* Correspondence: mjankajova@gmail.com; Tel.: +421-0557891410

**Abstract:** We present a case of a 31-year-old patient, smoker, with no previous medical history, presenting with acute limb ischemia and infarction of the spleen due to peripheral embolism. The source of embolism was thrombi formations in the left ventricular cavity, located in the area of the regional wall motions abnormalities. CT and coronary angiography confirmed the total occlusion of the left anterior descending artery with collateralization. The patient underwent acute bilateral embolectomy of the iliac, femoral, and popliteal arteries. Subsequently, cardiothoracic surgery was indicated with coronary bypass surgery and extirpation of left ventricular masses, later confirmed as thrombus by pathology characteristics. Hematological examinations proved homozygous thrombophilia, and the patient was indicated for lifelong anticoagulation therapy.

**Keywords:** myocardial infarction; thrombus; thrombophilia; embolism

## 1. Introduction

Myocardial infarction (MI) with thrombus formation in the left ventricular cavity is a rare source of embolism in a young patient. We describe the unique case of a young patient presenting with acute limb ischemia and spleen infarction due to peripheral embolism of a thrombus after MI.

## 2. Case Report

We report a case of a 31-year-old man, smoker, with no previous medical history, with negative family history of thrombotic and hemorrhagic events, who, in September 2021, was referred to the emergency department for pain and reduced sensitivity in his lower limbs. The pain appeared a month earlier and was preceded by chest pain radiating to his neck and arms. Angiological examination confirmed acute limb ischemia. Ultrasound and CT angiography showed subtotal occlusion in the distal part of bilateral femoral and popliteal arteries, subtotal occlusion of the superior mesenteric artery, infarction of the spleen, and post-infarction change in the kidneys. Blood pressure was 127/92 mmHg. An ECG showed sinus rhythm, 2 mm ST-segment elevations in leads V2–V3, and Q wave and negativization of T wave in leads V1–V5. Troponin I levels were elevated (374 ng/L), NT-pro-B-type natriuretic peptide was 8500 ng/L, and creatine kinase and myoglobin peaked at 92 ukat/L and 17,107 ug/L, respectively. The complete blood count was normal. The patient had a low-risk profile for atherosclerosis coronary artery disease.

When searching for a source of embolization, transthoracic and transesophageal echocardiograms (TTE and TOE) were performed. They revealed flowing structures in the

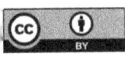

left ventricular apex with high embolic potential (Figures 1 and 2), reduced left ventricular ejection fraction (EF LV 38%), akinesis of the left ventricular apex, hypokinesis of adjacent segments of the lateral wall, interventricular septum, anterior and inferior wall, and no significant valvular disease.

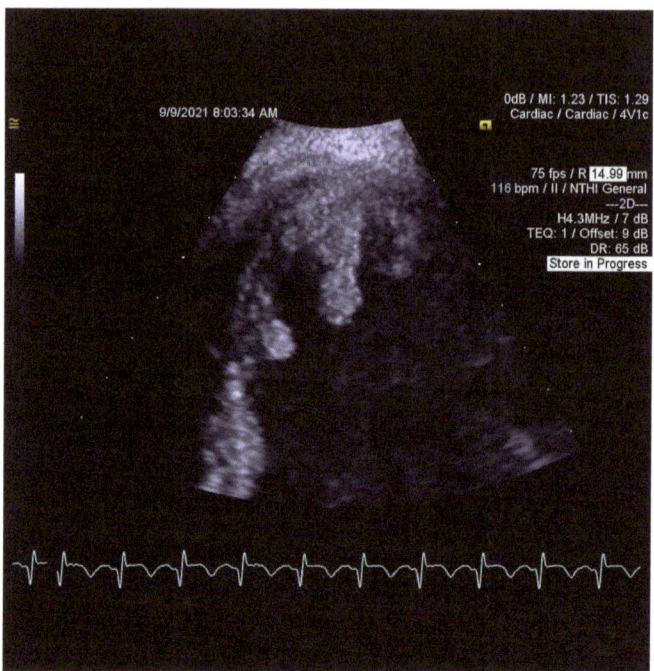

**Figure 1.** Thrombi in the left ventricular apex with high embolic potential.

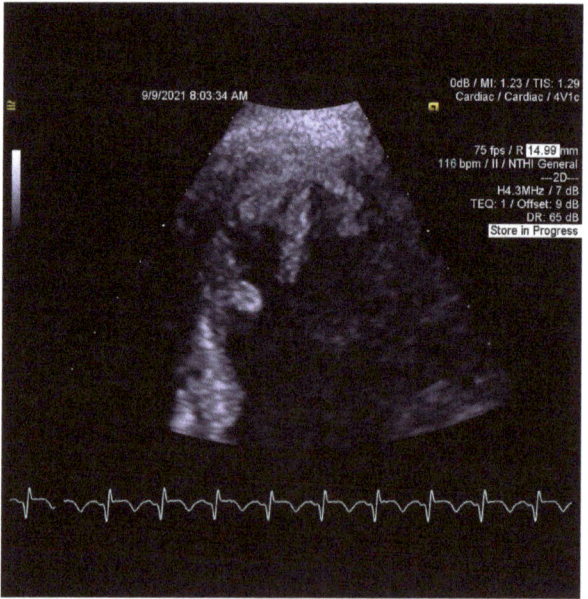

**Figure 2.** Another focus on thrombi in the left ventricular apex by TTE.

Emergent surgical revascularization was indicated, and the patient underwent bilateral embolectomy of iliac, femoral, and popliteal arteries. Additional CT angiography and subsequently selective coronary angiography showed total occlusion of the left anterior descending artery with collateralization (Figure 3).

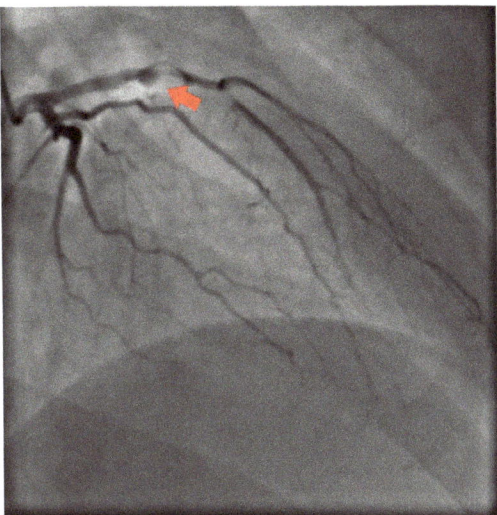

**Figure 3.** Selective coronary angiography showed total occlusion of left anterior descending artery with collateralization (red arrow).

CT examination confirmed two floating structures (20 × 16 × 8 mm and 27 × 11 × 15 mm) in the area of the interventricular septum and left ventricular apex (Figures 4 and 5).

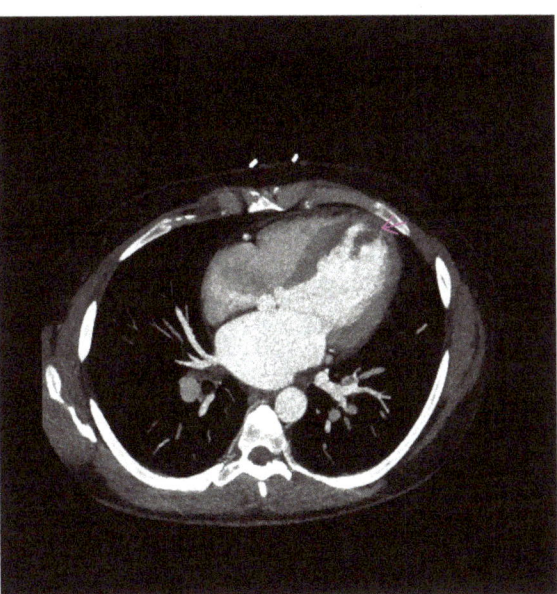

**Figure 4.** CT finding of first thrombus in the area of left ventricular apex (purple arrow).

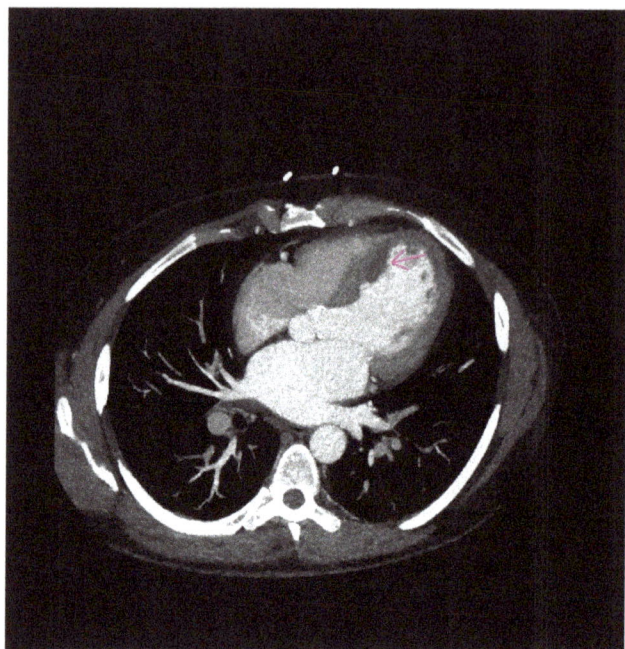

**Figure 5.** CT finding of second thrombus in the area of interventricular septum (purple arrow).

Cardiothoracic surgery was indicated by the Heart Team. Coronary artery bypass grafting (left internal mammary artery was used for revascularization of the left anterior descending artery) and removal of left ventricular masses were performed. Pathology characteristics confirmed the thrombus. Therefore, hematological screening was supplemented. The examinations positively proved antiphospholipid syndrome. The screening assay APTT–LA was used, and extended APTT was detected. The lupus anticoagulants testing was positive and repeated in 12 weeks with persistence of the antibody. Laboratory testing for anticardiolipin antibodies and anti-β2-glycoprotein I antibodies was not performed. Moreover, genetic testing assessed 4G/4G homozygosity for the PAI-1 gene. The control TTE revealed persistent regional wall motion abnormalities, reduced LV EF (38%), and no significant valvular diseases. The treatment of heart failure was boosted, and lifelong anticoagulation therapy was indicated. At the 5-month follow-up, there was no evidence of embolic recurrence.

## 3. Discussion

Thrombophilia is a common risk factor for venous thromboembolism. Arterial thrombosis and the risk of MI, particularly among young people with low atherosclerotic burden, are associated mainly with the presence of antiphospholipid syndrome. [1] In young patients with MI and conventional risk factors, the probability of thrombophilia is high. Thrombophilia may lead to MI in this specific group of patients. [2] The left anterior descending artery is more frequently the culprit artery of MI in young patients. [3] Previous studies have reported that atrial fibrillation is the underlying disease in patients with coronary embolism (CE). CE has also been detected in the case of concomitant cardiomyopathy, valvular heart disease, infective endocarditis, antiphospholipid antibody syndrome, autoimmune disorders, and malignancy. A total of 26.4% of cases were of unclear etiology [4]. CE is diagnosed with coronary angiography, concomitant CE in multiple locations, or evidence of systemic embolization. The source of embolism should be revealed. An important step is the identification of a thrombus or intracardiac shunt using echocardiography. CE is frequently associated with systemic embolism, which should be screened [5]. MI is caused by CE in 4% to 13% of cases [4,6]. Paradoxical embolism should also be considered in the presence of thrombophilia and a hypercoagulable risk factor [7–9].

We present a unique case of a young patient without previous medical history who overcame MI. The known risk factor was smoking. The first symptoms of MI and peripheral embolization appeared a month before hospitalization. We suppose that due to the total occlusion of the left anterior descending artery, the thrombi with high embolic potential were formed in the area of regional wall motions abnormalities. The patient was admitted to hospital presenting with acute limb ischemia. The source of embolism was with high probability the thrombi in the left ventricle. The cardiosurgical operation and removal of the floating thrombi, later confirmed by pathology characteristics, was indicated. Hematological screening revealed positivity of antiphospholipid syndrome, and genetic testing assessed 4G/4G homozygosity for the PAI-1 gene. Thrombectomy, sometimes aided by intracoronary glycoprotein IIb/ IIIa inhibitors or thrombolytic therapy, is performed if the diagnosis of CE is established during coronary angiography. Coronary stents are not commonly required. Oral anticoagulation therapy needs to be initiated. A search for risk factors needs to be conducted. There is no need for routine thrombophilia screening unless there is clinical suspicion [5].

In the presented case report, we suppose the CE related to thrombophilia and peripheral embolism was due to the thrombi formation in the left ventricle. According to the history of chest pain one month before hospitalization, overcomed MI was diagnosed. The culprit coronary artery, the left anterior descending artery, was in accordance with previous trials. The patient was indicated for lifelong anticoagulation therapy. The treatment of heart failure was also initiated.

In young patients with MI, routine thrombophilia screening is indicated in the case of clinical suspicion; that was also the case with our patient.

## 4. Conclusions

The main goal of this case report is to highlight the diagnostic approach in young patients with arterial thromboembolism. Up-to-date, routine thrombophilia screening is indicated in the case of clinical suspicion and should be considered in young patients presenting with myocardial infarction and peripheral embolism.

**Author Contributions:** All the authors contributed to this manuscript. The manuscript was prepared and written by M.V. Language corrections were made by K.A.S. M.J. (Monika Jankajová), M.J. (Marta Jakubová), T.P., G.V., P.Š., D.O. and J.P. were the attending physicians of this patient and made the revision of the text. The supervision of prepared manuscript was made by I.S. All authors have read and agreed to the published version of the manuscript.

**Funding:** This research was funded by KEGA grant: 007UPJŠ-4/2020 Detská obezita: tiopatogenéza, diagnostika a liečba.

**Institutional Review Board Statement:** This manuscript is Case report and patient signed informed consent.

**Informed Consent Statement:** Written informed consent has been obtained from the patient.

**Conflicts of Interest:** The authors declare no conflict of interest.

## References

1. Boekholdt, S.M.; Kramer, M.H. Arterial thrombosis and the role of thrombophilia. *Semin. Thromb. Hemost.* **2007**, *33*, 588–596. [CrossRef] [PubMed]
2. Segev, A.; Ellis, M.H.; Segev, F.; Friedman, Z.; Reshef, T.; Sparkes, J.D.; Tetro, J.; Pauzner, H.; David, D. High prevalence of thrombophilia among young patients with myocardial infarction and few conventional risk factors. *Int. J. Cardiol.* **2005**, *98*, 421–424. [CrossRef] [PubMed]
3. Zasada, W.; Bobrowska, B.; Plens, K.; Dziewierz, A.; Siudak, Z.; Surdacki, A.; Dudek, D.; Bartuś, S. Acute myocardial infarction in young patients. *Kardiol. Pol.* **2021**, *79*, 1093–1098. [CrossRef] [PubMed]

4. Shibata, T.; Kawakami, S.; Noguchi, T.; Tanaka, T.; Asaumi, Y.; Kanaya, T.; Nagai, T.; Nakao, K.; Fujino, M.; Nagatsuka, K.; et al. Prevalence, clinical features, and prognosis of acute myocardial infarction attributable to coronary artery embolism. *Circulation* **2015**, *132*, 241–250. [CrossRef] [PubMed]
5. Gulati, R.; Behfar, A.; Narula, J.; Kanwar, A.; Lerman, A.; Cooper, L.; Singh, M. Acute Myocardial Infarction in Young Individuals. *Mayo Clin. Proc.* **2020**, *95*, 136–156. [CrossRef] [PubMed]
6. Prizel, K.R.; Hutchins, G.M.; Bulkley, B.H. Coronary artery embolism and myocardial infarction. *Ann. Intern. Med.* **1978**, *88*, 155–161. [CrossRef]
7. Kanwar, S.M.; Noheria, A.; DeSimone, C.V.; Rabinstein, A.A.; Asirvatham, S.J. Coincidental impact of transcatheter patent foramen ovale closure on migraine with and without aura—A comprehensive meta-analysis. *Clin. Trials Regul. Sci. Cardiol.* **2016**, *15*, 7–13. [CrossRef] [PubMed]
8. Kleber, F.X.; Hauschild, T.; Schulz, A.; Winkelmann, A.; Bruch, L. Epidemiology of myocardial infarction caused by presumed paradoxical embolism via a patent foramen ovale. *Circ. J.* **2017**, *81*, 1484–1489. [CrossRef] [PubMed]
9. Chen, W.; Yu, Z.; Li, S.; Wagatsuma, K.; Du, B.; Yang, P. Concomitant acute myocardial infarction and acute pulmonary embolism caused by paradoxical embolism: A case report. *BMC Cardiovasc. Disord.* **2021**, *21*, 313. [CrossRef] [PubMed]

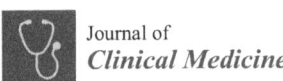 

*Systematic Review*

# Insights into the Role of Neutrophils and Neutrophil Extracellular Traps in Causing Cardiovascular Complications in Patients with COVID-19: A Systematic Review

**Francesco Nappi [1,*], Francesca Bellomo [2] and Sanjeet Singh Avtaar Singh [3]**

1 Department of Cardiac Surgery, Centre Cardiologique du Nord, 93200 Saint-Denis, France
2 Department of Clinical and Experimental Medicine, University of Messina, 98122 Messina, Italy; bellomofrancesca92@gmail.com
3 Department of Cardiothoracic Surgery, Aberdeen Royal Infirmary, Aberdeen AB25 2ZN, UK; sanjeetsinghtoor@gmail.com
* Correspondence: francesconappi2@gmail.com; Tel.: +33-1-4933-4104; Fax: +33-1-4933-4119

**Citation:** Nappi, F.; Bellomo, F.; Avtaar Singh, S.S. Insights into the Role of Neutrophils and Neutrophil Extracellular Traps in Causing Cardiovascular Complications in Patients with COVID-19: A Systematic Review. *J. Clin. Med.* **2022**, *11*, 2460. https://doi.org/10.3390/jcm11092460

Academic Editors: Lucia Stančiaková, Maha Othman and Peter Kubisz

Received: 14 April 2022
Accepted: 25 April 2022
Published: 27 April 2022

**Publisher's Note:** MDPI stays neutral with regard to jurisdictional claims in published maps and institutional affiliations.

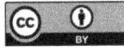

**Copyright:** © 2022 by the authors. Licensee MDPI, Basel, Switzerland. This article is an open access article distributed under the terms and conditions of the Creative Commons Attribution (CC BY) license (https:// creativecommons.org/licenses/by/ 4.0/).

**Abstract:** Background: The coronavirus disease 2019 (COVID-19) pandemic caused by the SARS-CoV-2 virus has resulted in significant mortality and burdening of healthcare resources. While initially noted as a pulmonary pathology, subsequent studies later identified cardiovascular involvement with high mortalities reported in specific cohorts of patients. While cardiovascular comorbidities were identified early on, the exact manifestation and etiopathology of the infection remained elusive. This systematic review aims to investigate the role of inflammatory pathways, highlighting several culprits including neutrophil extracellular traps (NETs) which have since been extensively investigated. Method: A search was conducted using three databases (MEDLINE; MEDLINE In-Process & Other Non-Indexed Citations and EMBASE). Data from randomized controlled trials (RCT), prospective series, meta-analyses, and unmatched observational studies were considered for the processing of the algorithm and treatment of inflammatory response during SARS-CoV-2 infection. Studies without the SARS-CoV-2 Infection period and case reports were excluded. Results: A total of 47 studies were included in this study. The role of the acute inflammatory response in the propagation of the systemic inflammatory sequelae of the disease plays a major part in determining outcomes. Some of the mechanisms of activation of these pathways have been highlighted in previous studies and are highlighted. Conclusion: NETs play a pivotal role in the pathogenesis of the inflammatory response. Despite moving into the endemic phase of the disease in most countries, COVID-19 remains an entity that has not been fully understood with long-term effects remaining uncertain and requiring ongoing monitoring and research.

**Keywords:** SARS-CoV-2 infection; COVID-19; coronary artery thrombosis; neutrophil extracellular traps (NETs)

## 1. Introduction

Since the first outbreak of the severe acute respiratory syndrome-coronavirus-2 infection (SARS-CoV-2), patients who developed coronavirus disease 2019 (COVID-19) frequently had cardiovascular involvement [1]. The myocardial injury was associated with high levels of troponin, especially among hospitalised COVID-19 patients [2]. However, the myocardial damage revealed by the increase in biomarkers was confirmed by echocardiography, which noted damage in 70% of hospitalized patients [3]. Therefore, cardiac involvement during COVID-19 was a truly probable event, despite the primary manifestation of disease within the lungs. Unfavourable outcome of the disease is likely in these subjects, which was immediately reported as sequelae of this complication [4]. Given these significant reports, the scientists' attention has focused on two main clinical-pathological entities.

First, it must be emphasized that only a few patients with COVID-19 have experienced fulminant myocarditis, suggesting that this complication is rare [5,6]. In the small number of cases in which clinically suspected myocarditis was diagnosed, infection with SARS-CoV-2 was associated with cardiac inflammation [7].

Second, myocardial ischaemia, attributable to thrombotic coronary obstruction, appears to be the most likely event at the origin of myocardial damage, however, other causes such as heart failure, pulmonary embolism, tachycardia, and sepsis cannot be excluded [8]. Acute cardiac injury occurs in patients who experienced severe COVID-19 and confers serious complications and patient mortality [9].

We know that SARS-CoV-2, in addition to causing severe acute respiratory syndrome, has been shown to predispose infected patients to thrombotic disease with the involvement of arterial and venous vascular districts [10]. This complication is assumed to be secondary to uncontrolled inflammatory process, platelet activation, endothelial dysfunction, and marked stasis [11].

Recently the attention of several reports has suggested that in patients with severe organ dysfunction, SARS-CoV-2 infection is associated with excessive formation of neutrophil extracellular traps (NETs) with consequent vascular damage [12]. Furthermore, the autopsies performed in patients with unfavorable outcomes revealed a vascular mechanical obstruction due to the aggregates of NET, identifying in this process a central moment that is decisive in the complex pathogenesis of COVID-19 [12,13].

The role of mononuclear cells is decisive, either during myocarditis or coronary thrombosis due to activation of NETs, thus unearthing the controversial presence of SARS-CoV-2 in myocardial tissue and its potential for replication within the heart structures (cells and extracellular matrix). However, the role of mononuclear cell infiltration that induces increased cytokine expression remains elusive, both in patients who died without the signs of clinically evident myocarditis and in those who died in the absence of ST-elevation that characterized the myocardial ischemia due to coronary obstruction [13,14]. Given the critical clinical context in which COVID-19 often occurs, burdened by a high percentage of deaths, the autopsies have contributed to unveiling many unsolved aspects related to its pathogenesis [13,15–19]. To foster a wider knowledge of mechanisms leading to myocardial injury and to provide a guide for clinicians, we herein debate the ongoing evidence basis on the role of NETs and propose an evidence-based algorithm for the prevention and control of inflammatory response during COVID-19 infections, Figure 1.

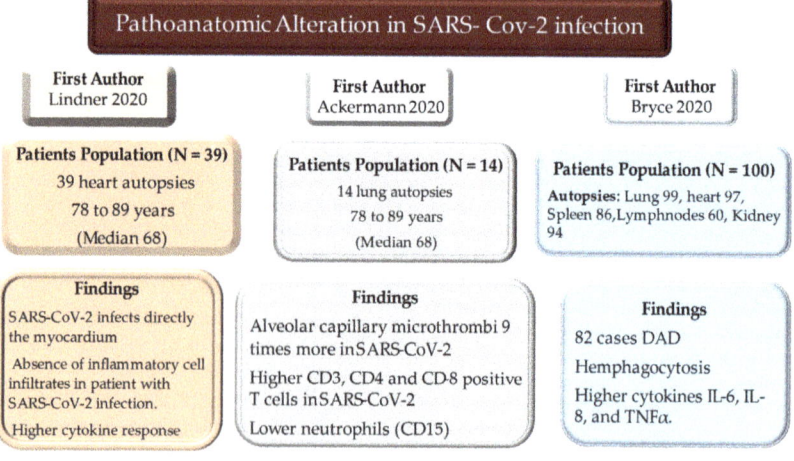

**Figure 1.** *Cont.*

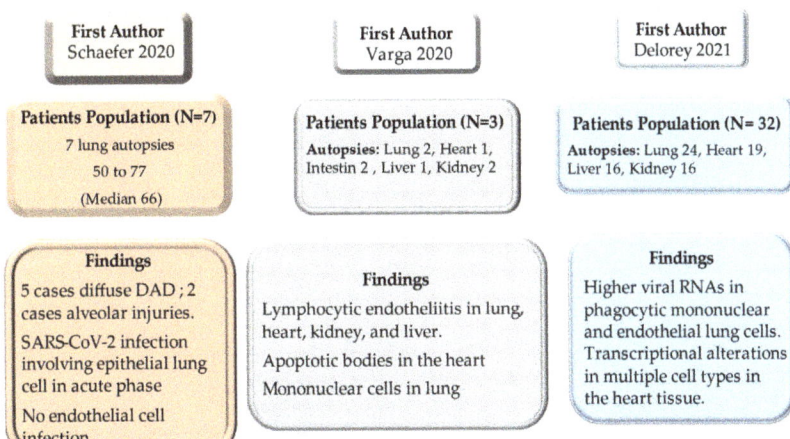

**Figure 1.** Autopsies substantially contributed to unveiling many unsolved aspects relating to the pathogenesis revealing the role of mononuclear cell infiltration leading to increased cytokine expression in patients who died with single or multi-failure organ pathologies. Abbreviations; DAD, diffuse alveolar damage; IL: interleukine; SARS-CoV-2, severe acute respiratory syndrome coronavirus 2; RNA, ribonucleic acid; TNF, tumor necrosis factor.

## 2. Search Method and Systematic Literature Review

In December 2021, databases (MEDLINE; MEDLINE In-Process & Other Non-Indexed Citations and EMBASE) were searched using the terms "SARS-CoV-2", "COVID-19", "myocarditis", "myocardial ischemia" and "neutrophil extracellular traps", coupled with "inflammation", mononuclear cell", "neutrophil cell", "cytokine", "cytokine storm". For this study, abstracts of included manuscripts were assessed and correlated. The present review focuses on data from randomized controlled trials (RCT), prospective series, meta-analyses, and unmatched observational studies that were considered for the processing of the algorithm and treatment of inflammatory response during SARS-CoV-2 infection. Data were extracted from the main publication, and searches were performed by two independent researchers (F.B, SSAS using blind method). A third independent reviewer estimated pertinence (FN). No funding was received for this study. The review was not formally registered. The protocol was not prepared. The authors have no conflicts of interest to declare. Prisma flow diagram for systematic review and Prisma checklist are reported in Figure 2, Tables 1 and 2.

**Table 1.** Characteristics of the included studies.

| Author/Year | Study Period | Total Number | COVID-19 Study Design | Hospitals/Centers | Type |
|---|---|---|---|---|---|
| Shi (2020) [1] JAMA | 20 January 2020 to 10 February 2020 | 416 | Clinical, laboratory, radiological, and treatment | Single Center Wuhan, China | Prospective |
| Guo (2020) [2] JAMA Cardiology | 20 January 2020 to 10 February 2020 | 187 | Clinical laboratory comorbidities, and treatments | Single Center Wuhan, China | Observational |
| Szekely (2020) [3] Circulation | 21 March 2020 to 16 April 2020 | 100 | Echocardiographic | Single Center Israel | Prospective |
| Lala (2020) [4] JACC | 27 February 2020 to 12 April 2020 | 506 | Clinical, laboratory, Echocardiographic | Single Center NYC, NY, USA | Prospective |
| Escher (2020) [7] ESC Heart Fail | 3 February 2020 to 26 March 2020 | 104 | Endomyocardial biopsies | Multicenter Germany | Prospective |
| Lindner (2020) [13] JAMA Cardiology | 8 April 2020 to 18 April 2020 | 39 | Autopsy | Multicenter Germany | Prospective |

Table 1. Cont.

| Author/Year | Study Period | Total Number | COVID-19 Study Design | Hospitals/Centers | Type |
|---|---|---|---|---|---|
| Blasco (2020) [14] JAMA Cardiology | 24 March 2020 to 11 April 2020 | 55 | PCI/Coronary aspirates, NETs | Single Center Spain | Prospective |
| Ackermann (2020) [15] NEJM | 2019 † 2009 †† | 24 | Pulmonary autopsy/ Immune profiling | Multicenter Germany/USA | Comparative study |
| Bryce (2021) [16] Mod. Pathol. | 20 March 2020 to 23 June 2020 | 100 | Pulmonary autopsy/ Immune profiling | Single Center NYC, NY, USA | Prospective |
| Schaefer (2020) [17] Mod. Pathol. | April 2020 | 7 | Pulmonary autopsy/ Immune profiling | Single Center Boston, MA, USA | Observational |
| Varga (2020) [18] Lancet | « « « | 3 | Autopsy/Immune profiling | Multicenter Switzerland/USA | Observational |
| Delorey (2021) [19] Nature | « « « | 17 | Autopsy/Immune profiling | Multicenter USA | Comparative study |
| Wang (2020) [20] JAMA | 1 January 2020 to 28 January 2020 | 138 | Clinical, laboratory, radiological, and treatment | Single Center Wuhan, China | Observational |
| Lucas (2020) [21] Nature | 18 March 2020 to 27 May 2020 | 113 | Immune profiling | Multicenter USA | Observational |
| Yang (2020) [22] J Allergy Clin. Immunol. | « « « | 50 | Immune profiling | Multicenter China | Observational |
| Huang (2020) [23] Lancet | 16 December 2019 to 2 January 2020 | 41 | Immune profiling | Multicenter China | Observational |
| Liu (2020) [24] J. Infect. | 11 January 2020 to 29 January 2020 | 245 | Immune profiling | Multicenter China/UK | Observational |
| Rodriguez (2021) [25] J. Exp. Med. | « « « | 124 | Autopsy/Immune profiling | Multicenter Brasil | Observational |
| Burkhard-Koren (2021) [26] J. Pathol. Clin. Res. | May 1918 to April 1919 2009–2020 Until 2020 | 411 | Autopsy/Immune profiling | Single center Switzerland | Comparative study |
| Sang (2021) [27] Cardiovasc. Pathol. | Until 2021 | 50 | Autopsy/Immune profiling | Single Center Birmingham, AL, USA | Observational |
| Melms (2021) [28] Nature | Until 2021 | 26 | Autopsy/Immune profiling | Multicenter USA | Comparative study |
| Qin (2020) [29] Clin. Infect. Dis. | 10 January 2020 to 12 February 2020 | 452 | Immune profiling | Single Center Wuhan, China | Observational |
| Wilk (2020) [30] Nat. Med. | March–April 2020 | 7 | Immune profiling | Single Center Stanford, CA, USA | Prospective |
| Wang (2020) [31] Front. Immunol. | 23 January 2020 to 15 March 2020 | 55 | Immune profiling/NETs | Multicenter China/Germany | Observational |
| Al-Aly (2021) [32] Nature | Until 2021 | 73,435 | Clinical, laboratory | Single Center Saint Louis, MO, USA | Observational |
| Xie (2020) [33] Br. Med. J. | 1 January 2017 to 31 January 2019 2 January 2020 to 17 June 2020 | 16,317 | Clinical, laboratory | Single Center Saint Louis, MO, USA | Comparative study |
| Piazza (2020) [34] JACC | 13 March 2020 to 3 April 2020 | 1114 | Clinical Thromboembolic Complication | Single Center Boston, MA, USA | Observational |
| Zhang (2020) [35] J. Thromb. Thrombolysis | 23 February 2020 to 3 March 2020 | 12 | Clinical Thromboembolic Complication | Multicenter China | Prospective |
| Liu (2020) [36] J. Transl. Med. | 1 February 2020 to 24 February 2020 | 61 | Immune profiling | Single Center Beijing, China | Prospective |

Table 1. Cont.

| Author/Year | Study Period | Total Number | COVID-19 Study Design | Hospitals/Centers | Type |
|---|---|---|---|---|---|
| Fu (2020) [37] *Thromb. Res.* | 20 January 2020 to 20 February 2020 | 75 | Immune profiling Thromboembolic Complication | Single Center Suzhou, China | Comparative study |
| Webb (2020) [38] *Lancet Rheumatol.* | 13 March 2020 to 5 May 2020 | 299 | Immune profiling | Multicenter USA | Observational |
| Ye (2020) [39] *Respir. Res.* | 1 January 2020 to 16 March 2020 | 349 | Immune profiling Thromboembolic Complication | Multicenter China | Prospective |
| Tatum (2020) [40] *Shock* | Until 2021 | 125 | Immune profiling | Multicenter USA | Multicenter Prospective Registry |
| Yang (2020) [41] *Int. Immunopharmacol.* | Until 20 February 2020 | 93 | Immune profiling | Multicenter China | Observational |
| Wang (2020) [42] *Int. Immunopharmacol.* | 15 January 2020 to 2 March 2020 | 95 | Immune profiling | Single Center Wuhan, China | Observational |
| Zhou (2020) [43] *Lancet* | 29 December 2019 to 30 January 2020 | 191 | Clinical, laboratory, radiological, and treatment | Multicenter China | Observational |
| Klok (2020) [44] *Thromb. Res.* | 7 March 2020 to 5 April 2020 | 184 | Thromboembolic Complication | Multicenter Netherlands | Prospective |
| Tang (2020) [45] *J. Thromb. Haemost.* | 1 January 2020 to 13 February 2020 | 448 | Thromboembolic Complication | Single Center Wuhan, China | Observational |
| Zuo (2020) [46] *Sci. Transl. Med.* | « « « « | 172 | Immune profiling Thromboembolic Complication/NETs | Multicenter China/USA | Prospective |
| Carsana (2020) [47] *Lancet Infect. Dis.* | 29 February 2020 to 24 March 2020 | 38 | Autopsy/Immune profiling | Multicenter Italy | Observational |
| Chen (2020) [48] *Lancet* | 1 January 2020 to 20 January 2020 | 99 | Clinical, laboratory, radiological, and treatment | Multicenter China | Observational |
| Guan (2020) [49] *NEJM* | 11 December 2019 to 29 January 2020 | 1099 | Clinical, laboratory, radiological, and treatment | Multicenter China | Observational |
| COVIDSurg Collaborative (2022) [50] *Anaesthesia* | 10 January 2020 to 30 January 2020 | 128,013 | Thromboembolic Complication | Multicenter | Prospective |
| COVIDSurg Collaborative (2021) [51] *Anaesthesia* | 10 January 2020 to 30 January 2020 | 96,454 | Clinical | Multicenter | Prospective |
| COVIDSurg Collaborative (2021) [52] *Br. J. Surg.* | 10 January 2020 to 30 January 2020 | 56,589 | Clinical/Vaccine effectiveness | Multicenter | Prospective |
| COVIDSurg Collaborative (2021) [53] *Anaesthesia* | 10 January 2020 to 30 January 2020 | 140,231 | Clinical | Multicenter | Prospective |
| Xie (2022) [54] *Nat. Med.* | 1 March 2020 to 15 January 2021 | 153,760 | Clinical | Multicenter USA | Observational |

Abbreviations: †, it refers to the flu pandemic; ††, it refers to the flu pandemic.

Table 2. Prisma checklist. n/a = not application.

| Section and Topic | Item # | Checklist Item | Location Where Item Is Reported |
|---|---|---|---|
| TITLE | | | |
| Title | 1 | Identify the report as a systematic review. | Title and introduction |
| ABSTRACT | | | |
| Abstract | 2 | See the PRISMA 2020 for Abstracts checklist. | Abstract |

Table 2. Cont.

| Section and Topic | Item # | Checklist Item | Location Where Item Is Reported |
|---|---|---|---|
| INTRODUCTION | | | |
| Rationale | 3 | Describe the rationale for the review in the context of existing knowledge. | Introduction |
| Objectives | 4 | Provide an explicit statement of the objective(s) or question(s) the review addresses. | Introduction |
| METHODS | | | |
| Eligibility criteria | 5 | Specify the inclusion and exclusion criteria for the review and how studies were grouped for the syntheses. | Methods |
| Information sources | 6 | Specify all databases, registers, websites, organisations, reference lists and other sources searched or consulted to identify studies. Specify the date when each source was last searched or consulted. | Methods/PRISMA statement |
| Search strategy | 7 | Present the full search strategies for all databases, registers and websites, including any filters and limits used. | Methods |
| Selection process | 8 | Specify the methods used to decide whether a study met the inclusion criteria of the review, including how many reviewers screened each record and each report retrieved, whether they worked independently, and if applicable, details of automation tools used in the process. | Methods |
| Data collection process | 9 | Specify the methods used to collect data from reports, including how many reviewers collected data from each report, whether they worked independently, any processes for obtaining or confirming data from study investigators, and if applicable, details of automation tools used in the process. | Methods |
| Data items | 10a | List and define all outcomes for which data were sought. Specify whether all results that were compatible with each outcome domain in each study were sought (e.g., for all measures, time points, analyses), and if not, the methods used to decide which results to collect. | Methods |
| | 10b | List and define all other variables for which data were sought (e.g. participant and intervention characteristics, funding sources). Describe any assumptions made about any missing or unclear information. | Methods |
| Study risk of bias assessment | 11 | Specify the methods used to assess risk of bias in the included studies, including details of the tool(s) used, how many reviewers assessed each study and whether they worked independently, and if applicable, details of automation tools used in the process. | n/a |
| Effect measures | 12 | Specify for each outcome the effect measure(s) (e.g., risk ratio, mean difference) used in the synthesis or presentation of results. | n/a |
| Synthesis methods | 13a | Describe the processes used to decide which studies were eligible for each synthesis (e.g., tabulating the study intervention characteristics and comparing against the planned groups for each synthesis (item #5)). | Methods |
| | 13b | Describe any methods required to prepare the data for presentation or synthesis, such as handling of missing summary statistics, or data conversions. | n/a |
| | 13c | Describe any methods used to tabulate or visually display results of individual studies and syntheses. | Methods |
| | 13d | Describe any methods used to synthesize results and provide a rationale for the choice(s). If meta-analysis was performed, describe the model(s), method(s) to identify the presence and extent of statistical heterogeneity, and software package(s) used. | n/a |
| | 13e | Describe any methods used to explore possible causes of heterogeneity among study results (e.g., subgroup analysis, meta-regression). | n/a |
| | 13f | Describe any sensitivity analyses conducted to assess robustness of the synthesized results. | n/a |

**Table 2.** *Cont.*

| Section and Topic | Item # | Checklist Item | Location Where Item Is Reported |
|---|---|---|---|
| Reporting bias assessment | 14 | Describe any methods used to assess risk of bias due to missing results in a synthesis (arising from reporting biases). | n/a |
| Certainty assessment | 15 | Describe any methods used to assess certainty (or confidence) in the body of evidence for an outcome. | n/a |
| RESULTS | | | |
| Study selection | 16a | Describe the results of the search and selection process, from the number of records identified in the search to the number of studies included in the review, ideally using a flow diagram. | Prisma diagram |
| | 16b | Cite studies that might appear to meet the inclusion criteria, but which were excluded, and explain why they were excluded. | Prisma diagram |
| Study characteristics | 17 | Cite each included study and present its characteristics. | Table 1 |
| Risk of bias in studies | 18 | Present assessments of risk of bias for each included study. | n/a |
| Results of individual studies | 19 | For all outcomes, present, for each study: (a) summary statistics for each group (where appropriate) and (b) an effect estimate and its precision (e.g., confidence/credible interval), ideally using structured tables or plots. | n/a |
| Results of syntheses | 20a | For each synthesis, briefly summarise the characteristics and risk of bias among contributing studies. | n/a |
| | 20b | Present results of all statistical syntheses conducted. If meta-analysis was carried out, present for each the summary estimate and its precision (e.g., confidence/credible interval) and measures of statistical heterogeneity. If comparing groups, describe the direction of the effect. | Table 1 |
| | 20c | Present results of all investigations of possible causes of heterogeneity among study results. | n/a |
| | 20d | Present results of all sensitivity analyses conducted to assess the robustness of the synthesized results. | n/a |
| Reporting biases | 21 | Present assessments of risk of bias due to missing results (arising from reporting biases) for each synthesis assessed. | n/a |
| Certainty of evidence | 22 | Present assessments of certainty (or confidence) in the body of evidence for each outcome assessed. | n/a |
| DISCUSSION | | | |
| Discussion | 23a | Provide a general interpretation of the results in the context of other evidence. | 3.2 |
| | 23b | Discuss any limitations of the evidence included in the review. | n/a |
| | 23c | Discuss any limitations of the review processes used. | n/a |
| | 23d | Discuss implications of the results for practice, policy, and future research. | 3.2 |
| OTHER INFORMATION | | | |
| Registration and protocol | 24a | Provide registration information for the review, including register name and registration number, or state that the review was not registered. | Methods |
| | 24b | Indicate where the review protocol can be accessed, or state that a protocol was not prepared. | Methods |
| | 24c | Describe and explain any amendments to information provided at registration or in the protocol. | n/a |
| Support | 25 | Describe sources of financial or non-financial support for the review, and the role of the funders or sponsors in the review. | Methods |
| Competing interests | 26 | Declare any competing interests of review authors. | Methods |
| Availability of data, code and other materials | 27 | Report which of the following are publicly available and where they can be found: template data collection forms; data extracted from included studies; data used for all analyses; analytic code; any other materials used in the review. | n/a |

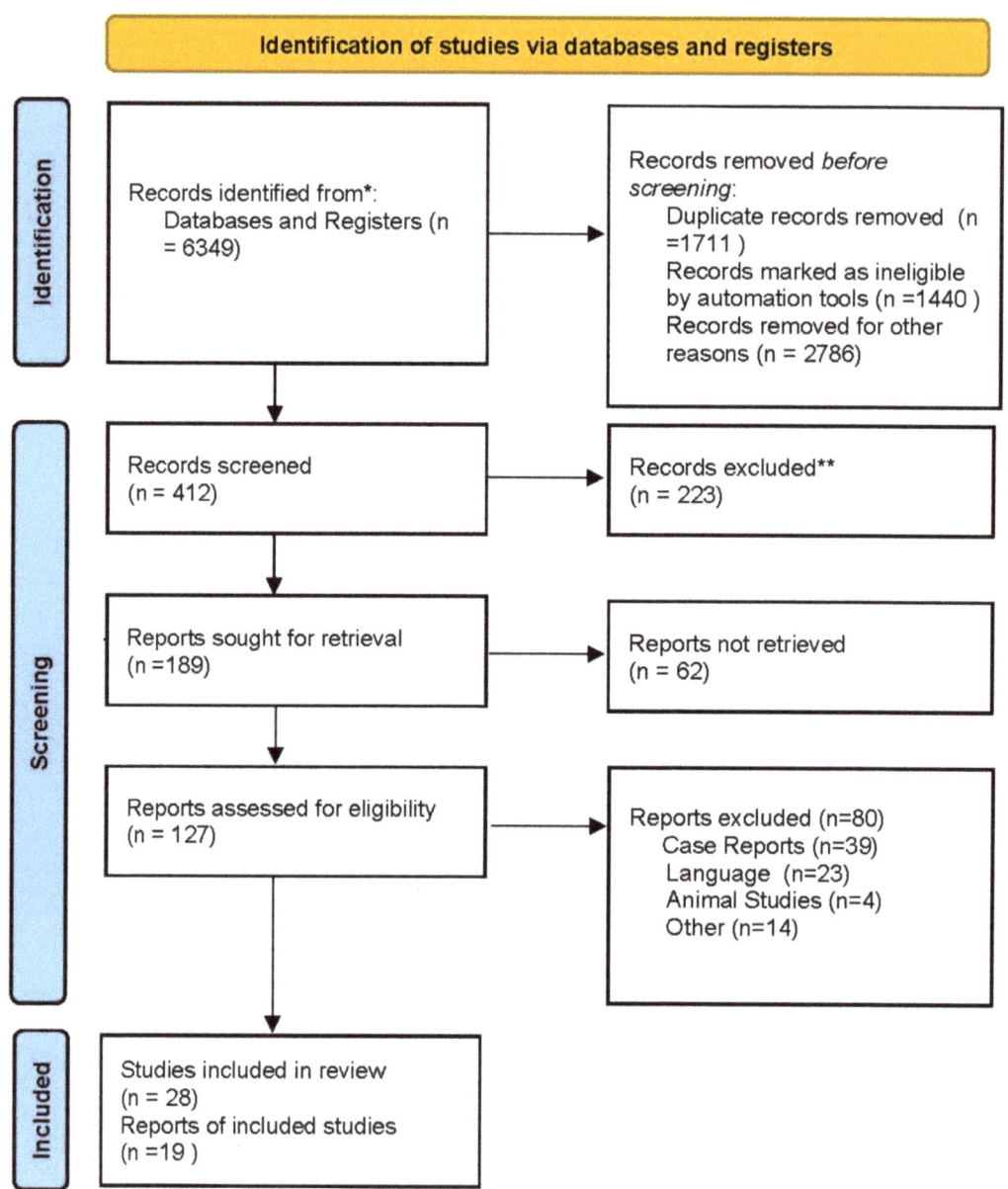

**Figure 2.** Prisma FloW Chart 2020 allowed to reach 47 determinant publications for the systematic review. * Search database; ** excluded for no meet criteria.

## 3. Results

*3.1. Description of the Included Studies and of the Population*

A total of 6349 studies was reported of which 412 studies were screened. 47 of these met the inclusion criteria and were included in the final systematic review (Flowchart). A total of 28 studies were international and/or multicentre of which 9 were from China and 6 from the USA; 3 prospective and 1 randomized multicenter clinical trial included approximately 116 countries. Most of the single-center studies were from China (Table 1). The number of patients in the individual studies ranged from 3 to 153,760. In clinical studies 99 to 153,760, autopsy studies 3 to 411, immune profile studies 7 to 349, and thromboembolism studies 12 to 1144 (Table 1).

*3.2. Evidence from Neutrophil Deployment: Target Organs and Mechanism of Action*

Pre-existing cardiovascular disease (CVD) represents a significant risk factor in patients with SARS-CoV-2 infection who develop COVID-19. Once SARS-CoV-2 infects the myocardium, it can cause direct or indirect damage. Likewise, in these patients, outcomes are worse than in patients without CVD [55]. A specific role favoring the post-inflammatory injury is played by neutrophils that work as major representative cells of the innate immune system. The formation of extracellular neutrophil traps (NETs) is included among the multiple functions that neutrophils perform [56]. Neutrophil extracellular traps (NETs) are released by neutrophils to counter infections through the formation of extracellular webs of chromatin, oxidizing enzymes, and microbiocidal proteins [56].

3.2.1. COVID-19 and Inflammation

The first phase of infection with the development of COVID-19 begins with exposure to micro-droplets found in the exhalations of infected individuals. SARS-CoV-2 subsequently progresses to the bronchioles and alveolar spaces [57], where it is trapped in host cells (e.g., endothelial, epithelial, and smooth muscle cells) using a metallopeptidase available on the cell surface as the gateway, which is represented by the angiotensin-converting enzyme 2 (ACE2) [20,58–60]. We know that reaching the lung, SARS-CoV-2 infects alveolar cells (type I and II pneumocytes and alveolar macrophages) triggering intracellular replication mechanism in lung tissue. First early defense against the viral attacker is constituted by the production of type I and III interferons (IFN) which therefore have the role of inducing a premature defense mechanism to ensure the functional integrity of alveolar cells [57]. Recently, investigators disclosed an inadequate expression of these cytokines, other than the upregulation of the expression of chemokines and interleukins [61,62]. In normal human bronchial epithelial cell cultures (NHBE), an inhomogeneous profile affects cytokines. IFN deficiency is countered by an elevated expression of CCL20, CXC-type chemokines, IL-1$\beta$, IL-6, and tumor necrosis factor (TNF) [63–65]. In cell cultures exposed to SARS-CoV-2, the lack of IFN types I and III was evident, as despite susceptibility to the antiviral effect of IFN, SARS-CoV-2 retained the ability to inhibit its induction [62–65].

Likewise, SARS-CoV-2 positivity in cardiac tissue as well as in CD3+, CD45+ and CD68+ cells in myocardium and gene expression of tumor necrosis growth factor $\alpha$, interferon $\gamma$, chemokine ligand 5, as well as interleukin-6, -8 and -18 were found in cell cultures from autopsy findings of patients who died from COVID-19 [13]. Regarding the production of interferon, it seems clear that the reduction may derive at least in part from the triggering of a mechanism that blocks the activation of the IFN signaling pathway. This process can occur at an early stage after the nuclear transport of the interferon regulatory factors (IRF) [66].

We learned that the different inflammation pattern in the involved tissues was related to the recruitment of leukocytes. This is an imprint of authentication of the inflammatory response which is firmly linked to the chemokine profile. Therefore, the inflammatory site can be affected by one cell type over another. This process depends on the profile of the chemokines that act as drivers, conditioning the different pathologies that characterize the SARS-CoV-2 infection [67]. The increased presence of monocytes/macrophages is due to the production of chemokine ligand 2 (CCL2) and CCL8 responsible for their recruitment while chemokine (C-X-C) ligand 16 (CXCL16) is a powerful chemoattractant for Natural Killer (NK) lymphocytes. Interleukine 8 (CXCL8) is the main chemoattractant of neutrophils whereas chemokine CXCL9 and CXCL10 can recruit T cells that recognize these molecules as specific chemoattractants [67].

A variation between moderate and severe COVID-19 was immediately noticeable and relies on the different immune characteristics of the patients. These features can change after ten days of infection whereby individuals with a trend towards worsening symptoms experience elevated levels of proinflammatory cytokines [21]. Furthermore, in the forms of COVID-19 marked by nefarious evolution, the dysregulation of the inflammatory response to the SARS-CoV-2 infection can be responsible for the cytokine storm syndrome [22,68]. Regarding heart involvement, although unusual cases of COVID-19 fulminant viral myocarditis have been revealed, recent evidence has suggested that some individuals can exhibit direct damage to the myocardial tissue, albeit in small percentages of cases [13,14].

The cytokine storm syndrome is distinguished by high levels of interleukins, TNF-α, G-CSF, monocyte chemoattractant protein-1 (MCP-1), and: macrophage inflammatory protein 1 (MIP-1α), which remain higher in patients needing admission to the intensive care unit (ICU) than in patients who require this degree of clinical observation [21,23,24]. Furthermore, several studies have revealed that the NOD-like receptor family, pyrin domain containing 3 (NLRP3) inflammasome, a multiprotein complex crucial for host defense, maintains a high level of activation in patients with COVID-19. It is important to underline that prolonged activation of NLRP3 leads to an increase in the levels of IL-1β and IL-18 which are associated with more severe forms of COVID-19 [25,69,70]. The cytokine environment orchestrates the recall of immune cells by activating the T helper 1 (Th1) response, which is configured as type-specific immune response involved in the inhibition of macrophage activation and stimulation of B cells to produce IgM, IgG1. The most important function of Th1 cells includes the production of IFN-γ, a signature cytokine that activates macrophages and DCs to present antigens to T lymphocytes. Th1 cells can also secrete tumor necrosis factor (TNF), lymphotoxin, and IL-2 which help to give a solid immunological response in the host. High levels of IL-6 production were recorded and reliant on the inflammatory monocytes' activation as the distinct functions of Th1 cells in the severe form of COVID-19. This interaction supports the cytokine storm event [71], Figure 3.

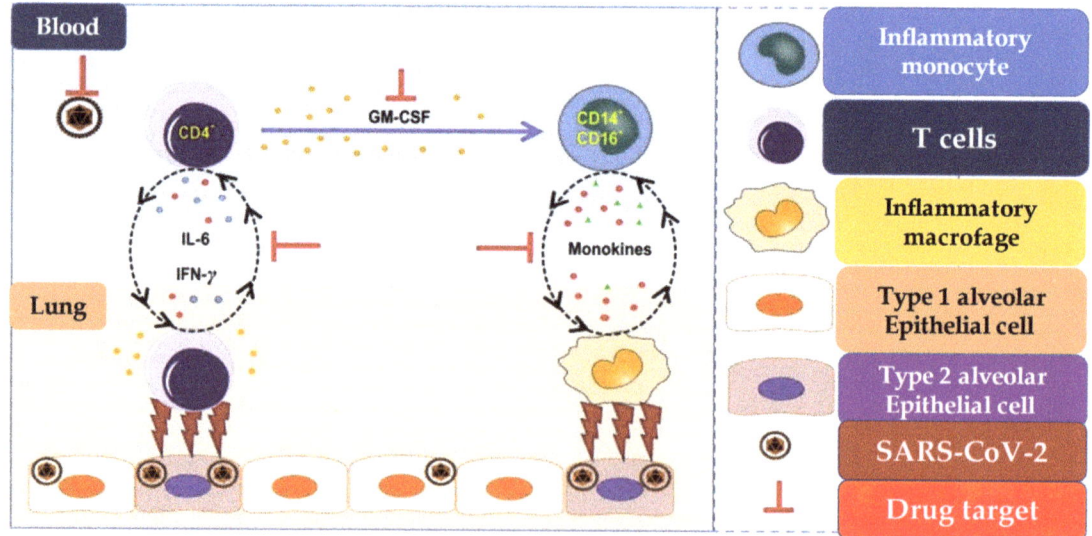

**Figure 3.** Pathogenic Th1 cells and inflammatory monocytes in severe COVID-19. Pathogenic CD4+ Th1 (GM-CSF+IFN-γ+) cells were rapidly activated to produce GM-CSF and other inflammatory cytokines to form a cascade signature of inflammatory monocytes (CD14+CD16+ with high expression of IL-6) and their progeny. These activated immune cells may enter the pulmonary circulation in large numbers and played an immune-damaging role in severe-pulmonary-syndrome patients. The monoclonal antibodies that target the GM-CSF or interleukin-6 receptor may potentially prevent or curb immunopathology caused by COVID-19. Abbreviations; GM-CSF, granulocyte-macrophage colony stimulating factor; IL, interleukine; IFN-γ, interféron gamma; SARS-CoV-2: severe acute respiratory syndrome-coronavirus-2.

Lindner et al. found high levels of IFN-γ and TNF in myocardiocytes of patients who died of COVID-19 suggesting that a Th1 response was elicited. Ref. [13] Huang et al. revealed that Th2 cytokine levels are detectable in patients with COVID-19 serum and their production can alter the response by modifying the Th1-inflammatory response [23]. Thus, as previously revealed by Lee et al. who reported that both inflammatory cytokine levels and a shift in Th1/Th2 balance worked as prognostic markers for hepatocellular carcinoma, ref. [72] the chemokine/cytokine environment coupled with the severe inflammatory response of the host may lead to potentially negative effects on the heart [13,14,55]. On the other hand, the environment where the chemokines/cytokines operate can constitute a possible target for the action of specific drugs used in the treatment of COVID-19 [73].

While awaiting the results from studies based on the pathoanatomical analysis of autopsy findings (heart, lung, kidney, and gastrointestinal system), which have demonstrated the occurrence of specific damage in the several tissues of deceased COVID-19 patients', ref. [13,26–28,74] the first reports have documented the substantial variation in the rate of peripheral blood immune cells (PBMC) in COVID-19 patients' [20,55]. Several convincing results have provided detailed answers on both the change in the percentage of cells of the immune response and the expression of HLA-DR genes [20,21,23,29,30,75]. Lucas et al. performed a longitudinal analysis from a large series of COVID-19 patients revealing an increased level of monocytes with a reduction of HLA-DR expression in the blood of infected individuals compared to that of the uninfected control cohort [23]. Evidence from other studies, involving patients with the severe form of COVID-19, disclosed a numerical reduction of B cells and NK cells associated with severe T-cell depletion. Instead, the neutrophil population recorded a considerable increase [21,23,29,30,75].

The increase in the rate of neutrophils varies with the worsening of clinical conditions and was generally observed after the seventh day from the onset of symptoms [31]. We recently reported a difference in the levels of immune response cells in the autopsy tissues of patients with poor outcomes [76].

3.2.2. Neutrophils Activation: Crucial in SARS-CoV-2 Cardiac Infection

Xie et al. analyzed data from nearly 154,000 U.S. veterans infected with SARS-CoV-2 providing evidence on the long-term cardiovascular outcomes of COVID-19 [32]. Patients were monitored during the following year after recovering from the severe form of the disease and noted to have an increased risk of developing a higher rate of cardiovascular complications. These included cases of heart rhythm abnormalities, inflammation of the heart muscles, blood clots, strokes, myocardial infarctions, and heart failure. The most relevant data emerged at 12-months, showed that the cohort of patients with COVID-19 compared to the control cohort had been associated with an additional 45.29 incidents for every 1000 people evaluated of any prespecified cardiovascular outcome [32].

The major concern related to the increased risk of long-term cardiovascular outcomes was the development of a cardiac inflammatory reaction sustained by the neutrophilic reaction. Neutrophils represent the most abundant immune cells in human blood (50–70% of all leukocytes). Given their function to serve as fundamental cells in counteracting a large number of infections, neutrophils play a critical homeostatic role working in the context of chronic inflammatory diseases [77]. Although these polymorphonuclear cells and NETs have the distinctive role of arousing a well-defined immune response against bacterial or fungal infections, their function in the context of viral infections is not entirely clear, especially with the development of the necroinflammation phenomenon [78,79].

The acute clinical manifestations of COVID-19 have been well characterized by a systemic inflammation leading to the development of sequelae in several organ systems, including cardiovascular disorders [20,33]. We learned, from limited evidence, that neutrophils improve antiviral response by interconnection with various immune cell populations. While fulfilling their tasks, the following specific actions have been taken into consideration: virus internalization and killing mechanism, cytokine release, degranulation, oxidative burst, and neutrophil extracellular traps (NETs) formation [79,80]. This sequence of events can lead to a series of accidents which in the first phase of the disease affect the respiratory system, but can subsequently extend as a pan-systemic inflammation favoring the onset of many other sequelae, which include cardiovascular disorders, gastrointestinal disorders, malaise, fatigue, musculoskeletal pain, nervous and neurocognitive system disorders, mental health disorders, metabolic disorders, and anemia [33].

The association between the presence of elevated levels of neutrophils at the site of infection and the development of pulmonary disease associated with acute respiratory distress syndrome (ARDS) is very frequent and has been documented in both influenza virus infection and SARS-CoV-1 [81]. Using a bioinformatics analysis method, Hemmat et al. revealed that neutrophil activation and degranulation were extremely powerful processes during SARS-CoV infection [82]. Likewise, the recruitment of polymorphonuclear (PMN) cells have been reported as a crucial hinge-point in the host immune response to COVID-19 associated with critical illness. Again, neutrophilia has been used to gauge the severity of ARDS and poor outcomes in patients with COVID-19.

In patients who exhibit the severe form of COVID-19, abnormal blood clots were described in association with pulmonary embolisms in the lungs and deep vein thromboses localized to the peripheral arterial and venous vascular branches of the legs. Dysregulated clot assembly leads to strokes or heart attacks [34,35,83]. This event is promoted by the formation of autoantibodies [84] and it is supported by an alteration of the neutrophil-to-lymphocyte ratio (NLR), which is one of the most relevant clinical inflammatory biomarkers. The increased NLR correlates and forecasts severe illness, especially when it emerges in the early stage of SARS-CoV-2 infection [36–38,85].

Some pooled data [24,39–41,86,87] have suggested that the emergence of severe COVID-19 was related to higher levels of D-dimer and C-reactive protein (CRP) that arises after the augmentation in NLR in critically ill COVID-19 cases [39,86]. Likewise, the corroboration of some comorbidities such as diabetes and CVD [87] associated with the increasing of NLR has been reported as an independent risk factor for mortality in hospitalized patients [24,40,41]. In particular, Liu et al. observed that the presence of diabetes with higher NLR in patients with COVID-19 leads to a more severe clinical picture with a longer hospital stay [88]. The conclusion of the investigators supported the idea that sustained chronic inflammation may favor a more severe COVID-19 [40,89].

Wang et al. and Varim et al. independently reported that the involvement of PMN cells leading to a substantial change in neutrophil/CD4+ lymphocyte index (NCD4LR) and the neutrophil count to albumin ratio (NAR), thus accounting for worsening progression of COVID-19 [42,90]. The first study found that although the fluctuation of the NLR ratio is a very selective diagnostic index of increased inflammatory response in patients with COVID-19, during SARS-CoV-2 infection the NCD4LR was associated with negative conversion time (NCT). The investigators have suggested that patients who exhibit elevated NCD4LR have a poorer immune function and prolonged virus clearance [42], which may be due to early cardiac complications such as ST elevation myocardial infarction (STEMI) [14]. The second study revealed that the NAR biomarker could be considered a new predictor of mortality in COVID-19 patients [90].

It may be speculated that NCD4LR and NAR values may also be used as clinical markers for COVID-19 progression in association with NLR [24] in patients with coronary artery disease and arterial hypertension, in which an increase of neutrophils is not only reported in the bloodstream, but also in the lungs and in the heart [18]. In patients with CVD who succumbed to deterioration of clinical condition following COVID-19 diagnosis, histological analyses revealed an accumulation of inflammatory cells associated with endothelium, as well as apoptotic bodies in the heart [18].

We learned that neutrophil infiltration is an unfavorable factor in patients with cardiovascular complications, the latter behaving readily as a key threat in COVID-19 in association with lung disease [43,91]. However, the role of neutrophils must be evaluated in a more organic context that involves angiotensin-converting enzyme 2 receptor (ACE2) and endothelial cells, since SARS-CoV-2 uses ACE2 as a gateway into the host. This receptor is expressed in several organs, including the heart, lung, kidneys, intestines, and endothelial cells [92]. Although PMN infiltrates are strongly associated with vascular derangements in COVID-19. However, whether this disequilibrium is due to endothelial cell involvement by the virus remains uncertain. Our current understanding suggests that human blood vessel organoids are directly infected by SARS-CoV-2 in vitro [93]. Varga et al. disclosed that circulatory failure due to myocardial infarction and ST-segment elevation complicated with right heart failure, cardiac arrest resulted in death were associated with PMN infiltration and lymphocytic endotheliitis in heart as well as lung, kidney, and liver with evidence of cell necrosis. The investigator pointed out that the emerged histological evidence of myocardial infarction was not associated with lymphocytic myocarditis. [18].

Another intriguing point is the discovery of immature phenotype and/or dysfunctional mature neutrophils that have been reported in the severe form of COVID-19 [94,95]. These studies indicate that increased infiltration of immature and/or dysfunctional neutrophils leads to an imbalance of the immune response of the lungs in severe cases of COVID-19, [96,97] in which cardiovascular atherosclerosis involvement and endothelitis occur [14,18], Figure 4.

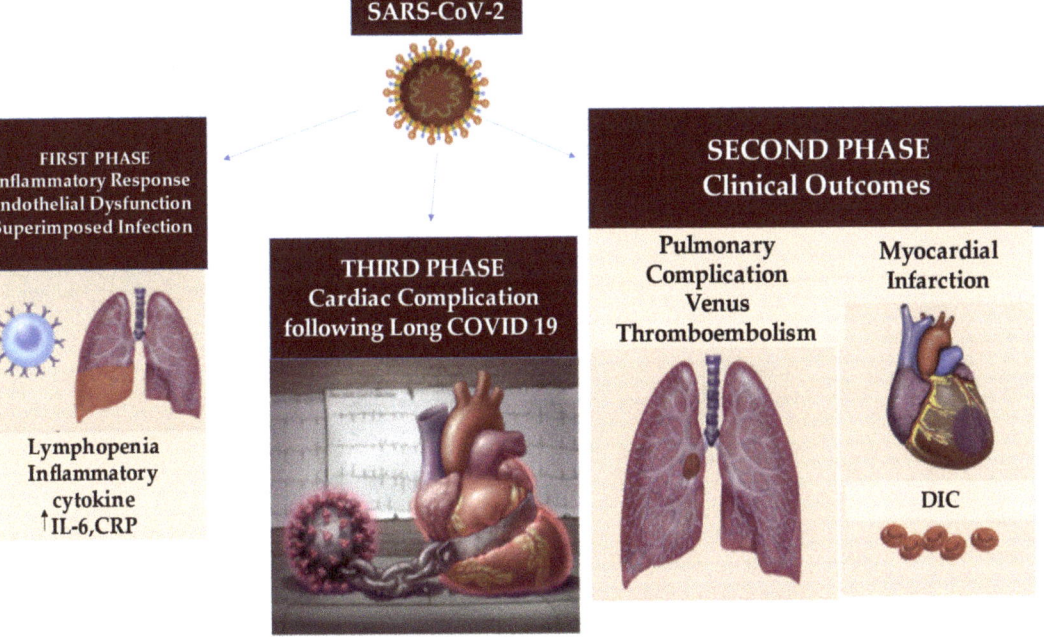

**Figure 4.** The acute clinical manifestations of COVID-19 are well characterized in the first and second phase, revealing an inflammatory response, endothelial dysfunction and overlapping infection that can evolve into thromboembolic and pulmonary complications, myocardial infarction and DIC. The third stage determines the COVID-19 heart condition after SARS-CoV-2 infection in which patients may reveal a range of increased cardiovascular risks. Abbreviations; CRP, C-reactive protein; DIC; disseminated intravascular coagulation. Other abbreviations in the previous figures. ↑, increase.

3.2.3. Neutrophils Extracellular Traps in COVID-19: The Hypothesis Takes Shape toward a Defined Role

Neutrophils extracellular traps are formed after the activation of neutrophils. The first description of the Nets was provided by Brinkman et al. who gave a new impetus to the investigation domain of granulocytes [56,98].

The structure of NETs is provided by nuclear chromatin to which nuclear histones and granular antimicrobial proteins are aggregated. NETs behave as scaffolds and this specificity makes them key elements to imprison microbes. Pathogens such as bacteria, fungi, viruses, and protozoa are killed once trapped [56,98]. This process is finalized inside the DNA fibers, avoiding the spread of pathogens and facilitating the concentration of antimicrobial factors at the site of infection [98].

NETosis orchestrates the entire process that leads to the formation of NETs and delineates a specific type of cell death, different from necrosis and apoptosis. Several studies have ascertained a very distinct role of NETosis in various infectious and non-infectious pathology such as the involvement in autoimmune diseases, cancer, venous thromboembolism, atherosclerosis, diabetes, etc. [99–101].

Briefly, NETosis is a cell death program that takes place in several stages which include the translocation of enzymes from the granules to the nucleus which facilitates chromatin decondensation. Importantly, the rupture of the internal membranes is recorded with the subsequent cytolysis and the release of the NETs. It should be pointed out that the main characteristic of NETosis is the disintegration of both the nuclear and granular membranes, but the integrity of the plasma membrane is preserved. This is a biological behavior that differentiates it from apoptosis or necrosis. The disruption of the nuclear wrapper during NETosis leads to the mixing of nuclear and cytoplasmic material, the loss of internal membranes, and the disappearance of cytoplasmic organelles. In detail, this process is marked by the absence of the peculiar signs of apoptosis such as the production of membrane bubbles, exposure to phosphatidylserine, condensation of nuclear chromatin, and DNA fragmentation [56].

In NETosis the intracellular proteins escape from the cells as both the nuclear and cytoplasmic membranes lose their integrity, thus delineating a process similar to that of cell necrosis. In inflammatory processes during the activation of neutrophils, specific biochemical mechanisms determine the production of reactive oxygen species (ROS), mediated by the activation of NADPH oxidase [102]. Nicotinamide adenine dinucleotide phosphate (NADPH) oxidase promotes the cell death process with the release of NETs. As regards the specific involvement of reactive oxygen species (ROS) in the release of NETs, it occurs through a process mediated by neutrophilic elastase and myeloperoxidase. Elastase translocates from cytoplasmic granules to the nucleus triggering the degradation of chromatin through histone cleavage [56,98,102]. Instead, myeloperoxidase contributes to the decondensation of nuclear DNA [56,98,102].

Since NETs participate in various pathological processes either by inhibiting or promoting damage, NETosis in oxidative stress has been carefully reconsidered [102,103]. There is evidence to reveal that this specific program, triggered during the life of neutrophils, is not just a path to death. So much so that a second mechanism biologically classified as "vital" NETosis has been proposed [104]. During the "vital" NETosis the release of NETs is also necessary. The difference between the two processes, « death » or « vital » NETosis, lies in the nature of the precipitate stimulus, in the timing and mechanisms used to induce the release of NETs [104].

Virologists explained this specific ability that viruses have in evading the host's immune response. This peculiar ability makes them particularly dangerous as promoters responsible for triggering the processes of NETosis [105–107]. Therefore, many viruses favor the production of NETs, after activating the neutrophils, with different modalities. First, the neutrophils release NETs according to the usual biological processes described above. On the other hand, neutrophils can produce antiviral agents or undertake the transition to apoptosis. It is important to underline that once the virus-induced NET production has taken place, with the constitution of double-stranded DNA complexes, histones, and granular proteins, they can circulate in an uncontrolled way. The resulting relative phenomenon is the organism's extreme systemic response to the production of immune complexes, cytokines, and chemokines, ultimately promoting inflammation. As emerges from recent studies that have revealed cardiac complications in patients with COVID-19, NETosis induced by the virus acts on two fronts. While on one front the mechanical entrapment of the virus is observed, on the other, the inflammatory and immunological reaction triggered by the release of the NETs with the induction of potential damage is highlighted [14].

With the advent of COVID-19, NETosis activity of infected patients has garnered interest to understand whether the clinical course of the disease is as a worsening evolution or as a clinical recovery, may be conditioned by NETosis, Figure 5.

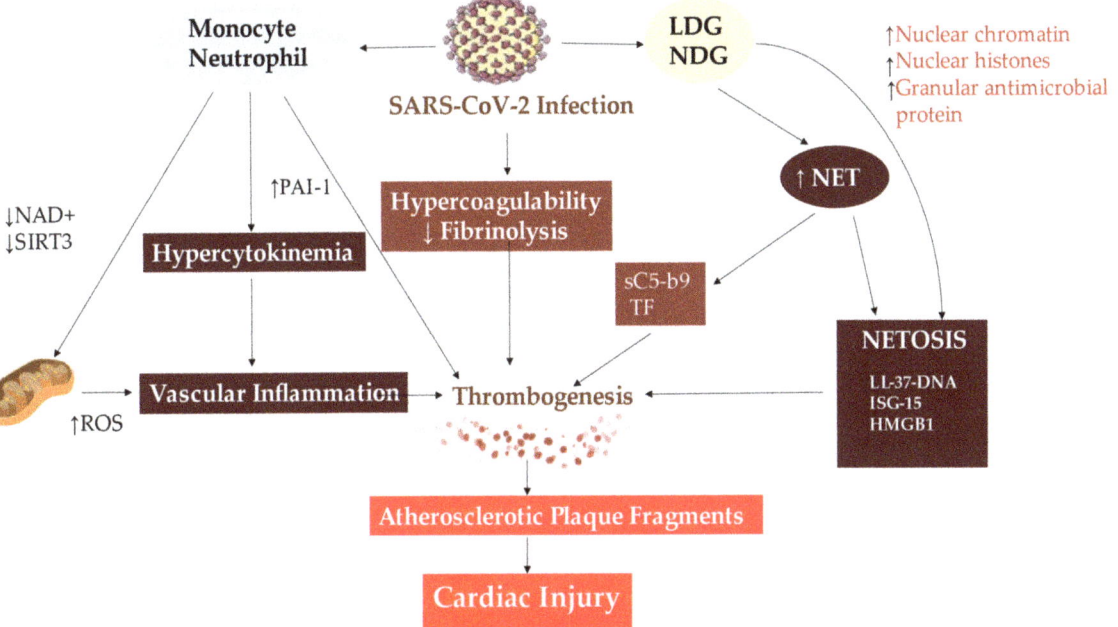

**Figure 5.** The mechanism leading to cardiac injury from NETs formation in patients with severe COVID-19 is determined by vascular inflammation, thrombogenesis and NETOSIS through the instability of the atherosclerotic plaque. Abbreviations: HMGB1, mobility group box; ISG-15; interferon-stimulated gene; LDG, low-density granulocytes; NDG, normal density granulocytes; NAD, nicotin adenin dinucleotide; ROS, reactive oxygen species; SIRT3, Sirtuin 3. Other abbreviations in previous figure. ↑, increase; ↓, decrease.

Two points should be underlined. The first concerns the fact that NETosis has been evoked as a well-defined process in the inflammatory response occurring in pulmonary diseases. In fact, evidence from bronchoalveolar lavage fluid suggested an increased level of NETs in patients with acute respiratory distress syndrome (ARDS) [108,109], as well as in patients who disclosed worse clinical condition after developing an acute respiratory failure secondary to chronic obstructive pulmonary disease (COPD) [110]. Likewise, patients with clinically severe forms of COVID-19 or who have exhibited worse progressive symptoms, sustained by the cytokine storm, develop an ARDS-like status with increased NETs [111]. The second point concerns the correlation between NETs release and thrombotic complications in COVID-19 infection, involving the arterial and venous districts [43,44]. Several studies have reported marked evidence of micro and macro thrombotic phenomena such as microangiopathy leading to pulmonary embolism [45], for which antithrombotic and/or coagulation prophylaxis was in short order initiated [43–45].

Histopathology from lung specimens disclosed fibrin-based blockages in the small blood vessels in COVID-19 patients' who died [13,15–19]. This pathoanatomic condition mimics acquired and potentially life-threatening thrombophilia such as the antiphospholipid syndrome, in which patients develop pathogenic autoantibodies targeting phospholipids and phospholipid-binding proteins (aPL antibodies) such as prothrombin and beta 2 glycoprotein I (beta 2GPI). These antibodies undertake cell surfaces leading to the activation of endothelial cells, platelets, and neutrophils [84,112,113]. Ultimately the antibodies affect the blood-endothelium interface toward thrombosis. These aPL antibodies have recently been reported in patients who experienced COVID-19 [114,115] as well as many patients admitted to hospital with the severe form of COVID-19 who displayed NETs in their blood which may also contribute to the prothrombotic milieu [84,116].

Zuo et al. found eight types of aPL antibodies in serum samples from 172 patients who required hospitalization for COVID-19 and with a rate ranging between 30% to 52%. These aPL antibodies included anticardiolipin IgG, IgM, and IgA; anti-β2 glycoprotein I IgG, IgM, and IgA; and anti-phosphatidylserine/prothrombin (aPS/PT) IgG and IgM. Three main findings were identified in this study [46]. The first revealed that neutrophil hyperreactivity was highly dependent on superior titers of aPL antibodies, including the release of extracellular neutrophil traps (NETs), greater platelet counts, more severe respiratory disease, and clinically estimated glomerular filtration rate. Second, as was observed with the presence of a specific IgG activity in patients with antiphospholipid antibody syndrome, the presence of isolated IgG fractions that favored the release of NETs from neutrophils isolated from healthy individuals was also recorded in patients with COVID-19. Third, IgG purified from serum from COVID-19 patients was injected into two mouse models of mice causing an acceleration of venous thrombosis. The authors concluded that half of the patients seeking admission for COVID-19 experienced a transient rise in aPL antibodies; these autoantibodies are potentially pathogenic and can lead to an increase in NETs [46].

These explained processes are of crucial importance as they outline the role of NETosis which appears to be substantial in all conditions characterized by venous and arterial thrombosis. Concerns related to the activity of DNAse I, an enzyme that catalyzes the digestion of NETs, and the phagocytic activity of macrophages, which profusely infiltrate the cardiac extracellular matrix in COVID-19 patients with cardiac complications [14], deserve a more in-depth evaluation. In fact, these are the two main mechanisms for regulating and self-limiting NETosis [20–43,56–98], show in Figure 6.

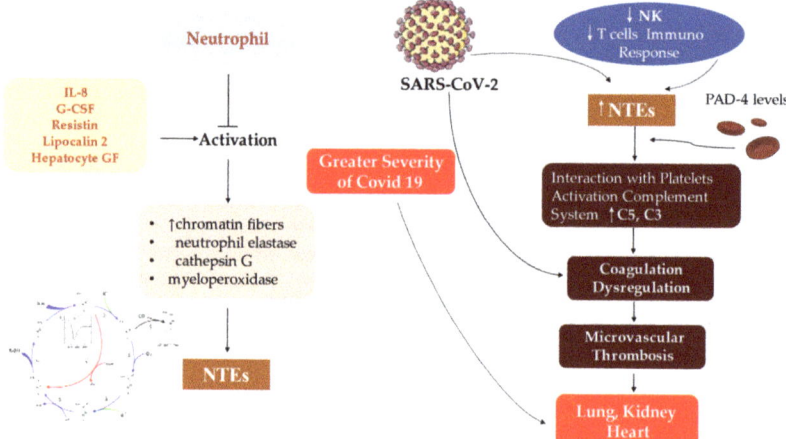

**Figure 6.** SARS-CoV-2 determines the activation of neutrophils mediated by IL-8, G-CSF, resistin, lipocalin-2, hepatocyte growth factor and NET release. The immune response of NK and T lymphocytes contributes to the formation of NETs with the increased level of a completement system (C5 and C3). The generated microvascular thrombosis leads to organ damage. Abbreviations: C, complement; GF, grow factor; IL, interleukine; NK; natural killer. Bottom left depict the biochemical reaction for the formation of NETs Other abbreviations in previous figure. ↑, increase; ↓, decrease.

## 4. Insights into the Role of Neutrophil Extracellular Traps and Their Interference in the Heart Inflammation Process from SARS-CoV-2 Infection

Myocardial injury has a crucial role as greater provider of mortality in COVID-19. The landmark study of Zhou et al. [43] from Wuhan reported a larger percentage of mortality reaching 70% of patients hospitalized with elevated cardiac troponin I plasma levels. Acute inflammation response precipitated by SARS-CoV-2 infection is fitted together atherosclerotic plaque development and progression. The concern related to SARS-CoV-2 heart infection is directly linked to acute inflammatory stimulus, prompted by virus localization in the cardiac tissue. The development and destabilization of atherosclerotic plaque may lead to acute myocardial infarction. Several studies [1,2,13,14,18,94] have confirmed these data thus highlighting the fundamental role offered by the phenomenon of the "cytokine storm" in determining ischemic heart disease [21,23,24,68,94]. Virologists and immunologists have learned that the proinflammatory cytokines elicited by endothelial cells lead to a change in homeostatic functions with the consequent endothelial damage, the subsequent destabilization of the atherosclerotic plaque and the evolution towards thrombosis. Cytokines such as IL-1 $\alpha$ and IL-1$\beta$, IL-6, and TNF-$\alpha$ can perturb all of the protective functions of the normal endothelium so as to enhance pathological processes [21,23,24,42,68,80–82,94].

Specifically, IL-1 can induce its own gene expression thus leading to an amplification of the levels of IL1 that trigger the cytokine storm [14,68]. Furthermore, IL-1 promotes the expression of other proinflammatory cytokines including TNF-$\alpha$. IL-1 and leukocyte migration can inspire the production of chemotactic molecules including chemokines that cause inflammatory cells to penetrate into tissues. Meanwhile, IL-1 stimulates the production of IL-6. The substantial role of IL-6, whose plasma levels are generally very low, is to promote a of immune and inflammatory responses. During acute infection, a wide kind of cells, including macrophages, B and T lymphocytes, work to determine an increase in the production of IL-6. In addition to local effects, IL-6 provides a proximal stimulus to the acute phase response [14,23–25,36,68–71,81,82,85].

Again, IL-6 works to support the production of fibrinogen which is the main precursor of clots and of PAI-1 which is an important inhibitor of endogenous fibrinolytic mediators. Finally, the action of IL-6 is aimed at increasing the levels of C-reactive protein, a biomarker of inflammation closely linked to COVID-19 infection. During the infection, a loss of the barrier function of the endothelium has been proved due to its activation, with a consequent increased expression of adhesion molecules such as soluble ICAM-1 (intercellular adhesion molecule 1), of soluble VCAM-1 (molecule vascular cell adhesion 1), and VWF release. The latter allows for platelet binding and TF expression which activates the coagulation system [11,34,36–40,86].

The evidence of NETs has been revealed in coronary thrombi from patients who exhibit STEMI and myocardial infarction as a complication of COVID-19 [14]. To date, there are no studies that have clarified precisely the intrinsic mechanism of coronary occlusion in patients with COVID-19 who develop STEMI. In this context, evidence resulting from a cohort of 55 patients who underwent primary coronary interventions for STEMI suggested that NETs play a decisive role in the pathogenesis of coronary thrombosis in COVID-19 and the onset of MI. The investigators disclosed NETs in all 5 patients with COVID-19 who received intracoronary aspirates compared to those (n = 50) without the infectious disease during the primary percutaneous coronary intervention (PCI) [14].

A relevant finding of this investigation disclosed that the median density of NET ranged at 61% (95%CI, 43–91%) and this value was remarkably higher than reported in a previous series. Rather, the investigators found that NETs reached 68% in the sampling of aspirated coronary thrombus during primary PCI from 34 patients with a median NET density reported at 19% (95% CI, 13–22%; $p < 0.001$) [117].

NETs are released by neutrophils and perform the function of trapping pathogens as they are made up of web-like structures of DNA and proteins (histones, microbicidal proteins, and oxidizing enzymes). However, dysregulation of NET function is critical in initiating and increasing inflammation and thrombosis [46,84]. Cersana et al. studied post mortem finding from a large series of pulmonary autopsy samples of COVID-19 patients' revealing an excessive NET formation, responsible for a quickly pulmonary microvessels occlusion and severe organ damage [47]. Importantly, Blasco et al. observed an abundant amount of NET in coronary thrombi of COVID-19 patients with complicated STEMI and MI [117]. Furthermore, the burden of NET was significantly higher than that reported in a previous series of patients with STEMI but without COVID-19 infection [14,117]. From the histochemical point of view, all thrombi were constituted by conglomerates of fibrin and polymorphonuclear cells. An interesting finding suggested the absence of atherosclerotic plaque fragments that were evident in 65% of the coronary clot aggregates of the control group who experienced STEMI without infection. The preponderance of atheromatous plaque fragments supported evidence that already emerged in a previous study by the same group in 142 patients with STEMI [117].

We learned that coagulation changes associated with COVID-19 suggested the existence of a hypercoagulable state that can lead to an increase in the risk of thromboembolic complications [14,46,84,114–117]. We also know that patients with COVID-19 typically experience an increase in D-dimer concentration, a relatively lowly decrease in platelet count, and a prolongation of prothrombin time [10]. These perturbations, except for an increase in Dimer D, are not found in patients showing NET release and STEMI [14,117]. Therefore, the idea is reinforced that neutrophils and NETs play an important role in causing thrombus formation in coronary arteries of patients with COVID-19 [12,56,98]. Once again, an association between NET and unfavorable clinical outcomes after STEMI is outlined, even if no definitive results are available on the specific components of the NET measured peripherally. NET may help to define an unfavorable prognostic picture in patients with COVID-19 to which a STEMI contributes to clinical manifestations [14,117].

Lindner et al. described the presence of the viral genome in myocardial tissue from 39 autopsy samples, in which fifteen (38.5%) did not disclose SARS-CoV-2 [13]. Pneumonia occurred as the cause of death with a rate of 89.7% of individuals (n = 35) and none of the patients revealed had clinically fulminant myocarditis [13]. This finding corroborates previous evidence to support the expression of the SARS-CoV-2 spike glycoprotein selective ACE2 receptor on the surface of myocardial cells [118] as well as the substantial involvement of myocardial tissue in infection [119]. The most revealing findings highlighted by Lindner after in situ hybridization of myocardial tissue suggests the most likely localization of SARS-CoV-2 was not found in cardiomyocytes but interstitial cells or macrophages invading myocardial tissue. The investigators reported the presence of CD3+, CD45+, and CD68+. However, the cohort that exhibited the viral genome did not record an increase in mononuclear cell infiltrates into the myocardium compared to the cohort without virus. [13] Particularly, 1/3 of patients with viral load greater than 1000 copies, deemed clinically significant, revealed signs of viral replication within myocardial tissue. Investigators documented increased expression in patients with a viral load greater than 1000 copies where cytokines are currently implicated in the modulation of the inflammatory process. 16 patients had an increased expression of 6 proinflammatory genes related to cytokine production (tumor necrosis growth factor α, interferon γ, chemokine ligand 5, interleukin-6, -8, and -18) compared with 15 patients without any SARS-CoV-2 in the heart [13].

This evidence is in line with the findings of Guzik et al. who linked cytokine-induced organ dysfunction to the disease process [6]. What emerges from Lindner's study is crucial in pointing out that patients with SARS-CoV-2 infection and viral replication did not show associated fulminant myocarditis. In fact, in this study, relevant data is offered by the lack of significant changes in the transendothelial migration of inflammatory cells in the myocardium of patients with high viral load compared to those who did not have any virus. Conversely, several studies reported a correlation between the occurrence of myocardial inflammation and evidence of clinical myocarditis. Lindner et al., therefore, offered an explanation supporting the idea that viral replication and myocarditis may not be two joint processes. Moreover, their results suggested no increased inflammatory cells in consecutive COVID-19 cases without clinical myocarditis [13].

The crucial point focuses on the long-term effects of the presence of the virus in myocardial tissue. Whether the presence of viral activity in the myocardium in the absence of clinical symptoms of myocarditis remains unknown. However, we know that the leukocytopenia that characterizes patients with COVID-19 could hinder the migration of activated mononuclear cells [120]. Among these cells, the scarce presence of macrophages, responsible for digesting NETs, could play a crucial role in maintaining a high NETs release level, Figure 7.

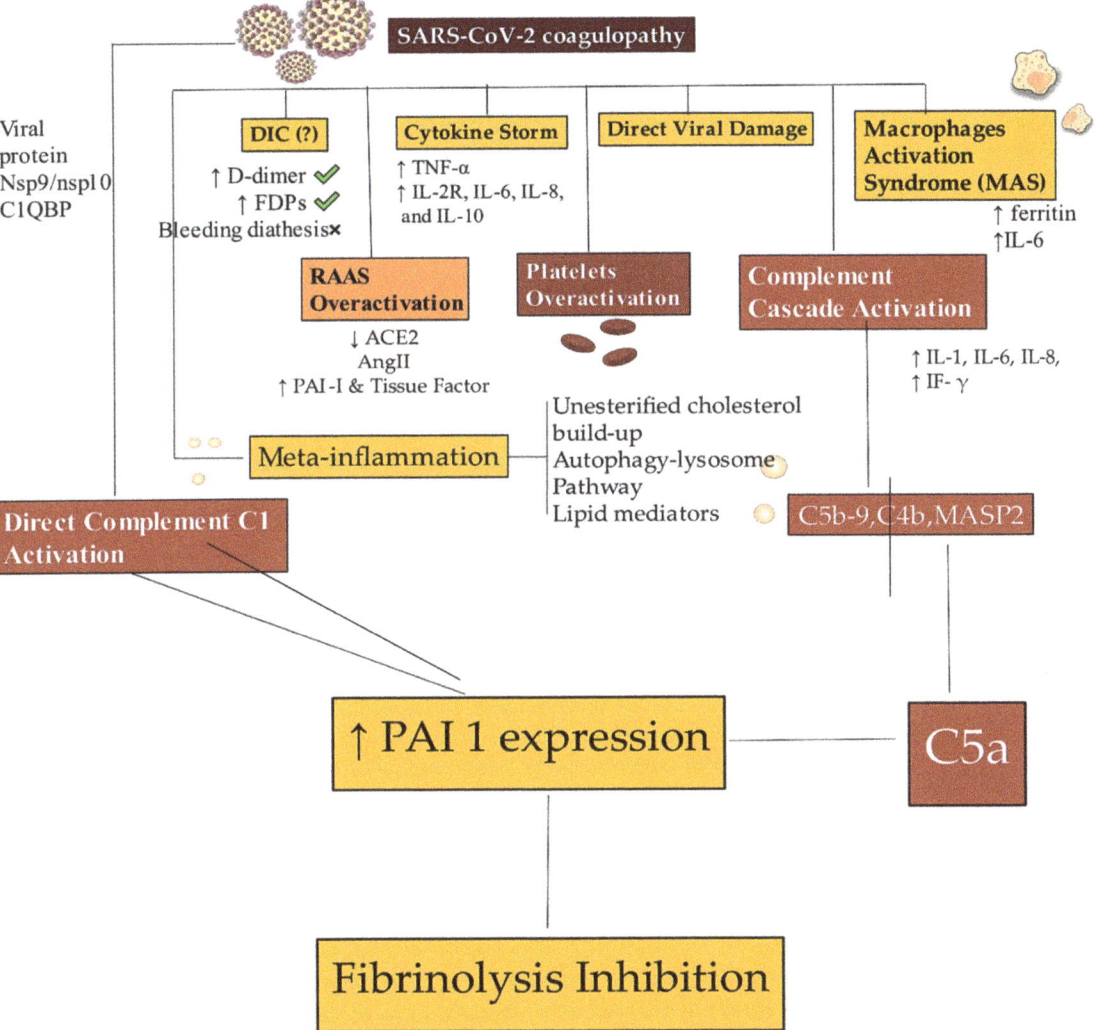

**Figure 7.** SARS-CoV-2 infection determines dysregulations in coagulation system. The coagulopathy is supported by the DIC, cytokine storm process, and direct action of the virus, inducing damage and activation of macrophages. RAAS overactivation associated with platelet and complement overactivation (direct and indirect) leads to fibrinolysis inhibition. Abbreviations are as shown in previous figures. Arrows explain the increase or decrease of relative component. ↑, increase; ↓, decrease.

## 5. Comment: Myocardial Injury and Mortality in Patients with COVID-19

The data available from China, Italy, in the United States are in favor of a COVID-19 which occurs in a relatively mild clinical form in most of the affected individuals, but in others, COVID-19 can be life-threatening. The experiences gained in these years of the pandemic support the evidence that the individuals at the highest risk of serious illness, such as requiring intensive care hospitalization and those at the greatest risk of mortality, are older individuals, with underlying comorbidities, including cardiovascular diseases [20,23,48–53,55,121–123]. However, even younger adults have disclosed serious illnesses for which hospitalization and surgery were necessary with deaths in this age group reported [50–53,123].

As previously observed in other epidemiological studies focused on the clinical evolution of influenza and other diseases supported by an acute inflammatory state, patients who develop COVID-19 in the presence of diagnosed coronary artery disease and those with risk factors for atherosclerotic cardiovascular disease have an increased risk of experiencing acute coronary syndromes during the disease [124–126]. Established acute coronary events, similar to type 2 myocardial infarction, could be related to the significant increase in myocardial demand directly related to infection that can lead to myocardial damage or infarction [127]. However, there is the possibility that an uncontrolled increase in the levels of circulating cytokines released during intense systemic inflammatory activity can lead to instability or even rupture of the atherosclerotic plaque. Another possible comparison with COVID-19 patients concerns patients with heart failure who can manifest an evolution towards haemodynamic decompensation during stressful conditions related to serious infectious diseases [50–53,123].

What emerged from the published reports found that patients with underlying cardiovascular disease, which are more prevalent in the elderly, are more prone to higher risks of adverse outcomes and death during the more aggressive forms of COVID-19 sustained by severe inflammatory states, compared to younger patients. It should be noted that similar to the Middle East Respiratory Syndrome coronavirus outbreak, acute/fulminant myocarditis associated with heart failure has been described in SARS-CoV-2 as well.

Two independent Chinese reports [1,2] describing hospital series from Wuhan, have corroborated these concepts while providing new evidence regarding the incidence and consequences of myocardial lesions associated with SARS-CoV-2. In the first study [1] investigators analyzed a cohort of 416 hospitalized patients with COVID-19, using the highly sensitive reverse transcriptase-polymerase chain reaction technique, confirmed that 19.7% (n = 82) of patients revealed myocardial damage from the increase in troponin I (TnI) levels. Patients with myocardial damage had a hospital stay with a significantly higher mortality rate of 51.2% (42 of 82) than 4.5% without myocardial damage (15 of 335). Furthermore, in patients with myocardial damage, higher levels of TnI elevation were associated with higher mortality rates.

The second report [2] supports the above with 11 in a cohort of 187 hospitalized patients with laboratory confirmed COVID-19, of which 27.8% (n = 52) revealed myocardial damage noted by elevated troponin T (TnT) levels, providing additional novel insights concerning levels of C-reactive protein and N-terminal pro-B-type natriuretic peptide (NT-proBNP). First, investigators pointed to a rate of in-hospital mortality of 59.6% (31 out of 52) in patients with high TnT levels compared to 8.9% (12 out of 135) in those with normal TnT levels. Other relevant evidence supported that the highest mortality rates of 69.4% (25 out of 36) were recorded in individuals with elevated TnT levels where the underlying cardiovascular disease was noted. Another crucial point suggested that mortality rates were lower in patients with high TnT levels without prior cardiovascular history. Second, patients with known cardiovascular disease without elevation of TnT levels disclosed a mortality rate that was relatively favorable despite a mortality rate of 13.3% (4 of 30). Third, TnT levels were significantly associated with levels of C-reactive protein and N-terminal pro-B-type natriuretic peptide (NT-proBNP), thus relating myocardial damage to the severity of the inflammatory state and ventricular dysfunction. Both

TnT and NT-proBNP levels recorded progressive serial increases during hospitalization in patients with progressively deteriorating clinical courses. Conversely, patients with a less severe form of the disease and more favorable outcomes with lower levels of these biomarkers [2].

The studies of Shi et al. and Guo et al. carried out at the beginning of the pandemic on the Wuhan population have offered us a picture with substantially similar characteristics in patients with COVID-19 and elevated levels of TnI or TnT, who develop myocardial damage with adverse outcomes [1,2]. Patients at risk of myocardial damage have more advanced age and higher comorbidities such as the increased prevalence of hypertension, coronary artery disease, heart failure, and diabetes compared to the cohorts with normal levels of TnI or TnT. Evidence of more severe systemic inflammation is indisputable in patients with myocardial damage, including substantial increases in PMNs, higher levels of C-reactive protein and procalcitonin as well as high levels of other myocardial biomarkers injury and stress, such as elevated creatine kinase, myoglobin, and NT-proBNP. A finding that emerges in patients with COVID-19 and associated myocardial injury concerns the presence of a greater acuity of the disease, with a higher incidence of acute respiratory distress syndrome and more frequent necessitation of mechanical ventilatory support compared to those without myocardial damage. Therefore, the picture that arises from these two studies, confirmed by other reports based on cardiac autopsy and PCI performed in patients with COVID-19, is consistent with the history of patients who experienced the disease. The picture offers older patients who have contracted SARS-CoV-2 with pre-existing cardiovascular comorbidities and diabetes who are most prone to developing the disease with greater clinical acuity. These individuals have an associated increased risk of developing myocardial damage and a significantly higher short-term mortality rate [1,2].

The first report carried out on the Wuhan population represents a window that opens to further evaluations. For example, Yang and Zin discussed the relationship between cardiovascular complications during the COVID-19 outbreak in China and the underlying cardiovascular outbreak that has been studied in China for decades [128]. Investigators agree with many recent observations that the occurrence of pre-existing cardiovascular comorbidity leads to the most adverse complications of COVID-19, including death [128]. However, it is important to point out that only with subsequent reports, highlighting systemic inflammation and an uncontrolled coagulopathy in COVID-19, was a more complete explanation offered those serious infections can destabilize patients with coronary artery disease or heart failure [49–53,122,123].

The important association between myocardial damage and adverse outcomes has focused its attention on possible complementary mechanisms such as intense systemic inflammatory stimuli that favors greater oxygen consumption resulting in demand ischemia which evolves into myocardial damage or plaque rupture stimulated by SARS-CoV-2 behaves similarly to other coronaviruses as it can elicit the intense release of multiple cytokine and chemokines [23–53,69–128]. This stage is decisive not only in favoring vascular inflammation, plaque instability, and inflammation of the myocardium but also in triggering the release of NETs.

In some patients with or without pre-existing cardiovascular comorbidities, myocarditis may occur as COVID-19 coupled myocardial damage [129]. Again, after the well-documented case of acute myocarditis following a respiratory infection associated with COVID-19 in a 53-year-old Italian woman, several studies have documented that direct viral infection of the myocardium is another possible causal pathway of myocardial damage [5]. However, in cardiac autopsies, the virus was found in interstitial myocardial tissue without the presence of replication in myocardial cells lacking unequivocal myocarditis [13].

We have learned the existence of the affinity of SARS-CoV-2 to the host angiotensin-converting enzyme 2 receptor [1,2,128], which has been shown previously for other coronaviruses [119], raising the possibility of direct viral infection of vascular endothelium and myocardium. Although the cardiovascular complications of acute COVID-19 disease are well described, the post-acute cardiovascular manifestations that characterize

COVID-19 have not yet been fully elucidated. Al-Aly et al. and Xie et al. using the national health care database of the United States Department of Veterans Affairs created a cohort of 153,760 individuals with COVID-19, to which two groups of control cohorts with 5,637,647 (contemporary controls) and 5,859,411 (historical controls) were added [32,54]. The authors using this large population estimated risks and 1-year charges of a set of pre-specified cardiovascular outcomes. Interestingly Xie et al. noted that beyond the first 30 days of the infectious incident, patients with COVID-19 had an increased risk of cardiovascular disease-related events affecting several categories, including cerebrovascular disorders, arrhythmias, ischemic and non-ischemic heart disease, pericarditis, myocarditis, heart failure, and thromboembolic disease [54].

The results reported by Xie et al. offer a crucial explanation of how these risks and charges were evident even among individuals for whom hospitalization was not required during the acute phase of the infection. The risk of developing a cardiovascular complication gradually increased based on the care setting in which patients were treated during the acute phase. The risk was lower in non-hospitalized patients, followed by hospitalized patients, and higher in ICU patients. The findings described in the report by Xie et al. support evidence that both the 1-year risk and burden of cardiovascular disease in acute COVID-19 survivors were considerable. COVID-19 is a disease with a high social impact and particular attention to the care pathways of those who survive the acute episode of COVID-19 is required. Attention to cardiovascular health and disease should be included among these [54], Figure 8.

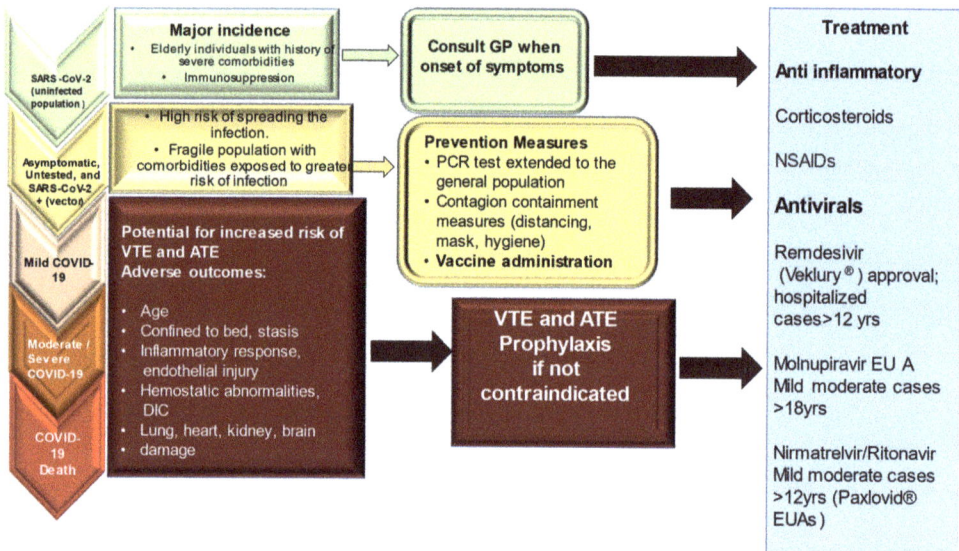

**Figure 8.** The infection from SARS-CoV-2 caused a variability in the manifestation of the disease. This explains the different population rates of infection and the distinct mortality rates of manifest cases in various regions and countries. Inflammatory response, increased age, and bed rest, which are most frequently seen in severe coronavirus disease 2019 (COVID-19), may contribute to thrombosis and adverse events resulting from multiorgan involvement. FDA timeline of antivirals approval and EUAs. Veklury® EUA was formalized in January 2020. Its definitive approval occurred in October, 2020. Molnupiravir and Paxlovid® EUAs followed in December 2021. Abbreviations: ATE, arterial thromboembolism.; COVID-19, coronavirus disease 2019; DIC, disseminated intravascular coagulation; EUA: Emergency Use Authorization; FDA: Food and Drug Administration; NSAIDs, non-steroid anti-inflammatory drugs; SARS-CoV-2, severe acute respiratory syndrome-coronavirus-2; VTE, venous thromboembolism.

## 6. Future Direction

New challenges await scientific community and among these the rewiring of granulopoiesis can offer a therapeutically relevant implication for trained immunity. In fact, a crucial role in successfully coping with SARS-CoV-2 infection can be offered by the trained innate immunity that is induced through the modulation of mature myeloid cells or their bone marrow progenitors. The bacillus of the Calmette-Guérin tuberculosis vaccine (BCG) has been shown to protect against certain heterologous infections through a process known as trained immunity. This type of immunity is probably achieved through the induction of innate nonspecific immune memory in monocytes and natural killer (NK) cells. Two recent independent studies revealed that induction of trained immunity is associated with a tendency to granulopoiesis in bone marrow hematopoietic progenitor cells [130–132].

The first study found that BCG vaccination of healthy humans induced long-lasting changes in the neutrophil phenotype, characterized by increased expression of activation markers and antimicrobial function. Evidence has suggested that enhanced human neutrophil function persists for at least 3 months after vaccination and is associated with genome-wide epigenetic modifications in histone 3 lysine 4 trimethylation [130].

In the second study promising evidence emerged on improving antitumor immunity that can be improved through the induction of trained immunity. Mouse models pretreated with β-glucan, a prototype of fungal-derived trained immunity agonist, revealed a substantial decrease in tumor growth. The antitumor effect of trained immunity induced by β-glucan, is associated with the transcriptomic and epigenetic rewiring of granulopoiesis and the reprogramming of neutrophils towards an antitumor phenotype. This process requires signaling of type I interferon, regardless of adaptive immunity in the host. Adoptive transfer of neutrophils from β-glucan-trained mice to untreated recipients suppressed tumor growth by ROS-dependent action [131,132].

## 7. Conclusions

The cardiovascular implications of the COVID-19 pandemic have caused significant morbidity and mortality. The process of understanding the mechanism for the manifestation of these adverse outcomes is crucial to permit treatment and management options for these patients. The adverse cardiovascular outcomes manifest in several different manners from demand-induced ischaemia, coronary obstruction, and direct myocardial infiltration alongside others. The long-term effects of this pandemic, however, remain uncertain and require ongoing monitoring and research as the endemic phase of the disease is embraced. Functional reprogramming of neutrophils by inducing trained immunity could offer original therapeutic strategies in clinical conditions that could benefit from modulation of neutrophil effector function.

**Author Contributions:** Conceptualization, F.N.; methodology, F.N., F.B. and S.S.A.S.; software, F.B. and S.S.A.S.; validation, F.N., F.B. and S.S.A.S.; formal analysis, F.N. and S.S.A.S.; investigation, F.N.; data curation, F.N., F.B. and S.S.A.S.; writing—original draft preparation, F.N.; writing—review and editing, F.N., F.B. and S.S.A.S.; visualization, F.N., F.B. and S.S.A.S.; supervision, F.N., F.B. and S.S.A.S. All authors have read and agreed to the published version of the manuscript.

**Funding:** This research received no external funding.

**Institutional Review Board Statement:** Not applicable.

**Informed Consent Statement:** Not applicable.

**Data Availability Statement:** Not applicable.

**Conflicts of Interest:** The authors declare no conflict of interest.

**Abbreviations**

| | |
|---|---|
| ACE1 | angiotensin I-converting enzyme |
| ACE2 | Angiotensin-Converting Enzyme 2 |
| ACEi | ACE–inhibitors |
| aPL | antiphospholipid |
| aPS/PT Ab | anti-phosphatidylserine/prothrombin autoantibodies |
| APS | antiphospholipid syndrome |
| ARDS | acute respiratory distress syndrome |
| AT1R | Angiotensin Type 1 Receptor |
| C | complement |
| CCL | chemokine ligand |
| COPD | Chronic Obstructive Pulmonary Disease |
| COVID-19 | Coronavirus disease-2019 |
| CRP | C-reactive protein |
| CXCL | chemokine ligand |
| CXCL8 | Interleukine 8 |
| CVD | cardiovascular disease |
| DAD | diffuse alveolar damage |
| DIC | disseminated intravascular coagulation |
| ECM | extracellular matrix |
| FDP | fibrinogen derived peptides |
| G-CSF | granulocytes colony-stimulating factor |
| GF | grow factor |
| GM-CSF | granulocyte-macrophage colony stimulating factor |
| HLA-DR | human leucocyte antigen- related D |
| ICAM-1 | intercellular adhesion molecule 1 |
| ICU | intensive care unit |
| IFN | interféron |
| IL | interleukine |
| IP-10 | interferon-gamma-induced protein |
| IRF | interferon regulatory factors |
| ISG-15 | interferon stimulated gene 15 |
| LDG | low-density granulocytes |
| mAb | monoclonal antibody |
| MASP2 | mannose-binding protein associated serine protease 2 |
| MAS | macrophage activation syndrome. |
| MCP-1 | monocyte chemoattractant protein-1 |
| M-CSF | macrophage colony-stimulating factor |
| MIP 1 | macrophage inflammatory protein 1 |
| NADPH | Nicotinamide adenine dinucleotide phosphate |
| NAR | neutrophil count to albumin ratio |
| NCD4LR | neutrophil/CD4 + lymphocyte index |
| NCT | negative conversion time |
| NDG | normal density granulocytes |
| NETs | neutrophil extracellular traps. |
| NHBE | human bronchial epithelial cell |
| NLR | neutrophil-to-lymphocyte ratio |
| NLRP3 | NOD-like receptor family, pyrin domain containing 3 |
| PAD | peptidyl arginine deaminase |
| PAI | platelet activator inhibitor |
| PBMC | peripheral blood immune cells |
| PMN | polymorphonuclear |
| RAAS | renin-angiotensin. -aldosterone system |
| RE | response element |
| ROS | reactive oxygen species |

| | |
|---|---|
| SARS-CoV-2 | severe acute respiratory syndrome-coronavirus-2 |
| Sirtuin 3 | SIRT3, |
| STEMI | ST elevation myocardial infarction |
| TF | tissue factor |
| TFPI | tissue factor pathway inhibitor |
| TGF beta-2 | transforming grow factor beta-2 |
| Th | T-helper |
| TNF | tumor necrosis factor |
| TRAP | thrombin receptor-activating peptide |
| β2GPI | β2 I glycoprotein |

## References

1. Shi, S.; Qin, M.; Shen, B.; Cai, Y.; Liu, T.; Yang, F.; Gong, W.; Liu, X.; Liang, J.; Zhao, Q.; et al. Association of Cardiac Injury with Mortality in Hospitalized Patients with COVID-19 in Wuhan, China. *JAMA Cardiol.* **2020**, *5*, 802–810. [CrossRef] [PubMed]
2. Guo, T.; Fan, Y.; Chen, M.; Wu, X.; Zhang, L.; He, T.; Wang, H.; Wan, J.; Wang, X.; Lu, Z. Cardiovascular implications of fatal outcomes of patients with Coronavirus disease 2019 (COVID-19). *JAMA Cardiol.* **2020**, *5*, 811–818. [CrossRef] [PubMed]
3. Szekely, Y.; Lichter, Y.; Taieb, P.; Banai, A.; Hochstadt, A.; Merdler, I.; Oz, A.G.; Rothschild, E.; Baruch, G.; Peri, Y.; et al. The spectrum of cardiac manifestations in coronavirus disease 2019 (COVID-19): A systematic echocardiographic study. *Circulation* **2020**, *142*, 342–353. [CrossRef] [PubMed]
4. Lala, A.; Johnson, K.W.; Januzzi, J.L.; Russak, A.J.; Paranjpe, I.; Richter, F.; Zhao, S.; Somani, S.; Van Vleck, T.; Vaid, A.; et al. Mount Sinai Covid Informatics Center. Prevalence and impact of myocardial injury in patients hospitalized with COVID-19 infection. *J. Am. Coll. Cardiol.* **2020**, *76*, 533–546. [CrossRef] [PubMed]
5. Inciardi, R.M.; Lupi, L.; Zaccone, G.; Italia, L.; Raffo, M.; Tomasoni, D.; Cani, D.S.; Cerini, M.; Farina, D.; Gavazzi, E.; et al. Cardiac involvement in a patient with coronavirus disease 2019 (COVID-19). *JAMA Cardiol.* **2020**, *5*, 819–824. [CrossRef]
6. Guzik, T.J.; Mohiddin, S.A.; Dimarco, A.; Patel, V.; Savvatis, K.; Marelli-Berg, F.M.; Madhur, M.S.; Tomaszewski, M.; Maffia, P.; D'Acquisto, F.; et al. COVID-19 and the cardiovascular system: Implications for risk assessment, diagnosis, and treatment options. *Cardiovasc. Res.* **2020**, *116*, 1666–1687. [CrossRef]
7. Escher, F.; Pietsch, H.; Aleshcheva, G.; Bock, T.; Baumeier, C.; Elsaesser, A.; Wenzel, P.; Hamm, C.; Westenfeld, R.; Schultheiss, M.; et al. Detection of viral SARS-CoV-2 genomes and histopathological changes in endomyocardial biopsies. *ESC Heart Fail.* **2020**, *7*, 2440–2447. [CrossRef]
8. Hartikainen, T.S.; Sörensen, N.A.; Haller, P.M.; Goßling, A.; Lehmacher, J.; Zeller, T.; Blankenberg, S.; Westermann, D.; Neumann, J.T. Clinical application of the 4th Universal Definition of Myocardial Infarction. *Eur. Heart J.* **2020**, *41*, 2209–2216. [CrossRef]
9. Bonow, R.O.; Fonarow, G.C.; O'Gara, P.T.; Yancy, C.W. Association of coronavirus disease 2019 (COVID-19) with myocardial injury and mortality. *JAMA Cardiol.* **2020**, *5*, 751–753. [CrossRef]
10. Levi, M.; Thachil, J.; Iba, T.; Levy, J.H. Coagulation abnormalities and thrombosis in patients with COVID-19. *Lancet Haematol.* **2020**, *7*, e438–e440. [CrossRef]
11. Bikdeli, B.; Madhavan, M.V.; Jiménez, D.; Chuich, T.; Dreyfus, I.; Driggin, E.; Nigoghossian, C.D.; Ageno, W.; Madjid, M.; Guo, Y.; et al. COVID-19 and Thrombotic or Thromboembolic Disease: Implications for Prevention, Antithrombotic Therapy, and Follow-Up: JACC State-of-the-Art Review. *J. Am. Coll. Cardiol.* **2020**, *75*, 2950–2973. [CrossRef] [PubMed]
12. Thierry, A.R.; Roch, B. Neutrophil extracellular traps and by-products play a key role in COVID-19: Pathogenesis, risk factors, and therapy. *J. Clin. Med.* **2020**, *9*, 2942. [CrossRef] [PubMed]
13. Lindner, D.; Fitzek, A.; Bräuninger, H.; Aleshcheva, G.; Edler, C.; Meissner, K.; Scherschel, K.; Kirchhof, P.; Escher, F.; Schultheiss, H.-P.; et al. Association of Cardiac Infection With SARS-CoV-2 in Confirmed COVID-19 Autopsy Cases. *JAMA Cardiol.* **2020**, *5*, 1281–1285. [CrossRef] [PubMed]
14. Blasco, A.; Coronado, M.J.; Hernández-Terciado, F.H.; Martín, P.; Royuela, A.; Ramil, E.; García, D.; Goicolea, J.; Del Trigo, M.; Ortega, J.; et al. Assessment of Neutrophil Extracellular Traps in Coronary Thrombus of a Case Series of Patients with COVID-19 and Myocardial Infarction. *JAMA Cardiol.* **2020**, *6*, 1–6. [CrossRef] [PubMed]
15. Ackermann, M.; Verleden, S.E.; Kuehnel, M.; Haverich, A.; Welte, T.; Laenger, F.; Vanstapel, A.; Werlein, C.; Stark, H.; Tzankov, A.; et al. Pulmonary vascular endothelialitis, thrombosis, and angiogenesis in COVID-19. *N. Engl. J. Med.* **2020**, *383*, 120–128. [CrossRef] [PubMed]
16. Bryce, C.; Grimes, Z.; Pujadas, E.; Ahuja, S.; Beasley, M.B.; Albrecht, R.; Hernandez, T.; Stock, A.; Zhao, Z.; AlRasheed, M.R.; et al. Pathophysiology of SARS-CoV-2: The Mount Sinai COVID-19 autopsy experience. *Mod. Pathol.* **2021**, *34*, 1456–1467. [CrossRef] [PubMed]
17. Schaefer, I.M.; Padera, R.F.; Solomon, I.H.; Kanjilal, S.; Hammer, M.M.; Hornick, J.L.; Sholl, L.M. In situ detection of SARS-CoV-2 in lungs and airways of patients with COVID-19. *Mod. Pathol.* **2020**, *33*, 2104–2114. [CrossRef]
18. Varga, Z.; Flammer, A.J.; Steiger, P.; Haberecker, M.; Andermatt, R.; Zinkernagel, A.S.; Mehra, M.R.; Schuepbach, R.A.; Ruschitzka, F.; Moch, H. Endothelial cell infection and endotheliitis in COVID-19. *Lancet* **2020**, *395*, 1417–1418. [CrossRef]

19. Delorey, T.M.; Ziegler, C.G.K.; Heimberg, G.; Normand, R.; Yang, Y.; Segerstolpe, Å.; Abbondanza, D.; Fleming, S.J.; Subramanian, A.; Montoro, D.T.; et al. COVID-19 tissue atlases reveal SARS-CoV-2 pathology and cellular targets. *Nature* **2021**, *595*, 107–113. [CrossRef]
20. Wang, D.; Hu, B.; Hu, C.; Zhu, F.; Liu, X.; Zhang, J.; Wang, B.; Xiang, H.; Cheng, Z.; Xiong, Y.; et al. Clinical characteristics of 138 hospitalized patients with 2019 novel coronavirus-infected pneumonia in Wuhan, China. *J. Am. Med. Assoc.* **2020**, *323*, 1061–1069. [CrossRef]
21. Lucas, C.; Wong, P.; Klein, J.; Castro, T.B.R.; Silva, J.; Sundaram, M.; Ellingson, M.K.; Mao, T.; Oh, J.E.; Israelow, B.; et al. Longitudinal analyses reveal immunological misfiring in severe COVID-19. *Nature* **2020**, *584*, 463–469. [CrossRef] [PubMed]
22. Yang, Y.; Shen, C.; Li, J.; Yuan, J.; Wei, J.; Huang, F.; Wang, F.; Li, G.; Li, Y.; Xing, L.; et al. Plasma IP-10 and MCP-3 levels are highly associated with disease severity and predict the progression of COVID-19. *J. Allergy Clin. Immunol.* **2020**, *146*, 119–127.e4. [CrossRef] [PubMed]
23. Huang, C.; Wang, Y.; Li, X.; Ren, L.; Zhao, J.; Hu, Y.; Zhang, L.; Fan, G.; Xu, J.; Gu, X.; et al. Clinical features of patients infected with, novel coronavirus in Wuhan, China. *Lancet* **2020**, *395*, 497–506. [CrossRef]
24. Liu, Y.; Du, X.; Chen, J.; Jin, Y.; Peng, L.; Wang, H.H.X.; Luo, M.; Chen, L.; Zhao, Y. Neutrophil-to-lymphocyte ratio as an independent risk factor for mortality in hospitalized patients with COVID-19. *J. Infect.* **2020**, *81*, e6–e12. [CrossRef]
25. Rodrigues, T.S.; de Sá, K.S.G.; Ishimoto, A.Y.; Becerra, A.; Oliveira, S.; Almeida, L.; Gonçalves, A.V.; Perucello, D.B.; Andrade, W.A.; Castro, R.; et al. Inflammasomes are activated in response to SARS-CoV-2 infection and are associated with COVID-19 severity in patients. *J. Exp. Med.* **2021**, *218*, e20201707. [CrossRef]
26. Burkhard-Koren, N.M.; Haberecker, M.; Maccio, U.; Ruschitzka, F.; Schuepbach, R.A.; Zinkernagel, A.S.; Hardmeier, T.; Varga, Z.; Moch, H. Higher prevalence of pulmonary macrothrombi in SARS-CoV-2 than in influenza A: Autopsy results from 'Spanish flu' 1918/1919 in Switzerland to Coronavirus disease 2019. *J. Pathol. Clin. Res.* **2021**, *7*, 135–143. [CrossRef]
27. Sang, C.J., 3rd; Burkett, A.; Heindl, B.; Litovsky, S.H.; Prabhu, S.D.; Benson, P.V.; Rajapreyar, I. Cardiac pathology in COVID-19: A single center autopsy experience. *Cardiovasc. Pathol.* **2021**, *54*, 107370. [CrossRef]
28. Melms, J.C.; Biermann, J.; Huang, H.; Wang, Y.; Nair, A.; Tagore, S.; Katsyv, I.; Rendeiro, A.F.; Amin, A.D.; Schapiro, D.; et al. A molecular single-cell lung atlas of lethal COVID-19. *Nature* **2021**, *595*, 114–119. [CrossRef]
29. Qin, C.; Zhou, L.; Hu, Z.; Zhang, S.; Yang, S.; Tao, Y.; Xie, C.; Ma, K.; Shang, K.; Wang, W.; et al. Dysregulation of immune response in patients with coronavirus, (COVID-19) in Wuhan, China. *Clin. Infect. Dis.* **2020**, *71*, 762–768. [CrossRef]
30. Wilk, A.J.; Rustagi, A.; Zhao, N.Q.; Roque, J.; Martínez-Colón, G.J.; McKechnie, J.L.; Ivison, G.T.; Ranganath, T.; Vergara, R.; Hollis, T.; et al. A single-cell atlas of the peripheral immune response in patients with severe COVID-19. *Nat. Med.* **2020**, *26*, 1070–1076. [CrossRef]
31. Wang, J.; Li, Q.; Yin, Y.; Zhang, Y.; Cao, Y.; Lin, X.; Huang, L.; Hoffmann, D.; Lu, M.; Qiu, Y. Excessive neutrophils and neutrophil extracellular traps in COVID-19. *Front. Immunol.* **2020**, *11*, 2063. [CrossRef]
32. Al-Aly, Z.; Xie, Y.; Bowe, B. High-dimensional characterization of post-acute sequelae of COVID-19. *Nature* **2021**, *594*, 259–264. [CrossRef] [PubMed]
33. Xie, Y.; Bowe, B.; Maddukuri, G.; Al-Aly, Z. Comparative evaluation of clinical manifestations and risk of death in patients admitted to hospital with COVID-19 and seasonal influenza: Cohort study. *BMJ* **2020**, *371*, m4677. [CrossRef] [PubMed]
34. Piazza, G.; Campia, U.; Hurwitz, S.; Snyder, J.E.; Rizzo, S.M.; Pferferman, M.B.; Morrison, R.B.; Leiva, O.; Fanikos, J.; Nauffal, V.; et al. Registry of arterial and venous thromboembolic complications in patients with COVID-19. *J. Am. Coll. Cardiol.* **2020**, *76*, 2060–2072. [CrossRef] [PubMed]
35. Zhang, Y.; Cao, W.; Jiang, W.; Xiao, M.; Li, Y.; Tang, N.; Liu, Z.; Yan, X.; Zhao, Y.; Li, T.; et al. Profile of natural anticoagulant, coagulant factor and anti-phospholipid antibody in critically ill COVID-19 patients. *J. Thromb. Thrombolysis* **2020**, *50*, 580–586. [CrossRef]
36. Liu, J.; Liu, Y.; Xiang, P.; Pu, L.; Xiong, H.; Li, C.; Zhang, M.; Tan, J.; Xu, Y.; Song, R.; et al. Neutro-philto-lymphocyte ratio predicts critical illness patients with 2019 coronavirus disease in the early stage. *J. Transl. Med.* **2020**, *18*, 206. [CrossRef]
37. Fu, J.; Kong, J.; Wang, W.; Wu, M.; Yao, L.; Wang, Z.; Jin, J.; Wu, D.; Yu, X. The clinical implication of dynamic neutrophil to lymphocyte ratio and D-dimer in COVID-19: A retroT, s.s.i.S.C.he clinical implication of dynamic neutrophil to lymphocyte ratio and D-dimer in COVID-19: A retrospective study in Suzhou China. *Thromb. Res.* **2020**, *192*, 3–8. [CrossRef]
38. Webb, B.J.; Peltan, I.D.; Jensen, P.; Hoda, D.; Hunter, B.; Silver, A.; Starr, N.; Buckel, W.; Grisel, N.; Hummel, E.; et al. Clinical criteria for COVID-19-associated hyperinflammatory syndrome: A cohort study. *Lancet Rheumatol.* **2020**, *2*, e754–e763. [CrossRef]
39. Ye, W.; Chen, G.; Li, X.; Lan, X.; Ji, C.; Hou, M.; Zhang, D.; Zeng, G.; Wang, Y.; Xu, C.; et al. Dynamic changes of D-dimer and neutrophil-lymphocyte count ratio as prognostic biomarkers in COVID-19. *Respir. Res.* **2020**, *21*, 169. [CrossRef]
40. Tatum, D.; Taghavi, S.; Houghton, A.; Stover, J.; Toraih, E.; Duchesne, J. Neutrophil-to-Lymphocyte ratio and outcomes in Louisiana COVID-19 Patients. *Shock* **2020**, *54*, 652–658. [CrossRef]
41. Yang, A.P.; Liu, J.P.; Tao, W.Q.; Li, H.M. The diagnostic and predictive role of N.L.R., d-NLR and PLR in COVID-19 patients. *Int. Immunopharmacol.* **2020**, *84*, 106504. [CrossRef] [PubMed]
42. Wang, H.; Zhang, Y.; Mo, P.; Liu, J.; Wang, H.; Wang, F.; Zhao, Q. Neutrophil to CD4+ lymphocyte ratio as a potential biomarker in predicting virus negative conversion time in COVID-19. *Int. Immunopharmacol.* **2020**, *85*, 106683. [CrossRef] [PubMed]

43. Zhou, F.; Yu, T.; Du, R.; Fan, G.; Liu, Y.; Liu, Z.; Xiang, J.; Wang, Y.; Song, B.; Gu, X.; et al. Clinical course and risk factors for mortality of adult in patients with COVID-19 in Wuhan, China: A retrospective cohort study. *Lancet* **2020**, *395*, 1054–1062. [CrossRef]
44. Klok, F.A.; Kruip, M.J.H.A.; van der Meer, N.J.M.; Arbous, M.S.; Gommers, D.A.M.P.J.; Kant, K.M.; Kaptein, F.H.J.; van Paassen, J.; Stals, M.A.M.; Huisman, M.V.; et al. Incidence of thrombotic complications in critically ill ICU patients with COVID-19. *Thromb. Res.* **2020**, *191*, 145–147. [CrossRef]
45. Tang, N.; Bai, H.; Chen, X.; Gong, J.; Li, D.; Sun, Z. Anticoagulant treatment is associated with decreased mortality in severe coronavirus disease 2019 patients with coagulopathy. *J. Thromb. Haemost.* **2020**, *18*, 1094–1099. [CrossRef]
46. Zuo, Y.; Estes, S.K.; Ali, R.A.; Gandhi, A.A.; Yalavarthi, S.; Shi, H.; Sule, G.; Gockman, K.; Madison, J.A.; Zuo, M.; et al. Prothrombotic autoantibodies in serum from patients hospitalized with COVID-19. *Sci. Transl. Med.* **2020**, *12*, eabd3876. [CrossRef]
47. Carsana, L.; Sonzogni, A.; Nasr, A.; Rossi, R.S.; Pellegrinelli, A.; Zerbi, P.; Rech, R.; Colombo, R.; Antinori, S.; Corbellino, M.; et al. Pulmonary post-mortem findings in a large series of COVID-19 cases from Northern Italy: A two-centre descriptive study. *Lancet Infect. Dis.* **2020**, *20*, 1135–1140. [CrossRef]
48. Chen, N.; Zhou, M.; Dong, X.; Qu, J.; Gong, F.; Han, Y.; Qiu, Y.; Wang, J.; Liu, Y.; Wei, Y.; et al. Epidemiological and clinical characteristics of 99 cases of 2019 novel coronavirus pneumonia in Wuhan, China: A descriptive study. *Lancet* **2020**, *395*, 507–513. [CrossRef]
49. Guan, W.J.; Ni, Z.Y.; Hu, Y.; Liang, W.H.; Qu, C.Q.; He, J.X.; Liu, L.; Shan, H.; Lei, C.L.; Hui, D.S.C.; et al. China Medical Treatment Expert Group for COVID-19. Clinical characteristics of coronavirus disease 2019 in China. *N. Engl. J. Med.* **2020**, *382*, 1708–1720. [CrossRef]
50. COVIDSurg Collaborative; GlobalSurg Collaborative. SARS-CoV-2 infection and venous thromboembolism after surgery: An international prospective cohort study. *Anaesthesia* **2022**, *77*, 28–39.
51. COVIDSurg Collaborative; GlobalSurg Collaborative. Effects of pre-operative isolation on postoperative pulmonary complications after elective surgery: An international prospective cohort study. *Anaesthesia* **2021**, *76*, 1454–1464.
52. COVIDSurg Collaborative; GlobalSurg Collaborative. SARS-CoV-2 vaccination modelling for safe surgery to save lives: Data from an international prospective cohort study. *Br. J. Surg.* **2021**, *108*, 1056–1063. [CrossRef] [PubMed]
53. COVIDSurg Collaborative; GlobalSurg Collaborative. Timing of surgery following SARS-CoV-2 infection: An international prospective cohort study. *Anaesthesia* **2021**, *76*, 748–758.
54. Xie, Y.; Xu, E.; Bowe, B.; Al-Aly, Z. Long-term cardiovascular outcomes of COVID-19. *Nat. Med.* **2022**, *28*, 583–590. [CrossRef] [PubMed]
55. Wu, Z.; McGoogan, J.M. Characteristics of and important lessons from the coronavirus disease 2019 (COVID-19) outbreak in China: Summary of a report of 72 314 cases from the Chinese Center for Disease Control and Prevention. *JAMA* **2020**, *323*, 1239–1242. [CrossRef]
56. Brinkmann, V.; Reichard, U.; Goosmann, C.; Fauler, B.; Uhlemann, Y.; Weiss, D.S.; Weinrauch, Y.; Zychlinsky, A. Neutrophil Extracellular Traps kill bacteria. *Science* **2004**, *303*, 1532–1535. [CrossRef]
57. García, L.F. Immune response, inflammation, and the clinical spectrum of COVID-19. *Front. Immunol.* **2020**, *11*, 1441. [CrossRef]
58. Zhou, P.; Yang, X.L.; Wang, X.G.; Hu, B.; Zhang, L.; Zhang, W.; Si, H.R.; Zhu, Y.; Li, B.; Huang, C.L.; et al. A pneumonia outbreak associated with a new coronavirus of probable bat origin. *Nature* **2020**, *579*, 270–273. [CrossRef]
59. Hamming, I.; Timens, W.; Bulthuis, M.L.; Lely, A.T.; Navis, G.; van Goor, H. Tissue distribution of ACE2 protein, the functional receptor for SARS coronavirus. A first step in understanding SARS pathogenesis. *J. Pathol.* **2004**, *203*, 631–637. [CrossRef]
60. Zou, X.; Chen, K.; Zou, J.; Han, P.; Hao, J.; Han, Z. Single-cell RNA-seq data analysis on the receptor ACE2 expression reveals the potential risk of different human organs vulnerable to 2019-nCoV infection. *Front. Med.* **2020**, *14*, 185–192. [CrossRef]
61. Chu, H.; Chan, J.F.; Wang, Y.; Yuen, T.T.; Chai, Y.; Hou, Y.; Shuai, H.; Yang, D.; Hu, B.; Huang, X.; et al. Comparative replication and immune activation profiles of SARS-CoV-2 and SARS-CoV in human lungs: An ex vivo study with implications for the pathogenesis of COVID-19. *Clin. Infect. Dis.* **2020**, *71*, 1400–1409. [CrossRef] [PubMed]
62. Blanco-Melo, D.; Nilsson-Payant, B.E.; Liu, W.C.; Uhl, S.; Hoagland, D.; Møller, R.; Jordan, T.X.; Oishi, K.; Panis, M.; Sachs, D.; et al. Imbalanced host response to SARS-CoV-2 drives development of COVID-19. *Cell* **2020**, *181*, 1036–1045.e9. [CrossRef] [PubMed]
63. Li, G.; Fan, Y.; Lai, Y.; Han, T.; Li, Z.; Zhou, P.; Pan, P.; Wang, W.; Hu, D.; Liu, X.; et al. Coronavirus infections and immune responses. *J. Med. Virol.* **2020**, *92*, 424–432. [CrossRef] [PubMed]
64. Perlman, S.; Dandekar, A.A. Immunopathogenesis of coronavirus infections: Implications for SARS. *Nat. Rev. Immunol.* **2005**, *5*, 917–927.
65. Shi, C.S.; Qi, H.Y.; Boularan, C.; Huang, N.N.; Abu-Asab, M.; Shelhamer, J.H.; Kehrl, J.H. SARS-coronavirus open reading frame-9b suppresses innate immunity by targeting mitochondria and the MAVS/TRAF3/TRAF6 signalosome. *J. Immunol.* **2014**, *193*, 3080–3089. [CrossRef]
66. Spiegel, M.; Pichlmair, A.; Martínez-Sobrido, L.; Cros, J.; García-Sastre, A.; Haller, O.; Weber, F. Inhibition of beta interferon induction by severe acute respiratory syndrome coronavirus suggests a two-step model for activation of interferon regulatory factor 3. *J. Virol.* **2005**, *79*, 2079–2086. [CrossRef]
67. Proudfoot, A.E. Chemokine receptors: Multifaceted therapeutic targets. *Nat. Rev. Immunol.* **2002**, *2*, 106–115. [CrossRef]
68. Vaninov, N. In the eye of the COVID-19 cytokine storm. *Nat. Rev. Immunol.* **2020**, *20*, 27. [CrossRef]

69. Freeman, T.L.; Swartz, T.H. Targeting the NLRP3 inflammasome in severe COVID-19. *Front. Immunol.* **2020**, *11*, 1518. [CrossRef]
70. van den Berg, D.F.; Te Velde, A.A. Severe COVID-19: NLRP3 inflammasome dysregulated. *Front. Immunol.* **2020**, *11*, 1580. [CrossRef]
71. Zhou, Y.; Fu, B.; Zheng, X.; Wang, D.; Zhao, C.; Qi, Y.; Sun, R.; Tian, Z.; Xu, X.; Wei, H. Pathogenic T-cells and inflammatory monocytes incite inflammatory storms in severe COVID-19 patients. *Natl. Sci. Rev.* **2020**, *7*, 998–1002. [CrossRef] [PubMed]
72. Lee, H.L.; Jang, J.W.; Lee, S.W.; Yoo, S.H.; Kwon, J.H.; Nam, S.W.; Bae, S.H.; Choi, J.Y.; Han, N.I.; Yoon, S.K. Inflammatory cytokines and change of Th1/Th2 balance as prognostic indicators for hepatocellular carcinoma in patients treated with transarterial chemoembolization. *Sci. Rep.* **2019**, *9*, 3260. [CrossRef] [PubMed]
73. Goodarzi, P.; Mahdavi, F.; Mirzaei, R.; Hasanvand, H.; Sholeh, M.; Zamani, F.; Sohrabi, M.; Tabibzadeh, A.; Jeda, A.S.; Niya, M.H.K.; et al. Coronavirus disease 2019 (COVID-19): Immunological ap-proaches and emerging pharmacologic treatments. *Int. Immunopharmacol.* **2020**, *88*, 106885. [CrossRef] [PubMed]
74. Goldsmith, C.S.; Miller, S.E.; Martines, R.B.; Bullock, H.A.; Zaki, S.R. Electron microscopy of SARS-CoV-2: A challenging task. *Lancet* **2020**, *395*, e99. [CrossRef]
75. Tan, M.; Liu, Y.; Zhou, R.; Deng, X.; Li, F.; Liang, K.; Shi, Y. Immunopathological characteristics of coronavirus disease, cases in Guangzhou China. *Immunology* **2020**, *160*, 261–268. [CrossRef]
76. Nappi, F.; Giacinto, O.; Ellouze, O.; Nenna, A.; Avtaar Singh, S.S.; Chello, M.; Bouzguenda, A.; Copie, X. Association between COVID-19 Diagnosis and Coronary Artery Thrombosis: A Narrative Review. *Biomedicines* **2022**, *10*, 702. [CrossRef]
77. Soehnlein, O.; Steffens, S.; Hidalgo, A.; Weber, C. Neutrophils as protagonists and targets in chronic inflammation. *Nat. Rev. Immunol.* **2017**, *17*, 248–261. [CrossRef]
78. Tomar, B.; Anders, H.J.; Desai, J.; Mulay, S.R. Neutrophils and neutrophil extracellular traps drive necroinflammation in COVID-19. *Cells* **2020**, *9*, 1383. [CrossRef]
79. Galani, I.E.; Andreakos, E. Neutrophils in viral infections: Current concepts and caveats. *J. Leukoc. Biol.* **2015**, *98*, 557–564. [CrossRef]
80. Naumenko, V.; Turk, M.; Jenne, C.N.; Kim, S.J. Neutrophils in viral infection. *Cell Tissue Res.* **2018**, *371*, 505–516. [CrossRef]
81. Camp, J.V.; Jonsson, C.B. A role for neutrophils in viral respiratory disease. *Front. Immunol.* **2017**, *8*, 550. [CrossRef] [PubMed]
82. Hemmat, N.; Derakhshani, A.; Bannazadeh Baghi, H.; Silvestris, N.; Baradaran, B.; De Summa, S. Neutrophils, crucial, or harmful immune cells involved in coronavirus infection: A bioinformatics study. *Front. Genet.* **2020**, *11*, 641. [CrossRef] [PubMed]
83. Shi, H.; Zheng, H.; Yin, Y.F.; Hu, Q.Y.; Teng, J.L.; Sun, Y.; Liu, H.L.; Cheng, X.B.; Ye, J.N.; Su, Y.T.; et al. Antiphosphatidylserine/prothrombin antibodies (aPS/PT) as potential diagnostic markers and risk predictors of venous thrombosis and obstetric complications in antiphospholipid syndrome. *Clin. Chem. Lab. Med.* **2018**, *56*, 614–624. [CrossRef] [PubMed]
84. Zuo, Y.; Shi, H.; Li, C.; Knight, J.S. Antiphospholipid syndrome: A clinical perspective. *Chin. Med. J.* **2020**, *133*, 929–940. [CrossRef] [PubMed]
85. Guan, J.; Wei, X.; Qin, S.; Liu, X.; Jiang, Y.; Chen, Y.; Chen, Y.; Lu, H.; Qian, J.; Wang, Z.; et al. Continuous tracking of COVID-19 patients' immune status. *Int. Immunopharmacol.* **2020**, *89 (Pt A)*, 107034. [CrossRef]
86. Ponti, G.; Maccaferri, M.; Ruini, C.; Tomasi, A.; Ozben, T. Biomarkers associated with COVID-19 disease progression. *Crit. Rev. Clin. Lab. Sci.* **2020**, *57*, 389–399. [CrossRef]
87. Azab, B.; Camacho-Rivera, M.; Taioli, E. Average values and racial differences of neutrophil lymphocyte ratio among a nationally representative sample of United States subjects. *PLoS ONE* **2014**, *9*, e112361. [CrossRef]
88. Liu, G.; Zhang, S.; Hu, H.; Liu, T.; Huang, J. The role of neutrophil-lymphocyte ratio and lymphocyte–monocyte ratio in the prognosis of type 2 diabetics with COVID-19. *Scott. Med. J.* **2020**, *65*, 154–160. [CrossRef]
89. Yang, P.; Wang, N.; Wang, J.; Luo, A.; Gao, F.; Tu, Y. Admission fasting plasma glucose is an independent risk factor for 28-day mortality in patients with COVID-19. *J. Med. Virol.* **2021**, *93*, 2168–2176. [CrossRef]
90. Varim, C.; Yaylaci, S.; Demirci, T.; Kaya, T.; Nalbant, A.; Dheir, H.; Senocak, D.; Kurt, R.; Cengiz, H.; Karacaer, C. Neutrophil count to albumin ratio as a new predictor of mortality in patients with COVID-19 infection. *Rev. Assoc. Med. Bras.* **2020**, *66* (Suppl. 2), 77–81. [CrossRef]
91. Horton, R. Offline: COVID-19—Bewilderment and candour. *Lancet* **2020**, *395*, 1178. [CrossRef]
92. Ferrario, C.M.; Jessup, J.; Chappell, M.C.; Averill, D.B.; Brosnihan, K.B.; Tallant, E.A.; Diz, D.I.; Gallagher, P.E. Effect of angiotensin-converting enzyme inhibition and angiotensin II receptor blockers on cardiac angiotensin-converting enzyme 2. *Circulation* **2005**, *111*, 2605–2610. [CrossRef] [PubMed]
93. Monteil, V.; Kwon, H.; Prado, P.; Hagelkrüys, A.; Wimmer, R.A.; Stahl, M.; Leopoldi, A.; Garreta, E.; del Pozo, C.H.; Prosper, F.; et al. Inhibition of SARS-CoV-2 infections in engineered human tissues using clinical-grade soluble human ACE2. *Cell* **2020**, *181*, 905–913.e7. [CrossRef] [PubMed]
94. Reusch, N.; De Domenico, E.; Bonaguro, L.; Schulte-Schrepping, J.; Baßler, K.; Schultze, J.L.; Aschenbrenner, A.C.A. Neutrophils in COVID-19. *Front. Immunol.* **2021**, *12*, 652470. [CrossRef]
95. Parackova, Z.; Zentsova, I.; Bloomfield, M.; Vrabcova, P.; Smetanova, J.; Klocperk, A.; Mesežnikov, G.; Casas Mendez, L.F.; Vymazal, T.; Sediva, A. Disharmonic inflammatory signatures in COVID-19 Augmented neutrophils' but impaired monocytes' and dendritic cells' responsiveness. *Cells* **2020**, *9*, 2206. [CrossRef]
96. Cicco, S.; Cicco, G.; Racanelli, V.; Vacca, A. Neutrophil Extracellular Traps (NETs) and Damage-Associated Molecular Patterns (DAMPs): Two potential targets for COVID-19 treatment. *Mediat. Inflamm.* **2020**, *2020*, 7527953. [CrossRef]

97. Xiong, Y.; Liu, Y.; Cao, L.; Wang, D.; Guo, M.; Jiang, A.; Guo, D.; Hu, W.; Yang, J.; Tang, Z.; et al. Transcriptomic characteristics of bronchoalveolar lavage fluid and peripheral blood mononuclear cells in COVID-19 patients. *Emerg. Microbes Infect.* **2020**, *9*, 761–770. [CrossRef]
98. Fuchs, T.A.; Abed, U.; Goosmann, C.; Hurwitz, R.; Schulze, I.; Wahn, V.; Weinrauch, Y.; Brinkmann, V.; Zychlinsky, A. Novel cell death program leads to neutrophil extracellular traps. *J. Cell Biol.* **2007**, *176*, 231–241. [CrossRef]
99. Demers, M.; Wagner, D.D. NETosis: A new factor in tumour progression and cancer associated thrombosis. *Semin. Thromb. Hemost.* **2014**, *40*, 277–283. [CrossRef]
100. Sangaletti, S.; Tripodo, C.; Chiodoni, C.; Guarnotta, C.; Cappetti, B.; Casalini, P.; Piconese, S.; Parenza, M.; Guiducci, C.; Vitali, C.; et al. Neutrophil Extracellular Traps mediate transfer of cytoplasmic neutrophil antigens to myeloid dendritic cells toward ANCA induction and associated autoimmunity. *Blood* **2012**, *120*, 3007–3018. [CrossRef]
101. Mozzini, C.; Garbin, U.; Fratta Pasini, A.M.; Cominacini, L. An exploratory look at NETosis in atherosclerosis. *Intern. Emerg. Med.* **2017**, *12*, 13–22. [CrossRef] [PubMed]
102. Almyroudis, N.G.; Grimm, M.J.; Davidson, B.A.; Röhm, M.; Urban, C.F.; Segal, B.H. NETosis and NADPH oxidase: At the intersection of host defence, inflammation, and injury. *Front. Immunol.* **2013**, *4*, 45. [CrossRef] [PubMed]
103. Stoiber, W.; Obermayer, A.; Steinbacher, P.; Krautgartner, W.D. The role of reactive oxygen species (ROS) in the formation of extracellular traps in humans. *Biomolecules* **2015**, *5*, 702–723. [CrossRef]
104. Yipp, B.G.; Kubes, P. NETosis: How vital is it? *Blood* **2013**, *122*, 2784–2794. [CrossRef] [PubMed]
105. Schönrich, G.; Raftery, M.J. Neutrophil Extracellular Traps go viral. *Front. Immunol.* **2016**, *7*, 366. [CrossRef]
106. Hiroki, C.H.; Toller-Kawahisa, J.E.; Fumagalli, M.J.; Colon, D.F.; Figueiredo, L.T.M.; Fonseca, B.A.L.D.; Franca, R.F.O.; Cunha, F.Q. Neutrophil Extracellular Traps effectively control acute Chikungunya virus infection. *Front. Immunol.* **2020**, *10*, 3108. [CrossRef] [PubMed]
107. Muraro, S.P.; de Souza, G.F.; Gallo, S.W.; de Silva, B.K.; de Oliveira, S.D.; Vinolo, M.A.R.; Saraiva, E.M.; Porto, B.N. Respiratory Syncytial Virus induces the classical ROS-dependent NETosis through PAD-4 and necroptosis pathways activation. *Sci. Rep.* **2018**, *8*, 14166. [CrossRef]
108. Mikacenic, C.; Moore, R.; Dmyterko, V.; West, T.E.; Altemeier, W.A.; Liles, W.C.; Lood, C. Neutrophil Extracellular Traps are increased in the alveolar spaces of patients with ventilator-associated pneumonia. *Crit. Care* **2018**, *22*, 358. [CrossRef]
109. Wong, J.J.M.; Leong, J.Y.; Lee, J.H.; Albani, S.; Yeo, J.G. Insights into the immune-pathogenesis of acute respiratory distress syndrome. *Ann. Transl. Med.* **2019**, *7*, 504. [CrossRef]
110. Grabcanovic-Musija, F.; Obermayer, A.; Stoiber, W.; Krautgartner, W.D.; Steinbacher, P.; Winterberg, N.; Bathke, A.C.; Klappacher, M.; Studnicka, M. Neutrophil extracellular trap (NET) formation characterises stable and exacerbated COPD and correlates with airflow limitation. *Respir. Res.* **2015**, *16*, 59. [CrossRef]
111. Baden, L.R.; Rubin, E.J. COVID-19: The search of effective therapy. *N. Engl. J. Med.* **2020**, *382*, 1851–1852. [CrossRef] [PubMed]
112. Madison, J.A.; Duarte-García, A.; Zuo, Y.; Knight, J.S. Treatment of thrombotic antiphospholipid syndrome in adults and children. *Curr. Opin. Rheumatol.* **2020**, *32*, 215–227. [CrossRef] [PubMed]
113. Yalavarthi, S.; Gould, T.J.; Rao, A.N.; Mazza, L.F.; Morris, A.E.; Núñez-Álvarez, C.; Hernández-Ramírez, D.; Bockenstedt, P.L.; Liaw, P.C.; Cabral, A.R.; et al. Release of neutrophil extracellular traps by neutrophils stimulated with antiphospholipid antibodies: A newly identified mechanism of thrombosis in the antiphospholipid syndrome. *Arthritis Rheumatol.* **2015**, *67*, 2990–3003. [CrossRef] [PubMed]
114. Zhang, Y.; Xiao, M.; Zhang, S.; Xia, P.; Cao, W.; Jiang, W.; Chen, H.; Ding, X.; Zhao, H.; Zhang, H.; et al. Coagulopathy and antiphospholipid antibodies in patients with COVID-19. *N. Engl. J. Med.* **2020**, *382*, e38. [CrossRef]
115. Siguret, V.; Voicu, S.; Neuwirth, M.; Delrue, M.; Gayat, E.; Stépanian, A.; Mégarbane, B. Are antiphospholipid antibodies associated with thrombotic complications in critically ill COVID-19 patients? *Thromb. Res.* **2020**, *195*, 74–76. [CrossRef]
116. Shi, H.; Zuo, Y.; Yalavarthi, S.; Gockman, K.; Zuo, M.; Madison, J.A.; Blair, C.; Woodward, W.; Lezak, S.P.; Lugogo, N.L.; et al. Neutrophil calprotectin identifies severe pulmonary disease in COVID-19. *J. Leukoc. Biol.* **2021**, *109*, 67–72. [CrossRef]
117. Blasco, A.; Bellas, C.; Goicolea, L.; Muñiz, A.; Abraira, V.; Royuela, A.; Mingo, S.; Oteo, J.F.; García-Touchard, A.; Goicolea, F.J. Immunohistological analysis of intracoronary thrombus aspirate in STEMI patients: Clinical implications of pathological findings. *Rev. Esp. Cardiol.* **2017**, *70*, 170–177. [CrossRef]
118. Nicin, L.; Abplanalp, W.T.; Mellentin, H.; Kattih, B.; Tombor, L.; John, D.; Schmitto, j.; Heineke, J.; Emrich, F.; Arsalan, M.; et al. Cell type-specific expression of the putative SARS-CoV-2 receptor ACE2 in human hearts. *Eur. Heart J.* **2020**, *41*, 1804–1806. [CrossRef]
119. Oudit, G.Y.; Kassiri, Z.; Jiang, C.; Liu, P.P.; Poutanen, S.; Penninger, J.; Butany, J. SARS-coronavirus modulation of myocardial ACE2 expression and inflammation in patients with SARS. *Eur. J. Clin. Investig.* **2009**, *39*, 618–625. [CrossRef]
120. Zhang, X.; Tan, Y.; Ling, Y.; Lu, G.; Liu, F.; Yi, Z.; Jia, X.; Wu, M.; Shi, B.; Xu, S.; et al. Viral and host factors related to the clinical outcome of COVID-19. *Nature* **2020**, *583*, 437–440. [CrossRef]
121. Nappi, F.; Iervolino, A.; Avtaar Singh, S.S. COVID-19 Pathogenesis: From Molecular Pathway to Vaccine Administration. *Biomedicines* **2021**, *9*, 903. [CrossRef] [PubMed]
122. Nappi, F.; Iervolino, A.; Avtaar Singh, S.S. Thromboembolic Complications of SARS-CoV-2 and Metabolic Derangements: Suggestions from Clinical Practice Evidence to Causative Agents. *Metabolites* **2021**, *11*, 341. [CrossRef] [PubMed]

123. Nappi, F. Incertitude Pathophysiology and Management During the First Phase of the COVID-19 Pandemic. *Ann. Thorac. Surg.* **2022**, *113*, 693. [CrossRef] [PubMed]
124. Madjid, M.; Miller, C.C.; Zarubaev, V.V.; Marinich, I.G.; Kiselev, O.I.; Lobzin, Y.V.; Filippov, A.E.; Casscells, S.W. Influenza epidemics and acute respiratory disease activity are associated with a surge in autopsy-confirmed coronary heart disease death: Results from years of autopsies in 34,892 subjects. *Eur. Heart J.* **2007**, *28*, 1205–1210. [CrossRef] [PubMed]
125. Nguyen, J.L.; Yang, W.; Ito, K.; Matte, T.D.; Shaman, J.; Kinney, P.L. Seasonal influenza infections and cardiovascular disease mortality. *JAMA Cardiol.* **2016**, *1*, 274–281. [CrossRef] [PubMed]
126. Kwong, J.C.; Schwartz, K.L.; Campitelli, M.A.; Chung, H.; Crowcroft, N.S.; Karnauchow, T.; Katz, K.; Ko, D.T.; McGeer, A.J.; McNally, D.; et al. Acute myocardial infarction after laboratory-confirmed influenza infection. *N. Engl. J. Med.* **2018**, *378*, 345–353. [CrossRef] [PubMed]
127. Smeeth, L.; Thomas, S.L.; Hall, A.J.; Hubbard, R.; Farrington, P.; Vallance, P. Risk of myocardial infarction and stroke after acute infection or vaccination. *N. Engl. J. Med.* **2004**, *351*, 2611–2618. [CrossRef]
128. Yang, C.; Jin, Z. An acute respiratory infection runs into the most common noncommunicable epidemic—COVID-19 and cardiovascular diseases. *JAMA Cardiol.* **2020**, *5*, 743–744. [CrossRef]
129. Madjid, M.; Safavi-Naeini, P.; Solomon, S.D.; Vardeny, O. Potential effects of coronaviruses on the cardiovascular system: A review. *JAMA Cardiol.* **2020**, *5*, 831–840. [CrossRef]
130. Moorlag, S.J.C.F.M.; Rodriguez-Rosales, Y.A.; Gillard, J.; Fanucchi, S.; Theunissen, K.; Novakovic, B.; de Bont, C.M.; Negishi, Y.; Fok, E.T.; Kalafati, L.; et al. BCG Vaccination Induces Long-Term Functional Reprogramming of Human Neutrophils. *Cell Rep.* **2020**, *33*, 108387. [CrossRef]
131. Kalafati, L.; Kourtzelis, I.; Schulte-Schrepping, J.; Li, X.; Hatzioannou, A.; Grinenko, T.; Hagag, E.; Sinha, A.; Has, C.; Dietz, S.; et al. Innate Immune Training of Granulopoiesis Promotes Anti-tumor Activity. *Cell* **2020**, *183*, 771–785.e12. [CrossRef] [PubMed]
132. Lajqi, T.; Köstlin-Gille, N.; Hillmer, S.; Braun, M.; Kranig, S.A.; Dietz, S.; Krause, C.; Rühle, J.; Frommhold, D.; Pöschl, J.; et al. Gut Microbiota-Derived Small Extracellular Vesicles Endorse Memory-like Inflammatory Responses in Murine Neutrophils. *Biomedicines* **2022**, *10*, 442. [CrossRef] [PubMed]

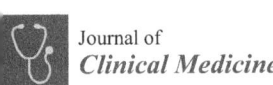

*Review*

# Risk Stratification in Patients with Acute Pulmonary Embolism: Current Evidence and Perspectives

Antonio Leidi [1,†], Stijn Bex [1,†], Marc Righini [2], Amandine Berner [1], Olivier Grosgurin [1] and Christophe Marti [1,*]

1. Division of General Internal Medicine, Department of Medicine, Geneva University Hospitals, 1205 Geneva, Switzerland; antonio.leidi@hcuge.ch (A.L.); stijn.bex@hcuge.ch (S.B.); amandine.berner@hcuge.ch (A.B.); olivier.grosgurin@hcuge.ch (O.G.)
2. Division of Angiology and Haemostasis, Department of Medicine, Geneva University Hospitals, 1205 Geneva, Switzerland; marc.righini@hcuge.ch
* Correspondence: christophe.marti@hcuge.ch; Tel.: +41-22-3723311
† These authors contributed equally to the manuscript.

**Abstract:** Risk stratification is one of the cornerstones of the management of acute pulmonary embolism (PE) and determines the choice of both diagnostic and therapeutic strategies. The first step is the identification of patent circulatory failure, as it is associated with a high risk of immediate mortality and requires a rapid diagnosis and prompt reperfusion. The second step is the estimation of 30-day mortality based on clinical parameters (e.g., original and simplified version of the pulmonary embolism severity index): low-risk patients without right ventricular dysfunction are safely managed with ambulatory anticoagulation. The remaining group of hemodynamically stable patients, labeled intermediate-risk PE, requires hospital admission, even if most of them will heal without complications. In recent decades, efforts have been made to identify a subgroup of patients at an increased risk of adverse outcomes (intermediate-high-risk PE), who might benefit from a more aggressive approach, including reperfusion therapies and admission to a monitored unit. The cur-rent approach, combining markers of right ventricular dysfunction and myocardial injury, has an insufficient positive predictive value to guide primary thrombolysis. Sensitive markers of circulatory failure, such as plasma lactate, have shown interesting prognostic accuracy and may play a central role in the future. Furthermore, the improved security of reduced-dose thrombolysis may enlarge the indication of this treatment to selected intermediate–high-risk PE.

**Keywords:** risk assessment; pulmonary embolism; thrombolysis

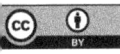

## 1. Introduction

Pulmonary embolism (PE) is the third most frequent cardiovascular disease and is associated with a high mortality burden, accounting for approximately 300,000 deaths in Europe every year [1,2]. PE is defined as the obstruction of a pulmonary artery, mostly resulting from the dislodgement of thrombotic material from the lower limbs. It has a wide variety of presentations, ranging from an asymptomatic incidental finding to circulatory collapse and sudden death. Diagnosis of PE often requires a sequential strategy combining a pre-test probability assessment, D-dimers measurement when indicated and thoracic imaging. Risk stratification immediately guides the management of acute PE, as it determines the need for urgent reperfusion therapy (high-risk PE) and identifies patients who can be safely treated as outpatients (low-risk PE). The remaining group of patients, called intermediate-risk PE, is highly heterogeneous with most of the patients recovering, but a significant proportion being at risk of complications. The present article will review the evidence supporting risk stratification and reperfusion strategies in the management of PE, with a particular focus on intermediate-risk pulmonary embolism.

## 2. Risk Stratification in Acute Pulmonary Embolism

Risk stratification is applied in various medical conditions to stratify patients' severity in therapeutic trials or guide specific diagnostic or therapeutic interventions. Risk stratification often relies on prognostic scores built on clinical or biological parameters. Traditional steps in the development of a prognostic tool include derivation, internal and external validation and impact studies (i.e., studies evaluating the benefit of a risk stratification strategy). While derivation and validation studies are plentiful, impact studies are scarce [3]. Risk stratification in the setting of acute PE includes three main steps: identification of patients at a high risk of early mortality, hence, requiring immediate reperfusion treatment; identification of patients at a low risk of complications who can be safely treated as outpatients; identification of patients with an increased risk of complications requiring hospitalization for close monitoring and potential primary or rescue reperfusion therapy (Figure 1) [4].

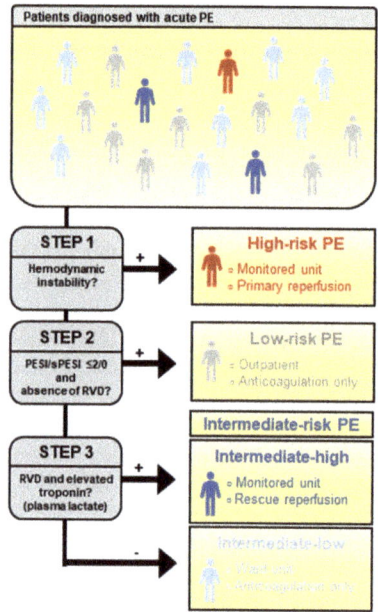

**Figure 1.** Step-by-step risk stratification in acute pulmonary embolism.

Nomenclature and definitions slightly differ between the European Society of Cardiology (ESC) and American Heart Association (AHA) guidelines; differences are highlighted in Table 1 [4,5]. This review mainly relies on the principles outlined in the 2019 ESC guidelines [4].

### 2.1. Step 1: Identification of High-Risk Patients

The first step in risk stratification of acute PE is the identification of patients at a high risk of early mortality. The most feared complication of acute PE is right ventricular overload and dysfunction which may lead to circulatory collapse and death. Therefore, patients with patent hemodynamic instability are considered as high-risk, according to the ESC criteria. Hemodynamic instability is defined by a systolic blood pressure (SBP) inferior to 90 mmHg for more than 15 min in the absence of hypovolemia, sepsis or arrhythmia; and/or the need of vasopressors in combination with end-organ hypoperfusion. In a recent systematic review including forty thousand patients with PE, 3.9% had high-risk PE. Short-term mortality was 19% among patients presenting with unstable PE versus 5.7% among patients with stable PE (OR 5.9; 95% CI 2.7 to 13.0) [6]. In a recent cohort of 7438 Chinese patients, the prevalence of unstable PE was 4.2% and mortality was 15.8% [7]. In high-risk acute PE, management relies on organ support and prompt reperfusion with thrombolytic therapies or percutaneous/surgical thrombectomy. The benefit of systemic thrombolysis has been demonstrated in small randomized controlled trials (RCTs) and large observational databases [6,8]. In the landmark study by Jerjes-Sanchez et al., eight patients with high-risk PE were randomized to anticoagulation (AC) alone or in combination with streptokinase [8]. The four patients randomized to AC died and the four patients randomized to thrombolysis survived. However, this small size, open-label trial was limited by an imbalance between groups. Recent RCTs evaluating thrombolytic therapy usually excluded high-risk PE [9–11], while older studies did not separately report outcomes for high-risk PE [12,13]. In a large North American database including more than two million patients with PE, in-hospital mortality was 15% among patients with unstable PE receiving TT and 47% among patients with unstable PE treated with AC alone. However, 70% of unstable patients did not receive TT [14,15]. This underutilization may be explained by the reluctance of physicians to administer TT because of its bleeding complications. Moreover, the definition of high-risk PE in previous ESC criteria, based exclusively on the presence of hypotension, was probably too simplistic as systolic blood pressure should probably be considered as a continuous risk marker rather than a dichotomized variable [16]. In the 2019 recommendations, they have been enriched by evidence of end-organ dysfunction and the exclusion of alternative contributors of shock [4,17].

**Table 1.** Nomenclature in current European and American guidelines.

| Nomenclature | Hemodynamic Instability | RVD | Elevated Troponin | PESI > Class II or sPESI > 0 |
|---|---|---|---|---|
| **European Society of Cardiology (ESC) 2019** | | | | |
| High risk | + | (+) | (+) | + |
| Intermediate–high risk | − | + | + | + * |
| Intermediate–low risk | − | One or none | | + * |
| Low risk | − | − | (−) | − |
| **American Heart Association (AHA) 2011** | | | | |
| Massive | + | (+) | (+) | NA |
| Submassive | − | One or both | | NA |
| Low risk | − | − | − | NA |

RVD: right ventricular dysfunction; PESI: pulmonary embolism severity index; sPESI: simplified pulmonary embolism severity index; NA: not assessed. * Presence of RVD despite PESI ≤ 2 or sPESI 0 classifies patients in intermediate-risk category.

In summary, identification of high-risk patients based on the presence of hemodynamic instability is recommended for rapid diagnosis and prompt reperfusion therapy.

*2.2. Step 2: Outpatient Management of Low-Risk Pulmonary Embolism*

Historically, all patients with acute PE were admitted to the hospital. Short-term mortality prediction rules have, therefore, been developed to identify patients at a low risk of mortality who could be treated as outpatients. The pulmonary embolism severity index (PESI) was derived and internally validated in 2005 in a cohort of 15,531 patients. The PESI score comprises 11 clinical variables and stratifies patients into five severity classes [18]. A simplified version of the PESI (sPESI) was derived including six clinical variables, each scoring one point (Supplementary Table S1) [19]. According to a 2012 meta-analysis including 50,021 patients, the area under the curve (AUC) of sPESI was 0.79 for all-cause mortality with a pooled sensitivity of 0.92 and a pooled specificity of 0.38, which is similar to the original PESI score. The pooled mortality was 2% among patients with PESI class I or II and 1.8% among patients with 0 points in sPESI (Table 2) [20]. A non-inferiority interventional study compared PESI-based outpatient management with hospital admission [21]. Three hundred and forty-four patients with low-risk PE (PESI class I-II) were randomly allocated to outpatient versus inpatient management. Ninety-day mortality was non-inferior in outpatients compared to patients admitted in-hospital (0.6% in both groups, upper confidence limit (UCL) for difference 2.1%) as well as PE recurrence (0.6% in outpatients versus 0% for inpatients, UCL 2.7%). At three months, three outpatients (1.8%), but no inpatients, developed major bleeding (UCL 4.5%).

Table 2. Operative characteristics of original and simplified pulmonary embolism severity index for early all-cause mortality [22].

| Prediction Index | Validation Cohorts (Patients) | Sensitivity (95% CI) | Specificity (95% CI) | PLR (95% CI) | NLR (95% CI) |
|---|---|---|---|---|---|
| PESI | 19 (23,997) | 0.89 (0.87–0.90) | 0.49 (0.44–0.53) | 1.72 (1.57–1.89) | 0.22 (0.18–0.25) |
| sPESI | 9 (26,610) | 0.92 (0.89–0.94) | 0.38 (0.32–0.44) | 1.47 (1.28–1.68) | 0.20 (0.13–0.31) |

PESI: pulmonary embolism severity index; sPESI: simplified pulmonary embolism severity index; CI: confidence interval; PLR: positive likelihood ratio; NLR: negative likelihood ratio.

Interestingly, when a low-risk PESI is combined with the absence of right ventricular dysfunction (RVD), 30-day mortality decreases even further (0.2–0.3%) [23,24]. In a single arm study evaluating the early discharge of low-risk PE (normotensive, absence of RVD and absence of serious comorbidities) treated with rivaroxaban, the rate of major bleeding at 3 months was low (1.2%) [25]. However, this increased sensitivity is obtained at the expense of a significantly lower proportion of patients identified as low risk [26]. An alternative approach to identify low-risk patients is the use of the Hestia criteria (Supplementary Table S2), consisting of a checklist of eleven criteria requiring hospital admission. Home treatment of patients without these criteria has been shown to be safe and non-inferior to sPESI-based home treatment [27–29].

In summary, outpatient treatment appears to be safe for low-risk PE patients identified by PESI, sPESI or Hestia criteria and absence of RVD.

## 3. Step 3: Further Classification of Intermediate-Risk Pulmonary Embolism

About 4% and 40% of acute pulmonary embolisms are categorized as high risk and low risk, respectively [30]. The remaining patients (i.e., normotensive patients with PESI III-V or sPESI $\geq$ 1) are classified as intermediate-risk PE with an overall 30-day mortality between 5% and 15% [18,19,31]. This group of patients is highly heterogeneous, with the vast majority experiencing a favorable outcome with AC alone, and a small, albeit significant, proportion requiring rescue reperfusion and cardiopulmonary resuscitation. For this reason, efforts have been made in recent decades to identify a subgroup of patients at risk of deterioration who might benefit from initial aggressive therapy and/or admission to a monitored unit. Clinical scores, biological and radiological markers of right ventricular overload and circulatory failure, alone or in combination, have been proposed to further stratify intermediate-risk acute PE.

### 3.1. Clinical Scores

Despite a high sensitivity and negative predictive value, PESI and sPESI lack specificity to predict early mortality (Table 2). Moreover, these scores rely heavily on demographic and co-morbid conditions rather than the severity of the acute PE event. PE-attributable mortality represents less than half of the overall 3-month mortality among patients with an acute PE [32,33]. Clinical scores alone are, therefore, inadequate to guide admission to monitored units or to initiate reperfusion therapies. Right ventricular dysfunction with circulatory collapse is the most common mechanism leading to fatal PE. Various markers of RVD and circulatory failure have been investigated as potential tools to further stratify normotensive patients; they are detailed in the following sections and summarized in Table 3.

**Table 3.** Prognostic value of markers of right ventricular dysfunction for short-term mortality.

| Marker | Sensitivity (95% CI) | Specificity (95% CI) | PLR (95% CI) | NLR (95% CI) |
| --- | --- | --- | --- | --- |
| Troponin [34] | 0.66 (0.61 to 0.70) | 0.66 (0.65 to 0.67) | 2.13 (1.84 to 2.47) | 0.51 (0.40 to 0.60) |
| BNP [35] | 0.88 (0.65 to 0.96) | 0.70 (0.64 to 0.75) | 2.13 (1.84 to 2.47) | 0.51 (0.40 to 0.60) |
| NT-proBNP [35] | 0.93 (0.14 to 1.00) | 0.58 (0.14 to 0.92) | 2.93 (2.28 to 3.77) | 0.17 (0.05 to 0.58) |
| RVD US [35] | 0.70 (0.46 to 0.86) | 0.57 (0.47 to 0.66) | 1.48 (1.05 to 2.08) | 0.82 (0.65 to 1.03) |
| RVD CT [35] | 0.65 (0.35 to 0.85) | 0.56 (0.39 to 0.71) | 1.63 (1.27 to 2.08) | 0.53 (0.31 to 0.89) |

CI: confidence interval; PLR: positive likelihood ratio; NLR: negative likelihood ratio; BNP: brain natriuretic peptide; NT-proBNP: N-terminal brain natriuretic peptide; RVD: right ventricular dysfunction; US: ultrasonography; CT: computer tomography.

### 3.2. Markers of Right Ventricular Dysfunction

- *Cardiac troponin*

The prognostic value of Troponin I and T has been evaluated in a meta-analysis including 1985 patients [36]. Elevated troponin was associated with increased short-term mortality in the whole cohort and in the subgroup of normotensive patients (OR 5.90, 95% CI 2.68 to 12.95, overall short-term mortality 17.9%). Subsequent meta-analyses questioned the prognostic value of elevated troponin in normotensive patients (positive likelihood ratio 2.13, negative likelihood ratio 0.51) and it has been suggested to combine it with other prognostic factors [34,37].

- *Brain natriuretic peptides*

Brain natriuretic peptide (BNP) and its N-terminal portion (NT-proBNP) are secreted by cardiomyocytes in response to ventricular stretching due to volume or pressure overload. The prognostic value of natriuretic peptides has been evaluated in at least eight studies [35,38]. In a meta-analysis, the pooled relative risk for 30-day mortality was 9.5 (95% CI 3.1 to 28.6) for BNP and 8.3 (95% CI 3.6 to 19.3) for NT-proBNP [35]. A meta-analysis of five more recent studies reported a relative risk for the complicated clinical course of 5.63 (95% CI 2.77 to 11.43) when the NT-proBNP value was over 1000 pg/mL [39]. Interestingly, troponin and brain natriuretic peptides seem to have an additive prognostic value [38,40,41].

Other biomarkers, such as serum creatinine, heart fatty acid-binding protein and copeptin, have been studied but are less extensively validated and/or not available in clinical practice [42–45].

- *Computer tomography pulmonary angiography*

CTPA signs of RVD include an elevated RV/left ventricular (LV) end diastolic diameter ratio (cut-off of 0.9 or 1.0), interventricular septum bowing, pulmonary artery enlargement, and retrograde reflux of contrast into the vena cava [46]. The right-to-left ventricular ratio can be easily estimated using the largest transverse diameters which may be measured on different CTPA slices. Septum bowing has an excellent specificity (98%) but poor sensitivity (31%), and inter-observer reproducibility limits its clinical utilization [46,47]. CT obstruction indexes have also been proposed by Qanadli et al. and [48] have shown to be associated with increased mortality, mostly among patients without comorbidities [49].

- *Bedside echocardiography*

Increased right-to-left ventricular ratio, hypokinesis of the free RV wall and the presence of pulmonary hypertension estimated from tricuspid regurgitation velocity have been reported to be associated with an increased risk of early complications. More advanced measures, such as the ratio of tricuspid annular plane systolic excursion to pulmonary arterial systolic pressure (TAPSE/PASP) are being investigated to stratify the risk among PE patients, but they are impractical for daily use and bedside stratification [50]. More recently, additional echocardiographic markers such as left or right ventricular outflow tract velocity time integral (LVOT and RVOT VTI) and stroke volume index have been reported to be associated with death or clinical deterioration, with interesting discriminative performance among intermediate-risk patients [51–54].

Despite a consistent association with short-term mortality, markers of RVD have poor diagnostic performances when they are used as a stand-alone test (Table 3) [17,35]. They have, therefore, been combined in current risk stratification guidelines.

### 3.3. Current Stratification of Intermediate-Risk Pulmonary Embolism

The ESC 2019 risk stratification of patients with acute PE relies on the three-step process described above, based on the presence of hemodynamic instability, clinical scores (PESI or sPESI) and the combined presence of two markers of RVD (Figure 1 and Table 1). This revision of the previously published 2014 criteria allows us to identify a subgroup of intermediate-risk PE patients at risk of short-term circulatory collapse or mortality, labelled as intermediate–high risk. These criteria were conceived following expert opinions, and no impact study has been published to date. In a prospective cohort of 1015 patients with normotensive acute PE, the ESC 2019 criteria classified 347 (34%), 571 (56%) and 97 (9.6%) of patients as low, intermediate–low and intermediate–high-risk PE, respectively. All cause 30-day mortality was significantly higher in intermediate–high-risk patients (10%) than in those with low risk or intermediate–low risk (4%) [55].

## 4. Reperfusion Therapy for Intermediate–High-Risk Pulmonary Embolism

Systemic thrombolysis using plasminogen activators is the most widely studied reperfusion strategy. Tissue plasminogen activators (tPA), such as urokinase, alteplase or tenecteplase, have a fibrinolytic effect, allowing clot dissolution and improvement of hemodynamic parameters in patients with high-risk PE [8,13]. Several randomized controlled trials aimed to evaluate their potential benefit among normotensive patients with elevated markers of RVD. The most informative evidence is provided by the European Pulmonary Embolism Trombolysis (PEITHO) trial [10]. This large RCT included 1005 patients with acute PE and RVD on imaging (CTPA or echocardiography) and myocardial injury (elevated troponin T or I), corresponding to the current intermediate–high-risk category. Patients were randomly assigned to unfractionated heparin (UFH) plus tenecteplase or UFH alone. The incidence of the primary outcome (death or hemodynamic collapse within 1 week) was significantly lower among patients allocated to tenecteplase than to UFH alone (2.6% vs. 5.6%, $p = 0.02$). This difference was mainly driven by an increased risk in hemodynamic decompensation among patients allocated to UFH (5.0% vs. 1.6%) while mortality was low and did not significantly differ (1.2% vs. 1.8%). This was counterbalanced by a significant increase in the risk of both major (11.5% vs. 2.4%) and intracranial bleeding (2.0% vs. 0.2%). When thrombolysis studies exclusively including acute PE with RVD are pooled, the uncertain benefit in overall mortality is mitigated by the significant increase in both major and intracranial bleeding [11]. Of note, the increased risk of major bleeding was more pronounced in studies using tenecteplase than in those using alteplase, but direct comparison studies are lacking to confirm this observation [56].

## 5. Toward a Better Identification of Thrombolysis Candidates among Intermediate-Risk Pulmonary Embolism

The current ESC classification seems to have an insufficient positive predictive value to identify a subgroup of intermediate-risk patients warranting more aggressive therapy. The benefits of a full-dose systemic thrombolysis are outweighed by bleeding risks, particularly when using tenecteplase. Two strategies have been identified by researchers to enhance the benefit-risk ratio: identifying patients at a higher basal risk and improving the safety of TT.

*Identifying Patients at Higher Basal Risk: Markers of Circulatory Failure and Alternative Scores*

Various alternative prediction rules, including early markers of circulatory failure, have been studied to identify normotensive patients with a higher risk of hemodynamic collapse.

- *Plasma lactate*

Plasma lactate is an important prognostic marker of organ dysfunction and is widely used in patients with sepsis or trauma [57]. Several studies evaluated the prognostic value of plasma lactate among patients with acute PE [58,59]. A retrospective study including 287 patients with acute PE reported a significant association between plasma lactate levels above 2 mmol/L and in-hospital mortality (OR 4.6; 95% CI 1.57 to 13.53) [58]. An association with 30-day mortality was subsequently observed in a prospective study (HR 11.67; 95% CI 3.32 to 41.03) [59]. Interestingly, this association was independent of shock state, hypotension, RVD or elevated troponin. A single center registry of 419 consecutive PE patients confirmed the association of elevated venous lactate with adverse outcomes, and found that levels above 3.3 mmol/L had the best predictive performance for in-hospital adverse events (PPV 0.27 and NPV 0.97) [60]. Moreover, adding venous lactate levels to the ESC 2019 risk criteria allowed us to further fine-tune stratification. Intermediate–high-risk patients with venous lactate $\geq$3.3 mmol/L had a 27.5% prevalence of adverse events, versus 6.8% if lactate was <3.3 mmol/L. Intermediate low-risk patients with lactate levels <2.3 mmol/L were at a low risk of adverse events (0.6%, versus 12.2% if $\geq$2.3 mmol/L) [60].

- *BOVA score*

The Bova score was derived from pooled results of six prospective studies, including 2874 patients with hemodynamically stable acute PE [61]. Model predictors included heart rate, SBP, biomarkers (cardiac troponin or BNP) and echocardiography (Table 4 and Supplementary Table S3) [61]. RVD was defined by the presence of RV/LV >0.9 or 1, RV free wall hypokinesis, RV end-diastolic diameter >30 mm or estimated systolic pulmonary artery pressure > 30 mmH. The primary composite outcome was PE-related death, hemodynamic collapse or recurrent PE at 30 days. Thirty-day complications differed significantly across categories of the model (0–2 points 4.2%; 3–4 points 10.8%; >4 points 29.2%). The area under the ROC curve was 0.73 (95% CI 0.68–0.77) and 5.8% of patients were classified in the stage III category. Recently, a meta-analysis including the derivation study and eight prospective and retrospective external validation cohort studies were conducted [62]. The pooled cumulative incidence of PE-related complications (PE-related death, hemodynamic collapse or recurrent PE) at 30 days was 3.8% for stage I, 10.8% for stage II and 19.9% for stage III (1.9, 5.5 and 12.1 for 30-day PE mortality) with an AUC of 0.73 (Table 4) [63]. In another retrospective cohort including 994 normotensive patients, 5.9% of patients were classified in the stage III category. Death or hemodynamic collapse at 7 days occurred in 18.6% of patients in the stage III category. When lactate elevation was incorporated into an extended Bova score, the proportion of patients in the stage III category increased to 11.2 %, with a primary outcome rate of 25.9 %. Hemodynamic collapse by day 7 occurred in 15.3% of patients in the class III category according to the standard BOVA score, compared to 24.1% in the model including lactate elevation [64].

Table 4. Components of the Bova score.

| Predictor | Points |
|---|---|
| SBP 90–100 mmHg | 2 |
| Elevated troponin | 2 |
| RV dysfunction | 2 |
| Heart rate > 100/min | 1 |

- *TELOS score*

The TELOS score was derived in a prospective cohort of 496 normotensive PE patients. The primary outcome was PE-related death or hemodynamic collapse within 7 days. A model including RVD, troponin and plasma lactate elevation resulted in a 17.9% PPV [65]. The TELOS rule was further validated by the same group in a prospective cohort of 994 normotensive patients. A total of 5.9% of patients were allocated to the intermediate–high-risk category according to the TELOS criteria, with a cumulative incidence of the primary outcome (death or hemodynamic collapse at 7 days) of 21.1% (Table 5) [64].

Table 5. Prognostic value of stratification scores dichotomized at an intermediate–high-risk level.

| Score | Sensitivity | Specificity | PLR | PPV | Outcome |
|---|---|---|---|---|---|
| Scores including Plasma Lactate | | | | | |
| ESC 2019 + lactate [60] | 0.33 (0.16 to 0.55) | 0.95 (0.92 to 0.97) | 6.27 (3.11 to 12.66) | 0.27 | In-hospital adverse outcome |
| Bova + lactate [64] | 0.46 (0.34 to 0.58) | 0.91 (0.90 to 0.92) | 5.16 (3.55 to 7.13) | 0.26 | Adverse 7-day outcome |
| TELOS [64] | 0.19 (0.11 to 0.30) | 0.95 (0.95 to 0.96) | 3.94 (2.04 to 7.15) | 0.21 | Adverse 7-day outcome |
| Scores without plasma lactate | | | | | |
| Bova [66] | 0.48 (0.30 to 0.67) | 0.86 (0.82 to 0.90) | 3.41 (2.11 to 5.52) | 0.19 | Adverse 30-day outcome |
| ESC 2014 [66] | 0.80 (0.61 to 0.91) | 0.69 (0.64 to 0.73) | 2.60 (2.00 to 3.30) | 0.15 | Adverse 30-day outcome |
| ESC 2019 [67] | 0.52 (0.34 to 0.70) | 0.79 (0.77 to 0.82) | 2.5 (1.7 to 3.7) | 0.07 | In-hospital adverse outcome |

ESC: European Society of Cardiology; PLR: positive likelihood ratio; PPV: positive predictive value.

- *SHIELD score*

The SHIELD score was derived from a retrospective monocentric cohort of 554 normotensive patients and was externally validated. Predictors of the model included shock index $\geq 1$, hypoxemia, lactate elevation and signs of RVD (i.e., elevated troponin, NT-pro BNP and RV/LV ratio >1 using CTPA) [68]. The risk of 30-day mortality or rescue thrombolysis for each tercile was 0.6%, 1.8% and 16.4% (AUC 0.90, 95% CI 0.85 to 0.94) in the derivation cohort and 0.6%, 1.9% and 15.3% (AUC 0.82; 95% CI 0.75 to 0.87) in the external validation cohort.

- *Other scores*

Lankeit et al. derived a clinical prediction rule including heart fatty acid-binding protein (H-FABP), syncope and heart rate (FAST score). The positive predictive value was 20.5% and the AUC was 0.85 (95% CI 0.75 to 0.95) [69]. This score was validated in another cohort of the same center with a positive predictive value of 18.9% and an AUC of 0.82 (95% CI 0.75 to 0.89) [66].

A prospective study including 268 normotensive PE patients showed an association between copeptin level >24 pmol/L and 30-day mortality or adverse outcome. The positive predictive value was 11% (95% CI 7 to 19%) and the negative predictive value was 98% (95% CI 95 to 99%), suggesting that this biomarker could be combined with markers of RVD such as NT-proBNP or highly sensitive troponin T [42].

Other scores combining clinical variables, imaging and biomarkers have been studied with less extensive validation [70,71].

- *Between score comparison*

Vanni et al. compared the prognostic accuracy of the ESC 2014 criteria, TELOS and Bova score in a cohort of 994 normotensive patients with PE. The Bova and TELOS scores classified the same proportion of patients in the intermediate–high-risk category (5.9 and 5.7%) with a similar rate of early adverse events (18.6 and 21.1% 7-day death or hemodynamic collapse), while the ESC criteria classified a higher proportion of patients in the intermediate–high-risk category (12.5%, $p < 0.001$) with a lower rate of events (13% $p = 0.18$) [54]. Diagnostic performances of several existing scores are summarized in Table 5. While the risk of adverse events was comprised between 7% and 15% in the intermediate–high-risk group according to the ESC criteria, recent prediction rules, including markers of circulatory dysfunction (plasma lactates) or adjunction of plasma lactates to the Bova or ESC 2019 criteria, appeared to have a promising positive predictive value with event rates of around 25%. However, some variation in their PPVs was observed across studies, which is partly explained by variations in the outcome definitions. Moreover, the plasma lactate cut-off varied across studies and the optimal cut-off remains to be determined.

## 6. Expected Benefits from a Better Identification of Intermediate–High-Risk Patients

As discussed above, recent prediction rules, including markers of circulatory dysfunction, might allow us to identify a subgroup of patients with a significantly increased (>25%) risk in adverse events who might benefit from a more aggressive therapy. Figure 2 illustrates the extrapolated benefits of thrombolytic therapy in a theoretical cohort of patients with a 17.1% basal risk of adverse outcomes. This basal risk was obtained by combining the basal risk observed in the PEITHO trial and the positive likelihood ratio of elevated blood lactates [9]. Net benefits and harms were computed based on the relative risks reported in our previous meta-analysis on thrombolytic therapy in PE [11]. These extrapolations are mainly illustrative and should be evaluated in interventional studies, as bleeding complication risks might also increase among patients with a higher basal risk of a PE-related adverse event.

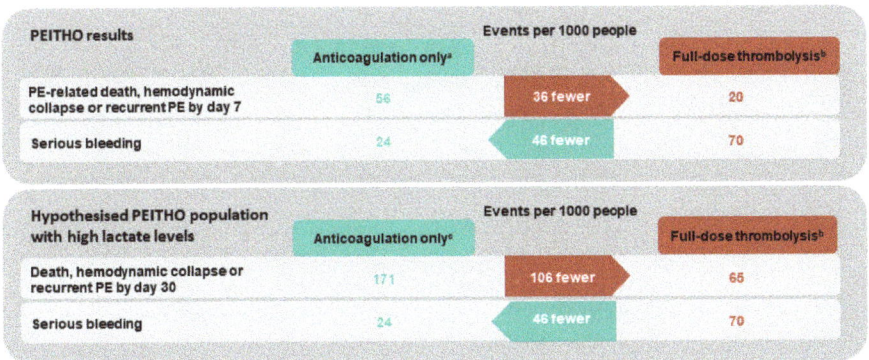

Figure 2. Extrapolated effect of full-dose thrombolysis in cohorts of patients with a different basal risk of an early adverse event. [a] Basal risk according to PEITHO trial [10], [b] relative effect according to Marti et al. [11]. [c] Basal risk obtained by combining the risk of the PEITHO population and the prognostic modulation obtained by adding lactate [60].

## 7. Improving the Safety Profile: Reduced-Dose Thrombolytic Therapy

Another strategy to optimize the risk-benefit ratio of TT among intermediate–high-risk PE is the reduction in TT bleeding complications. In this perspective, several trials investigated reduced-dose systemic thrombolysis regimens. In the Moderate Pulmonary Embolism Treated with Thrombolysis (MOPETT) trial, 121 patients with acute PE and a high thrombotic burden were randomized to half-dose tPA and heparin versus heparin alone. Half-dose thrombolysis was associated with a lower rate of pulmonary hypertension or recurrent PE at 28 months (16% versus 63% in the AC group) and no significantly increased risk of bleeding [72]. Similarly, a systematic review including 5 small-size randomized trials suggested a similar efficacy and reduced bleeding complications when half-dose was compared to standard dose thrombolysis [73]. These preliminary results based on a limited sample of patients need to be further confirmed.

Catheter-based thrombolytic therapies, including catheter-released thrombolysis (CRT), ultrasound-assisted thrombolysis and mechanical fragmentation or aspiration, alone or in combination, are alternative strategies to reduce bleeding risks associated with systemic TT [74,75]. Catheter-based therapies are an evolving technology and several devices have been shown to improve echocardiographic signs of RVD in single-arm studies [75,76]. Their impact regarding clinically relevant outcomes should be further evaluated in randomized controlled studies [77]. These alternatives may be proposed to high-risk patients at an increased risk of bleeding. More recently, circulatory support using extracorporeal membrane oxygenation (ECMO) in combination with surgical embolectomy has been proposed for high-risk patients with high in-hospital survival rates [78].

## 8. Evidence to Come: The PEITHO-3 Study

The ongoing PEITHO-3 study is expected to add further evidence for the management of intermediate–high-risk PE. This ongoing, multicentric, randomized controlled trial aims to combine the two previously discussed strategies. Identification of patients with a higher basal risk of adverse events will be obtained based on a retrospective analysis of the PEITHO population by adding clinical markers of severity (SBP $\leq$ 110 mmHg, respiratory rate > 20/min, history of chronic heart failure) to the ESC intermediate–high-risk criteria with an expected event rate of 11.2% [79,80]. At the same time, a reduced dose of alteplase (0.6 mg/kg) will be used. The PEITHO-3 trial plans to include 650 patients with, expected to be completed in September 2025 [80]. The expected benefits in the hypothesized PEITHO-3 population are illustrated in Figure 3, assuming a constant relative effect of treatment and a constant basal bleeding risk with important uncertainty regarding the increase in bleeding complications with reduced-dose TT.

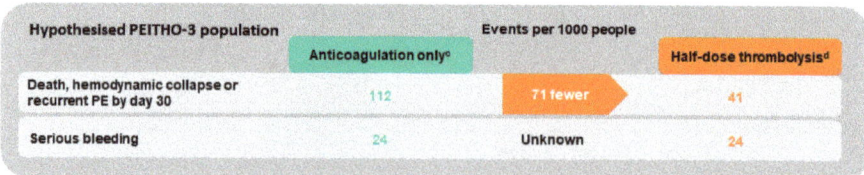

**Figure 3.** Extrapolated effect of half-dose thrombolysis in the hypothesized PEITHO-3 population. [c] Basal risk derived from applying the PEITHO-3 inclusion criteria and outcome to the PEITHO population [79]. [d] Relative treatment effect of full-dose thrombolysis is applied, and no increased risk of serious bleeding is assumed, according to a meta-analysis on half-dose thrombolysis [73].

## 9. Conclusions

The management of patients with acute PE requires an accurate step-by-step risk stratification. Hemodynamic instability allows to quickly detect high-risk patients who will benefit from TT; clinical prediction rules, such as PESI or sPESI, allow us to identify low-risk patients who can be safely treated as outpatients. The intermediate-risk group is composed of a highly heterogeneous group of patients, most of whom will experience favorable short-term outcomes. Individual evaluations by dedicated multidisciplinary PE response teams may be useful to decide the optimal treatment strategy [81,82]. Several prediction models combining clinical variables, biomarkers and medical imaging have been developed to identify the subgroup of patients with a significant risk of early adverse events who might benefit from early aggressive management. The inclusion of plasma lactate may increase the performance of risk stratification models, but it needs to be further validated in future studies. Optimization of reperfusion strategies by using reduced regimens of thrombolysis or catheter-directed reperfusion techniques might contribute to improving the prognosis of patients by limiting the side effects. Results of ongoing studies (NCT04430569) will clarify the benefits of initial reperfusion strategies in this subgroup of patients. While waiting for these results, current guidelines recommend admitting patients of the intermediate–high-risk category to a monitored unit for early detection of clinical deterioration and the potential need for rescue reperfusion.

**Supplementary Materials:** The following supporting information can be downloaded at: https://www.mdpi.com/article/10.3390/jcm11092533/s1, Supplementary Table S1. Original and simplified pulmonary embolism severity index (PESI and sPESI); Supplementary Table S2. The Hestia rule; Supplementary Table S3. Components of several prediction scores.

**Author Contributions:** Conceptualization, A.L., S.B., C.M.; methodology, A.L., S.B., C.M.; validation, A.L., S.B., C.M., A.B., O.G., M.R.; resources, A.L., C.M., S.B.; writing—original draft preparation, A.L., S.B., C.M.; writing—review and editing, A.L., S.B., C.M., M.R., O.G., A.B.; supervision, C.M., M.R.; Y. All authors have read and agreed to the published version of the manuscript.

**Funding:** This research received no external funding.

**Institutional Review Board Statement:** Not applicable.

**Informed Consent Statement:** Not applicable.

**Conflicts of Interest:** The authors declare no conflict of interest.

# References

1. ISTH Steering Committee for World Thrombosis Day. Thrombosis: A major contributor to the global disease burden. *J. Thromb. Haemost.* **2014**, *12*, 1580–1590. [CrossRef] [PubMed]
2. Cohen, A.T.; Agnelli, G.; Anderson, F.A.; Arcelus, J.I.; Bergqvist, D.; Brecht, J.G.; Greer, I.A.; Heit, J.A.; Hutchinson, J.L.; Kakkar, A.K. Venous thromboembolism (VTE) in Europe. The number of VTE events and associated morbidity and mortality. *Thromb. Haemost.* **2007**, *98*, 756–764. [PubMed]
3. Reilly, B.M.; Evans, A.T. Translating clinical research into clinical practice: Impact of using prediction rules to make decisions. *Ann. Intern. Med.* **2006**, *144*, 201–209. [CrossRef]
4. Konstantinides, S.V.; Meyer, G. The 2019 ESC Guidelines on the Diagnosis and Management of Acute Pulmonary Embolism. *Eur. Heart J.* **2019**, *40*, 3453–3455. [CrossRef] [PubMed]
5. Jaff, M.R.; McMurtry, M.S.; Archer, S.L.; Cushman, M.; Goldenberg, N.; Goldhaber, S.Z.; Jenkins, J.S.; Kline, J.A.; Michaels, A.D.; Thistlethwaite, P.; et al. Management of massive and submassive pulmonary embolism, iliofemoral deep vein thrombosis, and chronic thromboembolic pulmonary hypertension: A scientific statement from the American Heart Association. *Circulation* **2011**, *123*, 1788–1830. [CrossRef]
6. Quezada, C.A.; Bikdeli, B.; Barrios, D.; Barbero, E.; Chiluiza, D.; Muriel, A.; Casazza, F.; Monreal, M.; Yusen, R.D.; Jiménez, D. Meta-Analysis of Prevalence and Short-Term Prognosis of Hemodynamically Unstable Patients with Symptomatic Acute Pulmonary Embolism. *Am. J. Cardiol.* **2019**, *123*, 684–689. [CrossRef]
7. Zhai, Z.; Wang, D.; Lei, J.; Yang, Y.; Xu, X.; Ji, Y.; Yi, Q.; Chen, H.; Hu, X.; Liu, Z.; et al. Trends in risk stratification, in-hospital management and mortality of patients with acute pulmonary embolism: An analysis from the China pUlmonary thromboembolism REgistry Study (CURES). *Eur. Respir. J.* **2021**, *58*, 2002963. [CrossRef]
8. Jerjes-Sanchez, C.; Ramirez-Rivera, A.; de Lourdes Garcia, M.; Arriaga-Nava, R.; Valencia, S.; Rosado-Buzzo, A.; Pierzo, J.A.; Rosas, E. Streptokinase and heparin versus heparin alone in massive pulmonary embolism: A randomized controlled trial. *J. Thromb. Thrombolysis* **1995**, *2*, 227–229. [CrossRef]
9. Konstantinides, S.V.; Geibel, A.; Heusel, G.; Heinrich, F.; Kasper, W. Heparin plus Alteplase Compared with Heparin Alone in Patients with Submassive Pulmonary Embolism. *N. Engl. J. Med.* **2002**, *347*, 1143–1150. [CrossRef]
10. Meyer, G.; Vicaut, E.; Danays, T.; Agnelli, G.; Becattini, C.; Beyer-Westendorf, J.; Bluhmki, E.; Bouvaist, H.; Brenner, B.; Couturaud, F.; et al. Fibrinolysis for patients with intermediate-risk pulmonary embolism. *N. Engl. J. Med.* **2014**, *370*, 1402–1411. [CrossRef]

11. Marti, C.; John, G.; Konstantinides, S.; Combescure, C.; Sanchez, O.; Lankeit, M.; Meyer, G.; Perrier, A. Systemic thrombolytic therapy for acute pulmonary embolism: A systematic review and meta-analysis. *Eur. Heart J.* **2014**, *36*, 605–614. [CrossRef] [PubMed]
12. Dotter, C.T.; Seaman, A.J.; Rösch, J.; Porter, J.M. Streptokinase and Heparin in the Treatment of Pulmonary Embolism: A Randomized Comparison. *Vasc. Surg.* **1979**, *13*, 42–52. [CrossRef]
13. Urokinase Pulmonary Embolism Trial Study Group. Urokinase pulmonary embolism trial. Phase 1 results: A cooperative study. *JAMA* **1970**, *214*, 2163–2172. [CrossRef]
14. Stein, P.D.; Matta, F. Thrombolytic therapy in unstable patients with acute pulmonary embolism: Saves lives but underused. *Am. J. Med.* **2012**, *125*, 465–470. [CrossRef] [PubMed]
15. Stein, P.D.; Matta, F.; Hughes, P.G.; Hughes, M.J. Adjunctive Therapy and Mortality in Patients With Unstable Pulmonary Embolism. *Am. J. Cardiol.* **2020**, *125*, 1913–1919. [CrossRef]
16. Quezada, A.; Jiménez, D.; Bikdeli, B.; Moores, L.; Porres-Aguilar, M.; Aramberri, M.; Lima, J.; Ballaz, A.; Yusen, R.D.; Monreal, M. Systolic blood pressure and mortality in acute symptomatic pulmonary embolism. *Int. J. Cardiol.* **2019**, *302*, 157–163. [CrossRef]
17. Konstantinides, S.V. 2014 ESC Guidelines on the diagnosis and management of acute pulmonary embolism. *Eur. Heart J.* **2014**, *35*, 3145–3146. [CrossRef]
18. Aujesky, D.; Obrosky, D.S.; Stone, R.A.; Auble, T.E.; Perrier, A.; Cornuz, J.; Roy, P.-M.; Fine, M.J. Derivation and Validation of a Prognostic Model for Pulmonary Embolism. *Am. J. Respir. Crit. Care Med.* **2005**, *172*, 1041–1046. [CrossRef]
19. Jiménez, D.; Aujesky, D.; Moores, L.; Gómez, V.; Lobo, J.L.; Uresandi, F.; Otero, R.; Monreal, M.; Muriel, A.; Yusen, R.D. Simplification of the Pulmonary Embolism Severity Index for Prognostication in Patients With Acute Symptomatic Pulmonary Embolism. *Arch. Intern. Med.* **2010**, *170*, 1383–1389. [CrossRef]
20. Zhou, X.-Y.; Ben, S.-Q.; Chen, H.-L.; Ni, S.-S. The prognostic value of pulmonary embolism severity index in acute pulmonary embolism: A meta-analysis. *Respir. Res.* **2012**, *13*, 1–12. [CrossRef]
21. Aujesky, D.; Roy, P.-M.; Verschuren, F.; Righini, M.; Osterwalder, J.; Egloff, M.; Renaud, B.; Verhamme, P.; Stone, R.A.; Legall, C.; et al. Outpatient versus inpatient treatment for patients with acute pulmonary embolism: An international, open-label, randomised, non-inferiority trial. *Lancet* **2011**, *378*, 41–48. [CrossRef]
22. Kohn, C.G.; Mearns, E.S.; Parker, M.W.; Hernandez, A.V.; Coleman, C.I. Prognostic accuracy of clinical prediction rules for early post-pulmonary embolism all-cause mortality: A bivariate meta-analysis. *Chest* **2015**, *147*, 1043–1062. [CrossRef] [PubMed]
23. Barco, S.; Mahmoudpour, S.H.; Planquette, B.; Sanchez, O.; Konstantinides, S.V.; Meyer, G. Prognostic value of right ventricular dysfunction or elevated cardiac biomarkers in patients with low-risk pulmonary embolism: A systematic review and meta-analysis. *Eur. Heart J.* **2019**, *40*, 902–910. [CrossRef] [PubMed]
24. Becattini, C.; Maraziti, G.; Vinson, D.R.; Ng, A.C.C.; Exter, P.L.D.; Côté, B.; Vanni, S.; Doukky, R.; Khemasuwan, D.; Weekes, A.J.; et al. Right ventricle assessment in patients with pulmonary embolism at low risk for death based on clinical models: An individual patient data meta-analysis. *Eur. Heart J.* **2021**, *42*, 3190–3199. [CrossRef] [PubMed]
25. Barco, S.; Schmidtmann, I.; Ageno, W.; Bauersachs, R.M.; Becattini, C.; Bernardi, E.; Beyer-Westendorf, J.; Bonacchini, L.; Brachmann, J.; Christ, M.; et al. Early discharge and home treatment of patients with low-risk pulmonary embolism with the oral factor Xa inhibitor rivaroxaban: An international multicentre single-arm clinical trial. *Eur. Heart J.* **2019**, *41*, 509–518. [CrossRef] [PubMed]
26. Myc, L.A.; Richardson, E.D.; Barros, A.J.; Watson, J.T.; Sharma, A.M.; Kadl, A. Risk stratification in acute pulmonary embolism: Half of the way there? *Ann. Am. Thorac. Soc.* **2021**, *18*, 1066–1068. [CrossRef] [PubMed]
27. Roy, P.-M.; Penaloza, A.; Hugli, O.; Klok, F.A.; Arnoux, A.; Elias, A.; Couturaud, F.; Joly, L.-M.; Lopez, R.; Faber, L.M.; et al. Triaging acute pulmonary embolism for home treatment by Hestia or simplified PESI criteria: The HOME-PE randomized trial. *Eur. Heart J.* **2021**, *42*, 3146–3157. [CrossRef]
28. den Exter, P.L.; Zondag, W.; Klok, F.A.; Brouwer, R.E.; Dolsma, J.; Eijsvogel, M.; Faber, L.M.; van Gerwen, M.; Grootenboers, M.J.; Heller-Baan, R.; et al. Efficacy and Safety of Outpatient Treatment Based on the Hestia Clinical Decision Rule with or without N-Terminal Pro-Brain Natriuretic Peptide Testing in Patients with Acute Pulmonary Embolism. A Randomized Clinical Trial. *Am. J. Respir. Crit. Care Med.* **2016**, *194*, 998–1006. [CrossRef]
29. Zondag, W.; Hiddinga, B.I.; Crobach, M.J.; Labots, G.; Dolsma, A.; Durian, M.; Faber, L.M.; Hofstee, H.M.; Melissant, C.F.; Ullmann, E.F.; et al. Hestia criteria can discriminate high- from low-risk patients with pulmonary embolism. *Eur. Respir. J.* **2013**, *41*, 588–592. [CrossRef]
30. Elias, A.; Mallett, S.; Daoud-Elias, M.; Poggi, J.-N.; Clarke, M. Prognostic models in acute pulmonary embolism: A systematic review and meta-analysis. *BMJ Open* **2016**, *6*, e010324. [CrossRef]
31. Sanchez, D.; De Miguel, J.; Sam, A.; Wagner, C.; Zamarro, C.; Nieto, R.; Garcia, L.; Aujesky, D.; Yusen, R.D.; Jiménez, D. The effects of cause of death classification on prognostic assessment of patients with pulmonary embolism. *J. Thromb. Haemost.* **2011**, *9*, 2201–2207. [CrossRef] [PubMed]
32. Goldhaber, S.Z.; Visani, L.; De Rosa, M. Acute pulmonary embolism: Clinical outcomes in the International Cooperative Pulmonary Embolism Registry (ICOPER). *Lancet* **1999**, *353*, 1386–1389. [CrossRef]
33. Laporte, S.; Mismetti, P.; Décousus, H.; Uresandi, F.; Otero, R.; Lobo, J.L.; Monreal, M.; The RIETE Investigators. Clinical predictors for fatal pulmonary embolism in 15,520 patients with venous thromboembolism: Findings from the Registro Informatizado de la Enfermedad TromboEmbolica venosa (RIETE) Registry. *Circulation* **2008**, *117*, 1711–1716. [CrossRef] [PubMed]

34. Bajaj, A.; Saleeb, M.; Rathor, P.; Sehgal, V.; Kabak, B.; Hosur, S. Prognostic value of troponins in acute nonmassive pulmonary embolism: A meta-analysis. *Heart Lung* **2015**, *44*, 327–334. [CrossRef] [PubMed]
35. Sanchez, O.; Trinquart, L.; Colombet, I.; Durieux, P.; Huisman, M.V.; Chatellier, G.; Meyer, G. Prognostic value of right ventricular dysfunction in patients with haemodynamically stable pulmonary embolism: A systematic review. *Eur. Heart J.* **2008**, *29*, 1569–1577. [CrossRef] [PubMed]
36. Becattini, C.; Vedovati, M.C.; Agnelli, G. Prognostic value of troponins in acute pulmonary embolism: A meta-analysis. *Circulation* **2007**, *116*, 427–433. [CrossRef]
37. Jiménez, D.; Uresandi, F.; Otero, R.; Lobo, J.L.; Monreal, M.; Martí, D.; Zamora, J.; Muriel, A.; Aujesky, D.; Yusen, R.D. Troponin-based risk stratification of patients with acute nonmassive pulmonary embolism: Systematic review and metaanalysis. *Chest* **2009**, *136*, 974–982. [CrossRef]
38. Lankeit, M.; Jiménez, D.; Kostrubiec, M.; Dellas, C.; Kuhnert, K.; Hasenfuß, G.; Pruszczyk, P.; Konstantinides, S. Validation of N-terminal pro-brain natriuretic peptide cut-off values for risk stratification of pulmonary embolism. *Eur. Respir. J.* **2014**, *43*, 1669–1677. [CrossRef]
39. Nithianandan, H.; Reilly, A.; Tritschler, T.; Wells, P. Applying rigorous eligibility criteria to studies evaluating prognostic utility of serum biomarkers in pulmonary embolism: A systematic review and meta-analysis. *Thromb. Res.* **2020**, *195*, 195–208. [CrossRef]
40. Jiménez, D.; Kopecna, D.; Tapson, V.; Briese, B.; Schreiber, D.; Lobo, J.L.; Monreal, M.; Aujesky, D.; Sanchez, O.; Meyer, G.; et al. Derivation and validation of multimarker prognostication for normotensive patients with acute symptomatic pulmonary embolism. *Am. J. Respir. Crit. Care Med.* **2014**, *189*, 718–726. [CrossRef]
41. Santos, A.R.; Freitas, P.; Ferreira, J.; Félix-Oliveira, A.; Gonçalves, M.; Faria, D.; Augusto, J.; Simões, J.; Gago, M.; Oliveira, J.; et al. Risk stratification in normotensive acute pulmonary embolism patients: Focus on the intermediate–high risk subgroup. *Eur. Heart J. Acute Cardiovasc. Care* **2020**, *9*, 279–285. [CrossRef] [PubMed]
42. Hellenkamp, K.; Schwung, J.; Rossmann, H.; Kaeberich, A.; Wachter, R.; Hasenfuß, G.; Konstantinides, S.; Lankeit, M. Risk stratification of normotensive pulmonary embolism: Prognostic impact of copeptin. *Eur. Respir. J.* **2015**, *46*, 1701–1710. [CrossRef] [PubMed]
43. Kostrubiec, M.; Pływaczewska, M.; Jiménez, D.; Lankeit, M.; Ciurzynski, M.; Konstantinides, S.; Pruszczyk, P. The Prognostic Value of Renal Function in Acute Pulmonary Embolism—A Multi-Centre Cohort Study. *Thromb. Haemost.* **2019**, *119*, 140–148. [CrossRef] [PubMed]
44. Chopard, R.; Jimenez, D.; Serzian, G.; Ecarnot, F.; Falvo, N.; Kalbacher, E.; Bonnet, B.; Capellier, G.; Schiele, F.; Bertoletti, L.; et al. Renal dysfunction improves risk stratification and may call for a change in the management of intermediate- and high-risk acute pulmonary embolism: Results from a multicenter cohort study with external validation. *Crit. Care* **2021**, *25*, 1–11. [CrossRef]
45. Dellas, C.; Puls, M.; Lankeit, M.; Schäfer, K.; Cuny, M.; Berner, M.; Hasenfuss, G.; Konstantinides, S. Elevated heart-type fatty acid-binding protein levels on admission predict an adverse outcome in normotensive patients with acute pulmonary embolism. *J. Am. Coll. Cardiol.* **2010**, *55*, 2150–2157. [CrossRef]
46. John, G.; Marti, C.; Poletti, P.-A.; Perrier, A. Hemodynamic Indexes Derived from Computed Tomography Angiography to Predict Pulmonary Embolism Related Mortality. *BioMed Res. Int.* **2014**, *2014*, 1–8. [CrossRef]
47. Chornenki, N.L.J.; Poorzargar, K.; Shanjer, M.; Mbuagbaw, L.; Delluc, A.; Crowther, M.; Siegal, D.M. Detection of right ventricular dysfunction in acute pulmonary embolism by computed tomography or echocardiography: A systematic review and meta-analysis. *J. Thromb. Haemost.* **2021**, *19*, 2504–2513. [CrossRef]
48. Qanadli, S.D.; El Hajjam, M.; Vieillard-Baron, A.; Joseph, T.; Mesurolle, B.; Oliva, V.L.; Barré, O.; Bruckert, F.; Dubourg, O.; Lacombe, P. New CT index to quantify arterial obstruction in pulmonary embolism: Comparison with angiographic index and echocardiography. *AJR Am. J. Roentgenol.* **2001**, *176*, 1415–1420. [CrossRef]
49. Kay, F.U.; Abbara, S. Refining Risk Stratification in Nonmassive Acute Pulmonary Embolism. *Radiol. Cardiothorac. Imaging* **2020**, *2*, e200458. [CrossRef]
50. Lyhne, M.D.; Kabrhel, C.; Giordano, N.; Andersen, A.; Nielsen-Kudsk, J.E.; Zheng, H.; Dudzinski, D.M. The echocardiographic ratio tricuspid annular plane systolic excursion/pulmonary arterial systolic pressure predicts short-term adverse outcomes in acute pulmonary embolism. *Eur. Heart J. Cardiovasc. Imaging* **2020**, *22*, 285–294. [CrossRef]
51. Brailovsky, Y.; Lakhter, V.; Weinberg, I.; Porcaro, K.; Haines, J.; Morris, S.; Masic, D.; Mancl, E.; Bashir, R.; Alkhouli, M.; et al. Right Ventricular Outflow Doppler Predicts Low Cardiac Index in Intermediate Risk Pulmonary Embolism. *Clin. Appl. Thromb.* **2019**, *25*, 1076029619886062. [CrossRef] [PubMed]
52. Yuriditsky, E.; Mitchell, O.J.; Sibley, R.A.; Xia, Y.; Sista, A.; Zhong, J.; Moore, W.H.; Amoroso, N.E.; Goldenberg, R.; Smith, D.E.; et al. Low left ventricular outflow tract velocity time integral is associated with poor outcomes in acute pulmonary embolism. *Vasc. Med.* **2020**, *25*, 133–140. [CrossRef] [PubMed]
53. Yuriditsky, E.; Mitchell, O.J.; Sista, A.; Xia, Y.; Sibley, R.A.; Zhong, J.; Moore, W.H.; Amoroso, N.E.; Goldenberg, R.; Smith, D.E.; et al. Right ventricular stroke distance predicts death and clinical deterioration in patients with pulmonary embolism. *Thromb. Res.* **2020**, *195*, 29–34. [CrossRef] [PubMed]
54. Prosperi-Porta, G.; Solverson, K.; Fine, N.; Humphreys, C.J.; Ferland, A.; Weatherald, J. Echocardiography-Derived Stroke Volume Index Is Associated with Adverse In-Hospital Outcomes in Intermediate-Risk Acute Pulmonary Embolism: A Retrospective Cohort Study. *Chest* **2020**, *158*, 1132–1142. [CrossRef]

55. Mirambeaux, R.; León, F.; Bikdeli, B.; Morillo, R.; Barrios, D.; Mercedes, E.; Moores, L.; Tapson, V.; Yusen, R.D.; Jiménez, D. Intermediate-High Risk Pulmonary Embolism. *TH Open* **2019**, *03*, e356–e363. [CrossRef]
56. Guillermin, A.; Yan, D.J.; Perrier, A.; Marti, C. Safety and efficacy of tenecteplase versus alteplase in acute coronary syndrome: A systematic review and meta-analysis of randomized trials. *Arch. Med Sci.* **2016**, *12*, 1181–1187. [CrossRef]
57. Jones, A.E.; Shapiro, N.I.; Trzeciak, S.; Arnold, R.C.; Claremont, H.A.; Kline, J.A.; Emergency Medicine Shock Research Network (EMShockNet) Investigators. Lactate clearance vs central venous oxygen saturation as goals of early sepsis therapy: A randomized clinical trial. *JAMA* **2010**, *303*, 739–746. [CrossRef]
58. Vanni, S.; Socci, F.; Pepe, G.; Nazerian, P.; Viviani, G.; Baioni, M.; Conti, A.; Grifoni, S. High Plasma Lactate Levels Are Associated with Increased Risk of In-hospital Mortality in Patients With Pulmonary Embolism. *Acad. Emerg. Med.* **2011**, *18*, 830–835. [CrossRef]
59. Vanni, S.; Viviani, G.; Baioni, M.; Pepe, G.; Nazerian, P.; Socci, F.; Bartolucci, M.; Bartolini, M.; Grifoni, S. Prognostic Value of Plasma Lactate Levels Among Patients with Acute Pulmonary Embolism: The Thrombo-Embolism Lactate Outcome Study. *Ann. Emerg. Med.* **2013**, *61*, 330–338. [CrossRef]
60. Ebner, M.; Pagel, C.F.; Sentler, C.; Harjola, V.-P.; Bueno, H.; Lerchbaumer, M.H.; Stangl, K.; Pieske, B.; Hasenfuß, G.; Konstantinides, S.V.; et al. Venous lactate improves the prediction of in-hospital adverse outcomes in normotensive pulmonary embolism. *Eur. J. Intern. Med.* **2021**, *86*, 25–31. [CrossRef]
61. Bova, C.; Sanchez, O.; Prandoni, P.; Lankeit, M.; Konstantinides, S.; Vanni, S.; Jiménez, D. Identification of intermediate-risk patients with acute symptomatic pulmonary embolism. *Eur. Respir. J.* **2014**, *44*, 694–703. [CrossRef] [PubMed]
62. Chen, X.; Shao, X.; Zhang, Y.; Zhang, Z.; Tao, X.; Zhai, Z.; Wang, C. Assessment of the Bova score for risk stratification of acute normotensive pulmonary embolism: A systematic review and meta-analysis. *Thromb. Res.* **2020**, *193*, 99–106. [CrossRef] [PubMed]
63. Fernández, C.; Bova, C.; Sanchez, O.; Prandoni, P.; Lankeit, M.; Konstantinides, S.; Vanni, S.; Fernández-Golfín, C.; Yusen, R.D.; Jiménez, D. Validation of a Model for Identification of Patients at Intermediate to High Risk for Complications Associated With Acute Symptomatic Pulmonary Embolism. *Chest* **2015**, *148*, 211–218. [CrossRef]
64. Vanni, S.; Nazerian, P.; Bova, C.; Bondi, E.; Morello, F.; Pepe, G.; Paladini, B.; Liedl, G.; Cangioli, E.; Grifoni, S.; et al. Comparison of clinical scores for identification of patients with pulmonary embolism at intermediate–high risk of adverse clinical outcome: The prognostic role of plasma lactate. *Intern. Emerg. Med.* **2016**, *12*, 657–665. [CrossRef] [PubMed]
65. Vanni, S.; Jiménez, D.; Nazerian, P.; Morello, F.; Parisi, M.; Daghini, E.; Pratesi, M.; López, R.; Bedate, P.; Lobo, J.L.; et al. Short-term clinical outcome of normotensive patients with acute PE and high plasma lactate. *Thorax* **2015**, *70*, 333–338. [CrossRef] [PubMed]
66. Hobohm, L.; Hellenkamp, K.; Hasenfuß, G.; Münzel, T.; Konstantinides, S.; Lankeit, M. Comparison of risk assessment strategies for not-high-risk pulmonary embolism. *Eur. Respir. J.* **2016**, *47*, 1170–1178. [CrossRef]
67. Hobohm, L.; Becattini, C.; Konstantinides, S.V.; Casazza, F.; Lankeit, M. Validation of a fast prognostic score for risk stratification of normotensive patients with acute pulmonary embolism. *Clin. Res. Cardiol.* **2020**, *109*, 1008–1017. [CrossRef]
68. Freitas, P.; Santos, A.R.; Ferreira, A.M.; Oliveira, A.; Gonçalves, M.; Corte-Real, A.; Lameiras, C.; Maurício, J.; Ornelas, E.; Matos, C.; et al. Derivation and external validation of the SHIeLD score for predicting outcome in normotensive pulmonary embolism. *Int. J. Cardiol.* **2019**, *281*, 119–124. [CrossRef]
69. Lankeit, M.; Friesen, D.; Schäfer, K.; Hasenfuß, G.; Konstantinides, S.; Dellas, C. A simple score for rapid risk assessment of non-high-risk pulmonary embolism. *Clin. Res. Cardiol.* **2013**, *102*, 73–80. [CrossRef]
70. Skowrońska, M.; Skrzyńska, M.; Machowski, M.; Bartoszewicz, Z.; Paczyńska, M.; Ou-Pokrzewińska, A.; Kurnicka, K.; Ciurzyński, M.; Roik, M.; Wiśniewska, M.; et al. Plasma growth differentiation factor 15 levels for predicting serious adverse events and bleeding in acute pulmonary embolism: A prospective observational study. *Pol. Arch. Intern. Med.* **2020**, *130*, 757–765.
71. Kaeberich, A.; Seeber, V.; Jiménez, D.; Kostrubiec, M.; Dellas, C.; Hasenfuß, G.; Giannitsis, A.; Pruszczyk, P.; Konstantinides, S.; Lankeit, M. Age-adjusted high-sensitivity troponin T cut-off value for risk stratification of pulmonary embolism. *Eur. Respir. J.* **2015**, *45*, 1323–1331. [CrossRef] [PubMed]
72. Sharifi, M.; Bay, C.; Skrocki, L.; Rahimi, F.; Mehdipour, M. Moderate pulmonary embolism treated with thrombolysis (from the "MOPETT" Trial). *Am. J. Cardiol.* **2013**, *111*, 273–277. [CrossRef] [PubMed]
73. Zhang, Z.; Zhai, Z.-G.; Liang, L.-R.; Liu, F.-F.; Yang, Y.-H.; Wang, C. Lower dosage of recombinant tissue-type plasminogen activator (rt-PA) in the treatment of acute pulmonary embolism: A systematic review and meta-analysis. *Thromb. Res.* **2014**, *133*, 357–363. [CrossRef] [PubMed]
74. Avgerinos, E.D.; Jaber, W.; Lacomis, J.; Markel, K.; McDaniel, M.; Rivera-Lebron, B.N.; Ross, C.B.; Sechrist, J.; Toma, C.; Chaer, R. Randomized Trial Comparing Standard Versus Ultrasound-Assisted Thrombolysis for Submassive Pulmonary Embolism: The SUNSET sPE Trial. *JACC Cardiovasc. Interv.* **2021**, *14*, 1364–1373. [CrossRef] [PubMed]
75. Sista, A.K.; Horowitz, J.M.; Tapson, V.F.; Rosenberg, M.; Elder, M.D.; Schiro, B.J.; Dohad, S.; Amoroso, N.E.; Dexter, D.J.; Loh, C.T.; et al. Indigo Aspiration System for Treatment of Pulmonary Embolism: Results of the EXTRACT-PE Trial. *JACC Cardiovasc. Interv.* **2021**, *14*, 319–329. [CrossRef]
76. Tu, T.; Toma, C.; Tapson, V.F.; Adams, C.; Jaber, W.A.; Silver, M.; Khandhar, S.; Amin, R.; Weinberg, M.; Engelhardt, T.; et al. A Prospective, Single-Arm, Multicenter Trial of Catheter-Directed Mechanical Thrombectomy for Intermediate-Risk Acute Pulmonary Embolism: The FLARE Study. *JACC Cardiovasc. Interv.* **2019**, *12*, 859–869. [CrossRef]

77. Pei, D.T.; Liu, J.; Yaqoob, M.; Ahmad, W.; Bandeali, S.S.; Hamzeh, I.R.; Virani, S.S.; Hira, R.S.; Lakkis, N.M.; Alam, M. Meta-Analysis of Catheter Directed Ultrasound-Assisted Thrombolysis in Pulmonary Embolism. *Am. J. Cardiol.* **2019**, *124*, 1470–1477. [CrossRef]
78. Pasrija, C.; Kronfli, A.; Rouse, M.; Raithel, M.; Bittle, G.J.; Pousatis, S.; Ghoreishi, M.; Gammie, J.S.; Griffith, B.P.; Sanchez, P.G.; et al. Outcomes after surgical pulmonary embolectomy for acute submassive and massive pulmonary embolism: A single-center experience. *J. Thorac. Cardiovasc. Surg.* **2018**, *155*, 1095–1106.e2. [CrossRef]
79. Barco, S.; Vicaut, E.; Klok, F.A.; Lankeit, M.; Meyer, G.; Konstantinides, S.V. Improved identification of thrombolysis candidates amongst intermediate-risk pulmonary embolism patients: Implications for future trials. *Eur. Respir. J.* **2018**, *51*, 1701775. [CrossRef]
80. Sanchez, O.; Charles-Nelson, A.; Ageno, W.; Barco, S.; Binder, H.; Chatellier, G.; Duerschmied, D.; Empen, K.; Ferreira, M.; Girard, P.; et al. Reduced-Dose Intravenous Thrombolysis for Acute Intermediate-High-risk Pulmonary Embolism: Rationale and Design of the Pulmonary Embolism International THrOmbolysis (PEITHO)-3 trial. *Thromb. Haemost.* **2021**. [CrossRef]
81. Araszkiewicz, A.; Kurzyna, M.; Kopeć, G.; Sławek-Szmyt, S.; Wrona, K.; Stępniewski, J.; Jankiewicz, S.; Pietrasik, A.; Machowski, M.; Darocha, S.; et al. Pulmonary embolism response team: A multidisciplinary approach to pulmonary embolism treatment. Polish PERT Initiative Report. *Kardiologia Polska* **2021**, *79*, 1311–1319. [CrossRef] [PubMed]
82. Dudzinski, D.M.; Piazza, G. Jd Multidisciplinary Pulmonary Embolism Response Teams. *Circulation* **2016**, *133*, 98–103. [CrossRef] [PubMed]

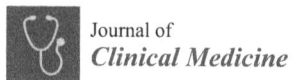

*Article*

# Prognostic Factors for Mortality in Acute Mesenteric Ischemia

Carlos Constantin Otto [1], Zoltan Czigany [1], Daniel Heise [1], Philipp Bruners [2], Drosos Kotelis [3,4], Sven Arke Lang [1], Tom Florian Ulmer [1], Ulf Peter Neumann [1,5], Christian Klink [1,6] and Jan Bednarsch [1,*]

1. Department of Surgery and Transplantation, University Hospital RWTH Aachen, 52074 Aachen, Germany; caotto@ukaachen.de (C.C.O.); zczigany@ukaachen.de (Z.C.); dheise@ukaachen.de (D.H.); svlang@ukaachen.de (S.A.L.); fulmer@ukaachen.de (T.F.U.); ulf.neumann@mumc.nl (U.P.N.); chirurgie-sp@diakonissen.de (C.K.)
2. Department of Diagnostic and Interventional Radiology, University Hospital RWTH Aachen, 52074 Aachen, Germany; pbruners@ukaachen.de
3. Department of Vascular Surgery, University Hospital RWTH Aachen, 52074 Aachen, Germany; dkotelis@ukaachen.de
4. Department of Vascular Surgery, University Hospital Bern, 3010 Bern, Switzerland
5. Department of Surgery, Maastricht University Medical Center (MUMC), 6229 HX Maastricht, The Netherlands
6. Department of Surgery, Diakonissen-Stiftungs-Krankenhaus Speyer, 67346 Speyer, Germany
* Correspondence: jbednarsch@ukaachen.de; Tel.: +49-241-80-89501

**Abstract:** Postoperative mortality in patients undergoing surgical and/or interventional treatment for acute mesenteric ischemia (AMI) has remained an unsolved problem in recent decades. Here, we investigated clinical predictors of postoperative mortality in a large European cohort of patients undergoing treatment for AMI. In total, 179 patients who underwent surgical and/or interventional treatment for AMI between 2009 and 2021 at our institution were included in this analysis. Associations between postoperative mortality and various clinical variables were assessed using univariate and multivariable binary logistic regression analysis. Most of the patients were diagnosed with arterial ischemia (AI; $n = 104$), while venous ischemia (VI; $n = 21$) and non-occlusive mesenteric ischemia (NOMI; $n = 54$) were present in a subset of patients. Overall inhouse mortality was 55.9% (100/179). Multivariable analyses identified leukocytes (HR = 1.08; $p = 0.008$), lactate (HR = 1.25; $p = 0.01$), bilirubin (HR = 2.05; $p = 0.045$), creatinine (HR = 1.48; $p = 0.039$), etiology (AI, VI or NOMI; $p = 0.038$) and portomesenteric vein gas (PMVG; HR = 23.02; $p = 0.012$) as independent predictors of postoperative mortality. In a subanalysis excluding patients with fatal prognosis at the first surgical exploration ($n = 24$), leukocytes (HR = 1.09; $p = 0.004$), lactate (HR = 1.27; $p = 0.003$), etiology (AI, VI or NOMI; $p = 0.006$), PMVG (HR = 17.02; $p = 0.018$) and intraoperative FFP transfusion (HR = 4.4; $p = 0.025$) were determined as independent predictors of postoperative mortality. Further, the risk of fatal outcome changed disproportionally with increased preoperative lactate values. The clinical outcome of patients with AMI was determined using a combination of pre- and intraoperative clinical and radiological characteristics. Serum lactate appears to be of major clinical importance as the risk of fatal outcome increases significantly with higher lactate values.

**Keywords:** acute mesenteric ischemia; lactate; morbidity; mortality

**Citation:** Otto, C.C.; Czigany, Z.; Heise, D.; Bruners, P.; Kotelis, D.; Lang, S.A.; Ulmer, T.F.; Neumann, U.P.; Klink, C.; Bednarsch, J. Prognostic Factors for Mortality in Acute Mesenteric Ischemia. *J. Clin. Med.* **2022**, *11*, 3619. https://doi.org/10.3390/jcm11133619

Academic Editor: Vanessa Bianconi

Received: 5 May 2022
Accepted: 20 June 2022
Published: 23 June 2022

**Publisher's Note:** MDPI stays neutral with regard to jurisdictional claims in published maps and institutional affiliations.

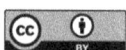

**Copyright:** © 2022 by the authors. Licensee MDPI, Basel, Switzerland. This article is an open access article distributed under the terms and conditions of the Creative Commons Attribution (CC BY) license (https://creativecommons.org/licenses/by/4.0/).

## 1. Introduction

Acute mesenteric ischemia (AMI) is a an often rapidly progressing clinical condition, which is commonly diagnosed late and associated with dismal outcome after surgical or endovascular therapy [1–3]. While a rapid diagnosis and subsequent treatment result in distinctively better outcomes [4,5], the overall mortality rates are high in comparison to other surgical emergencies [6]. Therefore, patients suspected of AMI should be diagnosed and treated with high priority to achieve acceptable outcomes [5,7]. Unfortunately, the lack of specific parameters and often vague early clinical symptoms frequently result in a notable delay in diagnostic measures and targeted treatment [8].

A variety of risk factors for adverse outcomes have been identified in the literature, with a prolonged duration of symptoms before specific treatment being the most prominent negative predictor, as described previously [9]. Additionally, individual patient characteristics as basic demographics and comorbidities as well as laboratory values have been under the spotlight of interest in recent decades [10–13]. Interestingly, the group of patients presenting with AMI is also heterogenous, as the underlying conditions and corresponding subtypes, e.g., arterial ischemia (AI), venous ischemia (VI) and non-occlusive mesenteric ischemia (NOMI), display different features and distinct outcomes [14].

Given the highly heterogenous nature of AMI and its relatively rare occurrence, only a limited number of monocentric series are available for investigating the disease. Moreover, those studies vary in design, endpoints, and findings [10,15,16], resulting in overall inconsistent and low-quality evidence. To further explore potential prognostic factors of surgical morbidity and mortality, we analyzed clinical outcomes in a European cohort of patients undergoing treatment for AMI.

## 2. Materials and Methods

### 2.1. Patients and Definitions

This study comprised one hundred seventy-nine ($n = 179$) consecutive patients diagnosed with AMI and treated with surgery between 2009 and 2021 at a large academic tertiary referral center (University Hospital RWTH Aachen (UH-RWTH)). Inclusion criteria were (a) patients undergoing surgical/endovascular treatment after the radiological diagnosis of AMI. Exclusion criteria were: (a) no present AMI during surgical exploration and (b) patients deceasing prior to surgical exploration and (c) patients refusing to undergo surgical/endovascular treatment. The study was further conducted in accordance with the requirements of the Institutional Review Board of the RWTH-Aachen University (EK 334/21), the current version of the Declaration of Helsinki, and the good clinical practice guidelines (ICH-GCP). In this retrospective study, AMI was defined as the occurrence of an abrupt cessation of the mesenteric blood flow leading to malperfusion of the bowel with associated and acute symptoms and eventually bowel necrosis [8]. AI was assumed in cases with arterial obstruction due to atherosclerotic disease, atherothrombosis, arterial dissection or arterial embolism, while VI was diagnosed in cases with thrombosis of the mesenterial veins. NOMI was present in patients with low blood states as a consequence of circulatory failure and no apparent vascular occlusion.

### 2.2. Standard Clinical Management of AMI Patients

AMI was diagnosed based on the clinical condition of the patient, blood values and cross-sectional imaging. After diagnosis, treatment was facilitated in terms of an interdisciplinary approach always involving a team of experienced visceral and vascular surgeons, as well as interventional radiologists. In cases of AI with acute arterial occlusions of the superior mesenteric artery (SMA) and/or the celiac trunk (TC), endovascular or open revascularization was carried out before or after subsequent bowel resection. The decision for endovascular or open revascularization and the therapeutic sequence was made on a case-by-case basis. In the endovascular approach, which was executed in the radiological department, the occluded vessel was recanalized via balloon angioplasty and balloon-expandable stenting (Formula® 535 Vascular Balloon-Expandable Stent, Cook Medical; Omnilink Elite Vascular Balloon-Expandable Stent System, MULTI-LINK VISION RX Coronary Stent System, Herculink Elite®, Abbott Vascular, Chicago, IL, USA) via a femoral or brachial artery access. In the case of two occluded vessels (usually SMA and TC), the SMA was preferably recanalized and the TC only if SMA was not possible to be recanalized, as previously described [17]. Dual antiplatelet therapy with acetylsalicylic acid and clopidogrel was administered after recanalization. Open revascularization was usually carried out using conventional thrombectomy via a Fogarty catheter and following intraoperative local heparin application and/or—if thrombectomy was unsuccessful—through surgical bypass utilizing autologous vein or prosthetic grafts in an antegrade or retrograde fashion on a case-by-case basis (Table 1). In VI, the therapy of choice was immediate therapeutic anticoagulation and surgical exploration.

**Table 1.** Patient characteristics with respect to disease etiology.

| Variables | Overall Cohort (n = 179) | Arterial (n = 104) | Venous (n = 21) | NOMI (n = 54) |
|---|---|---|---|---|
| Demographics | | | | |
| Gender, m/f, n (%) | 87 (48.6)/92 (51.4) | 46 (44.2)/58 (55.8) | 10 (47.6)/11 (52.4) | 31 (57.4)/23 (42.6) |
| Age, years | 71 (60–81) | 75 (63–82) | 65 (49–69) | 71 (59–78) |
| BMI, kg/m$^2$ | 26 (23–29) | 25 (22–28) | 29 (27–37) | 26 (24–29) |
| ASA, n (%) | | | | |
| I | 1 (0.6) | 0 | 1 (4.8) | 0 |
| II | 13 (7.3) | 8 (7.7) | 5 (23.8) | 0 |
| III | 126 (70.4) | 78 (75) | 13 (61.9) | 35 (64.8) |
| IV | 37 (20.7) | 17 (16.3) | 2 (9.5) | 18 (33.3) |
| Etiology, n (%) | | | | |
| Embolic | | 57 (54.8) | | |
| Thrombotic | | 41 (39.4) | | |
| Compression | | 4 (3.8) | | |
| Dissection | | 1 (1) | | |
| Unknown | | 1 (1) | | |
| Occluded vessel, n (%) | | | | |
| TC | | 3 (2.9) | | |
| SMA | | 66 (63.5) | | |
| IMA | | 8 (7.7) | | |
| TC+ SMA | | 19 (18.3) | | |
| TC+ IMA | | 1 (1) | | |
| SMA+ IMA | | 5 (4.8) | | |
| TC+ SMA+ IMA | | 2 (1.9) | | |
| Location of occlusion, n (%) * | | | | |
| Proximal | | 72 (69.2) | | |
| Distal | | 31 (29.8) | | |
| Refferal from another hospital, n (%) | 53 (29.6) | 35 (33.7) | 11 (52.4) | 7 (13.2) |
| Radiological characteristics | | | | |
| Pneumatosis intestinalis, n (%) | 48 (26.8) | 23 (22.1) | 1 (4.8) | 24 (44.4) |
| PMVG, n (%) | 20 (11.2) | 10 (9.6) | 0 | 10 (18.5) |
| Bowel distension, n (%) | 80 (44.7) | 42 (40.4) | 5 (23.8) | 33 (61.1) |
| Bowel wall thickening, n (%) | 99 (55.3) | 49 (47.1) | 18 (85.7) | 32 (59.3) |
| Pneumoperitoneum, n (%) | 21 (11.7) | 8 (7.7) | 0 | 13 (24.1) |
| Ascites, n (%) | 56 (31.3) | 16 (15.4) | 15 (71.4) | 25 (46.3) |

Table 1. Cont.

| Variables | Overall Cohort (n = 179) | Arterial (n = 104) | Venous (n = 21) | NOMI (n = 54) |
|---|---|---|---|---|
| Preoperative laboratory values | | | | |
| Leukocytes, 1/nL | 15.2 (10.9–23.5) | 14.9 (10.6–22.9) | 14.9 (10.9–26.9) | 17.4 (10.4–23.8) |
| C-Reactive-Protein, mg/L | 127 (37–230) | 127 (25–230) | 84 (53–161) | 157 (97–197) |
| Hemoglobin, g/dL | 12.0 (9.4–13.7) | 12.1 (10.8–14.0) | 13.9 (12.6–16.2) | 9.0 (8.2–12.0) |
| Thrombocytes, 1/nL | 228 (142–329) | 249 (160–354) | 294 (175–359) | 149 (113–239) |
| Prothrombin time, % | 70 (52–82) | 72 (55–85) | 71 (54–83) | 64 (49–78) |
| INR | 1.25 (1.12–1.53) | 1.24 (1.10–1.49) | 1.25 (1.10–1.47) | 1.30 (1.17–1.59) |
| Bilirubin, mg/dL | 0.7 (0.4–1.2) | 0.7 (0.5–1.1) | 0.9 (0.3–1.5) | 0.8 (0.4–1.5) |
| AP, U/L | 89 (69–129) | 87 (67–112) | 85 (72–120) | 116 (70–174) |
| GGT, U/l | 45 (24–93) | 38 (23–87) | 49 (23.3–114.3) | 59 (34–132) |
| Albumin, g/dL | 2.5 (1.8–3.4) | 3.3 (1.9–3.8) | 3.0 (2.5–3.6) | 2.0 (1.6–2.7) |
| AST, U/L | 44 (26–115) | 40 (25–111) | 28 (22–37) | 88 (37–208) |
| ALT, U/L | 38 (20–102) | 31 (18–105) | 25 (19–39) | 51 (26–216) |
| Creatinine, mg/dL | 1.3 (0.9–2.2) | 1.3 (0.9–2.1) | 1.1 (0.7–1.5) | 1.5 (1.0–3.2) |
| Lactate, mmol/L | 3.3 (1.8–6.5) | 3.3 (1.9–6.4) | 2.3 (1.2–3.6) | 4.0 (1.9–9.3) |
| Therapy Characteristics | | | | |
| Extent of bowel resection, n (%) | | | | |
| Small bowel | 57 (31.8) | 28 (26.9) | 20 (95.2) | 9 (16.7) |
| Colon | 56 (31.3) | 27 (26.0) | 0 | 29 (53.7) |
| Small bowel and colon | 30 (16.8) | 20 (19.2) | 0 | 10 (18.5) |
| No resection | 12 (6.7) | 11 (10.6) | 1 (4.8) | 0 |
| Fatal | 24 (13.4) | 18 (17.3) | 0 | 6 (11.1) |
| Technique of revascularization, n (%) | | | | |
| Endovascular | 27 (15.1) | | | |
| Open | 40 (22.3) | | | |
| Thrombectomy | 30 (17.8) | | | |
| Bypass, prosthetic, antegrade | 4 (2.2) | | | |
| Bypass, prosthetic, retrograde | 4 (2.2) | | | |
| Bypass, autologous vein, retrograde | 2 (1.2) | | | |
| Combination | 4 (2.2) | | | |

Table 1. Cont.

| Variables | Overall Cohort (n = 179) | Arterial (n = 104) | Venous (n = 21) | NOMI (n = 54) |
|---|---|---|---|---|
| Sequence of therapy | | | | |
| Revascularization before resection | 17 (9.5) | | | |
| Resection before revascularization | 20 (11.2) | | | |
| Simultaneous | 18 (10.1) | | | |
| Enterostomy, n (%) | 124 (69.3) | 68 (60.6) | 15 (71.4) | 46 (85.2) |
| Primary bowel anastomosis, n (%) | 14 (7.8) | 7 (6.7) | 5 (23.8) | 2 (3.7) |
| Intraoperative FFP transfusion, n (%) | 34 (19) | 12 (11.5) | 3 (14.3) | 19 (35.2) |
| Intraoperative blood transfusion, n (%) | 69 (38.5) | 38 (36.5) | 6 (28.6) | 25 (46.3) |
| Primary treatment time, minutes | 130 (99–180) | 129 (100–179) | 124 (99–179) | 140 (95–180) |
| Time to treatment, minutes | 191 (110–363) | 162 (100–269) | 593 (315–770) | 189 (113–339) |
| Intensive care stay, days | 4 (1–15) | 3.5 (1–14) | 8 (2–28) | 4 (1–16) |
| Postoperative data | | | | |
| Postoperative complications, n (%) | | | | |
| Clavien–Dindo I | 0 | 0 | 0 | 0 |
| Clavien–Dindo II | 13 (7.3) | 8 (7.7) | 4 (19.1) | 1 (1.9) |
| Clavien–Dindo IIIa | 9 (5) | 3 (2.9) | 2 (9.5) | 4 (7.4) |
| Clavien–Dindo IIIb | 17 (9.5) | 11 (10.6) | 4 (19.1) | 2 (3.7) |
| Clavien–Dindo IVa | 19 (10.6) | 10 (9.6) | 1 (4.8) | 8 (14.8) |
| Clavien–Dindo IVb | 19 (10.6) | 10 (9.6) | 6 (28.6) | 3 (5.6) |
| Clavien–Dindo V | 100 (55.9) | 61 (58.7) | 3 (14.3) | 36 (66.7) |

Data presented as median and interquartile range, if not noted otherwise. * Vessel occlusions proximal from the first branch of the vessel were defined as "proximal", while occlusions distal to the first branch were defined as "distal". ALT, alanine aminotransferase; AP, alkaline phosphatase: ASA, American Society of Anesthesiologists classification; AST, aspartate aminotransferase; BMI, body mass index; CCI, comprehensive complication index; FFP, fresh frozen plasma; GGT, gamma glutamyltransferase; IMA; inferior mesenteric artery; INR, international normalized ratio; NOMI, non-occlusive mesenteric ischemia; PMVG, portomesenteric vein gas; SMA, superior mesenteric artery; TC, celiac trunk.

In cases of AMI due to NOMI or VI (except for one case with conventional thrombectomy), no revascularization was carried out. Operative exploration was performed in every patient. All abdominal organs were carefully examined regarding signs of ischemia and were (partially) resected if no recovery was expected. Primary fascial closure was always preferred if feasible; however, in cases with elevated abdominal pressure, temporary abdominal closure with a prosthetic mesh in inlay position was conducted. Further, second look exploration was carried out per the protocol in every patient after 24 h to ensure sufficient radicality and treatment success.

2.3. Data Extraction and Quality Management

All relevant patient data were extracted from the electronical case records including preoperative characteristics, operative procedures, and postoperative outcome. Every cross-sectional imaging was also re-analyzed for signs of portomesenteric vein gas (PMVG), pneumatosis intestinalis (PI), ascites, bowel distension, bowel wall thickening and pneumoperitoneum by an experienced staff radiologist.

*2.4. Statistical Analysis*

The primary endpoint of this study was in-hospital mortality in AMI patients undergoing treatment. Categorial data are shown in the form of numbers and percentages. Data derived from continuous variables are presented as the median and inter-quartile range. Associations between perioperative variables and the primary endpoint were assessed by means of binary logistic regressions. Variables showing a $p$-value < 0.05 in univariate analysis were subsequently transferred into a multivariable model and analyzed with multivariable binary logistic regressions using backward elimination. For this purpose, nominal and categorical data were recoded into a scaled dummy variable. The level of significance was set to $p < 0.05$, and $p$-values are given for two-sided testing. Analyses were performed using SPSS Statistics 24 (IBM Corp., Armonk, NY, USA).

## 3. Results

*3.1. Preoperative, Operative and Postoperative Data*

A total of 179 patients with a median age of 71 years (range: 61–80) and median body mass index (BMI) of 26 kg/m$^2$ underwent surgery for AMI at our institution from 2009 to 2021. In the whole cohort, 104 patients (58.1%) presented with AI, 21 (11.7%) with VI and 54 (30.2%) with NOMI as underlying etiology. Of note, most patients (91.1%, 163/179) had a preoperative performance status of ASA III or higher, assessed by the attending anesthesiologist. While in most of the cohort (79.9%, 143/179), bowel resection was carried out, only 71 patients (39.6%) underwent open or endovascular revascularization. A total of 100 patients (55.9%) deceased during hospitalization, with 61 patients (58.7%) in the AI subgroup, 3 patients (14.3%) in the VI subgroup and 36 patients (66.7%) in the NOMI subgroup. Of note, a relevant subset of these patients (24/179, 13.4%) displayed a complete intestinal ischemia with a dismal prognosis during initial surgical exploration and were referred for palliative treatment. Almost all patients (177/179) showed postoperative complications, while a large proportion of the cohort (164/179; 91.6%) experienced major postoperative complications (Clavien Dindo $\geq$ 3). Further, a subanalysis comparing patients that had been revascularized to patients without revascularization showed no difference in major morbidity (Clavien Dindo $\geq$ 3, $p = 0.343$) or in-hospital mortality ($p = 0.963$, Supplementary Table S1). Detailed clinicopathological and perioperative characteristics are outlined in Table 1.

*3.2. Univariate and Multivariable Analysis of Postoperative Mortality*

A univariate binary logistic regression was carried out for postoperative mortality including all available pre- and intraoperative variables (Table 2). Here, age (HR = 1.02; $p = 0.04$), ASA (HR = 20.89; $p = 0.004$), leukocytes (HR = 1.04; $p = 0.025$), lactate (HR = 1.45; $p < 0.001$), hemoglobin (HR = 0.90; $p = 0.048$), bilirubin (HR = 1.60; $p = 0.026$), alkaline phosphatase (HR = 1.01; $p = 0.034$), prothrombine time (HR = 0.97; $p < 0.001$), INR (HR = 2.13; $p = 0.012$), etiology ($p = 0.001$), PI (HR = 2.74; $p = 0.007$), PMVG (HR = 18.25, $p = 0.005$), bowel distension (HR = 1.99, $p = 0.03$), extent of resection ($p = 0.003$) and FFP transfusion (HR = 3.75; $p = 0.001$) were associated with postoperative mortality (Table 2).

Variables showing a $p$-value < 0.05 in univariate analysis were further included in a multivariable binary logistic regression. In this multivariable model, leukocytes (HR = 1.08; $p = 0.008$), lactate (HR = 1.25; $p = 0.01$), bilirubin (HR = 2.05; $p = 0.045$), creatinine (HR = 1.48; $p = 0.39$), etiology ($p = 0.038$) and PMVG (HR = 23.02; $p = 0.012$) were determined as independent predictors of postoperative mortality.

To further explore the validity of predictors of postoperative mortality, a similar multivariable analysis regarding postoperative mortality was carried out excluding patients who presented with a dismal situation during initial surgical exploration and, therefore, referred to palliative care. In the corresponding multivariable model, leukocytes (HR = 1.09; $p = 0.004$), lactate (HR = 1.27; $p = 0.003$), etiology ($p = 0.006$), PMVG (HR = 17.02; $p = 0.018$) and intraoperative FFP transfusion (HR = 4.4; $p = 0.025$) showed independent significance (Table 3).

Table 2. Univariable and multivariable analysis of in-hospital mortality (overall cohort).

| Variable | n | Univariable | | | Multivariable | | |
|---|---|---|---|---|---|---|---|
| | | Hazard Ratio | 95% CI | p-Value | Hazard Ratio | 95% CI | p-Value |
| Sex | | | | 0.905 | | | |
| Age | | 1.02 | 1–1.05 | **0.040** | | | 0.961 |
| BMI, kg/m² | | | | 0.440 | | | |
| ASA | | | | **0.004** | | | 0.124 |
| I/II | 15 | 1 | | | | | |
| III/IV | 162 | 20.89 | 2.68–162.77 | | | | |
| Leukocytes, 1/nL | | 1.04 | 1.01–1.07 | **0.025** | 1.08 | 1.02–1.15 | **0.008** |
| C-Reactive-Protein, mg/L | | | | 0.808 | | | |
| Lactate, mmol/L | | 1.45 | 1.25–1.69 | **<0.001** | 1.25 | 1.05–1.47 | **0.010** |
| Hemoglobin, g/dL | | 0.90 | 0.81–0.99 | **0.048** | | | 0.361 |
| Albumin, g/L | | | | 0.832 | | | |
| AST, U/L | | | | 0.077 | | | |
| ALT, U/L | | | | 0.653 | | | |
| GGT, U/L | | | | 0.178 | | | |
| Bilirubin, mg/dL | | 1.6 | 1.06–2.41 | **0.026** | 2.05 | 1.02–4.12 | **0.045** |
| Alkaline phosphatase, U/L | | 1.01 | 1–1.01 | **0.034** | | | |
| Platelet count, 1/nL | | | | 0.290 | | | |
| Prothrombin time, % | | 0.97 | 0.96–0.98 | **<0.001** | | | 0.377 |
| INR | | 2.13 | 1.18–3.85 | **0.012** | | | 0.724 |
| Etiology | | | | **0.001** | | | **0.038** |
| Arterial | 104 | 1 | | | 1 | | |
| Venous | 21 | 0.12 | 0.03–0.42 | | 0.12 | 0.02–0.89 | |
| NOMI | 54 | 1.41 | 0.71–2.8 | | 0.97 | 0.32–2.97 | |
| Pneumatosis intestinalis | | | | **0.007** | | | 0.774 |
| No | 121 | 1 | | | | | |
| Yes | 48 | 2.74 | 1.32–5.68 | | | | |
| Portomesenteric vein gas | | | | **0.005** | | | **0.012** |
| No | 149 | 1 | | | 1 | | |
| Yes | 20 | 18.25 | 2.38–139.85 | | 23.02 | 2.01–263.11 | |
| Bowel Distension | | | | **0.030** | | | 0.838 |
| <6 cm | 89 | 1 | | | | | |
| ≥6 cm | 80 | 1.99 | 1.07–3.69 | | | | |
| Bowel wall thickening | | | | 0.074 | | | |
| Ascites | | | | 0.415 | | | |
| Pneumoperitoneum | | | | 0.575 | | | |
| Extent of resection | | | | **0.003** | | | 0.284 |

Table 2. Cont.

| Variable | n | Univariable | | | Multivariable | | |
|---|---|---|---|---|---|---|---|
| | | Hazard Ratio | 95% CI | p-Value | Hazard Ratio | 95% CI | p-Value |
| Small bowel | 57 | 1 | | | | | |
| Colon | 56 | 1.48 | 0.7–3.13 | | | | |
| Small bowel and colon | 30 | 4.38 | 1.66–11.53 | | | | |
| No resection in primary operation | 12 | 1.14 | 0.32–4.03 | | | | |
| Fatal | 24 | >10 | 0–n.a. | | | | |
| Treatment time, minutes | | | | 0.655 | | | |
| Blood transfusions | | | | 0.190 | | | |
| Intraoperative FFP transfusion | | | | **0.004** | | | 0.118 |
| No | 144 | 1 | | | | | |
| Yes | 34 | 3.75 | 1.54–9.16 | | | | |
| Time to treatment | | | | 0.128 | | | |
| Referral from another hospital | | | | 0.841 | | | |

Various parameters are associated with postoperative mortality. All variables showing statistical significance in univariate binary logistic regression were included in a multivariable logistic regression. Hazard ratios are shown for statistically significant variables. AP was excluded in the multivariable analysis due to low case numbers. Bold indicates statistical significance. ALT, alanine aminotransferase; AP, alkaline phosphatase: ASA, American Society of Anesthesiologists classification; AST, aspartate aminotransferase; BMI, body mass index; FFP, fresh frozen plasma; GGT, gamma glutamyltransferase; INR, international normalized ratio; NOMI, non-occlusive mesenteric ischemia.

Table 3. Multivariable analysis of in-hospital mortality (fatal situation in primary operation excluded).

| Variable | Mortality | | |
|---|---|---|---|
| | Hazard Ratio | 95% CI | p-Value |
| Age, years | | | 0.961 |
| ASA | | | 0.159 |
| Leucocytes, 1/nL | 1.09 | 1.03–1.15 | **0.004** |
| Lactate, mmol/L | 1.27 | 1.08–1.48 | **0.003** |
| Hemoglobin, g/dL | | | 0.361 |
| Bilirubin, mg/dL | | | 0.166 |
| Prothrombin time, % | | | 0.377 |
| INR | | | 0.724 |
| Creatinine, mg/dL | | | 0.710 |
| Etiology | | | **0.024** |
| AI | 1 | | |
| VI | 0.08 | 0.01–0.49 | |
| NOMI | 0.71 | 0.24–2.1 | |
| Pneumatosis intestinalis | | | 0.774 |
| PMVG | 17.02 | 1.62–178.58 | **0.018** |
| Bowel distension | | | 0.838 |
| Extent of resection | | | 0.233 |
| Intraoperative FFP transfusion | 4.4 | 1.2–16.11 | **0.025** |

All variables showing statistical significance in univariate binary logistic regression were included in a multivariable logistic regression. In this analysis, patients with a fatal result in the primary operation were excluded. Hazard ratios are shown for statistically significant variables. Bold values indicate statistical significance. AI, arterial ischemia; ASA, American Society of Anesthesiologists classification; INR, international normalized ratio; NOMI, non-occlusive mesenteric ischemia.; PMVG, portomesenteric vein gas; VI, venous ischemia.

As lactate showed significance in both multivariable models, we further analyzed its prognostic role in univariate analysis, dividing the cohort into subgroups according to preoperative lactate. Here, the preoperative lactate value was strongly associated with the likelihood of fatal outcome in our cohort (Table 4).

**Table 4.** Univariable analysis of in-hospital mortality divided in lactate subgroups.

| Variable | | Mortality | | |
|---|---|---|---|---|
| | n | Hazard Ratio | 95% CI | p-Value |
| Lactate, mmol/L | | | | |
| ≤2 | 48 | 1 | | <0.001 |
| >2; ≤4 | 57 | 2.52 | 1.09–5.80 | 0.030 |
| >4; ≤8 | 34 | 9.75 | 3.49–27.23 | <0.001 |
| >8 | 32 | 45 | 9.33–217.04 | <0.001 |

Statistical increasing risk of in-hospital mortality with increasing preoperative lactate values demonstrated in 4 subgroups.

All major risk factors for dismal outcome are also graphically presented in Figure 1.

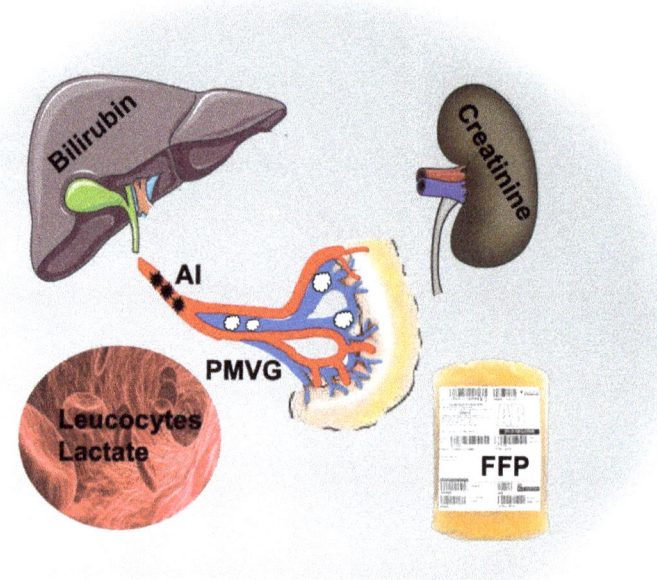

**Figure 1.** Major risk factors for mortality acute mesenteric ischemia. The graphical synopsis summarizes the major risk factors for mortality in acute mesenteric ischemia. Back dots indicate arterial occlusion, while white clouds indicate PMVG. AI, arterial ischemia; FFP, fresh frozen plasma; PMVG, portomesenteric vein gas.

## 4. Discussion

Despite a modern interdisciplinary treatment approach, the management and prevention of perioperative mortality are still challenging in AMI. Here, we aimed to evaluate the association of various clinico-pathological parameters with perioperative outcomes in patients with AMI undergoing surgical and/or interventional treatment. By conducting multivariate analyses, we identified leucocytes, bilirubin, creatinine and lactate, the presence of PMVG, AI and the intraoperative application of FFP as the most important predictors of outcome in our cohort.

In both multivariable models, the importance of lactate as a predictor of poor outcome was outlined. Although lactate levels have certain limitations for diagnosis purposes [7,8,18,19], an association between elevated lactate and inferior outcomes was described previously [11,20]. Here, we could demonstrate that postoperative mortality changes disproportionately with an increase in preoperative lactate levels (Table 4). Above 8 mmol/L at the time of initial diagnosis, a dismal in-house mortality of 95% was observed in our patients. However, our observation regarding lactate further underlines the prognostic and diagnostic dilemma in AMI patients. Almost one quarter of the cohort was diagnosed with AMI, despite lactate being within the physiological reference values and still displayed an in-house mortality of 25%. According to a meta-analysis from 2013, L-lactate, the isomer of lactate produced in anaerobic glycolysis, shows a pooled sensitivity of 86% and specificity of 44% in terms of diagnostic accuracy in patients with suspected AMI [18]. The latest guideline of the European Society of Vascular Surgery regarding the management of AMI rates L-lactate as too weak for diagnosing or ruling out an AMI [8]. In a further meta-analysis form 2017, D-lactate, produced due to bacterial fermentation, had a pooled sensitivity of 71.7%, but a specificity of 74.2% [19]. However, Nuzzo et al. showed, in a cross-sectional study from 2021, that D-lactate is not suitable for the differentiation of patients with AMI from patients with other acute abdominal pathologies [7]. In our cohort, lactate was measured preoperatively via venous blood gas analysis. Our findings underline that physiological serum lactate concentrations cannot be used to rule out neither an AMI nor a fatal outcome completely but if elevated, serum lactate provides a broadly available and feasible predictive marker.

Although this study did not aim to evaluate the diagnostic capabilities of radiological imaging for the diagnosis of AMI, we were still able to demonstrate a significant prognostic value of PVMG in our patients. The role of pathological signs within a CT scan for AMI has been examined previously. Emile et al. identified various radiological signs (PI, bowel distention, portomesenteric vein thrombosis and free intraperitoneal fluid) as predictors of existing bowel necrosis in AMI patients in a meta-analysis [21]. One larger multicenter study identified PMVG in combination with PI as a strong predictor for mortality independently from etiology [22]. In our univariate analysis, bowel distension and PI were also associated with mortality but did not achieve significance in the multivariable models. This might be explained by the notable morality in individuals presenting with PMVG (95.0%). However, the prognostic value is hampered by the relatively low prevalence (11.2%), indicating that PMVG is associated with a progressed AMI, subsequently resulting in fatal outcomes.

Despite the known role of lactate, also other laboratory parameters showed relevance in at least one of our multivariable models. The preoperative leukocyte count was an independent predictor for mortality in both multivariate analyses. Interestingly, the relevance of leukocyte count as prognostic parameter in AMI is not consistent throughout the literature. Although their prognostic value has been shown in some studies [12,13], other reports failed to show an association with mortality [23]. Furthermore, we were able to demonstrate serum creatinine and serum bilirubin as independent factors of postoperative mortality in our cohort. Renal impairment at initial diagnosis as prognostic factor was already shown in previous studies [16,24]; however, bilirubin has not been identified as a prognostic marker in AMI before. Of note, both parameters were not significant in the multivariable model excluding patients who deceased during primary surgery. This circumstance leads to the hypothesis, especially for bilirubin, that the elevation of these parameters is a sign of the onset of organ failure due to the septic constellation more likely than a direct malperfusion of the liver as a consequence of an accompanying occlusion of the TC. As part of the SOFA (sequential organ failure assessment) score, bilirubin and creatinine are commonly associated with higher mortality rates in septic patients independently from etiology [25].

Another prognostic factor in our analysis was the intraoperative administration of FFPs. During the study period, FFP was intraoperatively applied in cases of present coagulopathy. FFP transfusion is a known predictor of morbidity and mortality in gastrointestinal surgery [26]. One explanation might be the effect of transfusion-related immunomodulation. As such, Sarani et al. found a correlation between the transfusion of FFP and pulmonary or blood stream infections in critically ill surgical patients [27]. Some investigators speculated that soluble proteins in FFP may cause similar immunosuppressive effects, as seen in the case of red blood cell transfusions [27,28]. Potential mechanisms include diminished antigen processing by macrophages, the upregulation of both T suppressor/regulatory cells and humoral immunosuppressive mediators, impaired natural killer cell activity and the production of anti-idiotypic antibodies [28]. This is especially interesting as FFP was only significant in the secondary multivariable model after the exclusion of patients with fatal prognosis determined by the initial surgical exploration. Therefore, the above proposed effects of FFPs might in fact contribute to the inferior outcomes of initially treatable patients.

The importance of etiology subtypes as predictors for different outcomes was already identified by other groups [6,14]. As in our study, VI patients have a significantly better postoperative outcome compared to AI and NOMI. Interestingly, this better prognosis was observed, despite a higher median time to treatment in the VI group compared to other subtypes. It is, therefore, assumable that the time to irreversible bowel ischemia resulting in AI and NOMI patients is more rapid compared to the VI patients [29–31]. Interestingly, the time from diagnosis to treatment did not show prognostic value in our cohort at all, which is in contrast to previous reports underlining a short time to surgical treatment as a protective factor [4,5]. However, this might be explained by the small variety in time to treatment, limiting detectability within our used statical approach. Furthermore, AMI subtypes determine the extent of bowel resection in our cohort, which is line with the published literature [1]. In VI cases, the small bowel; in NOMI cases, mostly the colon; and in patients with AI, both the small intestine and colon in a similar distribution were evaluated as irreversibly damaged in the primary operation. Although no prognostic relevancy in multivariable analysis was observed in our patients, it must be considered that the extent of bowel resection is associated with long-term morbidity in surviving patients due to short bowel syndrome and high output enterostomies.

As with all retrospective clinical outcome studies, our analysis certainly has some obvious limitations, which have to be discussed. All data were collected in a retrospective fashion over a study period of more than ten years. Additionally, the patient treatment was carried out in accordance with our institutional clinical standards but not based on a defined study protocol, which carries an increased risk of selection bias and limits our conclusions. Due to the nature of AMI, a large set of patients deceased during the therapeutical process, with some patients considered palliative during initial exploration. To address the issue of these palliative patients within the dataset, we conducted two separate analyses including and excluding patients who did not undergo a curative treatment approach. Further, we are not able to elaborate on the time frame between the onset of symptoms and treatment as these data were not obtainable for a notable number of patients in this retrospective study. Additionally, our approach to include the full spectrum of AMI (AI, VI, and NOMI) combined with a limited dataset did not allow us to construct a valid preoperative risk score to predict outcome and guide treatment decisions.

Notwithstanding the limitations, we identified the degree of organ dysfunction (kidney and liver) and serum lactate, as well as radiological characteristics, of disease severity (PMVG), the underlying etiology (AI, NOMI) and intraoperative FFP administration to be of major importance for the prognosis of patients with AMI. As all these factors, except for FFP administration, are determined preoperatively and at the time of presentation, prognosis in these patients appears to be based on pretreatment characteristics. Furthermore, this underlines the importance of shortening the time to diagnosis of AMI. Unfortunately, the search for a valid biomarker has been and will be a challenge in upcoming years. In the above-mentioned cross-sectional study from 2021, D-lactate, intestinal fatty acid-binding protein and citrulline as three of the most promising biomarkers for early-stage AMI failed to distinguish patients with AMI from patients with acute abdominal pain of another origin [7]. The prevention and early diagnosis of AMI (e.g., through novel biomarkers and composite risk-assessment scores) seem to be of fundamental importance to improve outcomes in these patients and should be the focus of further research.

**Supplementary Materials:** The following supporting information can be downloaded at: https://www.mdpi.com/article/10.3390/jcm11133619/s1. Table S1. Sub-analysis for patients with arterial ischemia with respect to revascularization.

**Author Contributions:** All authors contributed significantly to this manuscript and are in agreement with the content. The authors contributed as follows: study conception and design: J.B. and C.C.O.; acquisition of data: C.C.O., Z.C., D.H., P.B., S.A.L. and J.B.; analysis and interpretation of data: C.C.O., D.K., T.F.U., U.P.N., C.K. and J.B.; drafting of manuscript: C.C.O.; critical revision of manuscript: Z.C., D.H., P.B., D.K., S.A.L., T.F.U., U.P.N., C.K. and J.B. All authors have read and agreed to the published version of the manuscript.

**Funding:** This research received no external funding.

**Institutional Review Board Statement:** The study was conducted according to the guidelines of the Declaration of Helsinki, and approved by the Institutional Review Board of RWTH Aachen University (protocol code: EK 334/21, date of approval: 2 February 2022).

**Informed Consent Statement:** Informed consent was obtained from all subjects involved in the study.

**Data Availability Statement:** The data presented in this study are available upon request from the corresponding author. The data are not publicly available due to privacy reasons.

**Conflicts of Interest:** The authors declare no conflict of interest.

# References

1. Bala, M.; Kashuk, J.; Moore, E.E.; Kluger, Y.; Biffl, W.; Gomes, C.A.; Ben-Ishay, O.; Rubinstein, C.; Balogh, Z.J.; Civil, I.; et al. Acute mesenteric ischemia: Guidelines of the World Society of Emergency Surgery. *World J. Emerg. Surg.* **2017**, *12*, 38. [CrossRef] [PubMed]
2. Renner, P.; Kienle, K.; Dahlke, M.H.; Heiss, P.; Pfister, K.; Stroszczynski, C.; Piso, P.; Schlitt, H.J. Intestinal ischemia: Current treatment concepts. *Langenbeck's Arch. Surg. Dtsch. Ges. Fur Chir.* **2011**, *396*, 3–11. [CrossRef] [PubMed]
3. Dahlke, M.H.; Asshoff, L.; Popp, F.C.; Feuerbach, S.; Lang, S.A.; Renner, P.; Slowik, P.; Stoeltzing, O.; Schlitt, H.J.; Piso, P. Mesenteric ischemia—Outcome after surgical therapy in 83 patients. *Dig. Surg.* **2008**, *25*, 213–219. [CrossRef] [PubMed]
4. Tilsed, J.V.T.; Casamassima, A.; Kurihara, H.; Mariani, D.; Martinez, I.; Pereira, J.; Ponchietti, L.; Shamiyeh, A.; al-Ayoubi, F.; Barco, L.A.B.; et al. ESTES guidelines: Acute mesenteric ischaemia. *Eur. J. Trauma Emerg. Surg.* **2016**, *42*, 253–270. [CrossRef]
5. Huang, H.H.; Chang, Y.C.; Yen, D.H.; Kao, W.F.; Chen, J.D.; Wang, L.M.; Huang, C.I.; Lee, C.H. Clinical factors and outcomes in patients with acute mesenteric ischemia in the emergency department. *J. Chin. Med. Assoc.* **2005**, *68*, 299–306. [CrossRef]
6. Adaba, F.; Askari, A.; Dastur, J.; Patel, A.; Gabe, S.M.; Vaizey, C.J.; Faiz, O.; Nightingale, J.M.D.; Warusavitarne, J. Mortality after acute primary mesenteric infarction: A systematic review and meta-analysis of observational studies. *Colorectal Dis.* **2015**, *17*, 566–577. [CrossRef]
7. Nuzzo, A.; Guedj, K.; Curac, S.; Hercend, C.; Bendavid, C.; Gault, N.; Tran-Dinh, A.; Ronot, M.; Nicoletti, A.; Bouhnik, Y.; et al. Accuracy of citrulline, I-FABP and d-lactate in the diagnosis of acute mesenteric ischemia. *Sci. Rep.* **2021**, *11*, 18929. [CrossRef]
8. Björck, M.; Koelemay, M.; Acosta, S.; Bastos Goncalves, F.; Kölbel, T.; Kolkman, J.J.; Lees, T.; Lefevre, J.H.; Menyhei, G.; Oderich, G.; et al. Editor's Choice—Management of the Diseases of Mesenteric Arteries and Veins: Clinical Practice Guidelines of the European Society of Vascular Surgery (ESVS). *Eur. J. Vasc. Endovasc. Surg.* **2017**, *53*, 460–510. [CrossRef]
9. Kougias, P.; Lau, D.; El Sayed, H.F.; Zhou, W.; Huynh, T.T.; Lin, P.H. Determinants of mortality and treatment outcome following surgical interventions for acute mesenteric ischemia. *J. Vasc. Surg.* **2007**, *46*, 467–474. [CrossRef]
10. Acosta-Merida, M.A.; Marchena-Gomez, J.; Hemmersbach-Miller, M.; Roque-Castellano, C.; Hernandez-Romero, J.M. Identification of risk factors for perioperative mortality in acute mesenteric ischemia. *World J. Surg.* **2006**, *30*, 1579–1585. [CrossRef]
11. Groteluschen, R.; Bergmann, W.; Welte, M.N.; Reeh, M.; Izbicki, J.R.; Bachmann, K. What predicts the outcome in patients with intestinal ischemia? A single center experience. *J. Visc. Surg.* **2019**, *156*, 405–411. [CrossRef] [PubMed]
12. Aliosmanoglu, I.; Gul, M.; Kapan, M.; Arikanoglu, Z.; Taskesen, F.; Basol, O.; Aldemir, M. Risk factors effecting mortality in acute mesenteric ischemia and mortality rates: A single center experience. *Int. Surg.* **2013**, *98*, 76–81. [CrossRef] [PubMed]
13. Paladino, N.C.; Inviati, A.; Di Paola, V.; Busuito, G.; Amodio, E.; Bonventre, S.; Scerrino, G. Predictive factors of mortality in patients with acute mesenteric ischemia. A retrospective study. *Ann. Ital. Chir.* **2014**, *85*, 265–270. [PubMed]

14. Schoots, I.G.; Koffeman, G.I.; Legemate, D.A.; Levi, M.; van Gulik, T.M. Systematic review of survival after acute mesenteric ischaemia according to disease aetiology. *Br. J. Surg.* **2004**, *91*, 17–27. [CrossRef] [PubMed]
15. Wu, W.; Liu, J.; Zhou, Z. Preoperative Risk Factors for Short-Term Postoperative Mortality of Acute Mesenteric Ischemia after Laparotomy: A Systematic Review and Meta-Analysis. *Emerg. Med. Int.* **2020**, *2020*, 1382475. [CrossRef]
16. Matthaei, H.; Klein, A.; Branchi, V.; Kalff, J.C.; Koscielny, A. Acute mesenteric ischemia (AMI): Absence of renal insufficiency and performance of early bowel resection may indicate improved outcomes. *Int. J. Colorectal Dis.* **2019**, *34*, 1781–1790. [CrossRef]
17. Pedersoli, F.; Schönau, K.; Schulze-Hagen, M.; Keil, S.; Isfort, P.; Gombert, A.; Alizai, P.H.; Kuhl, C.K.; Bruners, P.; Zimmermann, M. Endovascular Revascularization with Stent Implantation in Patients with Acute Mesenteric Ischemia due to Acute Arterial Thrombosis: Clinical Outcome and Predictive Factors. *Cardiovasc. Interv. Radiol.* **2021**, *44*, 1030–1038. [CrossRef]
18. Cudnik, M.T.; Darbha, S.; Jones, J.; Macedo, J.; Stockton, S.W.; Hiestand, B.C. The diagnosis of acute mesenteric ischemia: A systematic review and meta-analysis. *Acad. Emerg. Med.* **2013**, *20*, 1087–1100. [CrossRef]
19. Treskes, N.; Persoon, A.M.; van Zanten, A.R.H. Diagnostic accuracy of novel serological biomarkers to detect acute mesenteric ischemia: A systematic review and meta-analysis. *Intern. Emerg. Med.* **2017**, *12*, 821–836. [CrossRef]
20. Leone, M.; Bechis, C.; Baumstarck, K.; Ouattara, A.; Collange, O.; Augustin, P.; Annane, D.; Arbelot, C.; Asehnoune, K.; Baldési, O.; et al. Outcome of acute mesenteric ischemia in the intensive care unit: A retrospective, multicenter study of 780 cases. *Intensive Care Med.* **2015**, *41*, 667–676. [CrossRef]
21. Emile, S.H.; Khan, S.M.; Barsoum, S.H. Predictors of bowel necrosis in patients with acute mesenteric ischemia: Systematic review and meta-analysis. *Updates Surg.* **2021**, *73*, 47–57. [CrossRef] [PubMed]
22. Della Seta, M.; Kloeckner, R.; Pinto Dos Santos, D.; Walter-Rittel, T.C.; Hahn, F.; Henze, J.; Gropp, A.; Pratschke, J.; Hamm, B.; Geisel, D.; et al. Pneumatosis intestinalis and porto-mesenteric venous gas: A multicenter study. *BMC Med. Imaging* **2021**, *21*, 129. [CrossRef] [PubMed]
23. Destek, S.; Yabacı, A.; Abik, Y.N.; Gül, V.O.; Değer, K.C. Predictive and prognostic value of L-lactate, D-dimer, leukocyte, C-reactive protein and neutrophil/lymphocyte ratio in patients with acute mesenteric ischemia. *Ulus Travma Acil Cerrahi Derg.* **2020**, *26*, 86–94. [CrossRef] [PubMed]
24. Wu, W.; Yang, L.; Zhou, Z. Clinical Features and Factors Affecting Postoperative Mortality for Obstructive Acute Mesenteric Ischemia in China: A Hospital- Based Survey. *Vasc. Health Risk Manag.* **2020**, *16*, 479–487. [CrossRef]
25. Raith, E.P.; Udy, A.A.; Bailey, M.; McGloughlin, S.; MacIsaac, C.; Bellomo, R.; Pilcher, D.V. Prognostic Accuracy of the SOFA Score, SIRS Criteria, and qSOFA Score for In-Hospital Mortality Among Adults With Suspected Infection Admitted to the Intensive Care Unit. *JAMA* **2017**, *317*, 290–300. [CrossRef]
26. Bednarsch, J.; Czigany, Z.; Lurje, I.; Trautwein, C.; Ludde, T.; Strnad, P.; Gaisa, N.T.; Barabasch, A.; Bruners, P.; Ulmer, T.; et al. Intraoperative Transfusion of Fresh Frozen Plasma Predicts Morbidity Following Partial Liver Resection for Hepatocellular Carcinoma. *J. Gastrointest. Surg. Off. J. Soc. Surg. Aliment. Tract* **2020**, *25*, 1212–1223. [CrossRef]
27. Sarani, B.; Dunkman, W.J.; Dean, L.; Sonnad, S.; Rohrbach, J.I.; Gracias, V.H. Transfusion of fresh frozen plasma in critically ill surgical patients is associated with an increased risk of infection. *Crit. Care Med.* **2008**, *36*, 1114–1118. [CrossRef]
28. Refaai, M.A.; Blumberg, N. Transfusion immunomodulation from a clinical perspective: An update. *Expert. Rev. Hematol.* **2013**, *6*, 653–663. [CrossRef]
29. Haglund, U.; Bergqvist, D. Intestinal ischemia—The basics. *Langenbeck's Arch. Surg.* **1999**, *384*, 233–238. [CrossRef]
30. Rosenblum, J.D.; Boyle, C.M.; Schwartz, L.B. THE MESENTERIC CIRCULATION: Anatomy and Physiology. *Surg. Clin. N. Am.* **1997**, *77*, 289–306. [CrossRef]
31. van Petersen, A.S.; Kolkman, J.J.; Meerwaldt, R.; Huisman, A.B.; van der Palen, J.; Zeebregts, C.J.; Geelkerken, R.H. Mesenteric stenosis, collaterals, and compensatory blood flow. *J. Vasc. Surg.* **2014**, *60*, 111–119.e2. [CrossRef] [PubMed]

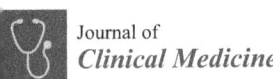

*Review*

# Non-Lipid Effects of PCSK9 Monoclonal Antibodies on Vessel Wall

Sabina Ugovšek [1] and Miran Šebeštjen [1,2,3,*]

[1] Faculty of Medicine, University of Ljubljana, 1000 Ljubljana, Slovenia; sabina.ugovsek@student.uni-lj.si
[2] Department of Cardiology, University Medical Centre Ljubljana, 1000 Ljubljana, Slovenia
[3] Department of Vascular Diseases, University Medical Centre Ljubljana, 1000 Ljubljana, Slovenia
* Correspondence: miran.sebestjen@guest.arnes.si

**Abstract:** Elevated low density lipoprotein (LDL) cholesterol and lipoprotein(a) (Lp(a)) levels have an important role in the development and progression of atherosclerosis, followed by cardiovascular events. Besides statins and other lipid-modifying drugs, PCSK9 monoclonal antibodies are known to reduce hyperlipidemia. PCSK9 monoclonal antibodies decrease LDL cholesterol levels through inducing the upregulation of the LDL receptors and moderately decrease Lp(a) levels. In addition, PCSK9 monoclonal antibodies have shown non-lipid effects. PCSK9 monoclonal antibodies reduce platelet aggregation and activation, and increase platelet responsiveness to acetylsalicylic acid. Evolocumab as well as alirocumab decrease an incidence of venous thromboembolism, which is associated with the decrease of Lp(a) values. Besides interweaving in haemostasis, PCSK9 monoclonal antibodies play an important role in reducing the inflammation and improving the endothelial function. The aim of this review is to present the mechanisms of PCSK9 monoclonal antibodies on the aforementioned risk factors.

**Keywords:** PCSK9 monoclonal antibodies; inflammation; endothelial dysfunction; haemostasis; thrombosis; coagulation; fibrinolysis

**Citation:** Ugovšek, S.; Šebeštjen, M. Non-Lipid Effects of PCSK9 Monoclonal Antibodies on Vessel Wall. *J. Clin. Med.* **2022**, *11*, 3625. https://doi.org/10.3390/jcm11133625

Academic Editors: Peter Kubisz, Lucia Stančiaková and Maha Othman

Received: 14 May 2022
Accepted: 21 June 2022
Published: 23 June 2022

**Publisher's Note:** MDPI stays neutral with regard to jurisdictional claims in published maps and institutional affiliations.

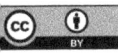

**Copyright:** © 2022 by the authors. Licensee MDPI, Basel, Switzerland. This article is an open access article distributed under the terms and conditions of the Creative Commons Attribution (CC BY) license (https://creativecommons.org/licenses/by/4.0/).

## 1. Introduction

Cardiovascular events remain the leading cause of morbidity and mortality in the Western countries despite new therapeutic options [1]. The underlying pathology of cardiovascular disease is atherosclerosis [2]. There are abundant epidemiological, genetic and clinical studies proving a causal link between the development of atherosclerotic plaques and low density lipoprotein (LDL) cholesterol [3]. LDL carries 60–70% of serum cholesterol [4]. It transports cholesterol from the liver to the peripheral tissues [4]. The LDL particle contains an apolipoprotein B-100 (apoB-100) which enables selective binding of LDL to its receptor [4]. By binding to the LDL receptor in the liver, more than 70% of LDL is removed from the circulation [4]. Therapies that lower elevated lipid levels slow the progression of atherosclerosis and reduce cardiovascular events and death [5]. Statins and ezetimibe are the standard of care for the management of high LDL cholesterol levels [6]. Promising results have been shown with PCSK9 monoclonal antibodies, inclisiran, bempedoic acid, angiopoietin-like 3 protein (ANGPTL3) inhibitors, peroxisome proliferator-activated receptor (PPAR) β/δ agonists and liver X receptor (LXR) agonists [6]. Regardless of statins and new lipid-modifying drugs to lower LDL cholesterol, only 54% of patients have achieved their risk-based LDL cholesterol goal [7]. The main reasons for failure to achieve LDL cholesterol goals are poor treatment adherence and suboptimal use of more efficacious lipid-lowering regimens.

Another modifiable risk factor associated with cardiovascular events is lipoprotein(a) (Lp(a)), a plasma protein that consists of LDL cholesterol, apoB-100 and plasminogen-like apolipoprotein(a) (apo(a)) [8]. Lp(a) levels are genetically determined by the LPA gene and have high inter-individually variability, but intra-individually are stable throughout life [8].

Considering the European guidelines, patients with Lp(a) concentration $\geq$ 50 mg/dL are at high risk of developing cardiovascular disease [9].

LDL cholesterol as well as Lp(a) internalize and accumulate in the arterial wall [10]. LDL cholesterol enters the intima via the LDL receptor, whereas Lp(a) are dependent on Lp(a) plasma concentrations, Lp(a) particle size, blood pressure, and arterial wall permeability [10,11]. The first one is found mainly in atherosclerotic lesions and the second accumulates all over the intima, respectively [10]. Both are taken up by macrophages to produce foam cells and thus promoting the development of atherosclerotic plaques [10]. Nevertheless, Lp(a) carries more atherogenic risk than LDL cholesterol because the former also consists of all the atherogenic components of LDL cholesterol and apo(a). [12,13]. Lp(a), due to the homology with plasminogen, competes with it for the same binding sites on endothelial cells, which promotes intravascular thrombosis and inhibits fibrinolysis [14,15]. PCSK9 induces inflammation in atherosclerosis independently from its hyperlipidemic effect. In addition to ox-LDL accumulation, PCSK9 can directly induce the expression of inflammatory cytokines [16].

In the last few years there have been therapies that lower LDL cholesterol as well as Lp(a), namely PCSK9 monoclonal antibodies and inclisiran. In this review we are focusing on the former since PCSK9 monoclonal antibodies are known to reduce levels of LDL cholesterol and Lp(a), and influence cardiovascular morbidity and mortality as well [17,18]. On the other hand, studies with inclisiran are in progress [19].

Various studies indicate that lipid-lowering agents not only reduce lipid levels, but also have non-lipid effects. They are mainly involved in inflammation, endothelial function and haemostasis. The latter begins with platelet adhesion and aggregation, followed by the activation cascade of clotting factors. Therefore, the aim of the present review is to describe the influence of PCSK9 monoclonal antibodies on the aforementioned risk factors.

## 2. Inflammation

Chronic inflammation plays an important role in the atherosclerotic process from endothelial dysfunction to plaque formation, its rupture and consequently arterial thrombosis, leading to acute cardiovascular events [20]. The most well studied biomarker for assessing inflammation and the most used in research and clinical practice is high sensitivity C-reactive protein (hsCRP) [21]. CRP is produced in the liver in response to proinflammatory cytokines such as interleukin (IL) 6, which is secreted by activated cells at the site of inflammation [22]. Other pro-inflammatory cytokines such as tumor necrosis factor-$\alpha$ (TNF-$\alpha$), IL 8 and IL 18 aggravate inflammatory responses including the expression of adhesion molecules in endothelial cells, whereas anti-inflammatory cytokines such as IL 10 attenuate the inflammatory response [23]. In general populations without known cardiovascular disease, CRP was an independent predictor of cardiovascular events [24]. On the other hand, in patients with stable coronary artery disease with optimal medical therapy, inflammatory cytokine IL 6, but not hsCRP, was independently associated with future coronary events [25]. Statins are known to have anti-inflammatory effects and decreased mortality rates in patients with coronary artery disease. Justification for the Use of Statins in Primary Prevention (JUPITER) was the first trial which prospectively assessed the effects of statin versus placebo on rates of cardiovascular events [26]. In more than 17,000 apparently healthy men and women with elevated levels of hsCRP, rosuvastatin significantly reduced the incidence of major cardiovascular events, despite the fact that nearly all study participants had lipid levels at baseline that were below the threshold for treatment according to current prevention guidelines. Statin therapy is associated with a significant increase in plasma PCSK9 concentrations, irrespective of the type of statin, dose and treatment duration [27]. PCSK9 plays a crucial role in the indirect regulation of serum LDL cholesterol concentration by regulating the number of LDL receptors on hepatic cell surfaces [28]. The role of PCSK9 in the atherosclerotic process is not limited just to lipids homeostasis, but is also involved in the inflammatory cascade (Figure 1) [29].

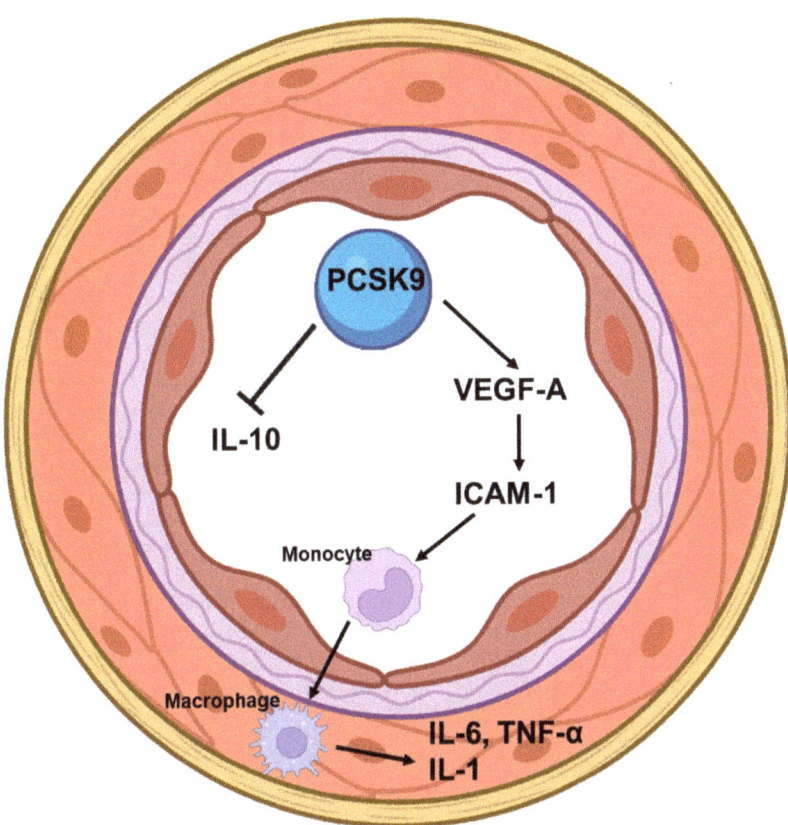

**Figure 1.** The role of PCSK9 in inflammation process. PCSK9 induces the expression of VEGF-A and ICAM-1 and, consequently, activates endothelial cells and stimulates monocyte/macrophage migration. The cascade promotes an inflammatory state and the progression of the atherosclerotic process. On the other hand, anti-inflammatory cytokines such as IL-10 attenuate the inflammatory response. PCSK9, proprotein convertase subtilisin/kexin type 9; VEGF-A, vascular endothelial growth factor A; ICAM-1, intracellular adhesion molecule-1; IL, interleukin; TNF-α, tumor necrosis factor-α.

Several epidemiological studies evaluated the association of PCSK9 with some inflammatory markers such as white blood cells and hsCRP [30,31]. In patients with stable coronary artery disease, PCSK9 was associated with monocyte subsets, especially with intermediate monocytes, which are characterized by CD14++CD16+ on their surface and express strong pro-inflammatory behaviors [5]. In patients treated with statins, these relationships were clear, while this was not the case in statin naïve patients, the second group being very small. In this study, no relationship was found between levels of PCSK9 and hsCRP. On the other hand, in patients with acute coronary syndrome, PCSK9 levels were associated with hsCRP [30]. They also found that PCSK9 levels did not predict future coronary events at one year, but it has to be pointed out that PCSK9 concentration increased over one year, and only 30% of patients were treated with statins at the time of the event. Contrary to their findings in association with the PCSK9 Serum Levels and Platelet Reactivity in Patients With Acute Coronary Syndrome Treated With Prasugrel or Ticagrelor (PCSK9-REACT) study [32], PCSK9 levels were found to predict future acute coronary events in patients with very similar baseline characteristics, including the proportion of patients treated with statins. We have to remember that hepatocytes are not the only source of PCSK9 and that PCSK9 is also produced in endothelial cells, monocytes and macrophages [29]. PSCK9 is not only produced locally, but it acts locally as it is linked to the chronic inflammatory state of the atherosclerotic plaque, what might be one of the factors involved in plaque progression and rupture [33]. PCSK9 monoclonal antibodies have no influence on hsCRP levels regardless of the PCSK9 inhibitor type, patient characteristics, concomitant treatment or treatment duration [34]. Similarly, in patients with elevated LDL and Lp(a) levels that were mostly already treated with statins, additional treatment with the PCSK9 inhibitor evolocumab did not alter either local inflammation in the arterial wall or systemic inflammation [35]. Contrary to this, in patients with coronary artery disease or familial hypercholesterolemia who do not take statins due to statin intolerance, treatment with alirocumab attenuates arterial wall inflammation without changing systemic hsCRP [36]. In both studies, local inflammation was measured using 18F-fluoro-deoxyglucose positron-emission tomography/computed tomography (18F-FDG PET/CT). Arterial 18F-FDG uptake correlates with arterial macrophage content [35]. The difference between these two studies was higher Lp(a) levels both at baseline and at the end of the study in the first study. Since Lp(a)-mediated cardiovascular risk is partly driven by pro-inflammatory oxidized phospholipids (OxPLs), which are abundant on the apo(a) tail of Lp(a) [12], we can assume that this difference may explain the persistent arterial wall inflammation. This is supported by ex vivo data that potent Lp(a)-lowering following AKCEA-APO(a)-LRx, but not modest Lp(a)-lowering combined with LDL cholesterol reduction following PCSK9 monoclonal antibodies treatment, reduced the pro-inflammatory state of circulating monocytes in patients with elevated Lp(a) [37]. The Global Assessment of Plaque Regression With a PCSK9 antibody in a Measured by Intravascular Ultrasound (GLAGOV) trial demonstrated that the addition of the evolocumab to patients with coronary artery disease already pretreated with statins had a favorable effect on progression of coronary atherosclerosis as measured by intravascular ultrasound (IVUS) [38]. The post hoc analysis evaluated the effect of evolocumab-treated patients according to the baseline hsCRP strata (i.e., patients were divided into three subgroups based on their hsCRP levels, <1, 1–3 and >3 mg/L) [39]. The ability of evolocumab to induce the regression of atherosclerotic plaque was not attenuated by the presence of enhanced systemic inflammation and was equal in all three hsCRP subgroups. The results showed that in patients treated with statins, which already have a positive effect on inflammatory parameters, regardless of residual inflammation, an additional reduction in LDL cholesterol, without affecting inflammatory parameters with evolocumab, had a positive effect on reducing atherosclerotic plaque. These results were further confirmed by the High-Resolution Assessment of Coronary Plaques in a Global Evolocumab Randomized Study (HUYGENS), which showed that evulocumab treatment increases the stability of the atherosclerotic bed by reducing the lipid core and increasing the fibrous cap thickness [40].

## 3. Endothelial Dysfunction

The endothelium is an active inner layer of the blood vessel and is indispensable for the regulation of vascular tone and the maintenance of vascular homeostasis [41]. Its functional impairment is characterized by an imbalance between vasodilators and contracting factors [41]. Endothelial dysfunction represents one of the first manifestations of atherosclerosis and is involved in plaque progression and atherosclerotic complications [41]. The most widely used non-invasive method for assessing endothelial function is with high-resolution external vascular ultrasound to measure flow-mediated dilatation (FMD) of the brachial artery during reactive hyperemia [41]. Given the fact that endothelial dysfunction represents a systemic disorder, the aforementioned technique correlates well with coronary FMD and strongly predicts future cardiovascular events [42]. The main reasons for endothelial dysfunction are exposure to oxidative stress and cardiovascular risk factors, including increased levels of cholesterol [43]. Several studies demonstrated an improvement in endothelial function after treatment with statins, independent of its lipid-lowering effects [41].

Besides statins, studies with PCSK9 monoclonal antibodies to evaluate the effects on endothelial function were performed. Maulucci et al. showed that in patients after myocardial infarction already treated with statins at high doses and ezetimibe, two-month therapy with evolocumab improves endothelial function proportional to LDL cholesterol reduction (r = 0.69; $p$ = 0.006) [44]. There is no data regarding Lp(a) values in their patients since it was found that increased Lp(a) values are associated with decreased FMD [45].

Furthermore, Di Minno et al. observed an improvement in endothelial function after treatment with 140 mg of evolocumab every 14 days for 12 weeks in patients with familial hypercholesterolemia on top of maximally tolerated lipid lowering therapy [46]. FMD significantly increased at week 12 (10.63% ± 5.89) from baseline values (4.78% ± 2.27) ($p < 0.001$) [46]. At the same time, a parallel improvement in the reactive hyperemia index and reduction in LDL cholesterol levels was seen [46]. In fact, a decrease of LDL cholesterol was the only independent predictor for FMD improvement (ß = −0.846; $p$ = 0.015). The decrease of Lp(a) in their study was 7%, which is statistically important ($p$ = 0.002), but not predictive for FMD improvement. On the other hand, treatment with alirocumab for 10 weeks in the ALIROCKS trial showed a nominal amelioration (+41%), but no significant change of flow-dependent dilatation of the brachial artery [47]. The sample size and duration of treatment with PCSK9 inhibitors were similar among the mentioned studies. Differences in the results in the ALIROCKS trial compared with the previously mentioned two studies may be due to lower baseline values of LDL cholesterol, although limitations of the FMD method cannot be ignored. In Evaluation of Cardiovascular Outcomes After an Acute Coronary Syndrome During Treatment With Alirocumab (ODYSSEY Outcomes) [48], baseline Lp(a) and LDL cholesterol levels and their reductions by alirocumab predicted the risk of future coronary events in patients after recent in secondary prevention. In their study, the mean decrease of Lp(a) was 23%, the decrease being the greatest in upper quartiles.

A noninvasive magnetic resonance imaging methodology can also be used to assess endothelial cell function [49]. Leucker et al. measured coronary endothelial function with magnetic resonance imaging after six weeks of treatment with evolocumab in people living with human immunodeficiency virus infection and in patients with dyslipidemia with no human immunodeficiency virus infection [49]. There was a significant increase in coronary endothelial function in both groups of patients [49]. In addition, LDL cholesterol levels significantly decreased, but there was no significant change in inflammatory markers in either group [49].

The exact mechanism by which the PCSK9 inhibitor improves endothelial function remains unknown. It is possible that its effect is mostly mediated by the reduction of LDL cholesterol levels, nevertheless other mechanisms can play the same role [44]. Lipid-lowering treatments ameliorate oxidative stress and improve endothelial nitric oxide synthase [44]. In addition, the inhibition of PCSK9 induces the up regulation of the LDL receptors [50]. This might increase the LDL cholesterol binding affinity for the LDL receptor, leading to an improvement of endothelial function [51]. On the other hand, PCSK9 is associated with a macrophage-mediated inflammatory response and treatment with PCSK9 monoclonal antibodies leads to decreased monocyte migratory capacity and reduced inflammatory response [52,53].

Marques et al. investigated the effects of alirocumab 150 mg every 14 days in patients with familiar hypercholesterolemia on subendothelial infiltration of leukocytes, a critical step in the atherogenic process [54]. After an eight-week regimen, the suppressed leukocyte adhesion to the dysfunctional arterial endothelium was observed [54].

PCSK9 monoclonal antibodies attenuate the proinflammatory activation of endothelial cells and reduce the apoptosis of endothelial cells, smooth muscle cells and macrophages [55]. Besides that, PCSK9 monoclonal antibodies may have an effect on circulating endothelial progenitor cells (cEPCs) [56]. The latter are characterized by positivity for CD34, CD133 and vascular endothelial growth factor receptor-2 (VEGFR-2), and are involved in the vascular repair as a response to the endothelial injury [56,57]. Itzhaki et al. in their study with the ePCSK9 inhibitor showed a decline in LDL cholesterol levels and the activation of cEPCs, evident by the elevated expression of CD34+/VEGFR-2+ cells [56]. Treatment with PCSK9 inhibitor promotes cECPs activation and differentiation into endothelial cells, independent of LDL cholesterol regulation [56].

## 4. Haemostasis

### 4.1. PCSK9 and Platelets' Function

It is well known hypercholesterolemia, in particular high native LDL cholesterol and oxidized LDL cholesterol (oxLDL) levels, is associated with an increased risk of atherosclerosis and thrombosis due to increased platelet biogenesis, turnover and activity [58]. Platelets interact with the thrombogenic subendothelial matrix of the ruptured atherosclerotic plaque and with subsequent activation and aggregation [32]. Platelet and endothelial cell activation results in increased P-Selectin expression (other name is CD62P), followed by increased levels of the soluble form of P-Selectin [59]. Besides P-Selectin, the soluble CD40 ligand and other platelet activation markers also play a role in inducing a procoagulant effect [60].

Studies implicate not only increased LDL cholesterol but also that PCSK9 levels are involved in promoting platelet activation and coagulation (Figures 2 and 3) independently of LDL cholesterol regulation [61–63].

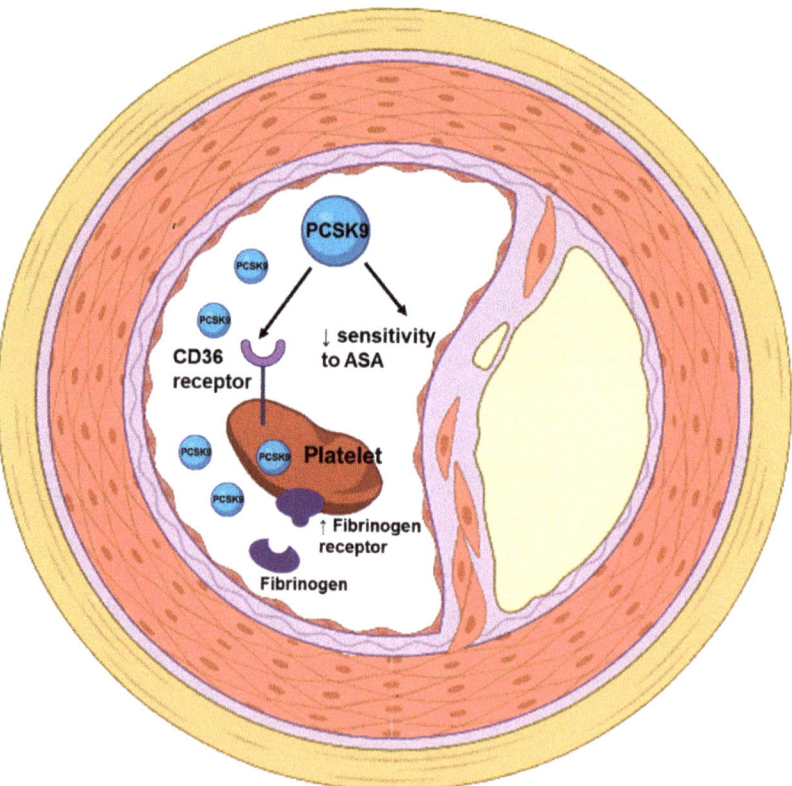

**Figure 2.** The role of PCSK9 in platelets' activity. High PCSK9 levels enhance platelet activation and reduce platelet responsiveness to acetylsalicylic acid, thus promoting atherosclerotic events. ASA, acetylsalicylic acid.

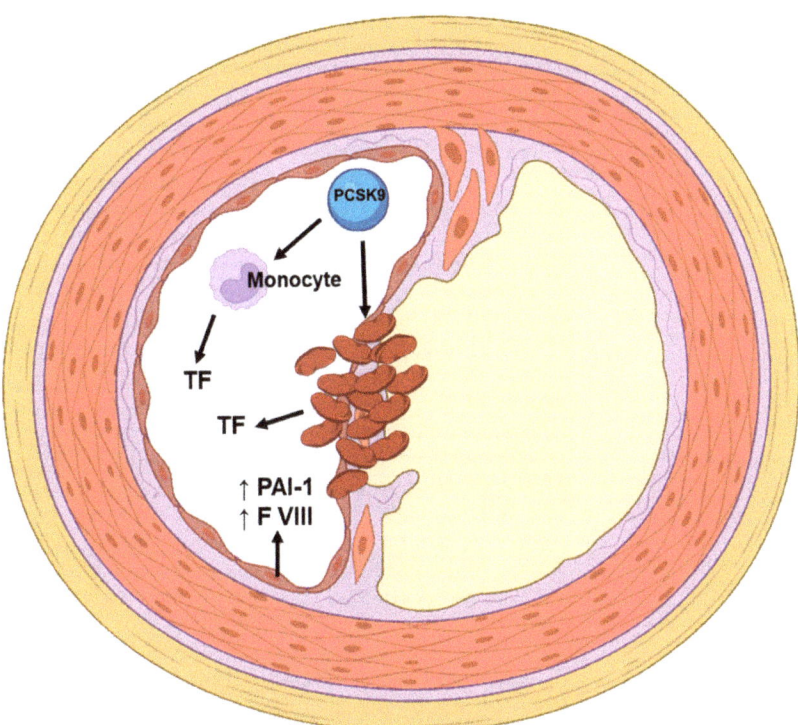

**Figure 3.** The role of PCSK9 in coagulation and fibrinolysis. PCSK9 induces the production of tissue factor, which is responsible for the activation of the extrinsic coagulation pathway and thrombus formation. TF, tissue factor; PAI-1, plasminogen activator inhibitor-1; F VIII, factor VIII.

In patients with stable coronary artery disease, a positive and independent relationship between plasma PCSK9 level and platelet count was observed [64]. Not only platelet count but also platelet activation was found to be associated with PCSK9 levels. In Pastori et al.'s study, the association between elevated PCSK9 and urinary 11-dehydro-thromboxane $B_2$ (11-dh-$TxB_2$), a stable metabolite of thromboxane A2 levels, suggested a role of PCSK9 in the regulation of platelet activation as well [65]. The potential mechanism underlying the connection between urinary 11-dh-$TxB_2$ and PCSK9 might lead to the possible involvement of cyclooxygenase (COX)-1, an essential enzyme for thromboxane A2 [66]. In PCSK9-REACT study, patients with acute coronary syndrome after percutaneous coronary intervention were treated with prasugrel or ticagrelor [32]. Those with higher PCSK9 levels had increased platelet reactivity, they were low platelet responders with no difference between antiplatelet agents used and had a higher incidence of atherothrombotic events after one year [32]. Increased PCSK9 levels have a role as a predictor of higher platelet activation and cardiovascular events [66]. PCSK9 directly enhance platelet activation by binding to platelet CD36 and thus activating the downstream signaling pathways independently of its effect on lipids [67]. Both PCSK9 inhibitors and aspirin abolish the enhancing effects of PCSK9 on platelet activation. This data supports the use of aspirin in patients with increased PCSK9, and on the other hand confirms the antithrombotic effects of PCSK9 monoclonal antibodies.

Beside PCSK9 from plasma platelets, derived PCSK9 plays a significant role in atherothrombosis as a modulator of platelet activation [41]. Platelets store and release PCSK9 upon activation, which is enhanced in the presence of LDL cholesterol, not only ex vivo but also in patients with coronary artery disease. In the presence of PCSK9 antibodies platelet aggregation was significantly attenuated. As a result, in presence of PSCK9 antibodies, platelet-dependent thrombus formations significantly reduced [68]. Many studies indicate that statins [69] and PCSK9 monoclonal antibodies [70] have an effect on the hemostatic system. In approximately a third of patients, platelets show suboptimal response to antithrombotic therapy that can be linked to hypercholesterolemia [71]. It was shown that treatment with statins in patients with hypercholesterolemia significantly increased the aspirin mediated inhibition of platelet aggregation and thrombus formation, and this was beyond the lipid-lowering effect [71]. Barale et al. showed that in patients with primary hypercholesterolemia on a background of maximal tolerated statin and in the presence of concomitant therapy with acetylsalicylic acid, treatment with alirocumab or evolocumab significantly decreased platelet aggregation and activation [58]. In all hypercholesterolemia patients, decreased platelet membrane expression of CD62P and plasma levels of the in vivo platelet activation markers (soluble CD40 Ligand, Platelet Factor-4, and soluble P-Selectin) were observed [58]. Barale et al. in their study claimed that in patients with hypercholesterolemia the inhibition of PCSK9 with alirocumab or evolocumab results in increased platelet responsiveness to acetylsalicylic acid [58]. In the same study, patients with hypercholesterolemia treated with ASA were shown to have reduced platelet aggregation when stimulated with adenosine diphosphate (ADP), arachidonic acid and collagen compared to healthy subjects. Hence, we can infer that ASA reduces platelet aggregation in statin-treated patients with hypercholesterolemia. Patients with hypercholesterolemia who were also treated with statins but not ASA had increased platelet response to ADP compared to healthy subjects [58]. Treatment with PCSK9 monoclonal antibodies in patients not treated with ASA did not affect the response of platelets to the aforementioned substances. In contrast, treatment with PCSK9 monoclonal antibodies in patients previously treated with ASA resulted in decreased platelet responsiveness to all three substances. Platelet aggregation in high shear stress was measured with platelet function analyzer PFA-100. Closure time (CT) with collagen plus epinephrine did not differ between patients with hypercholesterolemia not treated with ASA and their healthy peers, while it was prolonged in hypercholesterolemic patients treated with ASA [58]. Treatment with PCSK9 monoclonal antibodies prolonged CT only in patients treated with ASA. Since both therapies, statins [72] and PCSK9 monoclonal antibodies, [58] improve the platelet response to ASA, it could be that a decrease in LDL cholesterol concentration directly affects platelet aggregation, but we need to consider the option that this effect goes beyond LDL cholesterol reduction. In addition to sensitizing platelet activation, dyslipidemia also seems to result in thrombocytosis, which ultimately elevates the risk for adverse thrombotic events [73]. However, the lowering of LDL cholesterol, regardless of how it is achieved, followed by a consequent reduction in thrombocytopenic counts, may lead to a reduced risk of thrombocytopenic events.

*4.2. PCSK9 Monoclonal Antibodies and Coagulation and Fibrinolytic Parameters*

Thrombosis which is unwanted extension of a haemostasis reaction occurs in both arterial and venous beds by different mechanisms. In arteries it is due to the atherosclerotic plaque rupture and consequential platelets activation, while in veins due to clotting activation [74]. PCSK9 monoclonal antibodies beside their main effect on LDL cholesterol decrease also moderately decrease Lp(a), which can be a common risk factor for arterial and venous thrombosis. Lp(a) has an effect on the coagulation pathway through the promotion of the expression of tissue factor (TF). TF initiates activation of the extrinsic coagulation pathway, which leads to thrombus formation [75]. Lp(a) is believed to promote atherothrombosis due to its homology with plasminogen. Due to this structural homology, Lp(a) can bind to plasminogen receptors on the surface of platelets and prevent the interaction between plasminogen and tissue plasminogen activator (tPA). Therefore, tPA cannot convert plasminogen to plasmin [76]. In a prespecified analysis of both ODYSSEY Outcomes [77] and Further Cardiovascular Outcomes Research with

PCSK9 Inhibition in Subjects with Elevated Risk (FOURIER) [78] clinical trials, they sought to find an association between venous thromboembolism (VTE) and Lp(a) levels and the influence of PCSK9 monoclonal antibodies of future VTE. It was shown that patients with increased Lp(a) but not LDL cholesterol levels have an increased risk for VTE. In the ODYSSEY Outcomes randomized clinical trial, statin-treated patients with recent acute coronary syndrome received the PCSK9 inhibitor alirocumab [77]. In a prespecified analysis, a reduction of the risk of major peripheral artery disease events after treatment with alirocumab was observed (hazard ratio 0.69, 95% CI 0.54–0.89, $p = 0.004$) [77]. The effect was more evident among those with high levels of Lp(a) [77]. A similar but statistically nonsignificant relationship was observed between alirocumab and the occurrence of venous thromboembolism [77]. On the other hand, a post hoc analysis of the FOURIER trial treatment with PCSK9 inhibitor evolocumab demonstrated a 46% relative risk reduction in venous thromboembolism (hazard ratio 0.54, 95% CI 0.33–0.88, $p = 0.014$) [78]. Greater reductions in Lp(a) levels were associated with greater decreases in the risk of venous thromboembolism [78]. No relation between baseline LDL cholesterol levels and the magnitude of venous thromboembolism risk was observed [78]. In 685 consecutive patients with at least one episode of VTE and 266 sex- and age-matched healthy controls, serum levels of Lp(a) were found to be significantly higher in patients with previous VTE (49). No other established prothrombotic risk factors (activated protein C resistance, protein C, protein S, and antithrombin deficiency, and the factor V G1691A, MTHFR C677T, and prothrombin G20210A mutations) were found to be significantly combined with increased Lp(a). Elevated Lp(a) levels might contribute to the penetrance of thromboembolic disease in subjects being affected by other prothrombotic defects, such as FV G1691A mutation. Several case-control studies have shown increased VTE risk with elevated Lp(a) concentrations [79–81]. On the contrary, a population-based prospective study in 2180 middle-aged men without a history of VTE at the study entry showed no evidence of an association of circulating Lp(a) with the risk of VTE [82]. These results are similar to previous prospective studies in different populations [83–86]. No exact mechanism except lowering Lp(a) is known to be involved in the inhibition of coagulation or increasing of fibrinolysis by PCSK9 monoclonal antibodies. On the other hand, the potent reduction of Lp(a) with antisense oligonucleotides did not affect ex vivo fibrinolysis in humans [87], therefore, a decrease in Lp(a) is probably not the only factor influencing the reduction in VTE incidence. In order to determine the role of PCSK9 monoclonal antibodies in preventing VTE, we would need a study involving patients after VTE or at high risk of VTE. The research so far has included patients after a cardiovascular incident in the arterial system in which, although they share many common risk factors with patients with VTE, there are also significant differences.

In patients with familial hypercholesterolemia intolerant to statin treatment with either PCSK9 inhibitor did not decrease D-dimer or fibrinogen, which is one of the most robust clinical markers for decreased thrombogenicity [88]. An in vitro study showed that PCSK9 in a dose dependent manner induced TF production in peripheral blood mononuclear cells (PBMC), which can be inhibited with pretreatment with human anti-PCSK9 monoclonal antibody (mAb) [89]. Most importantly, the increase in TF procoagulant activity (TF PCA) is PCSK9 dose dependent without evidence of a plateau, and is also inhibited with PCSK9 mAB, while pretreatment with PCSK9 mAb has no effect on baseline TF PCA. The summary of the studies reviewed here is presented in Table 1.

Table 1. Overview of the studies that have evaluated the effects of PCSK9 monoclonal antibodies on inflammation, endothelial function and haemostasis. For full trial names and details, see main text.

| Study | Study Population (n) | Characteristics | Treatment | Primary Endpoint | Outcome |
|---|---|---|---|---|---|
| Cao et al. (2018) [34] | 4198 | FH or non-FH | A or E or LY3015014 or RG7652 | Change in hsCRP | No beneficial changes in hsCRP |
| Stiekema et al. (2019) [35] | 129 | Elevated Lp(a) | E vs. placebo | Change in arterial wall inflammation | No beneficial changes in arterial wall inflammation, assessed as MDS TBR of the index vessel |
| Hoogeveen et al. (2019) [36] | 50 | Atherosclerotic disease or FH | A vs. placebo | Change in arterial wall inflammation | Reduced arterial wall inflammation assessed as MDS TBR of the index carotid (−6.1%) |
| Stiekema et al. (2020) [37] | 18 | Elevated Lp(a) | E | Change in gene expression and function of monocytes | No beneficial changes in pro-inflammatory state of monocytes |
|  | 14 | CVD and elevated Lp(a) | AKCEA-APO(a)-L$_{Rx}$ |  | Reduced pro-inflammatory state of monocytes (−17%) |
| GLAGOV [38] | 968 | Angiographic coronary disease | E vs. placebo | Change in percent atheroma volume | Reduced percent atheroma volume (−0.95%), total atheroma volume |
| HUYGENS [40] | 161 | Non-ST-segment elevation myocardial infarction | E vs. placebo | Changes in plaque composition | Increased fibrous cap thickness, decreased atheroma volume, lipid arc and macrophage index |
| Maulucci et al. (2018) [44] | 14 | Myocardial infarction | E | Changes in endothelial function | Increased FMD (+40%), brachial artery diameter and velocity time integral |
| Di Minno et al. (2020) [46] | 25 | FH | E | Changes in endothelial function, lipid profile and oxidation markers | Increased FMD and RHI, reduced 11-dehydro-thromboxane (−18%) and 8-iso-prostaglandin F2α (−17%) |
| ALIROCKS [47] | 24 | Indication for treatment with PCSK9 antibodies | A | Changes in endothelial function | No beneficial changes in FMD carotid intima-media thickness, fractional anisotropy of carotid artery, P-selectin and VEGF |
| Leucker et al. (2020) [49] | 19 | Patients with HIV | E | Changes in coronary endothelial function at rest and during isometric handgrip exercise | Increased coronary CSA and CBF; no beneficial changes in CRP, IL-6, INFγ, TNFα and CD163 |
|  | 11 | Dyslipidemia |  |  |  |

Table 1. Cont.

| Study | Study Population (n) | Characteristics | Treatment | Primary Endpoint | Outcome |
|---|---|---|---|---|---|
| Marques et al. (2022) [54] | 14 | FH | A | Changes in inflammatory state, endothelial function and cardiovascular outcomes | Reduced activation of platelets and leukocytes, increased IL-10, reduced INFγ and soluble PCSK9 |
| Itzhaki et al. (2020) [56] | 26 | CVD | A or E | Change in cEPC | Increased CD34+/CD133+ (+0.98%), VEGF receptor-2+ (0.66%) and PCSK9 |
| Barale et al. (2019) [58] | 24 | Hyper-cholesterolemia | A or E | Change in platelet function | Reduced platelet aggregation and expression of CD62P, soluble CD40 ligand, platelet factor-4 and soluble P-selectin |
| Schwartz et al. (2020) [77] | 18,924 | ACS | A vs. placebo | Peripheral artery disease event or venous thromboembolism | Reduced risk of peripheral artery disease (hazard ratio 0.69), no beneficial changes in reducing the risk of venous thromboembolism |
| Marston (2020) [78] | 27,564 | Stable atherosclerosis, hyperlipidemia | E | Venous thromboembolism | Reduced risk of venous thromboembolism (hazard ratio 0.54) |
| Schol-Gelok et al. (2018) [88] | 30 | Statin-intolerant patients with FH | A or E | Change in D-dimer and fibrinogen | No beneficial changes in D-dimer and fibrinogen |

A, alirocumab; ACS, acute coronary syndrome; apoB, apolipoprotein B; CBF, coronary blood flow; CSA, cross sectional area; CVD, cardiovascular disease; E, evolocumab; FH, familial hypercholesterolemia; FMD, flow mediated dilation; HIV, human immunodeficiency virus; hsCRP, high sensitivity C-reactive protein; IL, interleukin; INFγ, interferon γ; LDL-C, low density lipoprotein cholesterol; Lp(a), lipoprotein(a); MDS TBR, most diseased segment target to background ratio; PCSK9, proprotein convertase subtilisin kexin type 9; RHI, reactive hyperemia index; TC, total cholesterol, TNFα, tumor necrosis factor α; VEGF, vascular endothelial growth factor.

## 5. Conclusions

A majority of the studies are focused on PCSK9 expressed in liver and its local function on LDLR. But we have to bear in mind that PCSK9 is also expressed in other cells and tissues [90]. It could be that the most important source of extrahepatic PCSK9 are cells in the arterial wall, in particular endothelial cells and smooth muscle cells, monocytes and macrophages. These cells are involved not only in the initiation and progression of atherosclerosis, but also in plaque rupture and consequent thrombus formation. Hence, not only local production, but mostly local utilization of PCSK9 is important. PCSK9 activates platelets, increases inflammation and prevails coagulation/fibrinolysis equilibrium to coagulation. On the other hand, Lp(a) possess the same properties in the atherosclerotic process. PCSK9 antibodies (alirocumab and evolocumab) that possess evidence on reducing cardiovascular morbidity and mortality decrease Lp(a) levels by the mechanisms not fully known and lower LDL cholesterol by increasing the number of LDLR. It was also found that both drugs decrease the incidence of VTE, which is associated with the decrease of Lp(a) values. One of the possible explanations would be that decreased levels of PCSK9 in circulation, and in particular in or near the atherosclerotic lesion or injured endothelium, are responsible for the lower incidence of acute arterial and VTE events. In the future it might be reasonable to measure the concentration of PCSK9 and not only levels of LDL cholesterol an Lp(a). Due to different mechanisms and the site of action of PCSK9 monoclonal antibodies and inclisiran in reducing PCSK9, the results of the ORION-4 study will be of particular interest [91]. ORION-4 is a double-blind randomized trial, which will answer the question of whether inclisiran reduces the risk of myocardial infarction and stroke in terms of safety and efficacy regarding hard clinical atherosclerotic cardiovascular disease endpoints. It would be most interesting to see if the results would be comparable to the results observed with both PCSK9 monoclonal antibodies. Since no direct comparison between inclisiran and PCSK9 monoclonal antibodies is to be expected, some answers could be obtained from the ORION-3 study. The ORION-3 study is an open-label, non-randomized, active comparator extension trial to assess the efficacy, safety, and tolerability of long-term dosing of inclisiran and evolocumab given as subcutaneous injections in participants with high cardiovascular risk and elevated LDL cholesterol (NCT03060577).

**Author Contributions:** Conceptualization, S.U. and M.Š.; writing—original draft preparation, S.U. and M.Š.; writing—review and editing, S.U. and M.Š.; visualization, S.U. and M.Š.; supervision, M.Š. All authors have read and agreed to the published version of the manuscript.

**Funding:** This study was funded by University Medical Centre Ljubljana (Funding number: 20210022).

**Institutional Review Board Statement:** Not applicable.

**Informed Consent Statement:** Not applicable.

**Data Availability Statement:** Not applicable.

**Acknowledgments:** Figures were created with BioRender.com, accessed on 10 May 2022.

**Conflicts of Interest:** The authors declare that they have no conflict of interest.

## References

1. Benjamin, E.J.; Muntner, P.; Alonso, A.; Bittencourt, M.S.; Callaaway, C.W.; Carson, A.P.; Chamberlain, A.M.; Chang, A.R.; Cheng, S.; Das, S.R.; et al. Heart disease and stroke statistics—2019 update: A report from the American Heart Association. *Circulation* **2019**, *139*, e1–e473. [CrossRef] [PubMed]
2. Krychtiuk, K.A.; Kastl, S.P.; Wojta, J.; Speidl, W.S. Inflammation and coagulation in atherosclerosis. *Hämostaseologie* **2013**, *33*, 269–282. [CrossRef] [PubMed]
3. Borén, J.; Chapman, M.J.; Krauss, R.M.; Packard, C.J.; Bentzon, J.F.; Binder, C.J.; Daemen, M.J.; Demer, L.L.; Hegele, R.A.; Nicholls, S.J.; et al. Low-density lipoproteins cause atherosclerotic cardiovascular disease: Pathophysiological, genetic, and therapeutic insights: A consensus statement from the European Atherosclerosis Society Consensus Panel. *Eur. Heart J.* **2020**, *41*, 2313–2330. [CrossRef] [PubMed]
4. Elshourbagy, N.A.; Meyers, H.V.; Abdel-Meguid, S.S. Cholesterol: The Good, the Bad, and the Ugly—Therapeutic Targets for the Treatment of Dyslipidemia. *Med. Princ. Pract.* **2013**, *23*, 99–111. [CrossRef] [PubMed]

8. Krychtiuk, K.A.; Lenz, M.; Hohensinner, P.; Distelmaier, K.; Schrutka, L.; Kastl, S.P.; Huber, K.; Dostal, E.; Oravec, S.; Hengstenberg, C.; et al. Circulating levels of proprotein convertase subtilisin/kexin type 9 (PCSK9) are associated with monocyte subsets in patients with stable coronary artery disease. *J. Clin. Lipidol.* **2021**, *15*, 512–521. [CrossRef]
9. Kosmas, C.E.; Pantou, D.; Sourlas, A.; Papakonstantinou, E.J.; Uceta, R.E.; Guzman, E. New and emerging lipid-modifying drugs to lower LDL cholesterol. *Drugs Context* **2021**, *10*, 1–22. [CrossRef]
10. Ray, K.K.; Molemans, B.; Schoonen, W.M.; Giovas, P.; Bray, S.; Kiru, G.; Murphy, J.; Banach, M.; De Servi, S.; Gaita, D.; et al. EU-Wide Cross-Sectional Observational Study of Lipid-Modifying Therapy Use in Secondary and Primary Care: The DA VINCI study. *Eur. J. Prev. Cardiol.* **2020**, *28*, 1279–1289. [CrossRef]
11. Cybulska, B.; Kłosiewicz-Latoszek, L.; Penson, P.E.; Banach, M. What do we know about the role of lipoprotein(a) in atherogenesis 57 years after its discovery? *Prog. Cardiovasc. Dis.* **2020**, *63*, 219–227. [CrossRef]
12. Nordestgaard, B.G.; Chapman, M.J.; Ray, K.; Borén, J.; Andreotti, F.; Watts, G.; Ginsberg, H.; Amarenco, P.; Catapano, A.L.; Descamps, O.S.; et al. Lipoprotein(a) as a cardiovascular risk factor: Current status. *Eur. Heart J.* **2010**, *31*, 2844–2853. [CrossRef]
13. Kiechl, S.; Willeit, J. The Mysteries of Lipoprotein(a) and Cardiovascular Disease Revisited. *J. Am. Coll. Cardiol.* **2010**, *55*, 2168–2170. [CrossRef]
14. Nordestgaard, B.G.; Nielsen, L.B. Atherosclerosis and arterial influx of lipoproteins. *Curr. Opin. Lipidol.* **1994**, *5*, 252–257. [CrossRef] [PubMed]
15. Tsimikas, S. A Test in Context: Lipoprotein(a): Diagnosis, prognosis, controversies, and emerging therapies. *J. Am. Coll. Cardiol.* **2017**, *69*, 692–711. [CrossRef] [PubMed]
16. Tsimikas, S.; Fazio, S.; Ferdinand, K.C.; Ginsberg, H.N.; Koschinsky, M.; Marcovina, S.M.; Moriarty, P.M.; Rader, D.J.; Remaley, A.T.; Reyes-Soffer, G.; et al. NHLBI Working Group Recommendations to Reduce Lipoprotein(a)-Mediated Risk of Cardiovascular Disease and Aortic Stenosis. *J. Am. Coll. Cardiol.* **2018**, *71*, 177–192. [CrossRef] [PubMed]
17. Stulnig, T.M.; Morozzi, C.; Reindl-Schwaighofer, R.; Stefanutti, C. Looking at Lp(a) and Related Cardiovascular Risk: From Scientific Evidence and Clinical Practice. *Curr. Atheroscler. Rep.* **2019**, *21*, 37. [CrossRef] [PubMed]
18. Ferretti, G.; Bacchetti, T.; Johnston, T.P.; Banach, M.; Pirro, M.; Sahebkar, A. Lipoprotein(a): A missing culprit in the management of athero-thrombosis? *J. Cell. Physiol.* **2017**, *233*, 2966–2981. [CrossRef] [PubMed]
19. Yurtseven, E.; Ural, D.; Baysal, K.; Tokgözoğlu, L. An Update on the Role of PCSK9 in Atherosclerosis. *J. Atheroscler. Thromb.* **2020**, *27*, 909–918. [CrossRef]
20. Sabatine, M.S.; Giugliano, R.P.; Keech, A.C.; Honarpour, N.; Wiviott, S.D.; Murphy, S.A.; Kuder, J.F.; Wang, H.; Liu, T.; Wasserman, S.M.; et al. Evolocumab and Clinical Outcomes in Patients with Cardiovascular Disease. *N. Engl. J. Med.* **2017**, *376*, 1713–1722. [CrossRef]
21. Robinson, J.G.; Farnier, M.; Krempf, M.; Bergeron, J.; Luc, G.; Averna, M.; Stroes, E.S.; Langslet, G.; Raal, F.J.; El Shahawy, M.; et al. Efficacy and Safety of Alirocumab in Reducing Lipids and Cardiovascular Events. *N. Engl. J. Med.* **2015**, *372*, 1489–1499. [CrossRef]
22. Stoekenbroek, R.M.; Kallend, D.; Wijngaard, P.L.; Kastelein, J.J. Inclisiran for the treatment of cardiovascular disease: The ORION clinical development program. *Futur. Cardiol.* **2018**, *14*, 433–442. [CrossRef]
23. Ross, R. Atherosclerosis as an inflammatory disease. *N. Engl. J. Med.* **1999**, *340*, 115–126. [CrossRef]
24. Aday, A.W.; Ridker, P.M. Targeting Residual Inflammatory Risk: A Shifting Paradigm for Atherosclerotic Disease. *Front. Cardiovasc. Med.* **2019**, *6*, 16. [CrossRef] [PubMed]
25. Gabay, C.; Kushner, I. Acute-Phase Proteins and Other Systemic Responses to Inflammation. *N. Engl. J. Med.* **1999**, *340*, 448–454. [CrossRef] [PubMed]
26. Levstek, T.; Podkrajšek, N.; Likozar, A.R.; Šebeštjen, M.; Podkrajšek, K.T. The Influence of Treatment with PCSK9 Inhibitors and Variants in the *CRP* (rs1800947), *TNFA* (rs1800629), and *IL6* (rs1800795) Genes on the Corresponding Inflammatory Markers in Patients with Very High Lipoprotein(a) Levels. *J. Cardiovasc. Dev. Dis.* **2022**, *9*, 127. [CrossRef] [PubMed]
27. Jeppesen, J.; Hansen, T.; Olsen, M.H.; Rasmussen, S.; Lbsen, H.; Torp-Pedersen, C.; Hildebrandt, P.R.; Madsbad, S. C-reactive protein, insulin resistance and risk of cardiovascular disease: A population-based study. *Eur. J. Cardiovasc. Prev. Rehabil.* **2008**, *15*, 594–598. [CrossRef] [PubMed]
28. Held, C.; White, H.D.; Stewart, R.A.H.; Budaj, A.; Cannon, C.P.; Hochman, J.S.; Koenig, W.; Siegbahn, A.; Steg, P.G.; Soffer, J.; et al. Inflammatory Biomarkers Interleukin-6 and C-Reactive Protein and Outcomes in Stable Coronary Heart Disease: Experiences from the STABILITY (Stabilization of Atherosclerotic Plaque by Initiation of Darapladib Therapy) Trial. *J. Am. Heart Assoc.* **2017**, *6*, e005077. [CrossRef]
29. Ridker, P.M.; Danielson, E.; Fonseca, F.A.; Genest, J.; Gotto, A.M., Jr.; Kastelein, J.J.; Koenig, W.; Libby, P.; Lorenzatti, A.J.; MacFadyen, J.G.; et al. Rosuvastatin to Prevent Vascular Events in Men and Women with Elevated C-Reactive Protein. *N. Engl. J. Med.* **2008**, *359*, 2195–2207. [CrossRef]
30. Sahebkar, A.; Simental-Mendía, L.E.; Guerrero-Romero, F.; Golledge, J.; Watts, G.F. Effect of statin therapy on plasma proprotein convertase subtilisin kexin 9 (PCSK9) concentrations: A systematic review and meta-analysis of clinical trials. *Diabetes Obes. Metab.* **2015**, *17*, 1042–1055. [CrossRef]
31. Roth, E.M.; Davidson, M.H. PCSK9 Inhibitors: Mechanism of Action, Efficacy, and Safety. *Rev. Cardiovasc. Med.* **2018**, *19*, 31–46. [CrossRef]

29. Barale, C.; Melchionda, E.; Morotti, A.; Russo, I. PCSK9 Biology and Its Role in Atherothrombosis. *Int. J. Mol. Sci.* **2021**, *22*, 5880. [CrossRef]
30. Gencer, B.; Montecucco, F.; Nanchen, D.; Carbone, F.; Klingenberg, R.; Vuilleumier, N.; Aghlmandi, S.; Heg, D.; Räber, L.; Auer, R.; et al. Prognostic value of PCSK9 levels in patients with acute coronary syndromes. *Eur. Heart J.* **2016**, *37*, 546–553. [CrossRef]
31. Li, S.; Zhang, Y.; Xu, R.-X.; Guo, Y.-L.; Zhu, C.-G.; Wu, N.-Q.; Qing, P.; Liu, G.; Dong, Q.; Li, J.-J. Proprotein convertase subtilisin-kexin type 9 as a biomarker for the severity of coronary artery disease. *Ann. Med.* **2015**, *47*, 386–393. [CrossRef] [PubMed]
32. Navarese, E.P.; Kołodziejczak, M.; Winter, M.-P.; Alimohammadi, A.; Lang, I.M.; Buffon, A.; Lip, G.Y.; Siller-Matula, J.M. Association of PCSK9 with platelet reactivity in patients with acute coronary syndrome treated with prasugrel or ticagrelor: The PCSK9-REACT study. *Int. J. Cardiol.* **2017**, *227*, 644–649. [CrossRef] [PubMed]
33. Punch, E.; Klein, J.; Diaba-Nuhoho, P.; Morawietz, H.; Garelnabi, M. Effects of PCSK9 Targeting: Alleviating Oxidation, Inflammation, and Atherosclerosis. *J. Am. Heart Assoc.* **2022**, *11*, e023328. [CrossRef] [PubMed]
34. Cao, Y.-X.; Li, S.; Liu, H.-H.; Li, J.-J. Impact of PCSK9 monoclonal antibodies on circulating hs-CRP levels: A systematic review and meta-analysis of randomised controlled trials. *BMJ Open* **2018**, *8*, e022348. [CrossRef]
35. Stiekema, L.C.A.; Stroes, E.S.G.; Verweij, S.L.; Kassahun, H.; Chen, L.; Wasserman, S.M.; Sabatine, M.S.; Mani, V.; Fayad, Z.A. Persistent arterial wall inflammation in patients with elevated lipoprotein(a) despite strong low-density lipoprotein cholesterol reduction by proprotein convertase subtilisin/kexin type 9 antibody treatment. *Eur. Heart J.* **2018**, *40*, 2775–2781. [CrossRef]
36. Hoogeveen, R.M.; Opstal, T.S.; Kaiser, Y.; Stiekema, L.C.; Kroon, J.; Knol, R.J.; Bax, W.A.; Verberne, H.J.; Cornel, J.; Stroes, E.S. PCSK9 Antibody Alirocumab Attenuates Arterial Wall Inflammation Without Changes in Circulating Inflammatory Markers. *JACC Cardiovasc. Imaging* **2019**, *12*, 2571–2573. [CrossRef]
37. Stiekema, L.C.A.; Prange, K.H.M.; Hoogeveen, R.M.; Verweij, S.L.; Kroon, J.; Schnitzler, J.G.; Dzobo, K.E.; Cupido, A.J.; Tsimikas, S.; Stroes, E.S.G.; et al. Potent lipoprotein(a) lowering following apolipoprotein(a) antisense treatment reduces the pro-inflammatory activation of circulating monocytes in patients with elevated lipoprotein(a). *Eur. Heart J.* **2020**, *41*, 2262–2271. [CrossRef]
38. Nicholls, S.J.; Puri, R.; Anderson, T.; Ballantyne, C.M.; Cho, L.; Kastelein, J.J.P.; Koenig, W.; Somaratne, R.; Kassahun, H.; Yang, J.; et al. Effect of Evolocumab on Progression of Coronary Disease in Statin-Treated Patients: The GLAGOV randomized clinical trial. *JAMA J. Am. Med. Assoc.* **2016**, *316*, 2373–2384. [CrossRef]
39. Nelson, A.J.; Puri, R.; Brennan, D.M.; Anderson, T.J.; Cho, L.; Ballantyne, C.M.; Kastelein, J.J.; Koenig, W.; Kassahun, H.; Somaratne, R.M.; et al. C-reactive protein levels and plaque regression with evolocumab: Insights from GLAGOV. *Am. J. Prev. Cardiol.* **2020**, *3*, 100091. [CrossRef]
40. Nicholls, S.J.; Kataoka, Y.; Nissen, S.E.; Prati, F.; Windecker, S.; Puri, R.; Hucko, T.; Aradi, D.; Herrman, J.-P.R.; Hermanides, R.S.; et al. Effect of Evolocumab on Coronary Plaque Phenotype and Burden in Statin-Treated Patients Following Myocardial Infarction. *JACC Cardiovasc. Imaging* **2022**, in press. [CrossRef]
41. Park, K.-H.; Park, W.J. Endothelial Dysfunction: Clinical Implications in Cardiovascular Disease and Therapeutic Approaches. *J. Korean Med. Sci.* **2015**, *30*, 1213–1225. [CrossRef] [PubMed]
42. Bonetti, P.O.; Lerman, L.O.; Lerman, A. Endothelial Dysfunction: A marker of atherosclerotic risk. *Arter. Thromb. Vasc. Biol.* **2003**, *23*, 168–175. [CrossRef] [PubMed]
43. Heitzer, T.; Schlinzig, T.; Krohn, K.; Meinertz, T.; Münzel, T. Cardiovascular events in patients with coronary artery disease. *Circulation* **2001**, *104*, 673–2678. [CrossRef] [PubMed]
44. Maulucci, G.; Cipriani, F.; Russo, D.; Casavecchia, G.; Di Staso, C.; Di Martino, L.F.M.; Ruggiero, A.; Di Biase, M.; Brunetti, N.D. Improved endothelial function after short-term therapy with evolocumab. *J. Clin. Lipidol.* **2018**, *12*, 669–673. [CrossRef] [PubMed]
45. Wu, H.D.; Berglund, L.; Dimayuga, C.; Jones, J.; Sciacca, R.R.; Di Tullio, M.R.; Homma, S. High lipoprotein(a) levels and small apolipoprotein(a) sizes are associated with endothelial dysfunction in a multiethnic cohort. *J. Am. Coll. Cardiol.* **2004**, *43*, 1828–1833. [CrossRef]
46. Di Minno, A.; Gentile, M.; Iannuzzo, G.; Calcaterra, I.; Tripaldella, M.; Porro, B.; Cavalca, V.; Di Taranto, M.D.; Tremoli, E.; Fortunato, G.; et al. Endothelial function improvement in patients with familial hypercholesterolemia receiving PCSK-9 inhibitors on top of maximally tolerated lipid lowering therapy. *Thromb. Res.* **2020**, *194*, 229–236. [CrossRef]
47. Metzner, T.; Leitner, D.R.; Dimsity, G.; Gunzer, F.; Opriessnig, P.; Mellitzer, K.; Beck, A.; Sourij, H.; Stojakovic, T.; Deutschmann, H.; et al. Short-Term Treatment with Alirocumab, Flow-Dependent Dilatation of the Brachial Artery and Use of Magnetic Resonance Diffusion Tensor Imaging to Evaluate Vascular Structure: An Exploratory Pilot Study. *Biomedicines* **2022**, *10*, 152. [CrossRef]
48. Bittner, V.A.; Szarek, M.; Aylward, P.E.; Bhatt, D.L.; Diaz, R.; Edelberg, J.M.; Fras, Z.; Goodman, S.G.; Halvorsen, S.; Hanotin, C.; et al. Effect of Alirocumab on Lipoprotein(a) and Cardiovascular Risk After Acute Coronary Syndrome. *J. Am. Coll. Cardiol.* **2020**, *75*, 133–144. [CrossRef]
49. Leucker, T.M.; Gerstenblith, G.; Schär, M.; Brown, T.T.; Jones, S.R.; Afework, Y.; Weiss, R.G.; Hays, A.G. Evolocumab, a PCSK9-Monoclonal Antibody, Rapidly Reverses Coronary Artery Endothelial Dysfunction in People Living with HIV and People with Dyslipidemia. *J. Am. Heart Assoc.* **2020**, *9*, e016263. [CrossRef]
50. Luquero, A.; Badimon, L.; Borrell-Pages, M. PCSK9 Functions in Atherosclerosis Are Not Limited to Plasmatic LDL-Cholesterol Regulation. *Front. Cardiovasc. Med.* **2021**, *8*, 639727. [CrossRef]

51. Luchetti, F.; Crinelli, R.; Nasoni, M.G.; Benedetti, S.; Palma, F.; Fraternale, A.; Iuliano, L. LDL receptors, caveolae and cholesterol in endothelial dysfunction: OxLDLs accomplices or victims? *J. Cereb. Blood Flow Metab.* **2020**, *178*, 3104–3114. [CrossRef] [PubMed]
52. Ricci, C.; Ruscica, M.; Camera, M.; Rossetti, L.; Macchi, C.; Colciago, A.; Zanotti, I.; Lupo, M.G.; Adorni, M.P.; Cicero, A.F.G.; et al. PCSK9 induces a pro-inflammatory response in macrophages. *Sci. Rep.* **2018**, *8*, 2267. [CrossRef] [PubMed]
53. Moens, S.J.B.; Neele, A.E.; Kroon, J.; Van Der Valk, F.M.; Bossche, J.V.D.; Hoeksema, M.A.; Hoogeveen, R.M.; Schnitzler, J.G.; Baccara-Dinet, M.T.; Manvelian, G.; et al. PCSK9 monoclonal antibodies reverse the pro-inflammatory profile of monocytes in familial hypercholesterolaemia. *Eur. Heart J.* **2017**, *38*, 1584–1593. [CrossRef] [PubMed]
54. Marques, P.; Domingo, E.; Rubio, A.; Martinez-Hervás, S.; Ascaso, J.F.; Piqueras, L.; Real, J.T.; Sanz, M.-J. Beneficial effects of PCSK9 inhibition with alirocumab in familial hypercholesterolemia involve modulation of new immune players. *Biomed. Pharmacother.* **2021**, *145*, 112460. [CrossRef] [PubMed]
55. Karagiannis, A.D.; Liu, M.; Toth, P.P.; Zhao, S.; Agrawal, D.K.; Libby, P.; Chatzizisis, Y.S. Pleiotropic Anti-atherosclerotic Effects of PCSK9 Inhibitors from Molecular Biology to Clinical Translation. *Curr. Atheroscler. Rep.* **2018**, *20*, 20. [CrossRef] [PubMed]
56. Ben Zadok, O.I.; Mager, A.; Leshem-Lev, D.; Lev, E.; Kornowski, R.; Eisen, A. The Effect of Proprotein Convertase Subtilisin Kexin Type 9 Inhibitors on Circulating Endothelial Progenitor Cells in Patients with Cardiovascular Disease. *Cardiovasc. Drugs Ther.* **2021**, *36*, 85–92. [CrossRef]
57. Hill, J.M.; Zalos, G.; Halcox, J.P.J.; Schenke, W.H.; Waclawiw, M.A.; Quyyumi, A.A.; Finkel, T. Circulating Endothelial Progenitor Cells, Vascular Function, and Cardiovascular Risk. *N. Engl. J. Med.* **2003**, *348*, 593–600. [CrossRef]
58. Barale, C.; Bonomo, K.; Frascaroli, C.; Morotti, A.; Guerrasio, A.; Cavalot, F.; Russo, I. Platelet function and activation markers in primary hypercholesterolemia treated with anti-PCSK9 monoclonal antibody: A 12-month follow-up. *Nutr. Metab. Cardiovasc. Dis.* **2019**, *30*, 282–291. [CrossRef]
59. Pawelczyk, M.; Kaczorowska, B.; Baj, Z. The impact of hyperglycemia and hyperlipidemia on plasma P-selectin and platelet markers after ischemic stroke. *Arch. Med. Sci.* **2017**, *13*, 1049–1056. [CrossRef]
60. Cipollone, F.; Mezzetti, A.; Porreca, E.; Di Febbo, C.; Nutini, M.; Fazia, M.; Falco, A.; Cuccurullo, F.; Davì, G. Association Between Enhanced Soluble CD40L and Prothrombotic State in Hypercholesterolemia: Effects of statin therapy. *Circulation* **2002**, *106*, 399–402. [CrossRef]
61. Camera, M.; Rossetti, L.; Barbieri, S.S.; Zanotti, I.; Canciani, B.; Trabattoni, D.; Ruscica, M.; Tremoli, E.; Ferri, N. PCSK9 as a Positive Modulator of Platelet Activation. *J. Am. Coll. Cardiol.* **2018**, *71*, 952–954. [CrossRef] [PubMed]
62. Hachem, A.; Hariri, E.; Saoud, P.; Lteif, C.; Lteif, L.; Welty, F. The Role of Proprotein Convertase Subtilisin/Kexin Type 9 (PCSK9) in Cardiovascular Homeostasis: A Non-Systematic Literature Review. *Curr. Cardiol. Rev.* **2017**, *13*, 274–282. [CrossRef] [PubMed]
63. Momtazi, A.A.; Sabouri-Rad, S.; Gotto, A.M.; Pirro, M.; Banach, M.; Awan, Z.; Barreto, G.E.; Sahebkar, A. PCSK9 and inflammation: A review of experimental and clinical evidence. *Eur. Heart J. Cardiovasc. Pharmacother.* **2019**, *5*, 237–245. [CrossRef] [PubMed]
64. Li, S.; Zhu, C.-G.; Guo, Y.-L.; Xu, R.-X.; Zhang, Y.; Sun, J.; Li, J.-J. The Relationship between the Plasma PCSK9 Levels and Platelet Indices in Patients with Stable Coronary Artery Disease. *J. Atheroscler. Thromb.* **2015**, *22*, 76–84. [CrossRef]
65. Pastori, D.; Nocella, C.; Farcomeni, A.; Bartimoccia, S.; Santulli, M.; Vasaturo, F.; Carnevale, R.; Menichelli, D.; Violi, F.; Pignatelli, P.; et al. Relationship of PCSK9 and Urinary Thromboxane Excretion to Cardiovascular Events in Patients with Atrial Fibrillation. *J. Am. Coll. Cardiol.* **2017**, *70*, 1455–1462. [CrossRef]
66. Puteri, M.U.; Azmi, N.U.; Kato, M.; Saputri, F.C. PCSK9 Promotes Cardiovascular Diseases: Recent Evidence about Its Association with Platelet Activation-Induced Myocardial Infarction. *Life* **2022**, *12*, 190. [CrossRef]
67. Qi, Z.; Hu, L.; Zhang, J.; Yang, W.; Liu, X.; Jia, D.; Yao, Z.; Chang, L.; Pan, G.; Zhong, H.; et al. PCSK9 (Proprotein Convertase Subtilisin/Kexin 9) Enhances Platelet Activation, Thrombosis, and Myocardial Infarct Expansion by Binding to Platelet CD36. *Circulation* **2021**, *143*, 45–61. [CrossRef]
68. Petersen-Uribe, Á.; Kremser, M.; Rohlfing, A.-K.; Castor, T.; Kolb, K.; Dicenta, V.; Emschermann, F.; Li, B.; Borst, O.; Rath, D.; et al. Platelet-Derived PCSK9 Is Associated with LDL Metabolism and Modulates Atherothrombotic Mechanisms in Coronary Artery Disease. *Int. J. Mol. Sci.* **2021**, *22*, 11179. [CrossRef]
69. Morofuji, Y.; Nakagawa, S.; Ujifuku, K.; Fujimoto, T.; Otsuka, K.; Niwa, M.; Tsutsumi, K. Beyond Lipid-Lowering: Effects of Statins on Cardiovascular and Cerebrovascular Diseases and Cancer. *Pharmaceuticals* **2022**, *15*, 151. [CrossRef]
70. Pęczek, P.; Leśniewski, M.; Mazurek, T.; Szarpak, L.; Filipiak, K.; Gąsecka, A. Antiplatelet Effects of PCSK9 Inhibitors in Primary Hypercholesterolemia. *Life* **2021**, *11*, 466. [CrossRef]
71. Luzak, B.; Boncler, M.; Rywaniak, J.; Wilk, R.; Stanczyk, L.; Czyz, M.; Rysz, J.; Watala, C. The effect of a platelet cholesterol modulation on the acetylsalicylic acid-mediated blood platelet inhibition in hypercholesterolemic patients. *Eur. J. Pharmacol.* **2011**, *658*, 91–97. [CrossRef] [PubMed]
72. Tirnaksiz, E.; Pamukcu, B.; Oflaz, H.; Nisanci, Y. Effect of high dose statin therapy on platelet function; statins reduce aspirin resistant platelet aggregation in patients with coronary heart disease. *J. Thromb. Thrombolysis* **2007**, *27*, 24–28. [CrossRef] [PubMed]
73. Wang, N.; Tall, A.R. Cholesterol in platelet biogenesis and activation. *Blood* **2016**, *127*, 1949–1953. [CrossRef] [PubMed]
74. Paciullo, F.; Momi, S.; Gresele, P. PCSK9 in Haemostasis and Thrombosis: Possible Pleiotropic Effects of PCSK9 Inhibitors in Cardiovascular Prevention. *Thromb. Haemost.* **2019**, *119*, 359–367. [CrossRef]
75. Ugovšek, S.; Šebeštjen, M. Lipoprotein (a)—The Crossroads of Atherosclerosis, Atherothrombosis and Inflammation. *Biomolecules* **2021**, *12*, 26. [CrossRef]

76. Boffa, M.; Koschinsky, M.L. Thematic review series: Lipoprotein (a): Coming of age at last: Lipoprotein (a): Truly a direct prothrombotic factor in cardiovascular disease? *J. Lipid Res.* **2016**, *57*, 745–757. [CrossRef]
77. Schwartz, G.G.; Steg, P.G.; Szarek, M.; Bittner, V.A.; Diaz, R.; Goodman, S.G.; Kim, Y.-U.; Jukema, J.W.; Pordy, R.; Roe, M.T.; et al. Peripheral Artery Disease and Venous Thromboembolic Events After Acute Coronary Syndrome: Role of lipoprotein(a) and modification by alirocumab: Prespecified analysis of the ODYSSEY OUTCOMES randomized clinical trial. *Circulation* **2020**, *141*, 1608–1617. [CrossRef]
78. Marston, N.A. The effect of PCSK9 inhibition on the risk of venous thromboembolism. *Circulation* **2020**, *141*, 1600–1607. [CrossRef]
79. von Depka, M.; Nowak-Gottl, U.; Eisert, R.; Dieterich, C.; Barthels, M.; Scharrer, I.; Ganser, A.; Ehrenforth, S. Increased lipo-protein (a) levels as an independent risk factor for venous thromboembolism. *Blood* **2000**, *96*, 3364–3368. [CrossRef]
80. Marcucci, R.; Liotta, A.A.; Cellai, A.P.; Rogolino, A.; Gori, A.M.; Giusti, B.; Poli, D.; Fedi, S.; Abbate, R.; Prisco, D. Increased plasma levels of lipoprotein(a) and the risk of idiopathic and recurrent venous thromboembolism. *Am. J. Med.* **2003**, *115*, 601–605. [CrossRef]
81. Grifoni, E.; Marcucci, R.; Ciuti, G.; Cenci, C.; Poli, D.; Mannini, L.; Liotta, A.A.; Miniati, M.; Abbate, R.; Prisco, D. The Thrombophilic Pattern of Different Clinical Manifestations of Venous Thromboembolism: A Survey of 443 Cases of Venous Thromboembolism. *Semin. Thromb. Hemost.* **2012**, *38*, 230–234. [CrossRef] [PubMed]
82. Kunutsor, S.K.; Mäkikallio, T.H.; Kauhanen, J.; Voutilainen, E.; Laukkanen, J.A. Lipoprotein(a) is not associated with venous thromboembolism risk. *Scand. Cardiovasc. J.* **2019**, *53*, 125–132. [CrossRef] [PubMed]
83. Kamstrup, P.R.; Tybjærg-Hansen, A.; Nordestgaard, B.G. Genetic Evidence That Lipoprotein(a) Associates with Atherosclerotic Stenosis Rather Than Venous Thrombosis. *Arter. Thromb. Vasc. Biol.* **2012**, *32*, 1732–1741. [CrossRef] [PubMed]
84. Tsai, A.W.; Cushman, M.; Rosamond, W.D.; Heckbert, S.R.; Polak, J.F.; Folsom, A.R. Cardiovascular Risk Factors and Venous Thromboembolism Incidence: The longitudinal investigation of thromboembolism etiology. *Arch. Intern. Med.* **2002**, *162*, 1182–1189. [CrossRef] [PubMed]
85. Danik, J.S.; Buring, J.E.; Chasman, D.I.; Zee, R.Y.L.; Ridker, P.M.; Glynn, R.J. Lipoprotein(a), polymorphisms in the *LPA* gene, and incident venous thromboembolism among 21 483 women. *J. Thromb. Haemost.* **2012**, *11*, 205–208. [CrossRef]
86. Mahmoodi, B.K.; Gansevoort, R.T.; Muntinghe, F.L.; Dullaart, R.P.; Kluin-Nelemans, H.C.; Veeger, N.J.; van Schouwenburg, I.M.; Meijer, K. Lipid levels do not influence the risk of venous thromboembolism. Results of a population-based cohort study. *Thromb. Haemost.* **2012**, *108*, 923–929. [CrossRef]
87. Boffa, M.B.; Marar, T.T.; Yeang, C.; Viney, N.J.; Xia, S.; Witztum, J.L.; Koschinsky, M.; Tsimikas, S. Potent reduction of plasma lipoprotein (a) with an antisense oligonucleotide in human subjects does not affect ex vivo fibrinolysis. *J. Lipid Res.* **2019**, *60*, 2082–2089. [CrossRef]
88. Schol-Gelok, S.; Galema-Boers, J.M.; van Gelder, T.; Kruip, M.J.; van Lennep, J.E.R.; Versmissen, J. No effect of PCSK9 inhibitors on D-dimer and fibrinogen levels in patients with familial hypercholesterolemia. *Biomed. Pharmacother.* **2018**, *108*, 1412–1414. [CrossRef]
89. Scalise, V.; Sanguinetti, C.; Neri, T.; Cianchetti, S.; Lai, M.; Carnicelli, V.; Celi, A.; Pedrinelli, R. PCSK9 Induces Tissue Factor Expression by Activation of TLR4/NFkB Signaling. *Int. J. Mol. Sci.* **2021**, *22*, 12640. [CrossRef]
90. Ragusa, R.; Basta, G.; Neglia, D.; De Caterina, R.; Del Turco, S.; Caselli, C. PCSK9 and atherosclerosis: Looking beyond LDL regulation. *Eur. J. Clin. Investig.* **2020**, *51*, e13459. [CrossRef]
91. The Official ORION-4 Study Website. Available online: https://www.orion4trial.org/homepage-uk (accessed on 10 May 2022).

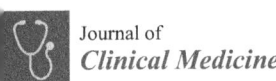 

Article

# The Ottawa Score Performs Poorly to Identify Cancer Patients at High Risk of Recurrent Venous Thromboembolism: Insights from the TROPIQUE Study and Updated Meta-Analysis

Corinne Frere [1,*], Benjamin Crichi [2], Clémentine Wahl [1], Elodie Lesteven [1], Jérôme Connault [3], Cécile Durant [3], Jose Antonio Rueda-Camino [4], Alexandra Yannoutos [5], Okba Bensaoula [6], Christine Le Maignan [2], Zora Marjanovic [7] and Dominique Farge [2,8,*]

1. INSERM UMRS-1166, Institute of Cardiometabolism and Nutrition, GRC 27 GRECO, Sorbonne Université, F-75013 Paris, France; clementine.wahl@aphp.fr (C.W.); elodie.lesteven@aphp.fr (E.L.)
2. Internal Medicine Unit (UF 04): CRMR MATHEC, Maladies Auto-Immunes et Thérapie Cellulaire, Saint-Louis Hospital, Assistance Publique-Hôpitaux de Paris, F-75010 Paris, France; benjamin.crichi@aphp.fr (B.C.); christine.lemaignan@aphp.fr (C.L.M.)
3. Department of Internal Medicine, CHU de Nantes, F-44093 Nantes, France; jerome.connault@chu-nantes.fr (J.C.); cecile.durant@chu-nantes.fr (C.D.)
4. Department of Internal Medicine, Hospital Rey Juan Carlos, Móstoles, 28933 Madrid, Spain; jose.rueda@hospitalreyjuancarlos.es
5. Vascular Medicine Department, Groupe Hospitalier Paris Saint-Joseph, F-75014 Paris, France; ayannoutsos@ghpsj.fr
6. Institut Curie, F-92210 Saint-Cloud, France; okbaibn-nafaa.bensaoula@curie.fr
7. Department of Hematology, Saint-Antoine Hospital, Assistance Publique-Hôpitaux de Paris, F-75012 Paris, France; zora.marjanovic@aphp.fr
8. Institut Universitaire d'Hématologie, Université de Paris, EA 3518, F-75010 Paris, France
* Correspondence: corinne.frere@aphp.fr (C.F.); dominique.farge-bancel@aphp.fr (D.F.)

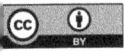

**Abstract:** The Ottawa score (OS) for predicting the risk of recurrent venous thromboembolism (VTE) in cancer patients with VTE may help to guide anticoagulant treatment decisions that will optimize benefit-risk ratios. However, data on its reliability are conflicting. We applied the OS to all cancer patients with VTE enrolled in the prospective multicenter TROPIQUE study who received low-molecular-weight heparin over a 6-month period. Of 409 patients, 171 (41.8%) had a high-risk OS. The 6-month cumulative incidence of recurrent VTE was 7.8% (95%CI 4.2–14.8) in the high-risk OS group versus 4.8% (95%CI 2.6–8.9) in the low-risk OS group (SHR 1.47; 95%CI 0.24–8.55). The Area Under the Receiver Operating Characteristic curve (AUROC) of the OS in identifying patients who developed recurrent VTE was 0.53 (95%CI 0.38–0.65), and its accuracy was 57.9%. Among individual variables included in the OS, only prior VTE was significantly associated with the 6-month risk of recurrent VTE (SHR 4.39; 95% CI 1.13–17.04). When pooling data from all studies evaluating this score for predicting VTE recurrence in cancer patients (7 studies, 3413 patients), the OS estimated pooled AUROC was 0.59 (95%CI 0.56–0.62), and its accuracy was 55.7%. The present findings do not support the use of the OS to assess the risk of recurrent VTE in cancer patients.

**Keywords:** cancer; venous thromboembolism; anticoagulants; recurrence; score

## 1. Introduction

Monotherapy with low-molecular-weight heparins (LMWHs) has been the standard of care for the treatment of cancer-associated thrombosis (CAT) for three decades [1,2]. Six recent randomized-control trials (RCTs) compared direct oral anticoagulants (DOACs) with LMWHs in this clinical setting [3–8]. A pooled analysis of these RCTs reported that DOACs decreased the 6-month risk of recurrent venous thromboembolism (VTE) by 33% compared with LMWHs without increasing the risk of major bleeding [9]. However, a significant increase in the risk of clinically relevant non-major bleeding was observed [9].

Current clinical practices guidelines (CPGs) reviewed these new pieces of evidence and now recommend monotherapy with LMWHs or DOACs for at least 3–6 months as first-line treatment of VTE in medical oncology patients [10–14].

Weight-adjusted LMWHs with a reduction to 75% of the full-dose after the first month of anticoagulation remain the preferred option in selected cancer patients, including those at high risk of bleeding, those with gastrointestinal or genitourinary cancers, and those having a significant risk of drug-drug interactions (DDIs) [10–14]. However, for patients at high risk of recurrent VTE, LMWHs without dose reduction or DOACs may be a more appropriate first-line option. Effective clinical tools to assess individual risk of VTE recurrence are needed to guide anticoagulant treatment decisions that will optimize benefit-risk ratios.

The Ottawa score is currently the only risk assessment model (RAM) available to assess the risk of recurrent VTE in patients with CAT [15]. This simple point-based RAM incorporates five readily available clinical variables and can be used dichotomously to classify patients into high (sum score $\geq 1$) versus low (sum score $\leq 0$) risk for recurrent VTE. A previous meta-analysis of four studies applying the original Ottawa score (1558 patients) assessed its ability to discriminate between high- and low-risk patients [16]. The Ottawa score was reported to have an estimated pooled Area Under the Receiver Operating Characteristic curve (AUROC) of 0.7 (95% confidence interval (95% CI) 0.6–0.8), a sensitivity of 70% (95%CI 60–80), and a specificity of 50% (95%CI 50–60) [16]. Patients with a high-risk Ottawa score (49.3%) had a 6-month pooled crude rate of recurrent VTE of 18.6% (95% CI 13.9–23.9) compared to 7.4% (95%CI 3.4–12.5) for those with a low-risk Ottawa score [16]. However, this score failed to identify patients at high risk of recurrent VTE in two recent large prospective studies [17,18], thereby questioning its reliability.

Herein, we applied the original Ottawa score to all cancer patient with VTE enrolled in the multicenter, prospective, observational TROPIQUE study, which was conducted in 65 French centers involved in the care of cancer patients. This analysis aimed to evaluate the overall discriminatory performance of the Ottawa score in identifying patients with CAT at high risk of recurrent VTE while receiving long-term treatment with LMWHs. We also performed an updated systematic review and meta-analysis of all studies evaluating this score in external validation sets.

## 2. Materials and Methods

*2.1. Study Design and Participants*

Full details of the TROPIQUE study design have been published previously [19]. Briefly, patients were eligible if they: (i) were over 18 years old; (ii) had a histologically or cytologically confirmed diagnosis of solid or hematological cancer; (iii) were receiving anti-neoplastic treatment or palliative care; (iv) had an objectively diagnosed recent index VTE including symptomatic deep vein thrombosis (DVT) of the upper or lower limbs, pulmonary embolism (PE), visceral vein thrombosis (VVT), or central venous catheter (CVC)-related thrombosis; (v) were initiating long-term treatment with LMWHs according to current CPGs. The index VTE diagnosis was established by the referring physician based on the following objective standard routine clinical practice criteria: (i) for DVT: a non-compressible proximal or distal vein on compression ultrasonography; (ii) for PE: an intraluminal filling defect in one or more subsegmental or proximal pulmonary arteries on the spiral computed tomography (CT) scan; an intraluminal filling defect or a sudden cut-off of vessels more than 2.5 mm in diameter on the pulmonary angiogram; a perfusion defect of at least 75% of a segment with a local normal ventilation result (high probability) on ventilation/perfusion lung scintigraphy; (iii) for VVT: a thrombus detected on a (staging) abdominal or pelvic CT. Exclusion criteria were: (i) patients already treated with anticoagulants more than 7 days; (ii) any contraindication to LMWHs' administration (hypersensitivity to LMWHs, active bleeding, previous heparin induced thrombocytopenia, severe renal impairment).

The study was approved by the Ile-de-France I Ethics Committee (Paris, France), and informed consent was obtained from all participants. The current report adheres to the

TRIPOD checklist for Prediction Model Validation [20] and to the PROBAST tool on risk of bias and applicability in prediction model studies [21].

*2.2. Data Collection and Study Outcomes*

Demographic and clinical data, risk factors for VTE, and ongoing treatments were collected at study enrollment and during the 3- and 6-month follow-up visits. The Ottawa score was calculated at study entry, as previously described [15], based on five items: female sex (+1 point), lung cancer (+1 point), breast cancer (−1 point), local disease (i.e., cancer TNM stage I, −2 points), and prior VTE (+1 point). An Ottawa sum score ≤0 classified a patient as being at low risk for recurrent VTE, while an Ottawa sum score ≥1 classified a patient as being at high-risk for recurrent VTE [15].

For the present analysis, the primary outcome measure was recurrent symptomatic or incidental objectively confirmed VTE or VTE-related death within 6 months. Recurrent VTE was defined as objectively documented DVT of upper or lower limbs, PE, VVT or CVC-related thrombosis. All VTE events were adjudicated based on radiology reports. Patients were followed-up from inclusion until 6 months (end of follow-up) or earlier if death or lost to follow-up.

*2.3. Statistical Analysis*

Statistical analysis was performed using NCSS 2022 (NCSS LLC, Kaysville, UT, USA) and R (https://www.R-project.org (accessed on 28 February 2022) with the "cmprisk," and "riskRegression" packages. All analyses were conducted on the intention-to-treat population (i.e., all included patients). Missing data were imputed using single imputation by predictive mean matching. Categorical variables were compared using the chi-square test or Fisher's exact test, and continuous variables were compared using the Mann–Whitney test. The Fine & Gray competing risk model, considering non-VTE-related death as a competing risk [22], was used to estimate the cumulative incidences of recurrent VTE in the high-risk and low-risk Ottawa score groups with their corresponding 95% CI. The individual variables included in the Ottawa score were assessed by estimating the subdistribution hazard ratios (SHRs) with 95% CI at 6 months in a multivariable model including all score variables. The overall discriminatory performance of the continuous Ottawa score to predict recurrent VTE at the 6-month follow-up was assessed by calculating the Area Under the Receiver Operating Characteristic curve (AUROC, Efron C-index) and its 95% CI. The variable of interest was the continuous Ottawa score, and the dichotomous outcome variable was recurrent venous thromboembolism within 6 months.

All tests were 2-sided, and a *p*-value lower than 0.05 was considered as statistically significant.

*2.4. Systematic Review and Pooled Analysis*

We then performed a literature search using MEDLINE and EMBASE and the following key words: "Ottawa score" AND "recurrent venous thromboembolism" AND "cancer" from 1 June 2012 (online publication of the Ottawa score was 7 June 2012) to 19 March 2022. We used the Covidence software for systematic reviews (Melbourne, Australia) for records screening. Briefly, 2 reviewers (C.F. and B.C.) independently screened all records identified in the literature search for study eligibility based on title and abstract. Eligible studies evaluated the predictive ability of the original Ottawa score for recurrent VTE in cancer patients treated with any anticoagulant for an index VTE. Any discrepancies in study selection were resolved by consensus and adjudicated by a third author (D.F.). In case of duplicate publications, only the most recent publication was considered. The same 2 reviewers independently assessed study quality and extracted clinical and outcomes data using dedicated forms. The method of the inverse variance on the arcsine-transformed proportions (random effects model) was used to calculate the pooled rate of recurrent VTE in each level of clinical probability (high-risk and low-risk Ottawa score groups). Heterogeneity among studies was assessed using the Cochran Q statistic, and study consistency was quantified with the $I^2$ statistics. Statistical analysis was performed using MetaXL (version 5.3).

## 3. Results

### 3.1. Performance of the Original Ottawa Score in the TROPIQUE Study Population

From November 2012 to August 2013, 409 out of 474 patients screened for eligibility were included in the TROPIQUE cohort at 65 participating centers in France (Appendix A) [19]. Patients' baseline characteristics are summarized in Table 1. No patient was lost to follow-up. During the 6-month follow-up period, 19 patients developed recurrent VTE. Of these 19 patients, 5 (26.3%) developed isolated PE; 5 (26.3%) developed isolated DVT; 1 developed PE and DVT (5.3%); 6 (31.6%) developed isolated CVC-associated thrombosis; 1 developed DVT and CVC-associated thrombosis (5.3%); and 1 (5.3%) developed isolated VVT. Overall, the 6-month cumulative incidence of recurrent VTE was 6.2% (95% CI 4.0–9.5). Death from any cause occurred in 146 (35.79% (95% CI 31.05–40.34)) patients. Most deaths were related to cancer progression (87.5%).

Table 1. Baseline characteristics of patients included in the TROPIQUE study.

| Patient Characteristics | All (n = 409) | Low-Risk Ottawa Score (n = 238) | High-Risk Ottawa Score (n = 171) | p |
|---|---|---|---|---|
| Age (years), mean ± SD | 65.0 ± 12.1 | 63.5 ± 12.9 | 65.9 ± 10.8 | ns |
| Women, no. (%) | 204 (49.8) | 90 (35.6) | 114 (73.1) | <0.0001 |
| BMI (kg/m$^2$), mean ± SD | 24.8 ± 5.1 | 25.2 ± 4.9 | 24.2 ± 5.3 | 0.0052 |
| ECOG > 2, no. (%) | 49 (11.9) | 23 (9.7) | 26 (17.1) | |
| Missing data | 3 | 2 | 1 | ns |
| **Estimated GFR, no. (%)** | | | | |
| <60 mL/min/1.73 m$^2$ | 65 (16.7) | 34 (15.4) | 31 (20.5) | ns |
| Missing data | 22 | 17 | 5 | |
| **Cancer type, no. (%)** | | | | |
| Gastrointestinal | 100 (24.4) | 60 (25.2) | 40 (23.4) | ns |
| Breast | 65 (15.9) | 57 (23.9) | 8 (4.7) | <0.0001 |
| Lung | 71 (17.4) | 7 (2.9) | 64 (37.4) | <0.0001 |
| Hematological | 54 (13.2) | 46 (19.3) | 8 (4.7) | <0.0001 |
| Genitourinaty | 38 (9.3) | 30 (12.6) | 8 (4.7) | 0.0088 |
| Other cancers | 81 (19.8) | 38 (16.0) | 43 (25.1) | 0.0239 |
| **Cancer Stage, no. (%)** | | | | |
| Stage I | 97 (23.7) | 97 (40.8) | 0 (0) | <0.0001 |
| Stage II | 61 (14.9) | 29 (12.2) | 32 (18.7) | ns |
| Stage III–IV | 251 (61.4) | 112 (47.1) | 139 (81.3) | <0.0001 |
| **Ongoing cancer treatment at time of diagnosis *, no. (%)** | | | | |
| Chemotherapy | 328 (80.2) | 186 (78.2) | 142 (83.0) | ns |
| Hormonal therapy | 26 (6.4) | 16 (6.7) | 10 (5.8) | ns |
| Radiotherapy | 37 (9.0) | 24 (10.1) | 13 (7.6) | ns |
| Antiangiogenics | 22 (5.4) | 13 (5.5) | 9 (5.3) | ns |
| Targeted therapy | 53 (13.0) | 34 (14.3) | 19 (11.1) | ns |
| Supportive care | 32 (7.8) | 17 (7.1) | 15 (8.8) | ns |
| **Risk factors for VTE, no. (%)** | | | | |
| Prior VTE | 54 (13.2) | 17 (7.1) | 37 (21.6) | <0.0001 |
| Major surgery in previous month | 100 (24.4) | 68 (28.6) | 32 (18.7) | 0.0265 |
| CVC | 303 (74.1) | 179 (75.2) | 124 (72.5) | ns |
| Immobilization in previous month | 47 (11.5) | 23 (9.7) | 24 (14) | ns |
| Thrombophilia | 6 (1.5) | 5 (2.1) | 1 (0.6) | ns |
| **Index VTE *, no. (%)** | | | | |
| PE | 145 (35.5) | 75 (31.5) | 70 (40.9) | 0.0264 |
| DVT of the lower limb | 193 (47.2) | 112 (47.1) | 81 (47.4) | ns |
| DVT of the upper limb | 45 (11.0) | 28 (11.8) | 17 (9.9) | ns |
| Visceral vein thrombosis | 16 (3.9) | 11 (4.6) | 5 (2.9) | ns |
| CVC-related thrombosis | 66 (16.1) | 45 (18.9) | 21 (66) | ns |

* One or more. Abbreviations: BMI, body mass index; CVC, central venous catheter; DVT, deep vein thrombosis; GFR, glomerular filtration rate; ns, not significant; PE, pulmonary embolism; VTE, venous thromboembolism.

At study enrollment, 171 patients (41.8% (95% CI 37.0–46.6)) were classified at high-risk for recurrent VTE and 238 (58.2% (95% CI 53.4–63.0)) patients at low risk. Nine recurrent VTE occurred in the high-risk Ottawa score group versus ten in the low-risk Ottawa score group. Six-month cumulative incidences of recurrent VTE did not significantly differ between the high-risk and the low-risk Ottawa score groups (7.8% (95% CI 4.2–14.8) versus 4.8% (95% CI 2.6–8.9), Gray test $p$ = 0.429; SHR 1.47 (95% CI 0.24–8.55) in competing risk analysis, $p$ = 0.670; Figure 1). The AUROC of the Ottawa score was 0.53 (95% CI 0.38–0.65; Figure 2). At the cutoff point defining high-risk (sum score $\geq$1), the model sensitivity was 47.4% (95% CI 24.4–71.1), and its specificity was 58.5.6% (95% CI 53.3–63.4). The corresponding positive and negative predictive values were 5.3% and 98.8%, respectively. The proportion of patients correctly classified (accuracy) was 57.9%. Excluding CVC-related thrombosis from the recurrent VTE events did not change the AUROC of the Ottawa score.

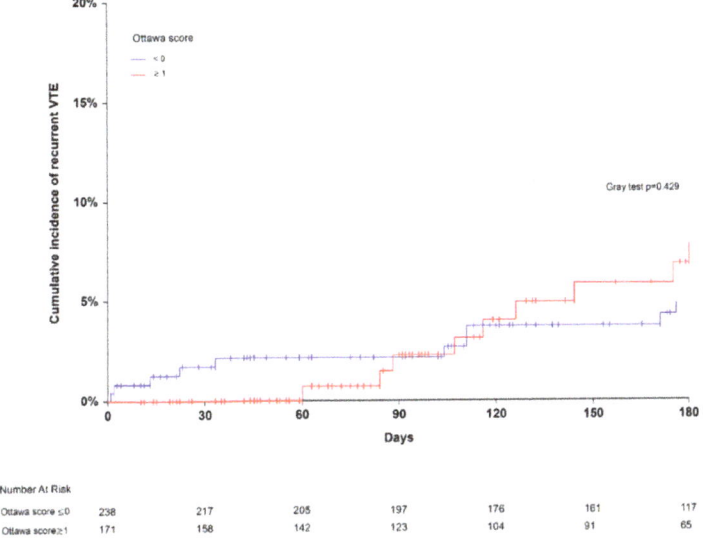

**Figure 1.** Six-month cumulative incidence of recurrent venous thromboembolism in patients with high- ($\geq$1) and low-risk Ottawa score ($\leq$0).

When evaluating the individual variables used in the Ottawa score in a multivariable model, only prior VTE was significantly associated with the 6-month risk of recurrent VTE (13.6% (95% CI 6.4–28.8) in patients with previous VTE versus 4.6% (95% CI 2.7–7.9) in patients without previous VTE, Gray test $p$ = 0.020; SHR 4.39 (95% CI 1.13–17.04) in competing risk analysis, $p$ = 0.033; Table 2 and Supplementary Figure S1). A classification based on previous VTE alone performed better than the Ottawa score in identifying patients who developed a recurrent VTE (AUROC 0.63 (95% CI 0.46–0.75); sensitivity 31.5% (95% CI 12.6–56.5); specificity 87.7% (95%CI 0.84–0.90); positive predictive value 11.1%; negative predictive value 96.3%; accuracy 85.1%). The 6-month cumulative incidence of recurrent VTE tended to be lower in women (3.3% (95% CI 1.4–7.9)) than in men (8.2% (95% CI 5.0–13.7), Gray test $p$ = 0.05871; SHR 0.50 (95%CI 0.16–1.52); Supplementary Figure S1 and Table S1). The 6-month cumulative incidence of recurrent VTE by primary tumor site is shown in Supplementary Figure S1 and Table S1 and tended to be higher in patients with lung (12.1% (95% CI 3.7–39.9)) and genitourinary (11.2% (95% CI 5.2–24.1)) cancers compared to other cancers. Finally, the 6-month cumulative incidence of recurrent VTE tended to be higher in patients with metastatic cancer (7.6% (95% CI 4.6–12.8)) compared to those with localized cancer (4.5% (95% CI 1.7–11.9), Gray test $p$ = 0.28339; Supplementary Figure S1 and Table S1).

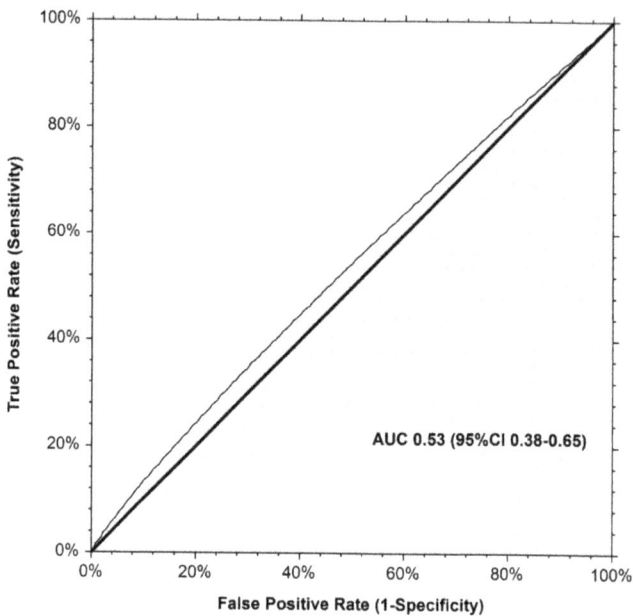

**Figure 2.** Receiver operating curve for the Ottawa score for prediction of recurrent venous thromboembolism in the TROPIQUE cohort.

**Table 2.** Multivariable analyses for recurrent VTE during the 6-month follow-up.

| Variables Included in the Ottawa Score | | SHR (95% CI) | $p$-Value |
|---|---|---|---|
| **Sex** | | - | |
| | Men | Ref | |
| | Women | 0.499 (0.164–1.52) | 0.220 |
| **Lung cancer** | | - | |
| | No | Ref | |
| | Yes | 2.172 (0.4296–10.98) | 0.350 |
| **Breast** | | - | |
| | No | Ref | |
| | Yes | 0.469 (0.0397–5.55) | 0.550 |
| **TNM Stage 1** | | - | |
| | No | Ref | |
| | Yes | 0.653 (0.1704–2.50) | 0.530 |
| **Prior venous thromboembolism** | | - | |
| | No | Ref | |
| | Yes | 4.395 (1.1300–17.09) | 0.033 |

*3.2. Pooled Analysis of Studies That Evaluated the Original Ottawa Score in Predicting CAT Recurrence*

We performed a systematic review and pooled analysis of all studies that evaluated the dichotomized original Ottawa score in predicting recurrent VTE in patients with CAT. The literature search identified 102 potentially relevant citations. Sixteen records were duplicates; 78 were excluded after title and abstract screening; and 12 were assessed for eligibility (Supplementary Figure S2). Six studies meeting the inclusion criteria [15,17,18,23–25] were added to the present post-hoc analysis of the TROPIQUE study resulting in a pooled analysis of 3413 patients (Supplementary Table S2). Patients with a high-risk Ottawa score (46.7%) had a pooled 6-month rate of recurrent VTE of 13.2% (95% CI 8.5–18.7%; $I^2 = 89\%$; $p < 0.001$, Figure 3) versus 6.8% (95% CI 4.4–9.6%; $I^2 = 77\%$; $p < 0.001$, Figure 3) for those with a low-risk Ottawa score. The dichotomized Ottawa score had an estimated pooled AU-

ROC of 0.59 (95% CI 0.56–0.62), with a sensitivity of 61.5% (95% CI 56.2–66.6), a specificity of 55.0% (95% CI 53.2–56.8), and an accuracy of 55.7%. When restricting the analysis to prospective studies including more than 200 patients, the pooled 6-month rate of recurrent VTE was 8.2% (95% CI 5.6–11.1%; $I^2 = 50\%$; $p = 0.14$) in patients with a high-risk Ottawa score versus 5.9% (95% CI 2.7–10.0%; $I^2 = 80\%$; $p = 0.01$) in those with a low-risk Ottawa score (Supplementary Figure S3). The corresponding estimated pooled AUROC was 0.53 (95% CI 0.48–0.57), with a sensitivity, specificity, and accuracy of 48.6% (95% CI 40.4–57.0), 55.82% (95% CI 53.4–58.2), and 55.2%, respectively.

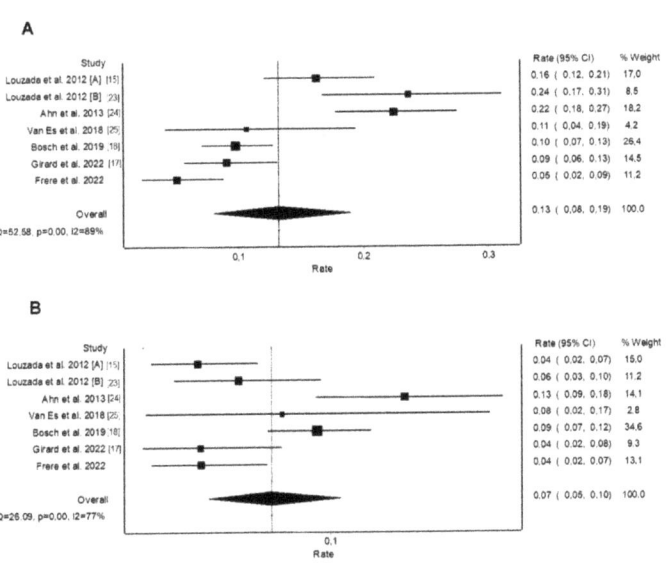

**Figure 3.** Pooled rates of recurrent venous thromboembolism for the original Ottawa score: (**A**) High-risk patients, (**B**) Low-risk patients.

## 4. Discussion

The Ottawa score is currently the only RAM available for predicting the risk of VTE recurrence in cancer patients. Developed by Louzada et al., in 2012 [15], this score has been assessed in several external validation studies with conflicting results [17,18,23–25]. Applying the Ottawa score to cancer patients enrolled in the prospective TROPIQUE study who were treated with LMWHs for a confirmed index VTE failed to identify accurately those who developed recurrent VTE within 6 months, as reflected by an AUROC of 0.53 and an accuracy of 57.9%.

Our results are in line with those from the recent prospective PREDICARE study [17]. In this cohort of 409 patients with CAT who received long-term treatment with LMWHs, the Ottawa score did not identify those who developed recurrent VTE within 6 months, as reflected by an AUROC of 0.60 (95% CI 0.55–0.65), a sensitivity of 75.0% (95% CI 55.1–89.3), and a specificity of 43.3% (95% CI 38.2–48.5). The original Ottawa score was initially derived to discriminate patients with an a priori risk of VTE recurrence under anticoagulation <7% from those with an a priori risk for VTE recurrence ≥7% [15]. In the TROPIQUE and PREDICARE studies, the rates of recurrent VTE were lower than in previous studies, i.e., 4.6% and 7.0% for TROPIQUE and PREDICARE, respectively, compared to approximately 10% in previous validation studies [16].

Similarly, in a post-hoc analysis of the HOKUSAI-VTE CANCER trial [18], which included 1046 patients with CAT receiving long-term treatment with either dalteparin or edoxaban, the Ottawa score had an overall AUROC of 0.52 (95% CI 0.46–0.58). The risk of recurrent VTE was 9.8% in patients with a high-risk Ottawa score compared to 9.4% in those with a low-risk Ottawa score (corresponding to a SHR of 1.20 (95% CI, 0.81–1.80)). A similar poor discriminatory performance was observed in both the dalteparin (AUROC 0.49 (95% CI, 0.42–0.57)) and the edoxaban groups (AUROC 0.55 (95% CI, 0.46–0.64)). When pooling the results from these three prospective studies (TROPIQUE, PREDICARE [17], HOKUSAI-VTE CANCER [18]), the estimated AUROC, sensitivity, specificity, and accuracy of the Ottawa score were 0.53 (95%CI 0.48–0.57), 48.6% (95%CI 40.4–57.0), 55.82% (95%CI 53.4–58.2), and 55.2%, respectively. Differences in study design (prospective versus retrospective), clinical setting, geographical locations, case-mix, follow-up periods, treatment regimens, and overall rates of recurrent VTE across cohorts may partly explain why these findings are inconsistent with previous validation studies [18,23–25]. Furthermore, most of these validation studies, except PREDICARE [17], did not consider the competing risk of death, which may have led to an overestimation of differences in risk estimates across high and low Ottawa score groups.

Numerous factors may influence the overall risk of recurrent VTE in patients with CAT. The original Ottawa score incorporates five items including female sex, lung cancer, breast cancer, cancer stage I, and prior VTE. In the present study, when these variables were evaluated individually in a multivariable model, only prior VTE was significantly associated with the risk of recurrent VTE.

The original Ottawa score derivation study reported that female sex was associated with a trend towards a lower risk of recurrent VTE (SHR 0.50 (95% CI 0.14–1.52)). Data regarding gender differences in CAT outcomes are conflicting. A retrospective analysis of the RIETE registry comparing the rates of recurrent VTE, major bleeding, and mortality in 5104 women and 5951 men with CAT did not report any gender difference in the rates of recurrent PE or DVT [26]. On the contrary, a recent analysis of the international, non-interventional PREFER in the VTE registry of patients with a first episode of acute symptomatic VTE reported that the rates of recurrent VTE within 12 months were higher in women with cancer (17.6%) compared to men with cancer (9.1%), with an absolute difference of 8.6% (95% CI 2.5–19.7%) [27].

It has been widely demonstrated that the site of primary cancer is a major determinant of the risk of developing a first CAT, but it is also associated with the risk of recurrent VTE. A post hoc analysis of the CLOT trial [28] first highlighted that lung cancer was associated with a significantly higher risk of recurrent VTE (HR 3.51, 95% CI 1.62–7.62) compared to other cancer types, while breast cancer tended to be associated with a lower risk (HR 0.59, 95% CI, 0.17–2.01). In the Ottawa score derivation study, lung and breast cancers were significantly associated with the risk of recurrent VTE in multivariate analysis. Consequently, presence of a lung cancer adds one point to the overall Ottawa score, while a breast cancer removes one point. A retrospective analysis of 3947 cancer patients included in the RIETE registry reported that the rate of recurrent VTE was 27 events per 100 patient-years (95% CI 22–33) in patients with lung cancer compared to 5.6 events per 100 patient-years (95% CI 3.8–8.1) in patients with breast cancer [29]. Similar to the results of the recent PREDICARE prospective study [17], we found that neither lung cancer nor breast cancer was significantly associated with the risk of recurrent VTE. We observed a trend towards a higher 6-month cumulative incidence of recurrent VTE in patients with lung (12.1% (95% CI 3.7–39.9)) and genitourinary (11.2% (95% CI 5.2–24.1)) cancers as compared to those with breast cancer (1.54% (95% 0.22–10.76)). Interestingly, a recent post hoc analysis of the CARAVAGGIO study found that the absolute risk difference in recurrent VTE in favor of apixaban was 5.5% in patients with lung cancer, 3.7% in those with genitourinary cancer, and 0.15% in those with breast cancer, suggesting that DOACs may be a more efficient option in lung cancer, provided the patients did not have a high risk of bleeding or of DDIs [30].

In the TROPIQUE study, metastatic cancer was associated with a trend towards a higher risk of recurrent VTE compared to locally advanced or localized cancers. A recent post-hoc analysis of the CARAVAGGIO study showed that patients with locally advanced (HR 2.8, 95% CI 1.1–6.9) and metastatic cancer (HR 3.3, 95% CI 1.4–7.7) have a higher rate of VTE recurrence than those with localized cancer [31]. However, any anticoagulant type should be used with caution in patients with metastases since they are at high risk of major bleeding [31].

With DOACs or LMWHs as possible first-line options for the treatment of CAT, clinicians are now faced with more complex anticoagulant treatment decisions. DOACs or a full dose of LMWHs can be used throughout the first 6 months of treatment when the risk of recurrent VTE is high, while in those with a low risk of recurrent VTE, dose de-escalation of LMWHs (75–80% of full dose) after 1 month, or Vitamin K antagonists (VKAs), may be more appropriate. Our data suggest that the Ottawa score does not provide sufficient predictive reliability to guide clinical decision making. Therefore, a personalized approach, based on individual patient risk factors, a benefit-risk ratio of each drug, physician's judgment, and patient values and preferences, remains essential in optimizing anticoagulant treatment decisions.

Major limitations of the present study relate to the population sample size and to the relatively small number of recurrent VTE events observed during the 6-month follow-up (4.6%). Since the TROPIQUE study was not initially designed to validate the Ottawa score [19], there was no sample size calculation for the present analysis. However, in the PREDICARE study [17], which was specifically designed to validate the Ottawa score in patients with CAT receiving LMWHs for 6 months, the calculated sample size was at least 392 patients to validate the score with an expect AUROC of 0.70 with a lower limit of its CI of 0.65. The TROPIQUE cohort included 409 patients [19].

## 5. Conclusions

The present findings do not support the use of the Ottawa score to personalize the treatment of CAT during the first 6 month of anticoagulant therapy. A multidisciplinary patient-centered approach, with close cooperation between oncologists and other specialists, balancing risk of benefit and harm for each individual patient, and taking account of patient values and preferences, is required to optimize anticoagulant therapy. According to current CPGs [10–14], anticoagulant treatment should be reassessed on a regular basis throughout the course of the disease and continued as long as the cancer is active.

**Supplementary Materials:** The following supporting information can be downloaded at: https://www.mdpi.com/article/10.3390/jcm11133729/s1, Figure S1: Six-month cumulative incidence of recurrent VTE according to sex, primary tumor site, cancer stage, and previous VTE; Figure S2: PRISMA Flow diagram for systematic review study selection; Figure S3: Pooled recurrence rates of recurrent VTE for the original Ottawa score in prospective studies including more than 200 patients; Table S1: Six-month cumulative incidence of recurrent VTE according to primary tumor site; Table S2: Characteristics of studies included in the pooled analysis; Table S3: TRIPOD Checklist: Prediction Model Validation.

**Author Contributions:** Conceptualization, C.F. and D.F.; Formal analysis, C.F., B.C. and D.F.; Methodology, C.F.; Supervision, D.F.; Writing—original draft, C.F. and D.F.; Writing—review & editing, C.W., E.L., J.C., C.D., J.A.R.-C., A.Y., O.B., C.L.M. and Z.M. C.F. and D.F. contributed equally to study conception and design. C.F. and B.C. analyzed the data and performed the statistical analysis. C.F. drafted the manuscript in close collaboration with B.C. and D.F. All authors have read and agreed to the published version of the manuscript.

**Funding:** The TROPIQUE study was funded by a grant from LEO PHARMA. The sponsor and funder of the study had no role in the study design, data collection, statistical analysis, writing of the manuscript, or decision to submit the manuscript.

**Institutional Review Board Statement:** The TROPIQUE study was approved by the Comité Consultatif sur le Traitement de l'Information en matière de recherche dans le domaine de la santé (CCTIRS) on 7 June 2012 (n°12.335), by the Commission Nationale de l'Informatique et des Libertés (CNIL) on 31 July 2012 (n°912315), and by the Ile-de-France I Ethics Committee (Paris, France, n°23/03/2013) on 3 March 2013.

**Informed Consent Statement:** Informed consent was obtained from all subjects involved in the study.

**Data Availability Statement:** The data that support the findings of this study are available from the corresponding author, C.F. and D.F., upon reasonable request.

**Conflicts of Interest:** C.F. reports receiving honoraria for participating as a speaker at satellite symposia organized by Bayer, Bristol Myers Squibb, and LEO Pharma; other authors have nothing to disclose.

## Appendix A

**TROPIQUE investigators:** F. Abbadie, E. Achille, S. Ahmed, A. Alibay, S. Antoun, S. Aquilanti, R. Belhadj Chaidi, C. Belizna, L. Bengrine-Lefevre, Y. Benhamou, H. Bennami, O. Bensaoula, J.F. Berdah, I. Bonnet, A. Bura Riviere, F. Cajfinger, J. Camuset, G. Catimel, A. Cattey-Javouhey, N. Caunes, O. Chiche, O. Cojocarasu, J. Connault, J. Constans, P. Cony-Makhoul, M. Couderier, F. Couturaud, S. Culine, J. Dauba, F. Del Piano, S. Dennetiere-Cluet, C. Desauw, A. Desplechin, L.M. Dourthe, C. Durant, B. Duvert, B. El sayadi, J. Ezenfis, C. Fabre, L. Falchero, N. Falvo, D. Farge, E. Ferrari, J.P. Fricker, A. Frikha, M.L. Garcia, G. Gerotziafas, F. Ghiringhelli, P. Girard, P. Goffette, A. Grenot-Mercier, A. Hamade, M. Hebbard, R. Hervé, L. Karlin, A. Khau Van Kien, P. Lanoye, S. Le Roy, F. Lecomte, G. Leftheriotis, E. Legac, I. Mahé, F. Maloisel, B. Maneglia, N. Mathe, B. Mennecier, G. Meyer, L. Moreau, M. Mousseau, M. Nae-Rejo, S. Nahon, H. Paradis, D. Péré-Veré, B. Peyrachon, G. Peyre, D. Pouessel, C. Pricaz, C. Quashie, S. Regina, C. Roncato, R. Rosario, S. Sadot-Lebouvier, A. Scherpereel, J. Schmidt, M.A. Sevestre, D. Spaeth, D. Stephan, D. Tavan, L. Vedrine, J.M. Vernejoux.

## References

1. Farge, D.; Debourdeau, P.; Beckers, M.; Baglin, C.; Bauersachs, R.M.; Brenner, B.; Brilhante, D.; Falanga, A.; Gerotzafias, G.T.; Haim, N.; et al. International Clinical Practice Guidelines for the Treatment and Prophylaxis of Venous Thromboembolism in Patients with Cancer. *J. Thromb. Haemost.* **2013**, *11*, 56–70. [CrossRef] [PubMed]
2. Farge, D.; Bounameaux, H.; Brenner, B.; Cajfinger, F.; Debourdeau, P.; Khorana, A.A.; Pabinger, I.; Solymoss, S.; Douketis, J.; Kakkar, A. International Clinical Practice Guidelines Including Guidance for Direct Oral Anticoagulants in the Treatment and Prophylaxis of Venous Thromboembolism in Patients with Cancer. *Lancet Oncol.* **2016**, *17*, e452–e466. [CrossRef]
3. Raskob, G.E.; van Es, N.; Verhamme, P.; Carrier, M.; Di Nisio, M.; Garcia, D.; Grosso, M.A.; Kakkar, A.K.; Kovacs, M.J.; Mercuri, M.F.; et al. Edoxaban for the Treatment of Cancer-Associated Venous Thromboembolism. *N. Engl. J. Med.* **2018**, *378*, 615–624. [CrossRef] [PubMed]
4. Young, A.M.; Marshall, A.; Thirlwall, J.; Chapman, O.; Lokare, A.; Hill, C.; Hale, D.; Dunn, J.A.; Lyman, G.H.; Hutchinson, C.; et al. Comparison of an Oral Factor Xa Inhibitor with Low Molecular Weight Heparin in Patients with Cancer with Venous Thromboembolism: Results of a Randomized Trial (SELECT-D). *J. Clin. Oncol.* **2018**, *36*, 2017–2023. [CrossRef]
5. McBane, R.D.; Wysokinski, W.E.; Le-Rademacher, J.G.; Zemla, T.; Ashrani, A.; Tafur, A.; Perepu, U.; Anderson, D.; Gundabolu, K.; Kuzma, C.; et al. Apixaban and Dalteparin in Active Malignancy-Associated Venous Thromboembolism: The ADAM VTE Trial. *J. Thromb. Haemost.* **2020**, *18*, 411–421. [CrossRef]
6. Agnelli, G.; Becattini, C.; Meyer, G.; Muñoz, A.; Huisman, M.V.; Connors, J.M.; Cohen, A.; Bauersachs, R.; Brenner, B.; Torbicki, A.; et al. Apixaban for the Treatment of Venous Thromboembolism Associated with Cancer. *N. Engl. J. Med.* **2020**, *382*, 1599–1607. [CrossRef]
7. Planquette, B.; Bertoletti, L.; Charles-Nelson, A.; Laporte, S.; Grange, C.; Mahé, I.; Pernod, G.; Elias, A.; Couturaud, F.; Falvo, N.; et al. Rivaroxaban vs. Dalteparin in Cancer-Associated Thromboembolism: A Randomized Trial. *Chest* **2022**, *161*, 781–790. [CrossRef]
8. Schrag, D.; Uno, H.; Rosovsky, R.P.G.; Rutherford, C.; Sanfilippo, K.M.; Villano, J.L.; Drescher, M.R.; Jayaram, N.H.; Holmes, C.E.; Feldman, L.E.; et al. The Comparative Effectiveness of Direct Oral Anti-Coagulants and Low Molecular Weight Heparins for Prevention of Recurrent Venous Thromboembolism in Cancer: The CANVAS Pragmatic Randomized Trial. *JCO* **2021**, *39*, 12020. [CrossRef]
9. Frere, C.; Farge, D.; Schrag, D.; Prata, P.H.; Connors, J.M. Direct Oral Anticoagulant versus Low Molecular Weight Heparin for the Treatment of Cancer-Associated Venous Thromboembolism: 2022 Updated Systematic Review and Meta-Analysis of Randomized Controlled Trials. *J. Hematol. Oncol.* **2022**, *15*, 69. [CrossRef]
10. Farge, D.; Frere, C.; Connors, J.M.; Ay, C.; Khorana, A.A.; Munoz, A.; Brenner, B.; Kakkar, A.; Rafii, H.; Solymoss, S.; et al. 2019 International Clinical Practice Guidelines for the Treatment and Prophylaxis of Venous Thromboembolism in Patients with Cancer. *Lancet Oncol.* **2019**, *20*, e566–e581. [CrossRef]
11. Key, N.S.; Khorana, A.A.; Kuderer, N.M.; Bohlke, K.; Lee, A.Y.Y.; Arcelus, J.I.; Wong, S.L.; Balaban, E.P.; Flowers, C.R.; Francis, C.W.; et al. Venous Thromboembolism Prophylaxis and Treatment in Patients with Cancer: ASCO Clinical Practice Guideline Update. *J. Clin. Oncol.* **2020**, *38*, 496–520. [CrossRef] [PubMed]

12. Lyman, G.H.; Carrier, M.; Ay, C.; Di Nisio, M.; Hicks, L.K.; Khorana, A.A.; Leavitt, A.D.; Lee, A.Y.Y.; Macbeth, F.; Morgan, R.L.; et al. American Society of Hematology 2021 Guidelines for Management of Venous Thromboembolism: Prevention and Treatment in Patients with Cancer. *Blood Adv.* **2021**, *5*, 927–974. [CrossRef] [PubMed]
13. Stevens, S.M.; Woller, S.C.; Kreuziger, L.B.; Bounameaux, H.; Doerschug, K.; Geersing, G.-J.; Huisman, M.V.; Kearon, C.; King, C.S.; Knighton, A.J.; et al. Antithrombotic Therapy for VTE Disease: Second Update of the CHEST Guideline and Expert Panel Report. *CHEST* **2021**, *160*, e545–e608. [CrossRef] [PubMed]
14. NCCN Guideline on Cancer-Associated Venous Thromboembolic Disease. Version 1. 2022. Available online: https://www.nccn.org/professionals/physician_gls/pdf/vte.pdf (accessed on 1 March 2022).
15. Louzada, M.L.; Carrier, M.; Lazo-Langner, A.; Dao, V.; Kovacs, M.J.; Ramsay, T.O.; Rodger, M.A.; Zhang, J.; Lee, A.Y.Y.; Meyer, G.; et al. Development of a Clinical Prediction Rule for Risk Stratification of Recurrent Venous Thromboembolism in Patients with Cancer-Associated Venous Thromboembolism. *Circulation* **2012**, *126*, 448–454. [CrossRef] [PubMed]
16. Delluc, A.; Miranda, S.; den Exter, P.; Louzada, M.; Alatri, A.; Ahn, S.; Monreal, M.; Khorana, A.; Huisman, M.V.; Wells, P.S.; et al. Accuracy of the Ottawa Score in Risk Stratification of Recurrent Venous Thromboembolism in Patients with Cancer-Associated Venous Thromboembolism: A Systematic Review and Meta-Analysis. *Haematologica* **2020**, *105*, 1436–1442. [CrossRef] [PubMed]
17. Girard, P.; Laporte, S.; Chapelle, C.; Falvo, N.; Falchero, L.; Cloarec, N.; Monnet, I.; Burnod, A.; Tomasini, P.; Boulon, C.; et al. Failure of the Ottawa Score to Predict the Risk of Recurrent Venous Thromboembolism in Cancer Patients: The Prospective PREDICARE Cohort Study. *Thromb. Haemost.* **2022**, *122*, 151–157. [CrossRef]
18. Bosch, F.T.M.; Van Es, N.; Di Nisio, M.; Carrier, M.; Segers, A.; Grosso, M.A.; Mulder, F.I.; Weitz, J.I.; Raskob, G.E. The Ottawa Score Does Not Predict Recurrent Venous Thromboembolism in Cancer Patients: Results from the Hokusai-VTE Cancer Study. *RPTH* **2019**, *3*, 717–718.
19. Cajfinger, F.; Debourdeau, P.; Lamblin, A.; Benatar, V.; Falvo, N.; Benhamou, Y.; Sevestre, M.A.; Farge-Bancel, D. TROPIQUE investigators Low-Molecular-Weight Heparins for Cancer-Associated Thrombosis: Adherence to Clinical Practice Guidelines and Patient Perception in TROPIQUE, a 409-Patient Prospective Observational Study. *Thromb. Res.* **2016**, *144*, 85–92. [CrossRef]
20. Collins, G.S.; Reitsma, J.B.; Altman, D.G.; Moons, K.G.M. Transparent Reporting of a Multivariable Prediction Model for Individual Prognosis or Diagnosis (TRIPOD): The TRIPOD Statement. *Ann. Intern. Med.* **2015**, *162*, 55–63. [CrossRef]
21. Moons, K.G.M.; Wolff, R.F.; Riley, R.D.; Whiting, P.F.; Westwood, M.; Collins, G.S.; Reitsma, J.B.; Kleijnen, J.; Mallett, S. PROBAST: A Tool to Assess Risk of Bias and Applicability of Prediction Model Studies: Explanation and Elaboration. *Ann. Intern. Med.* **2019**, *170*, W1–W33. [CrossRef]
22. Fine, J.P.; Gray, R.J. A Proportional Hazards Model for the Subdistribution of a Competing Risk. *J. Am. Stat. Assoc.* **1999**, *94*, 496–509. [CrossRef]
23. Louzada, M.L.; Bose, G.; Cheung, A.; Chin-Yee, B.H.; Wells, S.; Wells, P.S. Predicting Venous Thromboembolism Recurrence Risk in Patients with Cancer: A Validation Study. *Blood* **2012**, *120*, 394. [CrossRef]
24. Ahn, S.; Lim, K.S.; Lee, Y.-S.; Lee, J.-L. Validation of the Clinical Prediction Rule for Recurrent Venous Thromboembolism in Cancer Patients: The Ottawa Score. *Support. Care Cancer* **2013**, *21*, 2309–2313. [CrossRef] [PubMed]
25. van Es, N.; Louzada, M.; Carrier, M.; Tagalakis, V.; Gross, P.L.; Shivakumar, S.; Rodger, M.A.; Wells, P.S. Predicting the Risk of Recurrent Venous Thromboembolism in Patients with Cancer: A Prospective Cohort Study. *Thromb. Res.* **2018**, *163*, 41–46. [CrossRef]
26. Martín-Martos, F.; Trujillo-Santos, J.; Barrón, M.; Vela, J.; Javier Marchena, P.; Braester, A.; Hij, A.; Hernández-Blasco, L.; Verhamme, P.; Manuel, M.; et al. Gender Differences in Cancer Patients with Acute Venous Thromboembolism. *Thromb. Res.* **2015**, *135* (Suppl. S1), S12–S15. [CrossRef]
27. Giustozzi, M.; Valerio, L.; Agnelli, G.; Becattini, C.; Fronk, E.-M.; Klok, F.A.; Konstantinides, S.V.; Vedovati, M.C.; Cohen, A.T.; Barco, S. Sex-Specific Differences in the Presentation, Clinical Course, and Quality of Life of Patients with Acute Venous Thromboembolism According to Baseline Risk Factors. Insights from the PREFER in VTE. *Eur. J. Intern. Med.* **2021**, *88*, 43–51. [CrossRef]
28. Lee, A.; Parpia, S.; Julian, J.; Rickles, F.; Prins, M.; Levine, M. Predictors of Recurrent Thrombosis and Anticoagulant-Related Bleeding in Patients with Cancer. *JCO* **2009**, *27*, 9565. [CrossRef]
29. Mahé, I.; Chidiac, J.; Bertoletti, L.; Font, C.; Trujillo-Santos, J.; Peris, M.; Pérez Ductor, C.; Nieto, S.; Grandone, E.; Monreal, M.; et al. The Clinical Course of Venous Thromboembolism May Differ According to Cancer Site. *Am. J. Med.* **2017**, *130*, 337–347. [CrossRef]
30. Agnelli, G.; Muñoz, A.; Franco, L.; Mahé, I.; Brenner, B.; Connors, J.M.; Gussoni, G.; Hamulyak, E.N.; Lambert, C.; Suero, M.R.; et al. Apixaban and Dalteparin for the Treatment of Venous Thromboembolism in Patients with Different Sites of Cancer. *Thromb. Haemost.* **2021**, *122*, 796–807. [CrossRef]
31. Verso, M.; Agnelli, G.; Munoz, A.; Connors, J.M.; Sanchez, O.; Huisman, M.; Brenner, B.; Gussoni, G.; Cohen, A.T.; Becattini, C. Recurrent Venous Thromboembolism and Major Bleeding in Patients with Localised, Locally Advanced or Metastatic Cancer: An Analysis of the Caravaggio Study. *Eur. J. Cancer* **2022**, *165*, 136–145. [CrossRef]

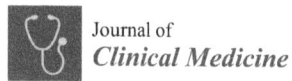 

Article

# Characteristics and Outcomes of Patients Consulted by a Multidisciplinary Pulmonary Embolism Response Team: 5-Year Experience

Arkadiusz Pietrasik [1,*], Aleksandra Gąsecka [1], Paweł Kurzyna [1], Katarzyna Wrona [2], Szymon Darocha [2], Marta Banaszkiewicz [2], Dariusz Zieliński [3], Dominika Zajkowska [1], Julia Maria Smyk [1], Dominika Rymaszewska [1], Karolina Jasińska [1], Marcin Wasilewski [1], Rafał Wolański [1], Grzegorz Procyk [1], Piotr Szwed [1], Michał Florczyk [2], Krzysztof Wróbel [3], Marcin Grabowski [1], Adam Torbicki [2] and Marcin Kurzyna [2]

[1] 1st Chair and Department of Cardiology, Medical University of Warsaw, 02-097 Warsaw, Poland; gaseckaa@gmail.com (A.G.); paw.kurzyna@gmail.com (P.K.); dominika_zajkowska@interia.pl (D.Z.); julia.lekarski@gmail.com (J.M.S.); dmnrymaszewska@gmail.com (D.R.); kari.jasinska@gmail.com (K.J.); marcin.vasilewski@wp.pl (M.W.); rafalwolanski7@gmail.com (R.W.); grzegorzprocyk@gmail.com (G.P.); szwedp12@gmail.com (P.S.); marcin.grabowski@wum.edu.pl (M.G.)

[2] Department of Pulmonary Circulation, Thromboembolic Diseases and Cardiology, Centre of Postgraduate Medical Education, European Health Centre Otwock, 05-400 Otwock, Poland; kasia.wrona18@gmail.com (K.W.); szymon.darocha@gmail.com (S.D.); marta.banaszkiewicz@gmail.com (M.B.); michal.florczyk@ecz-otwock.pl (M.F.); adam.torbicki@ecz-otwock.pl (A.T.); marcin.kurzyna@ecz-otwock.pl (M.K.)

[3] Department of Cardiac Surgery, Medicover Hospital, 02-972 Warsaw, Poland; farok@wp.pl (D.Z.); krzysztof.wrobel17@gmail.com (K.W.)

* Correspondence: apietrasik@o2.pl; Tel.: +48-22-599-19-51

**Abstract:** (1) Background: Pulmonary embolism (PE) is the third most frequent acute cardiovascular condition worldwide. PE response teams (PERTs) have been created to facilitate treatment implementation in PE patients. Here, we report on the 5-year experience of PERT operating in Warsaw, Poland, with regard to the characteristics and outcomes of the consulted patients. (2) Methods: Patients diagnosed with PE between September 2017 and December 2021 were included in the study. Clinical and treatment data were obtained from medical records. Patient outcomes were assessed in-hospital, at a 1- and 12-month follow-up. (3) Results: There were 235 PERT activations. The risk of early mortality was low in 51 patients (21.8%), intermediate–low in 83 (35.3%), intermediate–high in 80 (34.0%) and high in 21 (8.9%) patients. Anticoagulation alone was the most frequently administered treatment in all patient subgroups (altogether 84.7%). Systemic thrombolysis (47.6%) and interventional therapy (52%) were the prevailing treatment options in high-risk patients. The in-hospital mortality was 6.4%. The adverse events during 1-year follow-up included five deaths, two recurrent VTE and two minor bleeding events. (4) Conclusions: Our initial 5-year experience showed that the activity of the local PERT facilitated patient-tailored decision making and the access to advanced therapies, with subsequent low overall mortality and treatment complication rates, confirming the benefits of PERT implementation.

**Keywords:** pulmonary embolism; pulmonary embolism response team; PERT; catheter-based therapies

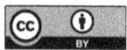

## 1. Introduction

Pulmonary embolism (PE) is the third most frequent acute cardiovascular condition worldwide [1]. The incidence is 100–200 per 100,000 inhabitants each year [2], generating annual costs ranging to EUR 8.5 billion in the European Union alone [3]. The major burden of PE to the public health implies the need to optimize the strategies of PE diagnosis and management.

Given the diversity of PE clinical manifestation and multiple therapeutic interventions available in the acute PE [3], implementation of the optimal patient-tailored treatment is of the utmost importance. The choice of the optimal therapy should take into account the risk of early mortality and the risk of treatment-associated complications [4]. Generally, systemic thrombolytic therapy is recommended for patients with high-risk PE. However, the rate of major bleeding during systemic thrombolysis ranges to 20%, with the rate of intracranial bleeding up to 3% [5,6]. In addition, there are numerous patients in whom thrombolysis is initially contraindicated or has failed. In such patients, surgical or percutaneous catheter-directed therapy are viable alternative treatment options.

Regarding the complex qualification of PE patients for interventional treatment and the delicate balance between the risk of death due to the disease itself and the risk of treatment-associated complications [6], the concept of multidisciplinary PE response teams (PERTs) emerged in 2012 at the Massachusetts General Hospital [5]. By gathering experts from various disciplines, including interventional cardiology, cardiothoracic surgery, emergency medicine and intensive care within a rapid real-time consultation, the aim of PERTs is to optimize and accelerate treatment implementation in PE patients at intermediate–high and high risk of mortality [5,7].

The first results indicate that the implementation of PERTs improved the efficiency of treatment initiation and decreased both the hospital length of stay and the generated costs [6,7], although the clear mortality benefit remains to be demonstrated [6–8]. Following the European Society of Cardiology (ESC) recommendation to set up the local interdisciplinary PERTs for PE management [1], the Centre for the Management of Pulmonary Embolism (CELZAT) in Warsaw was established in 2017. The main goal of CELZAT is to improve patient prognosis by developing a model of interdisciplinary, comprehensive care for patients with PE, with particular focus on the population of patients with contraindications to standard pharmacological treatment, who require complex qualification for the interventional treatment [9]. Here, we report on the characteristics and outcomes of patients consulted by CELZAT.

## 2. Materials and Methods

### 2.1. Algorithm of CELZAT Activation

CELZAT was created by experts from the Department of Pulmonary Circulation, Thromboembolic Diseases and Cardiology, European Health Center in Otwock, Poland; 1st Chair and Department of Cardiology, Medical University of Warsaw, Poland; and Department of Cardiac Surgery, Medicover Hospital, Warsaw, Poland. The CELZAT project has been implemented in collaboration with Professor Richard Channik from the Massachusetts General Hospital in Boston, the creator of the world's first interdisciplinary model of care for patients with pulmonary embolism, who acts as the Honorary Consultant.

An algorithm of the CELZAT activation consists of four stages (Figure 1). In the first stage, in patients with suspected acute PE, a thorough clinical assessment and risk stratification according to Pulmonary Embolism Severity Index (PESI) and simplified PESI (sPESI) is conducted by the treating physician. Based on the clinical picture, laboratory parameters and imaging finding, patients at high or intermediate–high-risk of mortality are identified.

The diagnosis of high- and intermediate–high-risk of mortality PE is followed by CELZAT activation via a phone call to an emergency number, operating 24 h per day, 7 days per week. Subsequently, an interdisciplinary teleconsultation is performed within 30 min, including the treating physician, interventional cardiologist, clinical radiologist, intensive care specialist, anesthesiologist and cardiothoracic surgeon. Depending on the patient's clinical condition and comorbidities, the expert panel may be extended by other specialists, such as a neurologist, general surgeon or vascular surgeon.

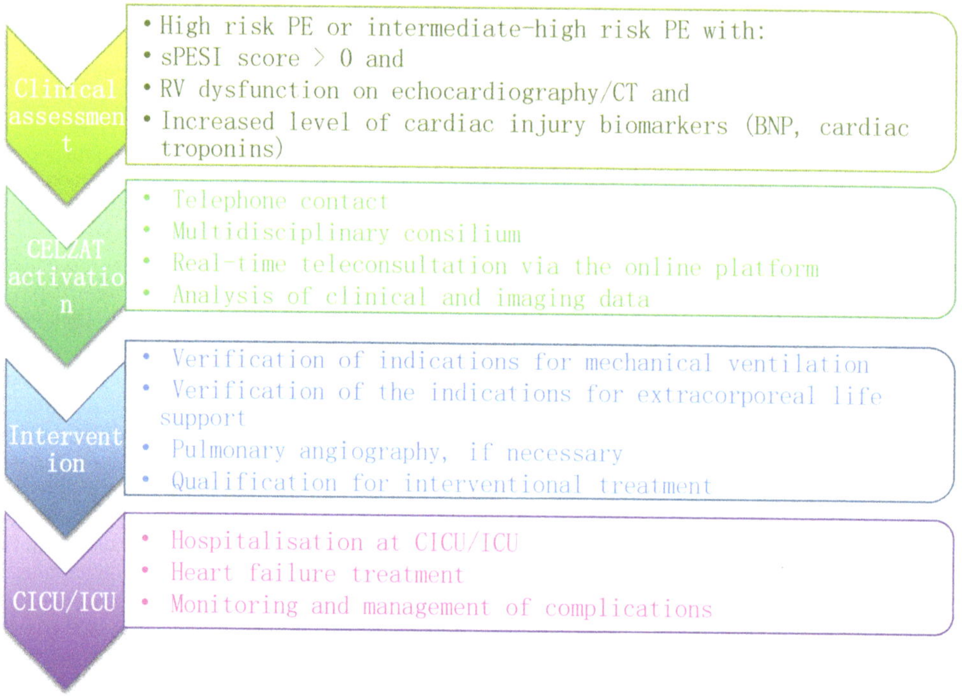

**Clinical assessment**
- High risk PE or intermediate-high risk PE with:
- sPESI score > 0 and
- RV dysfunction on echocardiography/CT and
- Increased level of cardiac injury biomarkers (BNP, cardiac troponins)

**CELZAT activation**
- Telephone contact
- Multidisciplinary consilium
- Real-time teleconsultation via the online platform
- Analysis of clinical and imaging data

**Intervention**
- Verification of indications for mechanical ventilation
- Verification of the indications for extracorporeal life support
- Pulmonary angiography, if necessary
- Qualification for interventional treatment

**CICU/ICU**
- Hospitalisation at CICU/ICU
- Heart failure treatment
- Monitoring and management of complications

**Figure 1.** Activation flowchart of CELZAT. PE—pulmonary embolism, sPESI—simplified Pulmonary Embolism Severity Index, RV—right ventricle, CT—computed tomography, BNP—brain natriuretic peptide, CICU—cardiac intensive care unit, ICU—intensive care unit.

The analysis of subsequent patients is conducted with the use of an online teleconsultation platform (Invisium MED, Ives-System, Warsaw, Poland). After logging in to the platform via a standard web browser, the analysis of clinical data and the results of additional examinations, which had previously been placed on the virtual drive, is performed during a real-time audiovisual consultation. The decisions made during the teleconsultation include (i) a possibility of pharmacological treatment optimization, (ii) indications for respiratory therapy, (iii) the use of extracorporeal membrane oxygenation (ECMO) and other forms of extra corporeal life support, (iv) indications for further invasive diagnostics (selective pulmonary angiography) and eventually percutaneous treatment and (v) indications for surgical treatment.

After the intervention, the patients are hospitalized in the Intensive Care Unit or the Cardiac Intensive Care Unit to stabilize the general condition, normalize hemodynamic parameters and monitor and treat the possible complications of the therapy. Particular emphasis is placed on the potential mechanical complications related to the percutaneous therapy, such as pulmonary dissection or perforation, cardiac tamponade and vascular access complications, as well as systemic complications, including contrast-induced acute kidney injury, arrhythmias, hypotension, hemolysis or bleeding.

*2.2. Patient Enrollment and Data Collection*

All patients diagnosed with PE who presented to any of the participating centers between September 2017 and December 2021 were included in the study. Information about clinical and treatment data was obtained from medical records, including (i) demographic data; (ii) symptoms and signs at presentation; (iii) risk factors of venous thromboembolism (VTE); (iv) comorbidities; (v) relevant laboratory and imaging findings (concentrations of cardiac troponins and natriuretic factors, features of RV overload on echocardiogram or computed tomography); (vi) VTE location, including the presence of deep vein thrombosis; (vii) in-hospital pharmacotherapy and interventional therapy; (vii) the need for endotracheal intubation, ECMO and admission to intensive care unit; and (viii) in-hospital and 1-month outcomes (mortality, recurrent PE or DVT and bleeding complications, as defined by the International Society of Thrombosis and Hemostasis, ISTH).

### 2.3. Assessment of PE Severity

The severity of PE was each time categorized into high, intermediate–high, intermediate–low or low, according to the most recent ESC guidelines [1]. In all patients, the PESI and sPESI were calculated. High-risk PE was defined as confirmed acute PE with hemodynamic instability, i.e., clinical symptoms of cardiogenic shock or persistent hypotension (systolic blood pressure (BP < 90 mmHg or systolic BP drop $\geq$ 40 mmHg, lasting longer than 15 min and not caused by new-onset arrhythmia, hypovolemia or sepsis). The intermediate–high-risk group included patients who were hemodynamically stable but had features of RV overload (dysfunction on echocardiography or dilation on computed tomography pulmonary angiogram, CTPA) and laboratory marker of myocardial damage (cardiac troponins level above the institution-specific cut-off values). Intermediate–low-risk was defined as the presence of RV overload on echocardiography or CTPA, or elevated level of troponins, or PESI class III or higher, or at least 1 point in sPESI. The low-risk category involved patients in the PESI class I or II, or 0 points in sPESI.

### 2.4. Treatment and Outcomes

Therapeutic interventions in hospital were recorded for each patient and involved: anticoagulation alone, systemic thrombolysis or interventional treatment. Anticoagulation was defined as the administration of the following: unfractionated heparin (UFH), low molecular weight heparin (LMWH), vitamin K antagonists (VKA) or direct oral anticoagulants (DOACs) without any additional therapies. Systemic thrombolysis referred to the intravenous administration of recombinant tissue plasminogen activator (rtPA). Catheter-directed procedures included catheter-directed thrombectomy (CDT), catheter-directed thrombolysis (CDL) and surgical embolectomy.

Interventional treatment was applied to patients with cardiogenic shock or significant hemodynamic instability who either were non-responsive or had contraindications to standard thrombolytic therapy. Catheter-directed thrombectomy or thrombolysis were preferred in patients at high perioperative risk of mortality and those who were disqualified from pulmonary embolectomy due to logistical reasons (lack of technical possibilities to transport the patient to the embolectomy-performing center, for example due to hemodynamic instability). Catheter-directed thrombectomy (CDT) was performed using the Angiojet™ Rheolytic Thrombectomy System (Boston Scientific, Marlborough, MA, USA), Cleaner XT™ Rotational Thrombectomy System (Argon Medical Devices, Athens, TX, USA), or Indigo CAT8 XTORQ system (Penumbra, Alameda, CA, USA), depending on the anatomical conditions and morphology of thromboembolic lesions. The rate of catheter-directed thrombolysis (CDL), surgical embolectomy, ECMO or inferior vena cava (IVC) filter placement was also recorded.

Patient outcomes were assessed in-hospital and at 1- and 12-month follow-ups. Follow-ups included (i) mortality, (ii) stroke, (iii) recurrent PE/DVT and (iv) bleeding complications as defined by the ISTH.

### 2.5. Statistical Analysis

Statistical analysis was conducted using IBM SPSS Statistics, version 27.0 (IBM, Sheffield, UK). Categorical variables were presented as number and percent. Continuous variables were presented as mean and standard deviation or median with interquartile range, depending on the distribution. A $p$-value below 0.05 was considered significant.

## 3. Results

### 3.1. Baseline Characteristics

During the 52-month enrollment period, there were 235 CELZAT activations: 104 in Medical University of Warsaw (44.3%), 116 in European Health Centre Otwock (49.3%) and 15 Medicover Hospital (6.4%). Patients' characteristics at admission are presented in Table 1. The mean age was $60.3 \pm 16.8$ years, and the majority of patients were men (53.6%). The most common symptom at admission was dyspnea at minimal exertion (New York Heart Association [NYHA] functional class III; 42.0%) or at rest (NYHA class IV; 33.3% patients). Other symptoms included chest pain, syncope, cough and pneumonia, which were present in 31.9%, 16.6%, 15.7% and 13.2% of patients, respectively. The least common symptom was hemoptysis in only 5.5% of cases. Malignancy was the most frequent PE risk factor (34.0%). Besides malignancy, obesity (27.2%) and recent hospitalization (25.5%) were the most common, followed by smoking (24.7%). Thirty-nine patients had a history of previous DVT (16.6%), and 13 patients had previous PE (5.5%). Previous COVID-19 infection was risk factor for PE in 14 cases (5.9%).

**Table 1.** Baseline characteristics of PE patients.

|  | Patients (n = 235) |
|---|---|
| **Baseline characteristics** |  |
| Age, years (mean ± SD) | 60.3 ± 16.8 |
| Sex, male (n, %) | 126 (53.6%) |
| **Symptoms on admission** |  |
| Dyspnea (NYHA; n, %) |  |
| I–II | 43 (24.7%) |
| III | 73 (42.0%) |
| IV | 58 (33.3%) |
| Chest pain (n, %) | 75 (31.9%) |
| Syncope (n, %) | 39 (16.6%) |
| Cough (n, %) | 37 (15.7%) |
| Pneumonia (n, %) | 31 (13.2%) |
| Hemoptysis (n, %) | 13 (5.5%) |
| **Comorbidities (n, %)** |  |
| Coronary artery disease | 24 (10.2%) |
| Congestive heart failure | 22 (9.4%) |
| Atrial fibrillation | 16 (6.8%) |
| Arterial hypertension | 113 (48.1%) |
| COPD | 11 (4.7%) |
| Diabetes mellitus | 41 (17.4%) |
| Obesity | 64 (27.2%) |
| Chronic kidney disease | 17 (7.2%) |
| Stroke | 15 (6.4%) |
| Depression | 12 (5.1%) |
| Malignancy | 80 (34.0%) |
| Thrombophilia | 12 (5.1%) |
| **Other VTE risk factors (n, %)** |  |
| Smoking | 58 (24.7%) |
| Indwelling catheter | 7 (3.0%) |
| Hormonal therapy | 13 (5.5%) |
| Reduced mobility | 27 (11.5%) |
| Recent hospitalization | 60 (25.5%) |
| Recent surgery | 28 (11.9%) |
| Recent trauma | 14 (6.0%) |
| Prior PE | 13 (5.5%) |
| Prior DVT | 39 (16.6%) |
| COVID-19 infection | 14 (6.0%) |

NYHA—New York Heart Association, COPD—chronic obstructive pulmonary disease, VTE—venous thromboembolism, DVT—deep vein thrombosis.

*3.2. Characteristics of Pulmonary Embolism*

The risk of early mortality was low in 51 patients (21.8%), intermediate–low in 83 (35.3%), intermediate–high in 80 (34.0%) and high in 21 (8.9%) patients (Figure 2). The vast majority of patients had thrombus located bilaterally (77.4%) and centrally (82.6%). The central location of the thrombus was defined as the saddle, main pulmonary artery, lobar artery and intracardiac location. Peripheral location was defined as the segmental and subsegmental artery. Patients with high-risk PE presented more often with bilateral PE (95.2%) and central PE (100.0%), compared to other risk categories (Figures 3 and 4). However, bilateral and central PE was also the most frequent phenotype in all other subgroups of patients.

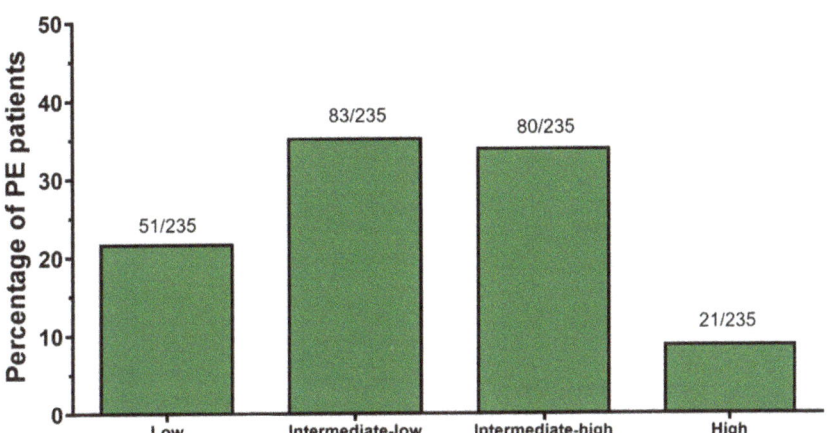

**Figure 2.** Distribution of the early mortality risk groups in the study population.

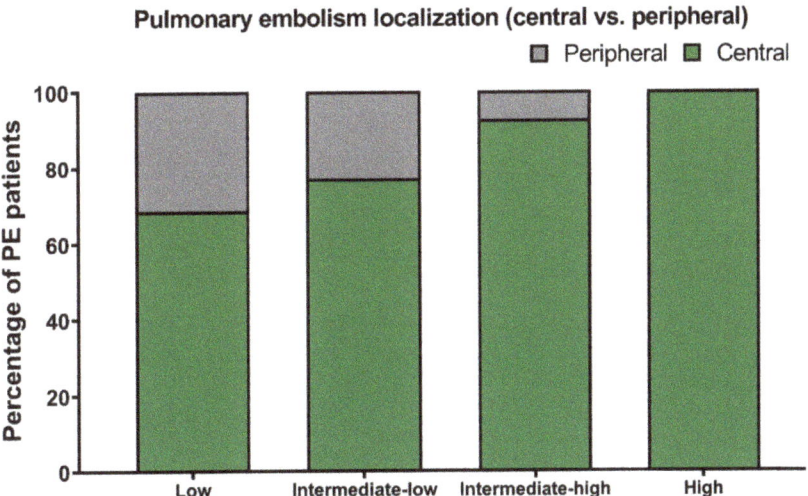

**Figure 3.** Pulmonary embolism localization (central vs. peripheral) according to the risk of early mortality.

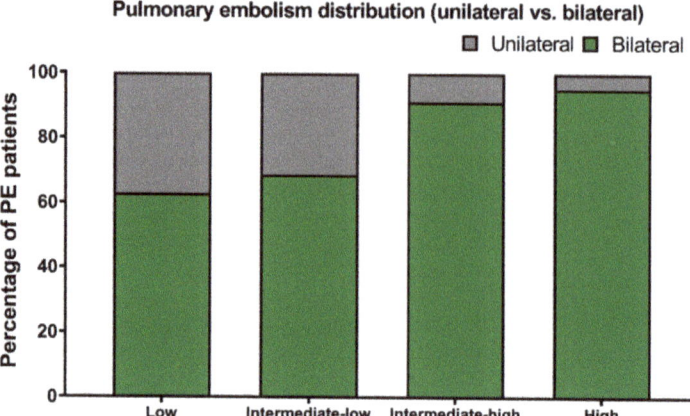

**Figure 4.** Pulmonary embolism distribution (unilateral vs. bilateral) according to the risk of early mortality.

The characteristics of PE categorized according to the risk of early mortality are showed in Table 2. The most common parameter of PE severity was RV overload on echocardiography or CTPA (67.2%), followed by elevated concentration of natriuretic peptides (73.6%) and troponins (55.7%). PE was accompanied by DVT in 51.1% of all patients. Twenty-six patients required endotracheal intubated (11.1%), fifteen high-risk patients required ECMO (6.4%) and eighty-four patients from intermediate–high and high-risk of mortality subgroups (83.2% of both subgroups) were admitted to the ICU. One hundred twenty-six patients were in the PESI class III or higher (53.6%). A high-risk score (at least 1 point on the sPESI scale) was present in 162 patients (68.9%).

**Table 2.** Characteristics of PE categorized according to the risk of early mortality.

| PE Risk Category | Low (n = 51) | | Intermediate–Low (n = 83) | | Intermediate–High (n = 80) | | High (n = 21) | | All (n = 235) | |
|---|---|---|---|---|---|---|---|---|---|---|
| PE location (n, %) | | | | | | | | | | |
| Bilateral | 32 | 62.7% | 57 | 68.7% | 73 | 91.3% | 20 | 95.2% | 182 | 77.4% |
| Unilateral | 19 | 37.3% | 26 | 31.3% | 7 | 8.7% | 1 | 4.8% | 53 | 22.6% |
| Central | 35 | 68.6% | 64 | 77.1% | 74 | 92.5% | 21 | 100.0% | 194 | 82.6% |
| Peripheral | 16 | 31.4% | 19 | 22.9% | 6 | 7.5% | 0 | 0.0% | 41 | 17.4% |
| Saddle | 1 | 2.0% | 8 | 9.6% | 26 | 32.5% | 9 | 42.9% | 44 | 18.7% |
| Main pulmonary artery | 19 | 37.3% | 28 | 33.7% | 61 | 76.3% | 16 | 76.2% | 124 | 52.8% |
| Lobar artery | 33 | 64.7% | 61 | 73.5% | 63 | 78.8% | 19 | 90.5% | 176 | 74.9% |
| Segmental artery | 43 | 84.3% | 70 | 84.3% | 51 | 63.8% | 14 | 66.7% | 178 | 75.7% |
| Intracardiac | 0 | 0.0% | 0 | 0.0% | 7 | 8.8% | 2 | 9.5% | 9 | 3.8% |
| Parameters of PE severity (n, %) PE location (n, %) | | | | | | | | | | |
| RV dysfunction (ECHO) | 0 | 0.0% | 21 | 25.3% | 70 | 87.5% | 16 | 76.2% | 107 | 45.5% |
| RV dilation (CTPA) | 0 | 0.0% | 10 | 12.0% | 31 | 38.8% | 10 | 47.6% | 51 | 21.7% |
| ↑ Troponin | 0 | 0.0% | 38 | 45.8% | 80 | 100.0% | 14 | 66.7% | 131 | 55.7% |
| ↑ Natriuretic peptides | 20 | 39.2% | 61 | 73.5% | 74 | 92.5% | 18 | 85.7% | 173 | 73.6% |
| DVT | 20 | 39.2% | 34 | 41.0% | 54 | 67.5% | 12 | 57.1% | 120 | 51.1% |
| PESI class (n, %) | | | | | | | | | | |

Table 2. Cont.

| PE Risk Category | | Low (n = 51) | | Intermediate–Low (n = 83) | | Intermediate–High (n = 80) | | High (n = 21) | | All (n = 235) | |
|---|---|---|---|---|---|---|---|---|---|---|---|
| | I–II | 36 | 70.6% | 38 | 45.8% | 34 | 42.5% | 1 | 4.8% | 109 | 46.4% |
| | III | 7 | 13.8% | 15 | 18.1% | 28 | 35.0% | 1 | 4.8% | 51 | 21.7% |
| | IV | 4 | 7.8% | 19 | 22.9% | 10 | 12.5% | 5 | 23.8% | 38 | 16.2% |
| | V | 4 | 7.8% | 11 | 13.2% | 8 | 10.0% | 14 | 66.6% | 37 | 15.7% |
| | Score (median, IQR) | 65 (49–88) | | 93 (74–113) | | 89 (71–105) | | 144 (123–195) | | 88 (69–114) | |
| sPESI (n, %) | | | | | | | | | | | |
| | Low risk | 32 | 62.7% | 21 | 25.3% | 20 | 25.0% | 0 | 0.0% | 73 | 31.1% |
| | High risk | 19 | 37.3% | 62 | 74.7% | 60 | 75.0% | 21 | 100.0% | 162 | 68.9% |
| Clinical severity (n, %) | | | | | | | | | | | |
| | Intubation | 0 | 0.0% | 1 | 1.2% | 13 | 16.3% | 12 | 57.1% | 26 | 11.1% |
| | ECMO support | 0 | 0.0% | 0 | 0.0% | 10 | 12.5% | 5 | 23.8% | 15 | 6.4% |
| | ICU admission | 24 | 47.1% | 37 | 44.6% | 63 | 78.8% | 21 | 100.0% | 145 | 61.7% |

RV—right ventricle, ECHO—echocardiography, CTPA—computed tomography pulmonary angiogram, ECMO—extracorporeal membrane oxygenation.

### 3.3. Treatment

The details of in-hospital and post-discharge treatment according to mortality risk groups are presented in Table 3. Anticoagulation alone was the most frequently administered treatment, received by 84.7% of patients and this trend applied to all risk subgroups, except for high-risk patients, where systemic thrombolysis (47.6%) and interventional therapy (52%; CDT/CDL 28.6% and surgical embolectomy 23.4%) were the prevailing treatment options.

Table 3. In-hospital and post-discharge treatment according to mortality risk groups.

| PE Risk Category | Low (n = 51) | | Intermediate–Low (n = 83) | | Intermediate–High (n = 80) | | High (n = 21) | | All (n = 235) | |
|---|---|---|---|---|---|---|---|---|---|---|
| **In-hospital (n, %) *** | | | | | | | | | | |
| Anticoagulation alone | 51 | 100.0% | 81 | 97.6% | 63 | 78.8% | 4 | 19.0% | 199 | 84.7% |
| Systemic thrombolysis | 0 | 0.0% | 1 | 1.2% | 4 | 5.0% | 10 | 47.6% | 15 | 6.4% |
| CDT/CDL | 0 | 0.0% | 1 | 1.2% | 2 | 5.0% | 6 | 28.6% | 11 | 4.7% |
| Surgical embolectomy | 0 | 0.0% | 0 | 0.0% | 10 | 12.5% | 5 | 23.4% | 15 | 6.4% |
| IVC filter | 1 | 2.0% | 8 | 9.6% | 7 | 8.8% | 3 | 14.3% | 19 | 8.1% |
| **At discharge (n, %) ** ** | n = 51 | | n = 80 | | n = 76 | | n = 13 | | n = 220 | |
| VKA | 3 | 5.9% | 5 | 6.3% | 12 | 15.8% | 2 | 15.4% | 22 | 10.0% |
| DOAC | 40 | 78.4% | 41 | 51.2% | 37 | 48.7% | 3 | 23.1% | 121 | 55.0% |
| LMWH | 8 | 15.7% | 34 | 42.5% | 27 | 35.5% | 8 | 61.5% | 77 | 35.0% |

* The number of patients might exceed 235 due to combined therapies applied to some patients (e.g., interventional therapy on top of anticoagulation or systemic thrombolysis). ** The number of patients at discharge is affected by in-hospital mortality. CDT—catheter directed thrombectomy, CDL—catheter directed thrombolysis, IVC—inferior vena cava, VKA—vitamin K antagonists, DOAC—direct oral anticoagulants, LMWH—low molecular weight heparin.

Systemic thrombolysis was administered in one intermediate–low-risk patient (1.2%) and four intermediate–high-risk patients (5.0%). Eleven patients (9.4%) were treated with catheter-directed procedures (seven patients with catheter-directed thrombectomy and four with catheter-directed thrombolysis. Fifteen patients (6.4%) with intermediate–high or high-risk PE underwent surgical embolectomy. Nineteen patients (8.1%) received IVC filter. The high rate of IVC use was due to the characteristics of the patients consulted by CELZAT. In addition to PE, the consulted patients had comorbidities that are contraindications to standard anticoagulant therapy. The most common indications for IVC filter were increased risk of bleeding in the context of malignancy and status after orthopedic surgery for massive trauma. In a few cases, the indication for IVC filter implantation was the recurrence of PE during standard anticoagulation treatment, which occurred most frequently in patients with oncological metastasis.

Combined therapy was performed in 10 patients. Four patients were treated by catheter-directed thrombectomy with subsequent transcatheter thrombolysis. Three of them received systemic thrombolysis followed by surgical embolectomy. In one case the transcatheter procedure was associated with further systemic thrombolysis and in one case the transcatheter procedure was followed by surgical embolectomy.

At discharge, the majority of all patients received DOACs (55.0%), followed by LMWH (35.0%) and VKA (10.0%). Among patients who received LMWH, 46 had a coexistent malignancy.

### 3.4. Outcomes

The in-hospital, 1-month follow-up and 12-month follow-up outcome events according to mortality risk groups are showed in Table 4. The rate of in-hospital mortality was 6.4% (15/235 patients: 8 in the high-risk subgroup, 4 in the intermediate–high-risk subgroup and 3 in the intermediate–low-risk subgroup). Three of them suffered from malignancy. All patients presented with dyspnea NYHA class IV (thirteen patients) or III (two patients). Thirteen patients were admitted to ICU and eight required endotracheal intubation. Nine patients received only anticoagulation, in two patients systemic thrombolysis was implemented, two patients underwent CDT and another two received combined therapy.

**Table 4.** In-hospital, 1-month and 12-month follow-up outcome events according to the mortality risk groups.

| PE Risk Category | Low (n = 51) | | Intermediate–Low (n = 83) | | Intermediate–High (n = 80) | | High (n = 21) | | All (n = 235) | |
|---|---|---|---|---|---|---|---|---|---|---|
| **In-hospital events (n, %)** | | | | | | | | | | |
| Death | 0 | 0.0% | 3 | 3.6% | 4 | 5.0% | 8 | 38.1% | 15 | 6.4% |
| Stroke | 0 | 0.0% | 1 | 1.2% | 0 | 0.0% | 2 | 9.5% | 3 | 1.3% |
| Major bleeding | 0 | 0.0% | 4 | 4.8% | 1 | 1.3% | 2 | 9.5% | 7 | 3.0% |
| Minor bleeding | 1 | 2.0% | 7 | 8.4% | 2 | 2.5% | 2 | 9.5% | 12 | 5.1% |
| Recurrent PE | 0 | 0.0% | 0 | 0.0% | 1 | 1.3% | 0 | 0.0% | 1 | 0.4% |
| Recurrent DVT | 0 | 0.0% | 1 | 1.2% | 0 | 0.0% | 0 | 0.0% | 1 | 0.4% |
| **1-month follow-up \*\*** | | | | | | | | | | |
| Death | 1 | 2.0% | 0 | 0.0% | 0 | 0.0% | 0 | 0.0% | 1 | 0.4% |
| Stroke | 1 | 2.0% | 0 | 0.0% | 0 | 0.0% | 0 | 0.0% | 1 | 0.4% |
| Major bleeding | 1 | 2.0% | 0 | 0.0% | 0 | 0.0% | 0 | 0.0% | 1 | 0.4% |
| Minor bleeding | 0 | 0.0% | 1 | 1.2% | 0 | 0.0% | 0 | 0.0% | 1 | 0.4% |
| Recurrent PE | 0 | 0.0% | 0 | 0.0% | 0 | 0.0% | 0 | 0.0% | 0 | 0.0% |
| Recurrent DVT | 0 | 0.0% | 0 | 0.0% | 0 | 0.0% | 0 | 0.0% | 0 | 0.0% |
| **12-month follow-up \*\*** | | | | | | | | | | |
| Death | 1 | 2.0% | 1 | 1.2% | 2 | 2.6% | 2 | 15.4% | 6 | 2.7% |
| Stroke | 0 | 0.0% | 0 | 0.0% | 0 | 0.0% | 0 | 0.0% | 0 | 0.0% |
| Major bleeding | 0 | 0.0% | 0 | 0.0% | 0 | 0.0% | 0 | 0.0% | 0 | 0.0% |
| Minor bleeding | 0 | 0.0% | 1 | 1.2% | 0 | 0.0% | 1 | 7.7% | 2 | 0.9% |
| Recurrent PE | 1 | 2.0% | 0 | 0.0% | 0 | 0.0% | 0 | 0.0% | 1 | 0.4% |
| Recurrent DVT | 0 | 0.0% | 1 | 1.2% | 0 | 0.0% | 0 | 0.0% | 1 | 0.4% |

\*\* The number of patients at follow-up is affected by in-hospital and follow-up mortality.

There were twelve minor bleeding events (5.1%) and four of them required reduced dosage of anticoagulant therapy. There were seven major bleeding events (3.0%), which required blood transfusion and the modification of anticoagulation treatment. There were three strokes (1.3%): one in the intermediate–low-risk patient treated with anticoagulation only and two in high-risk patients treated with thrombolysis. There was one fatal recurrence of PE in the intermediate–high patient treated with systemic full-dose thrombolysis and one recurrence of DVT, associated with major bleeding and the modification of anticoagulant treatment. In the last case, an IVC filter was applied to protect patients during the next weeks.

At 1-month follow-up, there was one death and one stroke. Two bleeding events were registered. One of them was minor and did not require future action. Another one was major and required medical attention. The latter patient died during the 1-year follow-up. Other adverse events during the 1-year follow-up included five deaths, one recurrent PE, one recurrent DVT and two minor bleeding events.

## 4. Discussion

The goal of PERT is to deliver rapid, interdisciplinary care to patients with PE to facilitate the access to advanced treatment and improve outcomes. Since the launch of the first PERT in 2012, the idea of PERT has spread worldwide. The results of hitherto published observational studies suggest that implementation of PERT increased patients' access to advanced therapies (systemic thrombolysis, catheter-directed procedures, surgery) without increasing the number of bleeding complications [6,7,10]. Moreover, recent studies comparing outcomes in the pre- and post-PERT era showed that the availability of multidisciplinary PERT was associated with decreased 30-day mortality, especially among high-risk patients, without incurring additional hospital costs or protracting hospital length-of-stay [11,12]. However, the clear benefits of PERT in terms of mortality have not been confirmed in all studies [6], which is likely due to the limited sample size and short follow-up time of patients included in these studies [6–8,10–18]. Hence, there is an unmet need to collect more data regarding the performance of PERT and share them with the medical community.

The current study is the first report concerning the activity of the local PERT, CELZAT. CELZAT operates in accordance with the standards outlined in the position paper of Polish PERT Initiative [19], with the primary objective to deliver care to intermediate–high and high-risk PE patients. However, in our cohort, less than half of patients presented with intermediate–high-risk PE (34.0%) and high-risk PE (8.9%). We registered numerous activations of PERT in the intermediate–low (35.4%) and low-risk (21.7%) subgroups, which might be due to two reasons. First, substantial efforts have been made to raise the awareness of the local PERT via journal publications [19], conference presentations and social media, which prompted the treating physicians to contact PERT experts in case of any acute PE. Second, the majority of intermediate–low and low-risk patients in our cohort presented with bilateral and central PE, raising concerns regarding the potential risk for sudden clinical deterioration and death despite normal hemodynamics at initial assessment. PERT activation in low-risk patients has been noticed in other papers reporting PERT activity [8,14], introducing the concept of a "high-risk patient with a low-risk PE" [8]. Further research is required to investigate the clinical benefits and economic efficacy of PERT activation in low-risk patients. For example, PERT activation might be rational in order to optimally manage the low-risk patients with contraindications to anticoagulation or with comorbidities requiring a multidisciplinary approach.

Anticoagulation was the most frequently administered treatment in all risk subgroups except for high-risk patients (approximately 85% of our cohort), in accordance with previous reports [8,14]. The most frequently administered anticoagulants at discharge were DOACs (55.0%), whereas only a minority of patients received VKA (10.0%). LMWH was received by a substantial number of patients at discharge (35.0%), the majority of whom presented with a co-existing malignancy. The choice of anticoagulation for cancer-associated VTE is a major therapeutic challenge due to a delicate balance between the recurrent thromboembolic and bleeding events in these patients [20]. LMWH has traditionally been the standard treatment for cancer-associated VTE due to higher efficacy and comparable safety, compared to VKA [21]. However, the results of recent trials comparing LMWH to DOAC showed that DOAC might be more effective than LMWH at preventing recurrent VTE in cancer patients but at the cost of increased bleeding, especially in patients with gastrointestinal (GI) and genitourinary (GU) tract cancer. Consequently, the ISTH International

Initiative on Thrombosis and Cancer (ITAC) guidelines state that DOACs can be used as first line treatment for cancer-associated thrombosis in non-GI/GU cancer patients at low bleeding risk. Among patients with GI/GU cancer-associated thrombosis, LMWH is still preferred [22]. Accordingly, the ESC guidelines recommend that edoxaban or rivaroxaban should be considered as an alternative to LMWH, with special caution for patients with GI cancer [1]. However, as demonstrated in our cohort, clinicians are still reluctant to prescribe DOAC in cancer patients and more evidence-based data are required to establish the optimal treatment regimen in this challenging population.

The proportion of patients receiving any advanced therapy (systemic thrombolysis, surgical embolectomy or catheter-directed procedures) in our study was 15.3% (81.0% of patients in the high-risk subgroup and 21.3% in the intermediate–high-risk group), confirming the widespread access of patients to the advanced treatment methods within PERT. As showed by the National PERT Consortium™ multicenter registry, this proportion varies between institutions, ranging from 16% to 46%, underlying the need to share the institutional PERT experiences [8,17]. In the entire cohort, systemic thrombolysis and surgical embolectomy were the most common advanced therapies (6.4% each group), followed by catheter-directed procedures (4.7%).

Although the evidence-based data regarding the effect of catheter-directed procedures on mortality are still pending, catheter-directed therapies has become an important and less-invasive treatment option both in intermediate–high and high-risk patients, either to temporarily stabilize the patient before surgical embolectomy or as a final therapy if hemodynamical stability is restored [23]. Although catheter-directed procedures are dedicated to intermediate–high and high-risk patients, they have also been applied to one intermediate–low-risk patient, who deteriorated hemodynamically following the initial assessment. Among eleven patients treated with catheter-directed procedures, there were four in-hospital deaths (one due to a stroke) and two major bleeding events. Although the efficacy and safety of catheter-directed procedures has been shown in other PERT reports, our data indicate the need for cautious patient qualification for these therapies, as they may be associated with complications [10,14–18].

The in-hospital mortality rate in our cohort was 6.4%, which is slightly lower than reported by other studies (8 and 14%) [10,14–18], likely due to the large percentage of low and intermediate–low-risk patients in our cohort. We registered only one death during the 1-month follow-up period, indicating the efficacy of rapid treatment implementation by PERT. The mortality rate in high-risk patients was high (38.1%), as compared to relatively low mortality in other subgroups (0.0% in low-risk, 3.6% in intermediate–low-risk and 5.0% in intermediate–high-risk). Although the mortality rate in high-risk PE patients remains unacceptably high, recent trend analyses showed a substantial decrease in mortality due to high-risk PE from 72.7% in 1999 to 49.8% in 2017 [24,25]. In high-risk PE, systemic thrombolysis is the first-line treatment and surgical embolectomy is recommended when systemic thrombolysis is contraindicated or has failed [1]. High-risk patients constituted approximately 9% of our cohort and were all treated with either systemic thrombolysis or, in the presence of contraindications, interventional treatment (surgical embolectomy or catheter-directed procedures). The detailed management of some of these patients has been previously published [26,27]. The high risk of mortality in high-risk PE patients, despite multidisciplinary PERT management, underlines the need for further treatment optimisation in this challenging population.

Any bleeding occurred in 8.1% and major bleeding in 3.0% of patients, which is lower than the previously reported bleeding rates, ranging from 11–13% for any bleeding and 4–13% for major events [10,13,15–18]. In our study, in-hospital bleeding events occurred in all risk groups, and five of the bleeding events occurred following systemic thrombolysis. These findings remain consistent with previous reports [8]. There were two bleeding episodes during the 1-month follow-up. However, these findings should be interpreted with caution due to a very low number of incidents.

Finally, we observed PERT activation cases in patients with non-thromboembolic embolism, such as those with iatrogenic PE [28,29]. In these situations, individualized risk stratification by PERT allowed the determination as to whether an interventional or conservative approach is more beneficial. Hence, although the primary goal of PERT is to consult patients with thromboembolism, the availability and expertise of PERT provided additional clinical benefits in non-thromboembolic, difficult clinical scenarios.

## 5. Limitations

Our analysis had several limitations. First, over 50% our cohort consisted of low- and intermediate–low-risk patients. Hence, the reported results are preliminary and should be confirmed in a larger cohort and in higher risk patients. The large proportion of low- and intermediate–low-risk patients does not allow an effective assessment of treatment complications and overall mortality. Further studies should specifically focus on patients in the intermediate–high- and high-risk groups. Second, we report on the activity of a single PERT, created at highly specialized academic medical centers with access to interdisciplinary care. Although different institutional PERTs have similar operating models, the local factors may affect the individual therapeutic choices, as reflected by different rates of advanced therapies, depending on the center [10,14–18]. Therefore, our results cannot be directly extrapolated to other institutions. Third, the efficacy and safety outcomes are limited to 12-month observation period, which does not allow the deriving of conclusions regarding the long-term benefits of PERT implementation. Since the goal of this study was to report on the characteristics and outcomes of patients consulted by the local PERT, CELZAT, our study design precluded comparison between some subgroups. It would be useful to compare patient outcomes before and after CELZAT implementation. Unfortunately, the lack of standardized reporting of patients with PE before CELZAT implementation made this analysis not feasible. In addition, subanalyses of outcomes in PE subgroups depend on the initial risk of mortality and/or comorbidities, such as malignancy. Fourth, because of the lack of data regarding the family history of VTE, we could not take this risk factor into account, which may be an important cause of VTE, especially in young patients. Finally, we did not evaluate the cost-efficacy of PERT implementation (length of hospital stay, costs of PERT activation, patient's quality of life following the PE episode). Hence, we cannot derive conclusions regarding the economic effects of PERT implementation in our institution.

## 6. Conclusions

We provide the initial experience regarding the 5-year activity of the local PERT (CELZAT). The implementation of a multidisciplinary PERT enabled patient-tailored decision making and facilitated the access to advanced therapies, with subsequent low overall mortality and treatment complication rates. Our findings add to the previously described experiences derived from other institutional PERTs, confirming the benefits of PERT implementation. There is a need for multicenter collaboration between the local PERTs to derive firm conclusions regarding the favorable effect of PERT activity on patient outcomes.

**Author Contributions:** Conceptualization, A.P., A.T. and M.K.; methodology, A.P., A.G. and M.K.; software, A.G.; validation, A.P. and M.K.; formal analysis, A.P. and A.G.; investigation, P.K., K.W. (Katarzyna Wrona), D.Z. (Dominika Zajkowska), J.M.S., D.R., K.J., M.W., R.W., G.P. and P.S.; resources, S.D., M.B., D.Z. (Dariusz Zieliński) and M.F.; data curation, A.P. and A.G.; writing—original draft preparation, A.P. and A.G.; writing—review and editing, M.G., A.T. and M.K.; visualization, P.K. and K.W. (Krzysztof Wróbel), D.Z. (Dominika Zajkowska), J.M.S., D.R., K.J., M.W., R.W., G.P. and P.S.; supervision, M.G., A.T. and M.K.; project administration, A.P., A.G. and P.K.; funding acquisition, M.K. All authors have read and agreed to the published version of the manuscript.

**Funding:** This manuscript was supported by the Centre of Postgraduate Medical Education, project number 501-1-054-25-22.

**Institutional Review Board Statement:** Not applicable.

**Informed Consent Statement:** Patient consent was waived due to the retrospective character of the study.

**Data Availability Statement:** Raw data are available upon request to the corresponding author.

**Conflicts of Interest:** The authors declare no conflict of interest. The funders had no role in the design of the study; in the collection, analyses, or interpretation of data; in the writing of the manuscript, or in the decision to publish the results.

## References

1. Konstantinides, S.V.; Meyer, G.; Becattini, C.; Bueno, H.; Geersing, G.-J.; Harjola, V.-P.; Huisman, M.V.; Humbert, M.; Jennings, C.S.; Jiménez, D.; et al. 2019 ESC Guidelines for the diagnosis and management of acute pulmonary embolism developed in collaboration with the European Respiratory Society (ERS): The Task Force for the diagnosis and management of acute pulmonary embolism of the European Society of Cardiology (ESC). *Eur. Heart J.* **2020**, *41*, 543–603. [PubMed]
2. Wendelboe, A.M.; Raskob, G.E. Global burden of thrombosis: Epidemiologic aspects. *Circ. Res.* **2016**, *118*, 1340–1347. [CrossRef] [PubMed]
3. Barco, S.; Woersching, A.L.; Spyropoulos, A.C.; Piovella, F.; Mahan, C.E. European Union-28: An annualised cost-of-illness model for venous thromboembolism. *Thromb. Haemost.* **2016**, *115*, 800–808. [CrossRef] [PubMed]
4. Stein, P.D.; Beemath, A.; Matta, F.; Weg, J.G.; Yusen, R.D.; Hales, C.A.; Hull, R.D.; Leeper, K.V.; Sostman, D.; Woodard, P.K.; et al. Clinical characteristics of patients with acute pulmonary embolism: Data from PIOPED II. *Am. J. Med.* **2007**, *120*, 871–879. [CrossRef]
5. Provias, T.; Dudzinski, D.M.; Jaff, M.R.; Rosenfield, K.; Channick, R.; Baker, J.; Weinberg, I.; Donaldson, C.; Narayan, R.; Rassi, A.N.; et al. The Massachusetts General Hospital Pulmonary Embolism Response Team (MGH PERT): Creation of a multidisciplinary program to improve care of patients with massive and submassive pulmonary embolism. *Hosp. Pract.* **2014**, *42*, 31–37. [CrossRef]
6. Rosovsky, R.; Chang, Y.; Rosenfield, K.; Channick, R.; Jaff, M.R.; Weinberg, I.; Sundt, T.; Witkin, A.; Rodriguez-Lopez, J.; Parry, B.A.; et al. Changes in treatment and outcomes after creation of a pulmonary embolism response team (PERT), a 10-year analysis. *J. Thromb. Thrombolysis* **2019**, *47*, 31–40. [CrossRef]
7. Liang, Y.; Nie, S.P.; Wang, X.; Thomas, A.; Thompson, E.; Zhao, G.Q.; Han, J.; Wang, J.; Griffiths, M.J.D. Role of Pulmonary Embolism Response Team in patients with intermediate- and high-risk pulmonary embolism: A concise review and preliminary experience from China. *J. Geriatr. Cardiol.* **2020**, *17*, 510–518. [CrossRef]
8. Schultz, J.; Giordano, N.; Zheng, H.; Parry, B.A.; Barnes, G.D.; Heresi, G.A.; Jaber, W.; Wood, T.; Todoran, T.; Courtney, D.M.; et al. EXPRESS: A Multidisciplinary Pulmonary Embolism Response Team (PERT)—Experience from a national multicenter consortium. *Pulm. Circ.* **2019**, *9*, 2045894018824563. [CrossRef]
9. Rosovsky, R.; Zhao, K.; Sista, A.; Rivera-Lebron, B.; Kabrhel, C. Pulmonary embolism response teams: Purpose, evidence for efficacy, and future research directions. *Res. Pract. Thromb. Haemost.* **2019**, *3*, 315–330. [CrossRef]
10. Carroll, B.J.; Beyer, S.E.; Mehegan, T.; Dicks, A.; Pribish, A.; Locke, A.; Godishala, A.; Soriano, K.; Kanduri, J.; Sack, K.; et al. Changes in Care for Acute Pulmonary Embolism Through a Multidisciplinary Pulmonary Embolism Response Team. *Am. J. Med.* **2020**, *133*, 1313–1321.e6. [CrossRef]
11. Chaudhury, P.; Gadre, S.K.; Schneider, E.; Renapurkar, R.D.; Gomes, M.; Haddadin, I.; Heresi, G.A.; Tong, M.Z.; Bartholomew, J.R. Impact of multidisciplinary pulmonary embolism response team availability on management and outcomes. *Am. J. Cardiol.* **2019**, *124*, 1465–1469. [CrossRef]
12. Myc, L.A.; Solanki, J.N.; Barros, A.J.; Nuradin, N.; Nevulis, M.G.; Earasi, K.; Richardson, E.D.; Tsutsui, S.C.; Enfield, K.B.; Teman, N.R.; et al. Adoption of a dedicated multidisciplinary team is associated with improved survival in acute pulmonary embolism. *Respir. Res.* **2020**, *21*, 159. [CrossRef]
13. Kabrhel, C.; Rosovsky, R.; Channick, R.; Jaff, M.R.; Weinberg, I.; Sundt, T.; Dudzinski, D.M.; Rodriguez-Lopez, J.; Parry, B.A.; Harshbarger, S.; et al. A Multidisciplinary Pulmonary Embolism Response Team: Initial 30-Month Experience with a Novel Approach to Delivery of Care to Patients with Submassive and Massive Pulmonary Embolism. *Chest* **2016**, *150*, 384–393. [CrossRef]
14. Sławek-Szmyt, S.; Jankiewicz, S.; Smukowska-Gorynia, A.; Janus, M.; Klotzka, A.; Puślecki, M.; Jemielity, M.; Krasiński, Z.; Żabicki, B.; Elikowski, W.; et al. Implementation of a regional multidisciplinary pulmonary embolism response team: PERT-POZ initial 1-year experience. *Kardiol. Pol.* **2020**, *78*, 300–310. [CrossRef]
15. Khaing, P.; Paruchuri, A.; Eisenbrey, J.R.; Merli, G.J.; Gonsalves, C.F.; West, F.M.; Awsare, B.K. First year experience of a pulmonary embolism response team with comparisons of outcomes between catheter directed therapy versus standard anticoagulation. *Hosp. Pract.* **2020**, *48*, 23–28. [CrossRef]
16. Sista, A.K.; Friedman, O.A.; Dou, E.; Denvir, B.; Askin, G.; Stern, J.; Estes, J.; Salemi, A.; Winokur, R.S.; Horowitz, J.M. A pulmonary embolism response team's initial 20-month experience treating 87 patients with submassive and massive pulmonary embolism. *Vasc. Med.* **2018**, *23*, 65–71. [CrossRef]
17. Mahar, J.H.; Haddadin, I.; Sadana, D.; Gadre, A.; Evans, N.; Hornacek, D.; Mahlay, N.F.; Gomes, M.; Joseph, D.; Serhal, M.; et al. A pulmonary embolism response team (PERT) approach: Initial experience from the Cleveland Clinic. *J. Thromb. Thrombolysis* **2018**, *46*, 186–192. [CrossRef]

8. Nouri, S.N.; Madhavan, M.; Lumish, H.S.; Lavelle, M.; Gavalas, M.; Brown, T.; Li, J.; Rosenzweig, E.B.; Parikh, S.; Einstein, A.; et al. Pulmonary embolism response teams: Do they result in better outcomes in severe pulmonary embolism (a single center retrospective analysis)? *JACC* **2019**, *73*, 1920. [CrossRef]
9. Araszkiewicz, A.; Kurzyna, M.; Kopeć, G.; Roik, M.; Darocha, S.; Pietrasik, A.; Puślecki, M.; Biederman, A.; Przybylski, R.; Stępniewski, J.; et al. Expert opinion on the creating and operating of the regional Pulmonary Embolism Response Teams (PERT). Polish PERT Initiative. *Cardiol. J.* **2019**, *26*, 623–632. [CrossRef]
20. Xiong, W. Current status of treatment of cancer-associated venous thromboembolism. *Thromb. J.* **2021**, *19*, 21. [CrossRef]
21. Lee, A.Y.; Levine, M.N.; Baker, R.I.; Bowden, C.; Kakkar, A.K.; Prins, M.; Rickles, F.R.; Julian, J.A.; Haley, S.; Gent, M.; et al. Low-molecular-weight heparin versus a coumarin for the prevention of recurrent venous thromboembolism in patients with cancer. *N. Engl. J. Med.* **2003**, *349*, 146–153. [CrossRef]
22. Farge, D.; Frere, C.; Connors, J.M.; Ay, C.; Khorana, A.A.; Munoz, A.; Brenner, B.; Kakkar, A.; Rafii, H.; Solymoss, S.; et al. 2019 international clinical practice guidelines for the treatment and prophylaxis of venous thromboembolism in patients with cancer. *Lancet Oncol.* **2019**, *20*, e566–e581. [CrossRef]
23. Dudzinski, D.M.; Giri, J.; Rosenfield, K. Interventional treatment of pulmonary embolism. *Circ. Cardiovasc. Interv.* **2017**, *10*, e004345. [CrossRef]
24. Stein, P.D.; Matta, F.; Hughes, P.G.; Hughes, M.J. Nineteen-Year Trends in Mortality of Patients Hospitalized in the United States with High-Risk Pulmonary Embolism. *Am. J. Med.* **2021**, *134*, 1260–1264. [CrossRef]
25. Hoskin, S.; Brieger, D.; Chow, V.; Kritharides, L.; Ng, A.C. Trends in Acute Pulmonary Embolism Admission Rates and Mortality Outcomes in Australia, 2002–2003 to 2017–2018: A Retrospective Cohort Study. *Thromb. Haemost.* **2021**, *121*, 1237–1245. [CrossRef]
26. Pietrasik, A.; Gąsecka, A.; Leśniewski, M.; Zieliński, D.; Darocha, S.; Kurzyna, M. Hybrid treatment of massive pulmonary embolism by catheter-directed and surgical embolectomy. *Adv. Interv. Cardiol.* **2021**, *17*, 236–238. [CrossRef]
27. Pietrasik, A.; Gąsecka, A.; Smyk, J.; Darocha, S.; Zieliński, D.; Kurzyna, M. Acute-on-chronic pulmonary embolism and concomitant paradoxical embolism: Two diseases, one intervention. *Pol. Arch. Intern. Med.* **2022**, *132*, 16155. [CrossRef]
28. Pietrasik, A.; Gąsecka, A.; Chojecka, D.; Pytlos, J.; Rymuza, B.; Główczyńska, R.; Banaszkiewicz, M.; Darocha, S.; Kurzyna, M. Iatrogenic pulmonary embolism with cyanoacrylate: To remove or to leave? *Kardiol. Pol.* **2021**, *79*, 706–707. [CrossRef] [PubMed]
29. Pietrasik, A.; Gąsecka, A.; Pieniak, K.; Karpiński, G.; Kochman, J.; Darocha, S.; Kurzyna, M. Iatrogenic embolism caused by fractured vascular port: Successful endovascular treatment. *Kardiol. Pol.* **2021**, *79*, 877–878. [CrossRef] [PubMed]

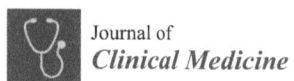 

## Article

# Tumor Necrosis Factor-Related Apoptosis-Inducing Ligand (TRAIL): A Novel Biomarker for Prognostic Assessment and Risk Stratification of Acute Pulmonary Embolism

Haixu Yu [1,2,†], Wei Rong [1,†], Jie Yang [1], Jie Lu [1], Ke Ma [1], Zhuohui Liu [1], Hui Yuan [1], Lei Xu [1], Yulin Li [1], Zhi-Cheng Jing [3,\*] and Jie Du [1,\*]

1. Beijing Anzhen Hospital of Capital Medical University and Beijing Institute of Heart Lung and Blood Vessel Diseases, Beijing 100029, China; yuhaixu6619@163.com (H.Y.); rongweiww@126.com (W.R.); yjyjlyang@163.com (J.Y.); jielu_0901@163.com (J.L.); make11191017@163.com (K.M.); lzh1540065015@163.com (Z.L.); 18911662931@189.cn (H.Y.); leixu2001@hotmail.com (L.X.); lyllyl_1111@163.com (Y.L.)
2. Department of Cardiology and Institute of Vascular Medicine, Peking University Third Hospital, Beijing 100191, China
3. Department of Cardiology, Peking Union Medical College Hospital, Chinese Academy of Medical Sciences and Peking Union Medical College, Beijing 100730, China
\* Correspondence: jingzhicheng@vip.163.com (Z.-C.J.); jiedu@ccmu.edu.cn (J.D.)
† These authors contributed equally to this work.

**Abstract:** Background: Tumor necrosis factor (TNF)-related apoptosis-inducing ligand (TRAIL) is associated with poor prognosis in cardiovascular diseases. However, the predictive value of TRAIL for the short-term outcome and risk stratification of acute pulmonary embolism (PE) remains unknown. Methods: This study prospectively included 151 normotensive patients with acute PE. The study outcome was a composite of 30-day adverse events, defined as PE-related death, shock, mechanical ventilation, cardiopulmonary resuscitation, and major bleeding. Results: Overall, nine of 151 (6.0%) patients experienced 30-day adverse composite events. Multivariable logistic regression showed that TRAIL was an independent predictor of study outcome (OR 0.19 per SD; 95% CI 0.04–0.90). An ROC curve revealed that TRAIL's area under the curve (AUC) was 0.83 (95% CI 0.76–0.88). The optimal cut-off value for TRAIL was 18 pg/mL, with a sensitivity, specificity, negative predictive value, positive predictive value, positive likelihood ratio, and negative likelihood ratio of 89%, 69%, 99%, 15%, 2.87, and 0.16, respectively. Compared with the risk stratification algorithm outlined in the 2019 ESC guidelines, our biomarker-based risk stratification strategy (combining TRAIL and hs-cTnI) has a similar risk classification effect. Conclusion: Reduced plasma TRAIL levels predict short-term adverse events in normotensive patients with acute PE. The combination of the 2019 ESC algorithm and TRAIL aids risk stratification in normotensive patients with acute PE.

**Keywords:** pulmonary embolism; TNF-related apoptosis-inducing ligand; prognosis; risk stratification

**Citation:** Yu, H.; Rong, W.; Yang, J.; Lu, J.; Ma, K.; Liu, Z.; Yuan, H.; Xu, L.; Li, Y.; Jing, Z.-C.; et al. Tumor Necrosis Factor-Related Apoptosis-Inducing Ligand (TRAIL): A Novel Biomarker for Prognostic Assessment and Risk Stratification of Acute Pulmonary Embolism. *J. Clin. Med.* 2022, 11, 3908. https://doi.org/10.3390/jcm11133908

Academic Editors: Peter Kubisz, Paolo P. Prandoni, Lucia Stančiaková and Maha Othman

Received: 10 April 2022
Accepted: 27 June 2022
Published: 5 July 2022

**Publisher's Note:** MDPI stays neutral with regard to jurisdictional claims in published maps and institutional affiliations.

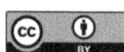

**Copyright:** © 2022 by the authors. Licensee MDPI, Basel, Switzerland. This article is an open access article distributed under the terms and conditions of the Creative Commons Attribution (CC BY) license (https://creativecommons.org/licenses/by/4.0/).

## 1. Introduction

Venous thromboembolism (VTE), including deep vein thrombosis and pulmonary embolism, contributes a significant burden on health and survival and ranks third among life-threatening cardiovascular diseases [1]. Acute pulmonary embolism (PE) is the most severe clinical manifestation of VTE. Most patients with acute PE are normotensive, and early mortality ranges from 3–7% [2–4]. Early prognostic assessment and risk stratification for normotensive patients with acute PE is essential for determining appropriate treatment management approaches. The 2019 European Society of Cardiology (ESC) guidelines suggested that the extensively validated and broadly used simplified pulmonary embolism severity index (sPESI), combined with right ventricular (RV) dysfunction and laboratory biomarkers, can be used to classify acute PE patients without hemodynamic instability into intermediate- or low-risk groups. In addition to clinical parameters and scores, patients in the intermediate-risk group who display RV dysfunction and elevated cardiac troponin levels are classified into the intermediate-high-risk category [5]. Previous evidence demonstrated that a subgroup of normotensive patients with acute PE (i.e., intermediate-risk group) might benefit from aggressive treatment strategies [6]. Thus, optimizing risk stratification in normotensive PE is essential to enhance clinical practice.

Tumor necrosis factor (TNF)-related apoptosis-inducing ligand (TRAIL), which is also known as Apo-2 ligand (Apo-2L) or TNF superfamily 10 (TNFSN10), is a member of the TNF superfamily of cytokines, which is broadly expressed in various tissues of the human body [7]. TRAIL is selectively expressed in vascular smooth muscle cells of the pulmonary artery and aorta [8]. Soluble TRAIL mainly appears to be released by activated leukocytes such as monocytes and neutrophils [9]. TRAIL is a pro-apoptotic protein which has broad biological functions. TRAIL may play a crucial role in the pathway linking coagulation and inflammation elicited by thrombin and mediates the amplification of pro-coagulant endothelial microparticles released by thrombin and the inflammatory process [10]. Several clinical studies have shown that reduced TRAIL levels are associated with poor prognosis in patients with acute myocardial infarction or heart failure, suggesting that TRAIL has predictive effects in cardiovascular diseases [11–13].

In this study, we hypothesized that TRAIL may be involved in the pathophysiological mechanism of PE through the interplay between coagulation and inflammation and might assist in the prognostic assessment of patients with acute PE. Thus, our study aimed to identify the short-term prognostic assessment and risk stratification of TRAIL in normotensive patients with acute PE.

## 2. Materials and Methods

### 2.1. Study Design and Setting

We conducted a prospective study of normotensive patients with acute pulmonary embolism from 2015 to 2017 at Beijing Anzhen Hospital in China (NCT 04118634). Based on the amended Declaration of Helsinki, the study protocol was approved by the Ethics Committee of Beijing Anzhen Hospital (No. 2018048X), and all patients provided written informed consent.

### 2.2. Selection of Participants

As shown in Figure 1, normotensive patients (defined as SBP $\geq$ 90 mmHg) were consecutively enrolled if they had acute PE, were aged $\geq$ 18 years, and the onset of the illness was $\leq$14 days ago. Patients with acute PE were objectively confirmed by computed tomography pulmonary angiography (CTPA) and a ventilation-perfusion lung scan. The exclusion criteria were the following: [14–16] (1) hemodynamic instability: (A) cardiac arrest: cardiopulmonary resuscitation required; (B) obstructive shock: systolic blood pressure (BP) < 90 mmHg or vasopressors required to achieve a BP $\geq$ 90 mmHg despite adequate filling status and end-organ hypoperfusion (altered mental status; cold, clammy skin; oliguria/anuria); (C) persistent hypotension: systolic BP < 90 mmHg or systolic BP drop $\geq$ 40 mmHg lasting longer than 15 min and not caused by new-onset arrhythmia, hypovolaemia, or sepsis; (2) recurrence of PE; (3) chronic thromboembolic pulmonary hypertension; (4) life expectancy <3 months (i.e., the end stage of diseases); (5) ongoing pregnancy; (6) renal insufficiency (estimated glomerular filtration rate <30 mL/min*1.73 m$^2$) or hepatic dysfunction (Child–Pugh class B or C); (7) withdrawal of written consent for participation in this study; and (8) missing blood samples and troponin data.

### 2.3. Methods of Measurement

The diagnosis of acute PE was assessed using the Wells clinical probability rule, D-dimer, and imaging tests by the diagnostic algorithm outlined in the 2019 ESC guidelines [5]. All patients underwent transthoracic echocardiography within 24 h after diagnosis of PE. The diagnosis of RV dysfunction was based on the following diagnostic criteria [5]: (1) RV dilatation at the apical four-chamber view (RV end-diastolic diameter/left ventricular end-diastolic diameter >1.0), (2) depressed contractility of the RV free wall, (3) tricuspid regurgitation velocity acceleration, and (4) decreased tricuspid annular systolic excursion (<17 mm). The electronic medical record system obtained other clinical data, laboratory findings, and treatment details. According to the risk stratification strategy proposed in the 2019 ESC guidelines, all normotensive patients with acute PE were classified into the intermediate-high-, intermediate-low-, and low-risk groups according to their sPESI score, RV dysfunction, and troponin level. The physicians made treatment decisions while being unaware of TRAIL levels after carefully considering each patient's clinical symptoms, laboratory findings, and imaging tests.

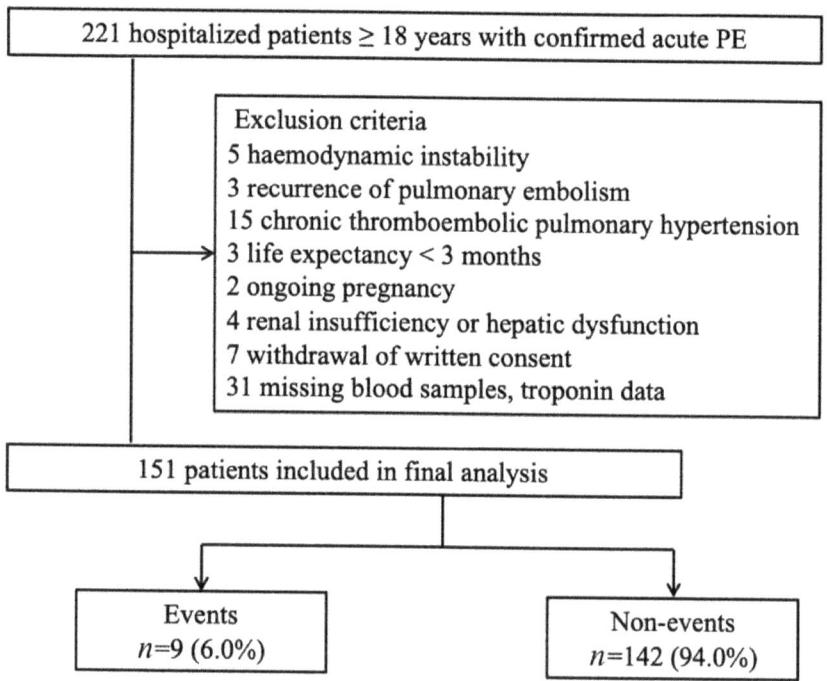

**Figure 1.** Study participants flow diagram. PE, pulmonary embolism.

Venous plasma samples were collected from patients within 24 h after admission in vacuum tubes and immediately frozen at −80 °C after centrifugation at 3000× $g$ for 10 min. Plasma TRAIL concentrations were determined using an ELISA kit (Ray Biotech, Inc. Norcross, GA, USA). Other laboratory tests were completed by the laboratory department of Beijing Anzhen Hospital.

*2.4. Outcome Measures*

The study outcome was 30-day adverse composite events, defined as PE-related death or at least one of the following complications: (1) the need for mechanical ventilation assistance, (2) the need for catecholamine administration for treatment or prevention, (3) cardiopulmonary resuscitation, or (4) major bleeding. PE-related death was determined by (1) autopsy, (2) clinically severe acute PE, and (3) in cases where other causes were excluded. Major bleeding was defined as clinically overt bleeding accompanied by at least one of the following: (1) fatal bleeding or bleeding that occurred at critical sites or organs (intracranial, intraspinal, retroperitoneal, intraocular, and pericardial bleeding); (2) hemodynamic instability due to bleeding and/or a fall in the hemoglobin level ≥20 g/L, or bleeding that led to the transfusion of at least two units of blood [17].

All patients were followed up by pre-trained research staff. We determined the occurrence of the study outcome by using data collected through a review of the electronic medical records, clinical visits, and telephone follow-up interviews for up to 30 days.

*2.5. Biomarker-Based Risk Algorithm*

In the 2019 ESC prognostic strategy, risk assessment for early mortality consists of seven clinical parameters (sPESI rule), two relevant imaging modalities (TTE or CTPA), and four cardiac biomarkers (troponin, NT-proBNP, H-FABP, and copeptin). Objective assessments are relatively time-consuming, labor-intensive, and cost-intensive. Thus, in this study, a biomarker-based risk algorithm was developed to evaluate the risk assessment of normotensive patients with acute PE. This biomarker-based stratification strategy was established using TRAIL combined with hs-cTnI levels. According to previous studies [18–20], hs-cTnI possessed superior negative predictive values (NPV) for short-term adverse events and could be used as the first step in risk stratification to classify patients with low-risk acute PE.

*2.6. Statistical Analyses*

The Kolmogorov–Smirnov test for normal distribution was used for continuous variables. Skewed continuous variables were expressed as medians (interquartile range [IQR]). Categorical variables were expressed as absolute numbers or percentages. Comparisons of continuous variables were analyzed using unpaired Student's *t*-tests or Mann–Whitney *U* tests, and comparisons of categorical variables were analyzed using Chi-squared or Fisher's exact tests. Correlations between continuous variables were analyzed using Spearman's rank correlation coefficient. The prognostic relevance of clinical variables, cardiac biomarkers, TRAIL levels, and sPESI scores for 30-day adverse events was calculated using univariate (unadjusted) and multivariate (adjusted) logistic regression analysis, producing odds ratios (OR) and 95% confidence intervals (CIs). Factors for inclusion in the multivariate analysis were determined after considering the findings from previous publications and the latest ESC guidelines and significant predictors ($p < 0.05$) from the univariate analysis. Receiver operating characteristic (ROC) curve analysis was performed to determine the area under the curve (AUC) of TRAIL cut-off values for the study outcomes. Youden's index was used to identify optimal cut-off values. Sensitivity, specificity, negative predictive values (NPV), positive predictive values (PPV), negative likelihood ratios (−LR), positive likelihood ratios (+LR), and the corresponding 95% CIs were calculated. The McNemar–Bowker test was used to compare the distribution of patients in different risk stratification strategies (2019 ESC algorithm and biomarker-based approach). Two-tailed *p* values < 0.05 were considered statistically significant. All statistical analyses were conducted using SPSS (version 25.0; IBM, Chicago, IL, USA).

## 3. Results

*3.1. Characteristics of Study Subjects*

Between January 2015 and December 2017, 221 patients were screened, of whom 70 met the exclusion criteria (flow chart shown as Figure 1). Among the 151 patients who participated in this study, nine (6%) experienced 30-day adverse composite events. One patient died directly due to PE; seven patients required catecholamine administration for treatment or prevention. Two patients required mechanical ventilation, two required cardiopulmonary resuscitation, and one suffered major bleeding. The clinical and demographic characteristics of study participants with and without study events are presented in Table 1. The event group more frequently experienced syncope, RV dysfunction, higher BNP and hs-cTnI concentrations, and sPESI scores $\geq 1$ compared to the non-event group. Additionally, nine (6.0%) patients received thrombolytic therapy and five (55.6%) experienced adverse outcomes.

**Table 1.** Baseline characteristics of normotensive patients with acute pulmonary embolism.

| | All Patients (n = 151) | Non-Events (n = 142) | Events (n = 9) | p Value |
|---|---|---|---|---|
| Age, years | 66 (60–73) | 66 (60–73) | 62 (48–72) | 0.453 |
| Male | 63 (41.7) | 60 (42.3) | 3 (33.3) | 0.735 |
| **Risk factors for VTE** | | | | |
| History of VTE | 19 (12.6) | 19 (13.4) | 0 | 0.603 |
| Immobility | 13 (8.6) | 12 (8.5) | 1 (11.1) | 0.566 |
| Recent surgery | 8 (5.3) | 7 (4.9) | 1 (11.1) | 0.396 |
| Recent long travel | 2 (1.3) | 2 (1.4) | 0 | 1.000 |
| Recent fracture | 9 (6.0) | 8 (5.6) | 1 (11.1) | 0.434 |
| **Comorbidities** | | | | |
| Cancer | 9 (6.0) | 9 (6.3) | 0 | 1.000 |
| COPD | 8 (5.3) | 7 (4.9) | 1 (11.1) | 0.396 |
| Coronary heart disease | 25 (16.6) | 24 (16.9) | 1 (11.1) | 1.000 |
| **Symptoms and signs** | | | | |
| Chest pain | 39 (25.8) | 38 (26.8) | 1 (11.1) | 0.448 |
| Dyspnea | 139 (92.1) | 130 (91.5) | 9 (100.0) | 1.000 |
| Syncope | 30 (19.9) | 24 (16.9) | 6 (66.7) | **0.002** |
| SBP, mmHg | 124 (114.5–124) | 124 (115–138) | 120 (113–134) | 0.691 |
| SBP < 100 mmHg | 4 (2.6) | 3 (2.1) | 1 (11.1) | 0.220 |
| Heart rate, bpm | 82 (73–98) | 82 (72–96) | 97 (84–102) | **0.010** |
| Heart rate ≥ 110 bpm | 9 (6.0) | 7 (4.9) | 2 (22.2) | 0.092 |
| SaO$_2$ < 90% | 15 (9.9) | 13 (9.2) | 2 (22.2) | 0.220 |
| Elevated PASP | 49 (32.5) | 45 (31.7) | 4 (44.4) | 0.473 |
| RV dysfunction (on TTE) | 15 (9.9) | 10 (7.0) | 5 (55.6) | **0.001** |
| LVEF, % | 63 (60–67) | 64 (60–68) | 60 (56–64) | 0.083 |
| **Laboratory biomarkers** | | | | |
| D-Dimer, ng/mL | 2166 (1076–3134) | 2114 (1056–3110) | 2823 (2389–3134) | 0.088 |
| Creatinine, μmol/L | 73.5 (61.1–83.7) | 73.2 (60.5–83.8) | 75.0 (62.6–83.1) | 0.75 |
| BNP, pg/mL | 141 (46–364) | 118 (44.0–310.0) | 1000 (653–2054) | **0.001** |
| hs-cTnI, ng/mL | 0.03 (0.01–0.15) | 0.02 (0.01–0.11) | 0.27 (0.09–0.91) | **0.001** |
| TRAIL, pg/mL | 23.1 (15.0–32.3) | 23.5 (16.1–32.6) | 10.1 (3.6–16.4) | **0.001** |
| sPESI ≥ 1 | 55 (36.4) | 47 (33.1) | 8 (88.9) | **0.001** |
| **Treatment** | | | | |
| Thrombolytic therapy | 9 (6.0) | 4 (2.8) | 5 (55.6) | **0.000** |

Data are presented as median (interquartile range) or number (%). VTE, venous thromboembolism; COPD, chronic obstructive pulmonary disease; SBP, systolic blood pressure; bpm, beats per minute; SaO$_2$, arterial oxyhemoglobin saturation; PASP, pulmonary artery systolic pressure; RV, right ventricular; TTE, transthoracic echocardiography; LVEF, left ventricular ejection fraction; BNP, brain natriuretic peptide; hs-cTnI, high-sensitivity cardiac troponin I; TRAIL, tumor necrosis factor-related apoptosis-inducing ligand; sPESI, simplified Pulmonary Embolism Severity Index.

## 3.2. Association between TRAIL Levels and Short-Term Prognosis

The median TRAIL concentration was 23.1 pg/mL (IQR 15.0–32.3) in all patients. Patients in the events group had significantly lower TRAIL levels (median, 10.1 pg/mL [IQR 3.6–16.4]) than patients in the non-event group (median 23.5 pg/mL [IQR 16.1–32.6], $p = 0.001$). The TRAIL concentrations were weakly correlated with BNP (r = $-0.28$, $p = 0.001$) and hs-cTnI (r = $-0.24$, $p = 0.003$). The predictors of 30-day adverse composite events were investigated using a univariate logistic regression analysis (Table 2). Significant predictors of 30-day adverse composite events in the univariate analysis included syncope (OR = 9.83; 95% CI 2.30–42.08, $p = 0.002$), RV dysfunction (OR = 16.5; 95% CI 3.82–71.30, $p = 0.000$), BNP (OR = 3.60 per SD; 95% CI 1.91–6.78, $p = 0.000$), TRAIL (OR = 0.18 per SD; 95% CI 0.06–0.56, $p = 0.003$), and a sPESI score $\geq 1$ (OR = 16.17; 95% CI 1.95–133.11, $p = 0.010$). Considering the findings from previous publications and the latest ESC guidelines, significant predictors from the univariate analysis and cardiac troponin (hs-cTnI) were included in the multivariate logistic regression analysis (Table 2). After adjustment, TRAIL was independently and significantly associated with 30-day adverse composite events in normotensive patients with acute PE (OR = 0.19 per SD; 95% CI 0.04–0.90, $p = 0.036$). As shown in Figure 2, ROC analysis revealed that the AUC of TRAIL was 0.83 (95% CI 0.76–0.88, $p < 0.001$) for the prediction of short-term adverse outcomes, and the optimal cut-off value for TRAIL based on Youden's index was 18 pg/mL, at which point the sensitivity, specificity, NPV, PPV, +LR, and $-$LR were 89%, 69%, 99%, 15%, 2.87, and 0.16, respectively.

**Table 2.** Predictors of an adverse 30-day outcome.

| | OR | 95%CI | p Value |
|---|---|---|---|
| Univariable analysis [a] | | | |
| Age > 80 years | 3.43 | 0.36–32.90 | 0.286 |
| Cancer | - | - | - |
| COPD | 2.41 | 0.26–22.05 | 0.436 |
| Syncope | 9.83 | 2.30–42.08 | 0.002 |
| SBP < 100 mmHg | 5.79 | 0.54–62.12 | 0.147 |
| Heart rate $\geq$ 110 bpm | 5.51 | 0.96–31.57 | 0.055 |
| SaO$_2$ < 90% | 2.84 | 0.53–15.09 | 0.222 |
| RV dysfunction (on TTE) | 16.5 | 3.82–71.30 | 0.000 |
| BNP, pg/mL, per SD | 3.60 | 1.91–6.78 | 0.000 |
| hs-cTnI, ng/mL, per SD | 1.25 | 0.85–1.85 | 0.254 |
| TRAIL, pg/mL, per SD | 0.18 | 0.06–0.56 | 0.003 |
| sPESI $\geq$ 1 | 16.17 | 1.96–133.11 | 0.010 |
| Multivariable analysis | | | |
| Syncope | 2.48 | 0.20–31.12 | 0.481 |
| RV dysfunction (on TTE) | 16.47 | 1.06–256.27 | 0.045 |
| BNP, pg/mL, per SD | 3.68 | 1.24–10.89 | 0.019 |
| hs-cTnI, ng/mL, per SD | 1.45 | 0.64–3.32 | 0.375 |
| TRAIL, pg/mL, per SD | 0.19 | 0.04–0.90 | 0.036 |
| sPESI $\geq$ 1 | 1.09 | 0.06–21.54 | 0.956 |

OR, odds ratio; SD, standard deviation; COPD, chronic obstructive pulmonary disease; SBP, systolic blood pressure; bpm, beats per minute; SaO$_2$, arterial oxyhemoglobin saturation; RV, right ventricular; TTE, transthoracic echocardiography; BNP, brain natriuretic peptide; hs-cTnI, high-sensitivity cardiac troponin I; TRAIL, tumor necrosis factor-related apoptosis-inducing ligand; sPESI, simplified Pulmonary Embolism Severity Index. [a] Variables found to significantly predict an adverse 30-day outcome in the univariate analysis are displayed. Additionally, hs-cTnI levels and all variables included in the sPESI are shown. The logistic regression analysis calculates odds ratios (ORs) and their respective 95% confidence intervals (CIs) for an adverse 30-day outcome.

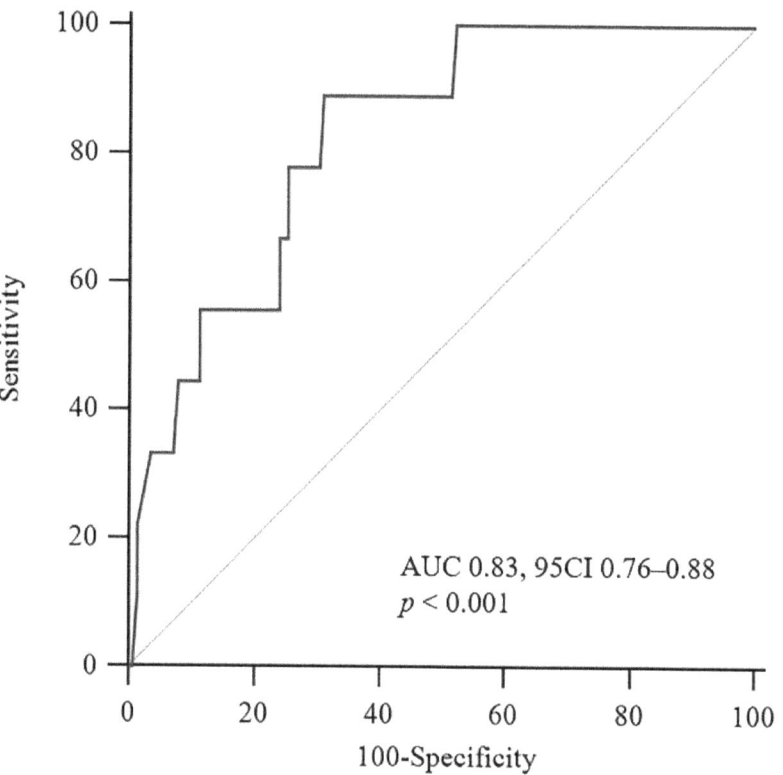

**Figure 2.** Receiver operating characteristic (ROC) curve for TRAIL concerning an adverse 30-day outcome. AUC: area under the curve; CI: confidence interval.

### 3.3. TRAIL's Role in Risk Stratification

According to the 2019 ESC risk algorithm (Figure 3), 10 (6.6%) patients were classified into the intermediate-high risk group, 78 (51.7%) into the intermediate-low risk group, and 63 (41.7%) into the low-risk group. During the follow-up, the 30-day adverse composite events occurred in 5 (50%), 4 (5.1%), and 0 (0%) patients, respectively. The risk assessment using the biomarker-based strategy based on hs-cTnI and TRAIL is shown in Figure 3. As with the 2019 ESC risk algorithm, the stepwise biomarker-based strategy demonstrated strong predictive performance in identifying intermediate-high- and low-risk group patients (Table 3). Both the biomarker-based strategy and the 2019 ESC algorithm showed high sensitivity (100%) and NPV (100%) in identifying low-risk patients, while the biomarker-based strategy had higher specificity than the 2019 ESC algorithm (65% vs. 44%, $p < 0.001$). When identifying intermediate-high-risk group patients, both strategies had high specificity (88% vs. 96%, $p < 0.001$) and the biomarker-based strategy had a superior trend of sensitivity (89% vs. 56%, $p = 0.375$). To combine the performance of the biomarker-based strategy and the 2019 ESC algorithm, we tested whether TRAIL may improve patients re-classified as belonging to the intermediate-high risk group, as shown in Figure 4. Using TRAIL < 18 pg/mL to further stratify patients in the intermediate-low risk group, 28 patients were identified as being at higher risk, with four adverse events. The prognostic performance of risk assessment using the 2019 ESC algorithm and TRAIL for the prediction of an adverse 30-day outcome is shown in Table 3, for which the sensitivity, specificity, NPV, PPV, +LR, and −LR were 100%, 80%, 100%, 24%, 5, and 0, respectively.

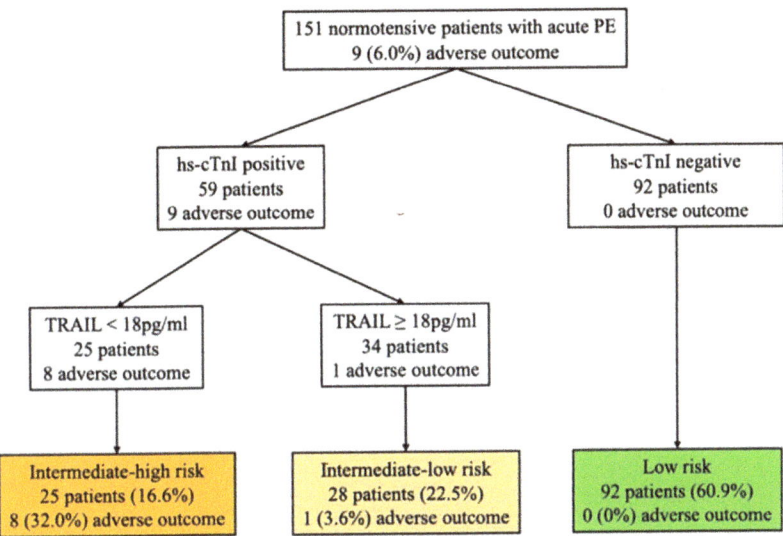

**Figure 3.** Risk assessment using the biomarker-based strategy based on hs-cTnI and TRAIL. The number (%) of patients with an adverse 30-day outcome is shown for each strategy. Hs-cTnI levels >0.04 ng/mL are defined as positive. PE: pulmonary embolism; hs-cTnI, high-sensitivity cardiac troponin I; TRAIL, tumor necrosis factor-related apoptosis-inducing ligand.

**Table 3.** Prognostic performance of risk assessment strategies for the prediction of an adverse 30-day outcome.

|  | Biomarker-Based Algorithm (95% CI) | 2019 ESC Algorithm (95% CI) | Combination of TRAIL and the 2019 ESC Algorithm (95% CI) |
|---|---|---|---|
| Low-risk vs. intermediate-low- and intermediate-high-risk ||||
| Sensitivity, % | 100 (66–100) | 100 (66–100) | 100 (66–100) |
| Specificity, % | 65 (56–73) | 44 (36–53) | 80 (72–86) |
| PPV, % | 15 (13–18) | 10 (9–12) | 24 (18–30) |
| NPV, % | 100 | 100 | 100 |
| +LR | 2.84 (2.3–3.5) | 1.80 (1.6–2.1) | 5 (3.5–6.8) |
| −LR | 0 | 0 | 0 |
| Low-risk and intermediate-low- vs. intermediate-high-risk ||||
| Sensitivity, % | 89 (52–100) | 56 (21–86) | - |
| Specificity, % | 88 (82–93) | 96 (92–99) | - |
| PPV, % | 32 (22–44) | 50 (26–74) | - |
| NPV, % | 99 (95–99) | 97 (94–99) | - |
| +LR | 7.42 (4.5–12.3) | 15.78 (5.6–44.7) | - |
| −LR | 0.13 (0.02–0.8) | 0.46 (0.2–1.0) | - |

ESC, european society of cardiology; CI, confidence interval; TRAIL, tumor necrosis factor (TNF)-related apoptosis-inducing ligand; PPV, positive predictive values; NPV, negative predictive values; +LR, positive likelihood ratios; -LR, negative likelihood ratios.

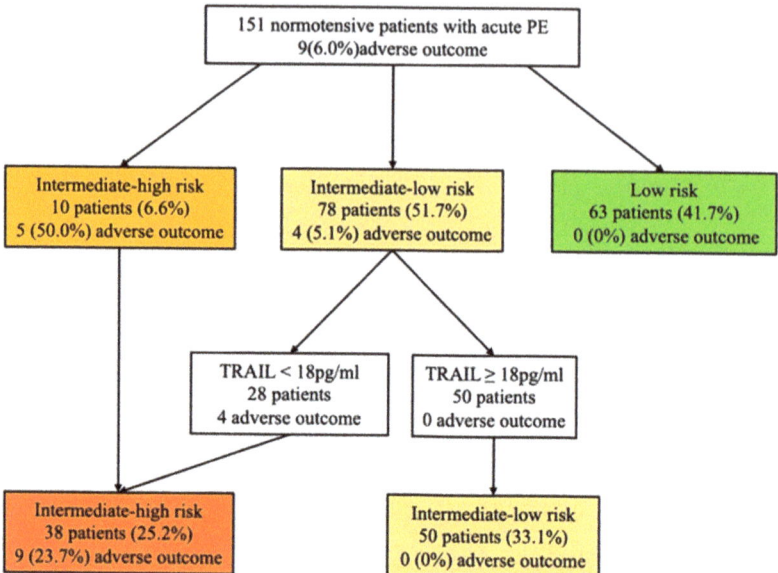

**Figure 4.** Risk assessment using the 2019 ESC algorithm and TRAIL. The number (%) of patients with an adverse 30-day outcome is shown for each strategy. Hs-cTnI levels > 0.04 ng/mL are defined as positive. PE: pulmonary embolism; TRAIL, tumor necrosis factor-related apoptosis-inducing ligand.

## 4. Discussion

This study investigated the relationship between plasma TRAIL concentrations and short-term adverse outcomes and whether TRAIL can optimize the current risk stratification. Using a cut-off value of 18 pg/mL, we found that decreased plasma TRAIL levels had an independently prognostic performance for 30-day adverse outcomes. A stepwise biomarker-based risk assessment strategy combining hs-cTnI and TRAIL improves predictive performance in identifying intermediate-high- and low-risk group patients. The combination of the 2019 ESC algorithm and TRAIL aids risk stratification in normotensive patients with acute PE.

### 4.1. The Potential Role of TRAIL in PE

TRAIL exists as either a type II membrane protein or a soluble protein. TRAIL receptors are expressed in the cardiovascular system in vascular smooth cells and cardiomyocytes, including osteoprotegerin (OPG). TRAIL has been found to play a role in ischemic vascular diseases and cardiovascular disease (CVD) [20–24]. Several prospective studies have demonstrated that lower TRAIL concentrations predicted poor prognosis in patients with CVD [13,25,26]. In our study, lower TRAIL concentrations were associated with short-term adverse outcomes. Low levels of TRAIL tend to represent poor prognosis. This is similar to the findings of several previous studies, in which serum TRAIL levels were negatively related to the severity of coronary heart disease [27], lower serum TRAIL levels were associated with worse outcomes in patients with acute myocardial infarction [28], and higher TRAIL levels in patients with advanced heart failure were associated with an improved prognosis [12,29]. Despite this, it is unclear how TRAIL can clinically influence the thrombosis and inflammation process during acute PE. However, it is plausible that the interaction between TRAIL and its receptors modulates the progression of thromboembolism. The role of inflammation-modulating maladaptive RV remodeling and dysfunction has been demonstrated. Acute PE leads to a cascade of inflammatory response which might be followed by leukocyte recruitment to the lesion. TRAIL recruits activated leukocytes to a particular tissue and initiates apoptosis to terminate the immune response. TRAIL promotes the proliferation of vascular smooth muscle cells and neovascularization [28,29]. TRAIL also enhances endothelial nitric oxide synthase phosphorylation, NOS activity, and NO synthesis; thus, it causes vasodilation [30,31]. Interestingly, there is a negative correlation between TRAIL and hsCRP, which provides further support for the protective role of TRAIL in the development of atherosclerosis and acute coronary disease [32].

*4.2. The Combination of TRAIL and the 2019 ESC Algorithm for Risk Assessment in Normotensive Patients with Acute PE*

Based on the 2019 ESC guidelines, treatment decisions for normotensive patients with acute PE need to be based on a risk stratification strategy, with low-risk patients being considered for early discharge and home treatment, intermediate-low or intermediate-high risk patients being closely monitored and offered reperfusion therapy if deterioration occurs. Recent cohort studies developed combination models for the identification of intermediate-high-risk PE patients (e.g., PREP score, FAST score, and Bova score) [33–35], and several studies investigated the prognostic value of biomarkers on risk stratification (e.g., Copeptin and Lipocalin-2) [16,19]. Due to the relatively limited performance of the 2019 ESC algorithm, we developed a novel and simple stepwise biomarker-based strategy using TRAIL and hs-cTnI. More patients were re-classified into the low-risk and intermediate-high risk groups using a biomarker-based algorithm. To combine the performance of the biomarker-based strategy and the 2019 ESC algorithm, we also tested whether TRAIL may improve patients re-classified as belonging to the intermediate-high risk group. As shown in Table 3 and Figure 4, the prognostic performance of risk assessment was improved using the 2019 ESC algorithm and TRAIL to predict an adverse 30-day outcome.

There are some limitations in this study that merit mentioning here. First, the included population came from a single center, and the number of people who experienced an outcome was low. However, adverse outcomes (6%) were similar to those reported in other studies [14,15,18,19]. Second, of the 221 patients screened, 31 (14.0%) were excluded due to missing data. Given the small size and the low event rate of this study, we could not evaluate if TRAIL has additional value on top of the existing risk stratification. Further large-scale studies are required in future using independent study cohorts. This study also lacked multiple consecutive measurements for TRAIL. The mechanism and pathophysiological process throughout the pulmonary embolism need to be further explored and validated.

## 5. Conclusions

In conclusion, reduced plasma TRAIL levels predict short-term adverse events in normotensive patients with acute PE. The combination of the 2019 ESC algorithm and TRAIL aids risk stratification to assist physicians in the making of treatment decisions and care of patients.

**Author Contributions:** H.Y. (Haixu Yu) and W.R. contributed equally as the first authors. Y.L., Z.-C.J. and J.D. conceived the study and its design. Y.L. and J.D. obtained research funding. H.Y. (Hui Yuan), L.X., Y.L., Z.-C.J. and J.D. supervised the conducting of the trial and data collection. J.Y., J.L., K.M. and Z.L. undertook the recruitment of patients and managed the data, including quality control. H.Y. (Haixu Yu), W.R. and J.Y. provided statistical advice on the study design and analyzed the data. H.Y. (Haixu Yu) and W.R. drafted the manuscript. All authors contributed substantially to article revisions and approved the final version for submission. J.D. and Z.-C.J. take responsibility for the paper as a whole. All authors have read and agreed to the published version of the manuscript.

**Funding:** This study was funded by the Natural Science Foundation of China (grant number 81930014) and the Beijing Collaborative Innovative Research Centre for Cardiovascular Diseases, Beijing, China.

**Institutional Review Board Statement:** This was a prospective study in a single center in China from 2015 to 2017. (NCT 04118634). The study protocol was approved by the Ethics Committee of Beijing Anzhen Hospital (No. 2018048X), and all patients provided written informed consent.

**Informed Consent Statement:** Informed consent was obtained from all subjects involved in the study.

**Data Availability Statement:** The data underlying the results presented in the study are available from Beijing Anzhen Hospital.

**Acknowledgments:** We would like to thank the Natural Science Foundation and Beijing Collaborative Innovative Research Centre for Cardiovascular Diseases for their funding support to the studies.

**Conflicts of Interest:** The authors declare no conflict of interest.

## References

1. Raskob, G.E.; Angchaisuksiri, P.; Blanco, A.N.; Buller, H.; Gallus, A.; Hunt, B.J.; Hylek, E.M.; Kakkar, T.L.; Konstantinides, S.V.; McCumber, M.; et al. Thrombosis: A major contributor to global disease burden. *Semin. Thromb. Hemost.* **2014**, *40*, 724–735. [CrossRef] [PubMed]
2. Naess, I.A.; Christiansen, S.C.; Romundstad, P.; Cannegieter, S.C.; Rosendaal, F.R.; Hammerstrom, J. Incidence and mortality of venous thrombosis: A population-based study. *J. Thromb. Haemost.* **2007**, *5*, 692–699. [CrossRef]
3. Alotaibi, G.S.; Wu, C.; Senthilselvan, A.; McMurtry, M.S. Secular Trends in Incidence and Mortality of Acute Venous Thromboembolism: The AB-VTE Population-Based Study. *Am. J. Med.* **2016**, *129*, 879.e19–879.e25. [CrossRef] [PubMed]
4. Zhang, Z.; Lei, J.; Shao, X.; Dong, F.; Wang, J.; Wang, D.; Wu, S.; Xie, W.; Wan, J.; Chen, H.; et al. Trends in Hospitalization and In-Hospital Mortality From VTE, 2007 to 2016, in China. *Chest* **2019**, *155*, 342–353. [CrossRef] [PubMed]
5. Konstantinides, S.V.; Meyer, G.; Becattini, C.; Bueno, H.; Geersing, G.J.; Harjola, V.P.; Huisman, M.V.; Humbert, M.; Jennings, C.S.; Jimenez, D.; et al. 2019 ESC Guidelines for the diagnosis and management of acute pulmonary embolism developed in collaboration with the European Respiratory Society (ERS). *Eur. Heart J.* **2020**, *41*, 543–603. [CrossRef] [PubMed]
6. Piazza, G. Advanced Management of Intermediate- and High-Risk Pulmonary Embolism: JACC Focus Seminar. *J. Am. Coll. Cardiol.* **2020**, *76*, 2117–2127. [CrossRef]
7. Wiley, S.R.; Schooley, K.; Smolak, P.J.; Din, W.S.; Huang, C.P.; Nicholl, J.K.; Sutherland, G.R.; Smith, T.D.; Rauch, C.; Smith, C.A.; et al. Identification and characterization of a new member of the TNF family that induces apoptosis. *Immunity* **1995**, *3*, 673–682. [CrossRef]
8. Gochuico, B.R.; Zhang, J.; Ma, B.Y.; Marshak-Rothstein, A.; Fine, A. TRAIL expression in vascular smooth muscle. *Am. J. Physiol. Lung Cell Mol. Physiol.* **2000**, *278*, L1045–L1050. [CrossRef]
9. Tecchio, C.; Huber, V.; Scapini, P.; Calzetti, F.; Margotto, D.; Todeschini, G.; Pilla, L.; Martinelli, G.; Pizzolo, G.; Rivoltini, L.; et al. IFNα-stimulated neutrophils and monocytes release a soluble form of TNF-related apoptosis-inducing ligand (TRAIL/Apo-2 ligand) displaying apoptotic activity on leukemic cells. *Blood* **2004**, *103*, 3837–3844. [CrossRef]
10. Simoncini, S.; Njock, M.S.; Robert, S.; Camoin-Jau, L.; Sampol, J.; Harle, J.R.; Nguyen, C.; Dignat-George, F.; Anfosso, F. TRAIL/Apo2L mediates the release of procoagulant endothelial microparticles induced by thrombin in vitro: A potential mechanism linking inflammation and coagulation. *Circ. Res.* **2009**, *104*, 943–951. [CrossRef]
11. Secchiero, P.; Corallini, F.; Ceconi, C.; Parrinello, G.; Volpato, S.; Ferrari, R.; Zauli, G. Potential prognostic significance of decreased serum levels of TRAIL after acute myocardial infarction. *PLoS ONE* **2009**, *4*, e4442. [CrossRef] [PubMed]
12. Niessner, A.; Hohensinner, P.J.; Rychli, K.; Neuhold, S.; Zorn, G.; Richter, B.; Hulsmann, M.; Berger, R.; Mortl, D.; Huber, K.; et al. Prognostic value of apoptosis markers in advanced heart failure patients. *Eur. Heart J.* **2009**, *30*, 789–796. [CrossRef] [PubMed]
13. Richter, B.; Koller, L.; Hohensinner, P.J.; Zorn, G.; Brekalo, M.; Berger, R.; Mortl, D.; Maurer, G.; Pacher, R.; Huber, K.; et al. A multi-biomarker risk score improves prediction of long-term mortality in patients with advanced heart failure. *Int. J. Cardiol.* **2013**, *168*, 1251–1257. [CrossRef]
14. Lankeit, M.; Jimenez, D.; Kostrubiec, M.; Dellas, C.; Hasenfuss, G.; Pruszczyk, P.; Konstantinides, S. Predictive value of the high-sensitivity troponin T assay and the simplified Pulmonary Embolism Severity Index in hemodynamically stable patients with acute pulmonary embolism: A prospective validation study. *Circulation* **2011**, *124*, 2716–2724. [CrossRef] [PubMed]
15. Vanni, S.; Jimenez, D.; Nazerian, P.; Morello, F.; Parisi, M.; Daghini, E.; Pratesi, M.; Lopez, R.; Bedate, P.; Lobo, J.L.; et al. Short-term clinical outcome of normotensive patients with acute PE and high plasma lactate. *Thorax* **2015**, *70*, 333–338. [CrossRef]
16. Yu, H.; Liu, Z.; Lu, J.; Yang, X.; Yan, X.X.; Mi, Y.; Hua, L.; Li, Y.; Jing, Z.C.; Du, J. Lipocalin-2 Predicts Long-Term Outcome of Normotensive Patients with Acute Pulmonary Embolism. *Cardiovasc. Toxicol.* **2020**, *20*, 101–110. [CrossRef]
17. Schulman, S.; Kearon, C.; Subcommittee on Control of Anticoagulation of the Scientific and Standardization Committee of the International Society on Thrombosis and Haemostasis. Definition of major bleeding in clinical investigations of antihemostatic medicinal products in non-surgical patients. *J. Thromb. Haemost.* **2005**, *3*, 692–694. [CrossRef]
18. Hellenkamp, K.; Schwung, J.; Rossmann, H.; Kaeberich, A.; Wachter, R.; Hasenfuß, G.; Konstantinides, S.; Lankeit, M. Risk stratification of normotensive pulmonary embolism: Prognostic impact of copeptin. *Eur. Respir. J.* **2015**, *46*, 1701–1710. [CrossRef]
19. Hellenkamp, K.; Pruszczyk, P.; Jimenez, D.; Wyzgal, A.; Barrios, D.; Ciurzynski, M.; Morillo, R.; Hobohm, L.; Keller, K.; Kurnicka, K.; et al. Prognostic impact of copeptin in pulmonary embolism: A multicentre validation study. *Eur. Respir. J.* **2018**, *51*, 1702037. [CrossRef]
20. Nash, M.; McGrath, J.P.; Cartland, S.P.; Patel, S.; Kavurma, M.M. Tumour necrosis factor superfamily members in ischaemic vascular diseases. *Cardiovasc. Res.* **2019**, *115*, 713–720. [CrossRef]
21. Harper, E.; Forde, H.; Davenport, C.; Rochfort, K.D.; Smith, D.; Cummins, P.M. Vascular calcification in type-2 diabetes and cardiovascular disease: Integrative roles for OPG, RANKL and TRAIL. *Vascul. Pharmacol.* **2016**, *82*, 30–40. [CrossRef] [PubMed]

2. Forde, H.; Harper, E.; Davenport, C.; Rochfort, K.D.; Wallace, R.; Murphy, R.P.; Smith, D.; Cummins, P.M. The beneficial pleiotropic effects of tumour necrosis factor-related apoptosis-inducing ligand (TRAIL) within the vasculature: A review of the evidence. *Atherosclerosis* **2016**, *247*, 87–96. [CrossRef] [PubMed]
3. D'Auria, F.; Centurione, L.; Centurione, M.A.; Angelini, A.; Di Pietro, R. Tumor Necrosis Factor Related Apoptosis Inducing Ligand (Trail) in endothelial response to biomechanical and biochemical stresses in arteries. *J. Cell. Biochem.* **2015**, *116*, 2427–2434. [CrossRef] [PubMed]
4. Rochette, L.; Meloux, A.; Rigal, E.; Zeller, M.; Cottin, Y.; Vergely, C. The role of osteoprotegerin in the crosstalk between vessels and bone: Its potential utility as a marker of cardiometabolic diseases. *Pharmacol. Ther.* **2018**, *182*, 115–132. [CrossRef] [PubMed]
5. Volpato, S.; Ferrucci, L.; Secchiero, P.; Corallini, F.; Zuliani, G.; Fellin, R.; Guralnik, J.M.; Bandinelli, S.; Zauli, G. Association of tumor necrosis factor-related apoptosis-inducing ligand with total and cardiovascular mortality in older adults. *Atherosclerosis* **2011**, *215*, 452–458. [CrossRef]
6. Osmancik, P.; Teringova, E.; Tousek, P.; Paulu, P.; Widimsky, P. Prognostic value of TNF-related apoptosis inducing ligand (TRAIL) in acute coronary syndrome patients. *PLoS ONE* **2013**, *8*, e53860. [CrossRef]
7. Ajala, O.; Zhang, Y.; Gupta, A.; Bon, J.; Sciurba, F.; Chandra, D. Decreased serum TRAIL is associated with increased mortality in smokers with comorbid emphysema and coronary artery disease. *Respir. Med.* **2018**, *145*, 21–27. [CrossRef]
8. Di Bartolo, B.A.; Cartland, S.P.; Prado-Lourenco, L.; Griffith, T.S.; Gentile, C.; Ravindran, J.; Azahri, N.S.; Thai, T.; Yeung, A.W.; Thomas, S.R.; et al. Tumor Necrosis Factor-Related Apoptosis-Inducing Ligand (TRAIL) Promotes Angiogenesis and Ischemia-Induced Neovascularization Via NADPH Oxidase 4 (NOX4) and Nitric Oxide-Dependent Mechanisms. *J. Am. Heart Assoc.* **2015**, *4*, e002527. [CrossRef]
9. Cartland, S.P.; Genner, S.W.; Zahoor, A.; Kavurma, M.M. Comparative Evaluation of TRAIL, FGF-2 and VEGF-A-Induced Angiogenesis In Vitro and In Vivo. *Int. J. Mol. Sci.* **2016**, *17*, 2025. [CrossRef]
10. Liu, M.; Xiang, G.; Lu, J.; Xiang, L.; Dong, J.; Mei, W. TRAIL protects against endothelium injury in diabetes via Akt-eNOS signaling. *Atherosclerosis* **2014**, *237*, 718–724. [CrossRef]
11. Manuneedhi Cholan, P.; Cartland, S.P.; Dang, L.; Rayner, B.S.; Patel, S.; Thomas, S.R.; Kavurma, M.M. TRAIL protects against endothelial dysfunction in vivo and inhibits angiotensin-II-induced oxidative stress in vascular endothelial cells in vitro. *Free Radic. Biol. Med.* **2018**, *126*, 341–349. [CrossRef] [PubMed]
12. Michowitz, Y.; Goldstein, E.; Roth, A.; Afek, A.; Abashidze, A.; Ben Gal, Y.; Keren, G.; George, J. The involvement of tumor necrosis factor-related apoptosis-inducing ligand (TRAIL) in atherosclerosis. *J. Am. Coll. Cardiol.* **2005**, *45*, 1018–1024. [CrossRef] [PubMed]
13. Bova, C.; Sanchez, O.; Prandoni, P.; Lankeit, M.; Konstantinides, S.; Vanni, S.; Jimenez, D. Identification of intermediate-risk patients with acute symptomatic pulmonary embolism. *Eur. Respir. J.* **2014**, *44*, 694–703. [CrossRef] [PubMed]
14. Sanchez, O.; Trinquart, L.; Caille, V.; Couturaud, F.; Pacouret, G.; Meneveau, N.; Verschuren, F.; Roy, P.M.; Parent, F.; Righini, M.; et al. Prognostic factors for pulmonary embolism: The prep study, a prospective multicenter cohort study. *Am. J. Respir. Crit. Care Med.* **2010**, *181*, 168–173. [CrossRef]
15. Lankeit, M.; Friesen, D.; Schafer, K.; Hasenfuss, G.; Konstantinides, S.; Dellas, C. A simple score for rapid risk assessment of non-high-risk pulmonary embolism. *Clin. Res. Cardiol.* **2013**, *102*, 73–80. [CrossRef]

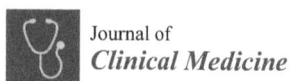 

*Review*

# Primary Thrombophilia XVII: A Narrative Review of Sticky Platelet Syndrome in México

Claudia Minutti-Zanella [1], Laura Villarreal-Martínez [2] and Guillermo J. Ruiz-Argüelles [3,*]

1. Laboratorios RUIZ-Escuela de Ciencias Médicas, Universidad Popular Autónoma del Estado de Puebla (UPAEP), Puebla 72530, Mexico; claudia.minutti@upaep.edu.mx
2. Facultad de Medicina, Hospital Universitario de Nuevo León, Monterrey 64460, Mexico; drlaura.villarrealmtz@gmail.com
3. Centro de Hematología y Medicina Interna, Clínica RUIZ, Puebla 72530, Mexico
* Correspondence: gruiz1@clinicaruiz.com

**Abstract:** Sticky Platelet Syndrome (SPS) is a disorder characterized by platelet hyperaggregability, diagnosed by studying in vitro platelet aggregation with ADP and epinephrine. It is the second most common cause of thrombophilia in Mexican Mestizos and manifests as an autosomal dominant trait which, combined with other coagulopathies, contributes significantly to the morbidity and mortality of patients with primary thrombophilia. It is easily treatable with antiplatelet drugs; however, the methods for diagnosis are not readily available in all clinical laboratories and the disorder is often overlooked by most clinicians. Herein, we present the results of more than 20 years of Mexican experience with the study of SPS in a Mestizo population.

**Keywords:** thrombophilia; sticky platelet syndrome; hyperaggregability

## 1. Introduction

In 1995, Mammen and colleagues studied a hereditary condition of hyper adhesive platelets that clump upon standard surface contact, after studying a family whose members suffered from rare arterial thrombotic events without identifiable risk factors such as diabetes or atherosclerosis to predispose them and otherwise normal coagulation laboratory parameters. Later, they observed the same condition in more than 200 patients who, as named by Holiday and colleagues, suffer from "Sticky Platelet Syndrome (SPS)". The condition is associated with angina pectoris, acute myocardial infarction, cerebral ischemic attacks or strokes, ischemic optic neuropathy, and recurrent venous thromboembolism, even while on optimal anticoagulant therapy [1].

We know now that SPS is a qualitative platelet disorder with familial occurrence that appears to have an autosomal dominant component as well, although not all patients have relatives with the disorder. It is characterized by increased platelet aggregation in response to ADP and epinephrine in vitro, and it is one of the most common causes of arterial thrombosis and pregnancy complications. Patients with SPS usually have their first thrombotic episode before age 40 and may or not have other acquired risk factors for thrombophilia. Anticoagulants such as vitamin K antagonists are inefficient, but some antiplatelet drugs have been shown to be effective at preventing rethrombosis and diminishing aggregation. An excellent review of the history of the disease and future perspectives was published by Kubisz and colleagues [2].

It has been considered that the glycoprotein receptors on the platelet surface may be involved in the pathogenesis of SPS; however, a specific cause of the condition has not been found [3]. Nonetheless, significant mortality and morbidity occur from these thrombotic events, such as paralysis, cardiac disability from repeated coronary events, miscarriages, and loss of vision and mobility. Rodger Bick (1998) mentioned that early diagnosis and treatment can prevent arterial and venous thrombotic events; however, clinicians and

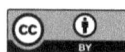

laboratories were unaware of the prevalence of the syndrome and thus failed to direct their diagnosis towards it. After studying 78 patients with said characteristics over a two year-period, he established that SPS is a common cause for arterial and venous thrombotic events in otherwise healthy patients [4]. These studies set the precedent for us to pioneer the study of the Mexican Mestizo population to determine the prevalence, incidence, and genetic background of SPS, aiming to determine its impact on morbidity and mortality in our country compared to other ethnic cohorts.

### 1.1. Primary Thrombophilia and Sticky Platlet Syndrome: The Mexican Experience

Pons-Estel and colleagues defined "mestizo" as those individuals born in Latin America who had both Amerindian and white ancestors, opposed to whites who have all white European ancestors and Amerindians, who have full autochthonous ancestry [5]. In 2005, Silva-Zolezzi and colleagues published the results of the first Mexican Genome Diversity Project (MGDP), which aimed to assess genetic ancestry in Mexicans to develop genomic medicine and genetic analysis in our country and Latin America. The study showed the great genetic diversity of Mexicans given by "mestizaje", which aside from adding to the cultural richness and beauty of our country, poses a clinical challenge on the study of diseases and raises a question on whether results obtained from studies on Caucasian or other populations are truly applicable to ours [6].

Our first study related to the investigation of the primary causes of thrombophilia in Mexican Mestizos was carried out on 102 persons with clinical features of inherited thrombophilia, who were tested for the activated protein C resistance (APCr) genotype and phenotype as well as levels of coagulation proteins C and S, antithrombin, plasminogen, tissue type plasminogen activator activity, plasminogen activator inhibitor activity, plasminogen activator inhibitor type I, anti-phospholipid antibodies and lupus anticoagulants. While 46% of the patients fit within the normal range for all tests, 39.2% were consistent with the APCr phenotype and only 4% with the factor V Leiden mutation. This finding is relevant because studies on Caucasian groups report that 20–60% of cases present such mutation, whereas in Mexican Indian groups it is almost nonexistent. In this cohort, most of the cases were acquired or unrelated to the factor V mutation, which led to conclude that the ethnic composition of Mexican Mestizo ancestry plays an important role in the etiology of primary thrombophilia [7].

In a continuing study, 37 Mexican Mestizo patients and 50 normal controls were tested under the same criteria to investigate prevalence of known mutations associated with primary thrombophilia. Four were heterozygous for the factor V Leiden mutation, 16 for the MTHFR 677 mutation, and 5 for the prothrombin 20,210 mutation. 6 were homozygous for the MTHFR 677 defect. It was also found that four individuals were compound heterozygotes for combinations of these mutations. MTHFR mutation alone is not sufficient to cause thrombophilia unless it is associated with other thrombophilia-causing conditions. Again, this study showed that the prevalence of mutations in Mexican Mestizos differs from that reported in Caucasians and paved the way for further analysis of these genetic differences and their implications on the diagnosis and prognosis of primary thrombophilia in Mexico [8].

In 2002, 10 patients with clinical characteristics of primary thrombophilia from the same ethnic group were prospectively studied to assess the prevalence of SPS. Platelet aggregation was measured from peripheral blood samples with increasing concentrations of ADP and epinephrine, while other coagulation and hemostasis parameters were measured as in previous studies [7,8]. Six out of ten patients fit within the SPS abnormality: five of them displayed other thrombophilia conditions linked to the genetic mutations previously studied, whereas only one presented SPS as a sole condition. Four of these six patients had a family history of thrombophilia. The study showed that SPS is frequently found in Mexican Mestizos with clinical characteristics of thrombophilia along with other genetic conditions that contribute to a multifactorial disease, changing the way clinicians approach diagnosis and treatment due to the implications on the health of patients and their families [9].

Given that few Mexican Mestizo patients with APCr-linked thrombophilia were affected by the FV Leiden mutation, the prevalence of other mutations such as HR2 haplotype, FV Cambridge, Hong Kong, and Liverpool was also looked at. Thirty-nine patients, regardless of their APCr phenotype status, were accrued for the study; inclusion criteria considered early-age and recurrent thrombosis, thrombosis at unusual anatomic sites, resistance to conventional therapy, and at least one episode of venous thrombosis, confirmed by phlebography or Doppler. Overall, 10% of patients were heterozygous for the FV Leiden mutation, 28% displayed the HR2 haplotype, one patient presented the Hong Kong mutation, and none presented the Cambridge or Liverpool mutations. This study yet again evidenced the differences in the genetic background of thrombophilia patients across ethnicities and concluded that the studied polymorphisms are nor relevantly implicated in thrombophilia in Mexican Mestizos [10].

In 2005, 46 Mexican Mestizo patients were accrued to assess the prevalence of SPS, protein C resistance, protein C activity and antigen, protein S, antithrombin, plasminogen, tissue type plasminogen activator activity, IgG and IgM isotypes of antiphospholipid antibodies, Factor V gene mutations, MTHFR 677 mutation and G20210A polymorphism. A total of 8% of individuals did not display any abnormality and thus were not counted for the final evaluation; 12% showed one abnormality and 88% percent presented two to five co-existing abnormalities; 48% of patients had SPS, 24% aPCR phenotype, 11% the FV Leiden mutation, 24% antiphospholipid antibodies, 9% protein S deficiency, and 13% protein C deficiency; 24% patients presented the HR2 haplotype and only one patient presented the Hong Kong mutation, supporting the results of the previous study [11]. Abnormalities in APCr were not significantly associated with the SPS phenotype in another study [12].

*1.2. Multifactorial Thrombophilia*

Hypercoagulability is a major health problem and has a high mortality and morbidity around the world. Inherited hypercoagulable states are associated with venous thrombosis rather than arterial problems, which are mostly due to the increased activation of platelets in the endothelial surface. Although genetic predisposition is unlikely to be the sole cause of a thrombotic event, people who have inherited more than one thrombophilia are at greater risk of thrombosis than those who are affected only by a single factor. Other "triggers" are needed to develop a thrombotic event, for example, atherosclerosis, pregnancy, or the use of oral contraceptives. This poses a model of "thrombosis threshold", which is based on a combination of inherited hypercoagulable states and patient lifestyle [13]. Based on this, in 2007 we investigated the relationship between clinical markers and thrombophilia in 100 patients. Overall, 19% of patients presented only one abnormality, while 81% presented two or more. SPS was found in 57 patients and the presence of other mutations was consistent with previous studies. Results also showed an association between the FV Leiden mutation and resistance to activated protein C; meaning that 94% of Mexican Mestizos that had at least one clinical marker of thrombophilia develop a thrombophilic condition. However, it is yet more common that the development of these pathologies is enhanced by two or more coexisting thrombophilia conditions [14].

Moreover, thrombophilia is often concomitant in myeloproliferative disorders (MPDs) such as polycythemia vera, essential thrombocythemia, idiopathic myelofibrosis, and chronic leukemias. Since myeloproliferative diseases arise from acquired genetic mutations, the group studied 77 Mexican Mestizos with primary thrombophilia to look for the JAK2 V617F mutation (commonly associated with MPDs) aiming to find whether underlying MPDs could be the precipitating factor of thrombotic episodes. None of the patients carried the mutation and only four were found to have splanchnic thrombosis, concluding that MPDs are an improbable cause of thrombophilia in this population. It is also noteworthy that the prevalence of MPDs in Mexican Mestizos is lower than in Caucasians [15].

Later on, we studied the effect of SPS in pregnancy. A total of 268 Mexican Mestizo patients were studied, of which 108 female patients were selected for further analysis; 71% of these patients had been pregnant at some point, and 37% had experienced at least one spontaneous abortion. Within the subset of patients who suffered from a spontaneous abortion, 86% had SPS, while the remaining percentage were heterozygous the MTHFR mutation. At the time, data in Mexico indicated that 12–13% of pregnancies in the general population end in a spontaneous abortion, meaning that the relative risk of having a miscarriage is 2.66 times higher in women with SPS. Timely and efficient treatment with antiplatelet drugs in these patients could reduce the risk of obstetric complications significantly. This study evidenced the necessity of further investigating complications and treatment of SPS in pregnant women [16]. Sokol and colleagues mentioned that SPS is especially relevant in the clinical management of patients with recurrent abortion [17].

*1.3. Subtypes of SPS and Inheritance*

It has been proposed that SPS is an autosomal dominant inherited disease that can manifest in one of three ways: type I, characterized by platelet hyperaggregability with ADP and epinephrine; type II, where aggregation happens only with epinephrine; and type III, only with ADP. To further study this observation, the group studied 5 kindreds of patients with known SPS and previous thrombotic episodes. A complete laboratory workup for thrombophilia was performed and in all five kindreds, where other relatives presented SPS. Results showed that family members of patients who carried the MTHFR mutation also had the mutation, and in one kindred, it was found in members of different generations [18]. Further on, the group aimed to establish a correlation between SPS phenotype and the GPIIIa PL A1/A2 polymorphism, a known marker of hyperaggregability and thromboembolism. A total of 160 patients with a clinical marker of primary thrombophilia were studied, of which 95 presented SPS (61 patients with type 1, 6 and 28 with type 2 and type 3, respectively). Of these patients, 79 had the PL A1/A2 genotype, 15 displayed the A1/A2 genotype, and 1 showed the PL A1/A2 genotype. In healthy controls, the frequencies were similar; thus, it was inferred that there is no significant association between PL A1/A2 polymorphisms and SPS phenotype [19].

In another study performed on 86 patients, we found that 65% of the cases were SPS type I, 10% type II, and 25% type III. Venous thrombosis was more frequent than arterial with 70% of cases, presenting in the lower limbs, CNS, upper limbs, mesenterial veins, and retina. There was no association between SPS type and localization of the thrombi, and no correlation between gender and localization of the episode nor subtype of SPS. Once again, this showed that there are important epidemiological differences between SPS in Mexican Mestizos and Caucasians. Caucasians suffer from SPS type II more frequently [20], whereas type I is more frequently seen in Mexican Mestizos. SPS is also the second most common cause of thrombophilia in this ethnic group [21]. We also conducted a study to define the identification of SPS worldwide and found that patients with the condition have been identified and reported in the five continents [12].

*1.4. Insights on the Treatment of SPS*

Treatment of SPS consists of diminishing platelet hyperaggregability with antiplatelet drugs such as aspirin. To evaluate the efficacy of this treatment on the prevention of rethrombosis and hyperaggregability, 55 patients with at least two assessments of SPS phenotype were treated and followed for up to 129 months with platelet aggregation studies. A total of 40 patients were treated with aspirin, 13 with a combination of aspirin and clopidogrel, and 2 with clopidogrel only. Two of these patients developed another vaso-occlusive episode in the retinal central artery despite treatment after 52 and 129 months; however, they showed no additional thrombophilia-causing conditions besides SPS after a full laboratory workup (Velázquez-Sanchez-de-Cima et al., 2013). Since SPS can contribute to "multifactorial thrombophilia", it is important that key laboratory tests are performed. Nevertheless, it was observed that treatment with common antiplatelet drugs such as aspirin and/or clopidogrel was effective in 96.4% of patients with SPS, regardless of the subtype. The results are in concordance with those obtained in a larger cohort ($n = 270$) by Kubisz and colleagues [22]. The findings of this study and observations made in the Mexican Mestizo population were presented at the 18th International Meeting of the Danubian League against Thrombosis and Haemorrhagic Disorders in 2015 and this continues to be the treatment of choice nowadays [23].

To further analyze the features of the treatment of SPS worldwide, we conducted a meta-analysis of 108 papers containing the term "Sticky Platelet" in the title or the abstract obtained from PubMed; of these, 43 were selected and 1783 patients with the condition were identified. We found that 332 patients received antiplatelet drugs, of which 303 were given aspirin only, 29 received combinations of heparin or coumadin with aspirin, and 2 patients received heparin + alteplase or abciximab. The rate of rethrombosis on these patients was 1.5%, showing that physicians around the world are aware that the use of antiplatelet drugs in SPS patients is beneficial. Although the treatment has been proven to be effective to control the condition, the importance of investigating its pathophysiology and epidemiology around the world has been deemed extremely important [24].

*1.5. Concluding Remarks*

Since the first description of Sticky Platelet Syndrome, it has been within our uttermost interest to contribute to the study of the genetic factors, clinical management, and diagnosis of the disease; especially given that it seems to be the second most common cause of thrombophilia in our country. SPS does not usually lead to thrombosis on its own, but rather needs association with another thrombophilia-causing condition to manifest itself, such as estrogen use, mutations, other alterations in blood coagulation, and in most recent times, COVID-19 [25,26]. In some patients, SPS can be so insidious that clinicians often mislabel thrombotic events as idiopathic. However, in patients with a high level of baseline genetic hypercoagulability, simple triggers could initiate thrombotic episodes and make them more likely to recur [11].

Even though the exact pathophysiology of SPS is not fully understood to date, a detailed review of known platelet function and molecular and genetic features associated with this syndrome was recently published by García-Villaseñor and colleagues. Some studies have been performed to assess the implications of microRNAs in platelet function, as well as to establish the relationship of polymorphisms with SPS complications, most of which are related to chronic degenerative diseases and infertility [27].

There is an urgent need to identify the cause of SPS, given that it is the most frequent cause of hereditary thrombophilia in México and probably in other countries as well. The gold standard to diagnose SPS is aggregometry; but since this technique is not readily available in most clinical laboratories, it is important to study more specific markers that could be studied with ease [28]. Many clinical professionals believe that SPS is only a reflection of "laboratory artifacts"; however, this is not due to lack of proof, but rather lack of understanding and availability of diagnostic methods. Given that SPS testing needs recently collected blood specimens, it is not possible to refer samples for testing, highlighting the need to standardize laboratory protocols and provide trustworthy information to make it more readily available for patients and clinicians. In Mexico, the topic is worthy of study since SPS has been proven to go hand-in-hand with other causes of thrombophilia, the most frequent cause of spontaneous miscarriages in thrombophilic women, and an important cause of venous thromboembolism. Nonetheless, SPS is an easily treatable condition given that antiplatelet drugs are cheap, available, and effective. Therefore, knowledge of the condition implies improving the quality of life for patients with this and other concomitant disorders; see Box 1 and Figure 1.

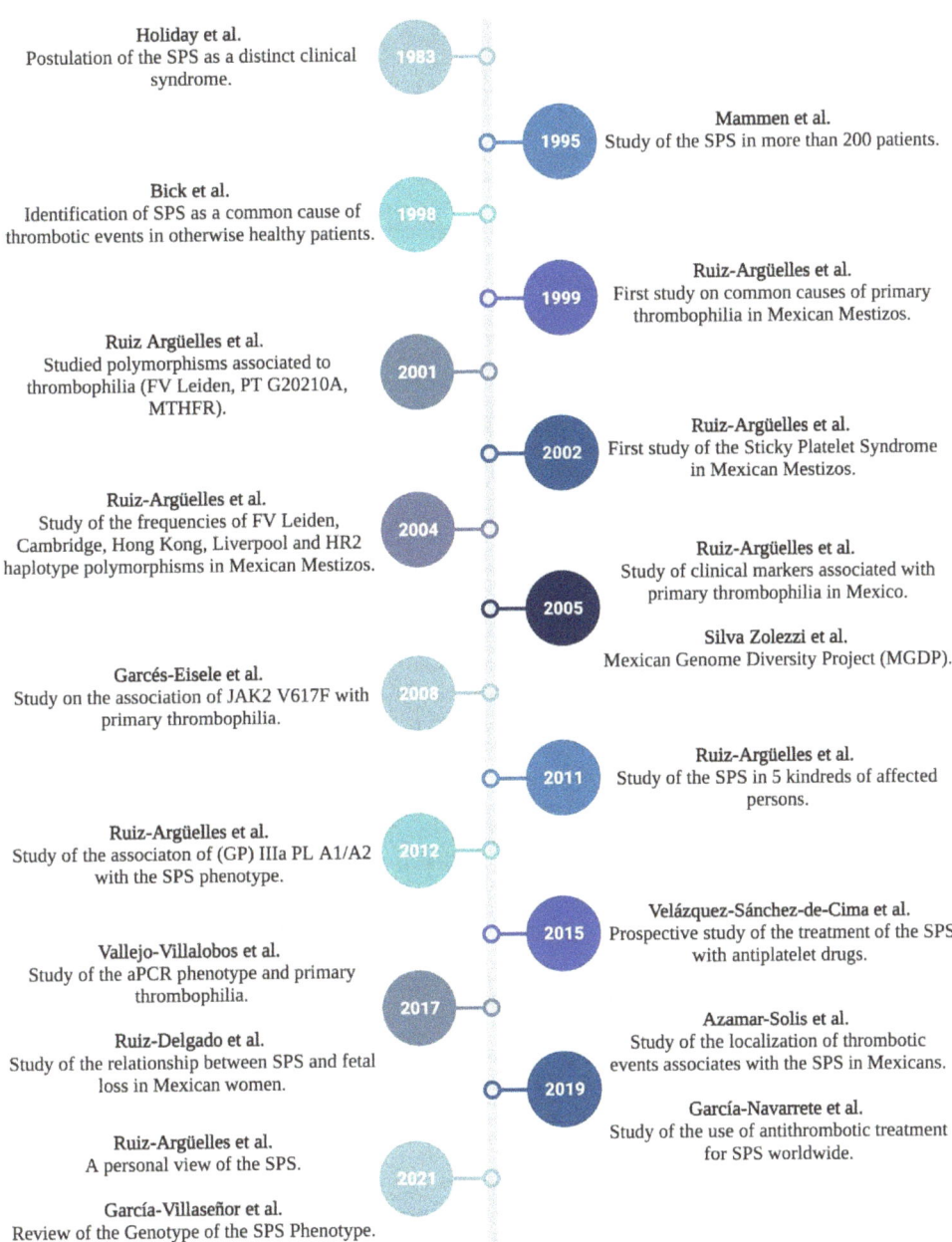

**Figure 1.** Timeline of the initial studies on Sticky Platelet Syndrome, and subsequent studies conducted and published in México. SPS: Sticky Platelet Syndrome. MTHFR: Methylenetetrahydrofolatereductase. (GP)IIIa PL A1/A2: Glycoprotein IIIa. aPCR: activated protein C resistance. Created in Biorender.com (accessed on 2 July 2022).

Box 1. Salient features of Sticky Platelet Syndrome.

(1) SPS is a phenotype of platelet hyperaggregability, defined by increased in vitro platelet aggregation after the addition of very low concentrations of adenosine diphosphate and/or epinephrine. The concentrations and dilutions of the agents are relatively well standardized.
(2) The genotype is currently unknown, but several observations on the genes of platelets proteins are being studied: platelet glycoprotein IIIa PLA1/A2; platelet glycoprotein 6, growth arrest specific 6, coagulation factor V, integrin subunit beta 3, platelet endothelial aggregation receptor 1, serpin family C member 1, serpin family E member 1.
(3) The SPS phenotype is probably the expression of genetic conditions interacting with other medical conditions or environmental factors, such as diabetes mellitus, hormonal therapy, and pregnancy.
(4) SPS may lead into both arterial and venous thrombosis, the latter being more frequent.
(5) SPS is a hereditary autosomal dominant trait.
(6) SPS is the most frequent cause of hereditary thrombophilia in México, and probably in other countries.
(7) Patients with SPS have been identified and treated in all continents of the world.
(8) SPS is a frequent cause of miscarriages and obstetric complications.
(9) SPS usually needs another thrombophilic condition to fully express as a thrombotic episode. It has recently been described as a risk factor for thrombosis during COVID-19.
(10) The hyperaggregability of SPS reverts to employing antiplatelet drugs and the re-thrombosis rate of persons with the syndrome is very low while being on treatment. Most patients revert the hyperaggregability with aspirin, but around one quarter need two antiplatelet drugs. It is therefore advisable to assess the SPS phenotype after starting the antiplatelet drug, in order to define further treatment. Treating persons with SPS with oral anticoagulants does not reduce the re-thrombosis rate
(11) Claiming that SPS is a non-entity indicates that it is not being assessed properly and may also be detrimental for patients. The treatment is cheap, available and effective, as well as tolerated by most persons, which is the use of low-doses of aspirin and other antiplatelet drugs.

**Funding:** This research received no external funding.

**Institutional Review Board Statement:** Not applicable.

**Informed Consent Statement:** Not applicable.

**Data Availability Statement:** Not applicable.

**Conflicts of Interest:** The authors declare no conflict of interest.

# References

1. Mammen, E.F. Ten Years' Experience with the "Sticky Platelet Syndrome". *Clin. Appl. Thromb.* **1995**, *1*, 66–72. [CrossRef]
2. Kubisz, P.; Ruiz-Argüelles, G.J.; Stasko, J.; Holly, P.; Ruiz-Delgado, G.J. Sticky Platelet Syndrome: History and Future Per-spectives. *Semin. Thromb. Hemost.* **2014**, *40*, 526–534.
3. Velázquez-Sánchez-de-Cima, S.; Zamora-Ortiz, G.; Hernández-Reyes, J.; Vargas-Espnosa, J.; García-Chavez, J.; Rosa-les-Padrón, J. Primary Thrombophilia in México X: A Prospective Study of the Treatment of the Sticky Platelet Syndrome. *Clin. Appl. Thromb. Hemost.* **2015**, *21*, 91–95. [CrossRef] [PubMed]
4. Bick, R.L. Sticky Platelet Syndrome: A Common Cause of Unexplained Arterial and Venous Thrombosis. *Clin. Appl. Thromb.* **1998**, *4*, 77–81. [CrossRef]
5. Pons-Estel, B.A.; Catoggio, L.J.; Cardiel, M.H.; Soriano, E.R.; Gentiletti, S.; Villa, A.R.; Abadi, I.; Caeiro, F.; Alvarellos, A.; Alarcón-Segovia, D. The GLADEL Multinational Latin American Prospective Inception Cohort of 1214 Patients with Systemic Lupus Erythematosus: Ethnic and disease heterogeneity among "Hispanics". *Medicine* **2004**, *83*, 1–17. [CrossRef]
6. Silva-Zolezzi, I.; Hidalgo-Miranda, A.; Estrada-Gil, J.; Fernandez-Lopez, J.C.; Uribe-Figueroa, L.; Contreras, A.; Balam-Ortiz, E.; del Bosque-Plata, L.; Velazquez-Fernandez, D.; Lara, C.; et al. Analysis of genomic diversity in Mexican Mestizo populations to develop genomic medicine in Mexico. *Proc. Natl. Acad. Sci. USA* **2009**, *106*, 8611–8616. [CrossRef] [PubMed]
7. Ruiz-Argüelles, G.J.; González-Estrada, S.; Garcés-Eisele, J.; Ruiz-Argüelles, A. Primary Thrombophilia in Mexico: A Pros-pective Study. *Am. J. Hematol.* **1999**, *60*, 1–5. [CrossRef]
8. Ruiz-Argüelles, G.J.; Garcés-Eisele, J.; Reyes-Núñez, V.; Ramírez-Cisneros, F.J. Primary Thrombophilia in Mexico. II. Factor V G1691A (Leiden), Prothrombin G20210A, and Methylenetetrahydrofolate Reductase C677T Polymorphism in Thrombophilic Mexican Mestizos. *Am. J. Hematol.* **2001**, *66*, 28–31. [CrossRef]

9. Ruiz-Argüelles, G.J.; López-Martinez, B.; Cruz-Cruz, D.; Esparza-Silva, L.; Reyes-Aulis, M.B. Primary Thrombophilia in Mexico III: A Prospective Study of the Sticky Platelet Syndrome. *Clin. Appl. Thromb.* **2002**, *8*, 273–277. [CrossRef] [PubMed]
10. Ruiz-Argüelles, G.J.; Poblete-Naredo, I.; Reyes-Núñez, V.; Garcés-Eisele, J.; López-Martínez, B.; Gómez-Rangel, J.D. Primary thrombophilia in Mexico IV: Frequency of the Leiden, Cambridge, Hong Kong, Liverpool and HR2 haplotype polymorphisms in the factor V gene of a group of thrombophilic Mexican Mestizo patients. *Rev. Investig. Clin.* **2004**, *56*, 600–604.
11. Ruiz-Argüelles, G.J.; López-Martínez, B.; Valdés-Tapia, P.; Gómez-Rangel, J.D.; Reyes-Núñez, V.; Garcés-Eisele, J. Primary thrombo-philia in Mexico. V. A comprehensive prospective study indicates that most cases are multifactorial: Multifactorial Throm-bophilia in Mexicans. *Am. J. Hematol.* **2005**, *78*, 21–26. [CrossRef] [PubMed]
12. Vallejo-Villalobos, M.F.; Gomez-Cruz, G.B.; Cantero-Fortiz, Y.; Olivares-Gazca, J.C.; Olivares-Gazca, M.; Murrieta-Alvarez, I.; Reyes-Nuñez, V.; Ruiz-Argüelles, G.J. Primary Thrombophilia XIV: Worldwide Identification of Sticky Platelet Syndrome. *Semin. Thromb. Hemost.* **2019**, *45*, 423–428. [CrossRef] [PubMed]
13. Schafer, A.I.; Levine, M.N.; Konkle, B.A.; Kearon, C. Thrombotic Disorders: Diagnosis and Treatment. *Hematology* **2003**, *2003*, 520–539. [CrossRef]
14. Ruiz-Argüelles, G.J.; González-Carrillo, M.L.; Estrada-Gómez, R.; Valdés-Tapia, P.; Parra-Ortega, I.; Porras-Juárez, A. Trombofilia primaria en México Parte VI: Falta de asociación estadística entre las condiciones trombofílicas heredadas. *Gac. Méd. Méx.* **2007**, *4*, 317–322.
15. Garcés-Eisele, J.; González-Carrillo, M.L.; Reyes-Núñez, V.; Ruiz-Argüelles, G.J. Primary thrombophilia in México VII: The V617F mutation of JAK2 is not a frequent cause of thrombosis. *Hematology* **2008**, *13*, 244–246. [CrossRef]
16. Ruiz-Delgado, G.J.; Cantero-Fortiz, Y.; Mendez-Huerta, M.A.; Leon-Gonzalez, M.; Nuñez-Cortes, A.K.; Leon-Peña, A.A.; Olivares-Gazca, J.C.; Ruiz-Argüelles, G.J. Primary Thrombophilia in Mexico XII: Miscarriages are More Frequent in People with Sticky Platelet Syndrome. *Turk. J. Hematol.* **2017**, *34*, 239–243.
17. Sokol, J.; Kubisz, P.; Stasko, J. Comment on: Inherited Thrombophilia and Pregnancy Complications: Should We Test? *Semin. Thromb. Hemost.* **2019**, *46*, 501. [CrossRef]
18. Ruiz-Argüelles, G.J.; Alarcón-Urdaneta, C.; Calderón-García, J.; Ruiz-Delgado, G.J. Primary thrombophilia in México VIII: De-scription of five kindreds of familial platelet syndrome phenotype. *Rev. Hematol. Mex.* **2011**, *12*, 73–78.
19. Ruiz-Argüelles, G.J.; Garcés-Eisele, J.; Camacho-Alarcón, C.; Moncada-Gonzalez, B.; Valdés-Tapia, P.; León-Montes, N.; Ruiz-Delgado, G.J. Primary thrombophilia in Mexico IX: The Glycoprotein IIIa PL A1/A2 Polymorphism is Not Associated With the Sticky Platelet Syndrome Phenotype. *Clin. Appl. Thromb. Hemost.* **2013**, *19*, 689–692. [CrossRef]
20. Skerenova, M.; Jedinakova, Z.; Simurda, T.; Skornova, I.; Stasko, J.; Kubisz, P.; Sokol, J. Progress in the Understanding of Sticky Platelet Syndrome. *Semin. Thromb. Hemost.* **2016**, *43*, 8–13. [CrossRef] [PubMed]
21. Azamar-Solis, B.; Cantero-Fortiz, Y.; Olivares-Gazca, J.C.; Olivares-Gazca, J.M.; Gomez-Cruz, G.B.; Murrieta-Álvarez, I.; Ruiz-Delgado, G.J.; Ruiz-Argüelles, G.J. Primary Thrombophilia in Mexico XIII: Localization of the Thrombotic Events in Mexican Mestizos with the Sticky Platelet Syndrome. *Clin. Appl. Thromb.* **2019**, *25*, 1–4. [CrossRef]
22. Kubisz, P. Response to "Comment on Sticky Platelet Syndrome". *Semin. Thromb. Hemost.* **2014**, *40*, 274. [CrossRef] [PubMed]
23. Mikovic, D.; Stanciakova, L.; Sinzinger, H.; Kubisz, P. Meeting Report: 18th International Meeting of the Danubian League against Thrombosis and Haemorrhagic Disorders. *Semin. Thromb. Hemost.* **2015**, *41*, 903–906. [CrossRef] [PubMed]
24. García-Navarrete, Y.I.; Vallejo-Villalobos, M.F.; Olivares-Gazca, J.M.; Cantero-Fortiz, Y.; León-Peña, A.A.; Olivares-Gazca, J.C.; Murrieta-Álvarez, I.; Ruiz-Delgado, G.J.; Ruiz-Argüelles, G.J. Primary thrombophilia XV: Antithrombotic treatment of sticky platelet syndrome worldwide. *Ann. Blood* **2019**, *4*, 15. [CrossRef]
25. Ruiz-Argüelles, G.J. A personal view of the sticky platelet syndrome. *Rev. Hematol. Mex.* **2021**, *22*, 199–201.
26. Ruiz-Argüelles, G.J.; Ruiz-Delgado, G.J. Algunas reflexiones sobre el síndrome de plaquetas pegajosas en 2019. *Rev. Hematol. Mex.* **2019**, *20*, 243–246. [CrossRef]
27. García-Villaseñor, E.; Bojalil-Álvarez, L.; Murrieta-Álvarez, I.; Cantero-Fortiz, Y.; Ruiz-Delgado, G.J.; Ruiz-Argüelles, G.J. Primary Thrombophilia XVI: A Look at the Genotype of the Sticky Platelet Syndrome Phenotype. *Clin. Appl. Thromb.* **2021**, *27*, 1076029619841700. [CrossRef] [PubMed]
28. Moncada, B.; Ruíz-Arguelles, G.J.; Castillo-Martínez, C. The sticky platelet syndrome. *Hematology* **2013**, *18*, 230–232. [CrossRef]

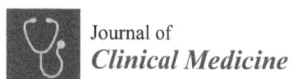 

*Systematic Review*

# Endovascular Treatment of Intracranial Vein and Venous Sinus Thrombosis—A Systematic Review

Philipp Bücke [1,*], Victoria Hellstern [2], Alexandru Cimpoca [2], José E. Cohen [3], Thomas Horvath [1], Oliver Ganslandt [4], Hansjörg Bäzner [5] and Hans Henkes [2,6]

1. Department of Neurology, Inselspital, Bern University Hospital, University of Bern, 3010 Bern, Switzerland; thomas.horvath@insel.ch
2. Neuroradiologische Klinik, Klinikum Stuttgart, 70174 Stuttgart, Germany; v.hellstern@klinikum-stuttgart.de (V.H.); a.cimpoca@klinikum-stuttgart.de (A.C.); h.henkes@klinikum-stuttgart.de (H.H.)
3. Department of Neurosurgery, Hadassah Medical Center, Hebrew University Jerusalem, Jerusalem 9103401, Israel; jcohenns@yahoo.com
4. Neurochirurgische Klinik, Klinikum Stuttgart, 70174 Stuttgart, Germany; o.ganslandt@klinikum-stuttgart.de
5. Neurologische Klinik, Klinikum Stuttgart, 70174 Stuttgart, Germany; h.baezner@klinikum-stuttgart.de
6. Medical Faculty, Universität Duisburg-Essen, 45147 Essen, Germany
* Correspondence: philipp.buecke@insel.ch

**Abstract:** Background: Cerebral venous sinus or vein thromboses (SVT) are treated with heparin followed by oral anticoagulation. Even after receiving the best medical treatment, numerous patients experience neurological deterioration, intracerebral hemorrhage or brain edema. Debate regarding whether endovascular treatment (EVT) is beneficial in such severe cases remains ongoing. This systematic review summarizes the current evidence supporting the use of EVT for SVT on the basis of case presentations, with a focus on patient selection, treatment strategies and the effects of the COVID-19 pandemic. Methods: This systemic literature review included randomized controlled trials (RCTs) and retrospective observational data analyzing five or more patients. Follow-up information (modified Rankin scale (mRS)) was required to be provided (individual patient data). Results: 21 records ($n$ = 405 patients; 1 RCT, 20 observational studies) were identified. EVT was found to be feasible and safe in a highly selected patient cohort but was not associated with an increase in good functional outcomes (mRS 0–2) in RCT data. In observational data, good functional outcomes were frequently observed despite an anticipated poor prognosis. Conclusion: The current evidence does not support the routine incorporation of EVT in SVT treatment. However, in a patient cohort prone to poor prognosis, EVT might be a reasonable therapeutic option. Further studies determining the patients at risk, choice of methods and devices, and timing of treatment initiation are warranted.

**Keywords:** cerebral venous sinus thrombosis; endovascular therapy; thrombolysis; thrombectomy; intracerebral hemorrhage; anticoagulation; VITT

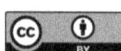

## 1. Introduction

Cerebral venous sinus or venous thrombosis (SVT) is a rare but potentially severe cause of cerebral hemorrhage or cerebral venous infarction (incidence: 1.32 per 100,000 person-years (2.78 per 100,000 person-years in women 31–50 years of age)) accounting for approximately 0.5% of all stroke cases [1–3]. Various factors are associated with the development of SVT [1,4]. Recent publications have reported a considerably higher incidence of SVT in the COVID-19 pandemic because both COVID-19 (reported incidence: 8.8 per 10,000 infections over 3 months) and COVID-19 vaccination (leading to vaccine-induced immune thrombotic thrombocytopenia (VITT)) appear to increase the risk of SVT [5,6]. Figure 1 illustrates the anatomy of the cerebral dural sinus and the deep cerebral veins.

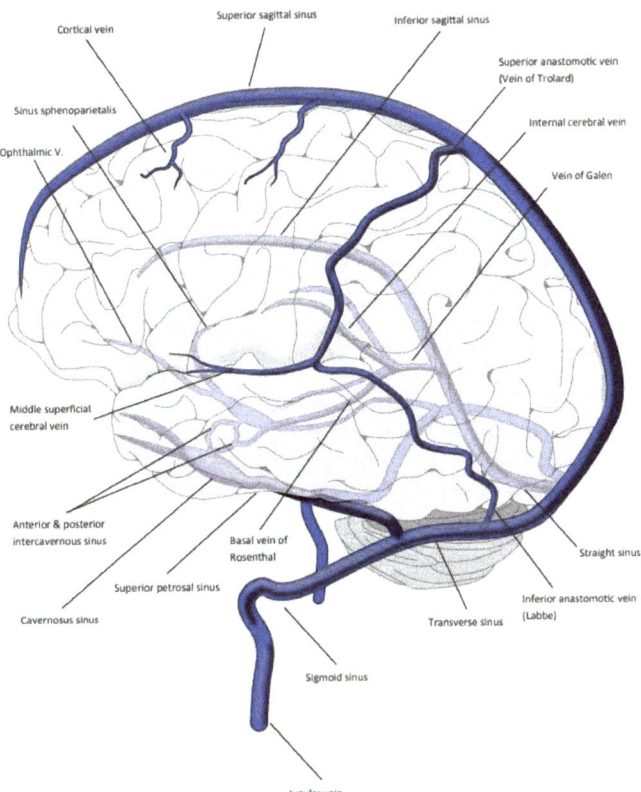

**Figure 1.** Illustration of the anatomy of the cerebral sinus and veins [7].

Outcomes after SVT in general are favorable assuming early diagnosis and treatment initiation [8]. Treatment is challenging, and its success highly depends on rapid anticoagulation with unfractionated or low-molecular-weight heparin, even in cases of intracerebral hemorrhage [9,10]. However, probably because of a limited capacity to dissolve an extensive intravenous thrombus load, many patients show deterioration, and as many as 13% eventually die or remain severely disabled despite sufficient anticoagulation therapy [11–13]. Patients with coma or altered mental status, intracerebral hemorrhage (ICH), underlying malignancy or an infection of the central nervous system appear to be at risk [12]. Pregnant or postpartum women, chronic hypertension as well as superior sagittal sinus and cortical vein involvement seem to be associated with ICH complications in SVT [14].

Endovascular treatment (EVT) strategies have been proposed to increase the frequency of good functional outcomes in high-risk or deteriorating patients [15–25]. Initially, endovascular thrombolysis with application of the thrombolytic agent locally and at the site of the occluded sinus was described [15,16]. Occasionally, the catheter is left in situ for 24 h or more [16,17]. In addition, several endovascular techniques have been discussed and investigated: rheolytic catheter thrombectomy, direct aspiration thrombectomy, balloon-guided thrombectomy or angioplasty and stent retriever thrombectomy [18–37]. Information on EVT in SVT is sparse and is based primarily on case series and anecdotal data and only a single published randomized controlled trial (RCT) [19,38–57]. Therefore, the current guideline recommendations remain vague. Whereas the American Heart Association and the American Stroke Association have together stated that endovascular therapy "may be considered if deterioration occurs despite intensive anticoagulation treatment," the European Stroke Organisation has not given any advice at all [58,59].

The goal of this systematic review is to provide an overview on the current evidence supporting EVT strategies in patients with SVT. We aimed to identify potential selection criteria for patients who might benefit from an additional EVT. Furthermore, the roles of SARS-CoV-2 infections and VITT are discussed.

## 2. Materials and Methods

We performed a systematic literature search in the PubMed (20 May 2022) and Medline (20 May 2022) databases by using the following search terms: "sinus thrombosis AND endovascular," "sinus thrombosis AND thrombectomy," "[cerebral] venous thrombosis AND endovascular" and "[cerebral] venous thrombosis AND thrombectomy." For the sub-analysis of patients with SVT caused by SARS-CoV-2 infection or after COVID-19 vaccination, additional search phrases were identified: "COVID-19 AND endovascular (AND thrombosis)," "COVID-19 AND thrombectomy (AND thrombosis)," "vaccination AND endovascular" and "vaccination AND thrombectomy." All articles published online until 20 May 2022 were screened. Two independent raters performed the literature search (P.B. and H.H.). This review follows the Preferred Reporting Items for Systematic Reviews and Meta-Analyses (PRISMA 2020) recommendations [60].

All identified publications were required to meet the following predefined inclusion criteria: (1) RCTs or retrospective studies, case series/case reports including more than five patients 18 years of age or older; (2) reported information on functional outcomes (modified Rankin scale (mRS) after discharge (not at the time of discharge)), death and complications (e.g., symptomatic intracranial hemorrhage or procedural complications); (3) inclusion of individual patient or study data only once (screening for repeated publications including identical cases); and (4) publication in English. In the analysis of EVT in patients with COVID-19 and VITT, only articles and manuscripts evaluating endovascular procedures (and the respective indications to treat patients) were eligible. We, therefore, did not consider registry data and meta-analyses reporting the frequency and the number of interventions without mentioning procedure-specific outcome parameters.

## 3. Results

A total of 456 records were identified and screened on the basis of the predefined search criteria (Figure 2). Only 92 were eligible for full-text evaluation. Eventually, 21 records were eligible for inclusion (reasons for exclusion of records: $n = 56$—case reports or case series with fewer than five reported events; $n = 14$—no follow-up data or data on functional outcomes; $n = 3$—not written in English).

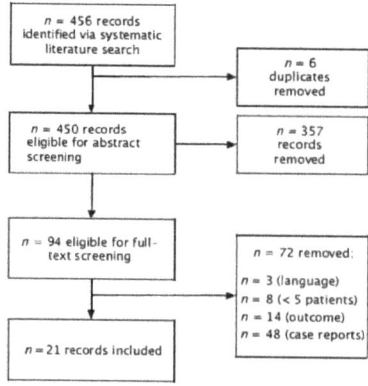

**Figure 2.** Flow diagram visualizing the selection process for the included publications.

One RCT (Thrombolysis or Anticoagulation for Cerebral Venous Thrombosis; TO-ACT) compared EVT ($n$ = 33) and standard care (i.e., anticoagulation; $n$ = 34) in patients with anticipated poor outcomes (Table 1) [38], which were defined as at least one of the following risk factors: mental status disorder, coma state (Glasgow coma scale (GCS) < 9), ICH or thrombosis of the deep cerebral venous system. Patients with more than 10 days from diagnosis to potential randomization, pregnancy (women in the puerperium were eligible), thrombocytopenia (platelet count < 100 × $10^9$/L), as well as clinical or radiological signs of impending trans-tentorial herniation were excluded. EVT (mechanical thrombectomy with an AngioJet (Boston Scientific, Marlborough, MA, USA), stent retriever, aspiration techniques or microcatheter) in combination with local thrombolytic treatment (urokinase administered continuously for up to 72 h) did not differ from standard care in terms of functional outcomes (mRS, 0–1 at 12 months; 67% vs. 68%; risk ratio, 0.99 (95% CI, 0.71–1.18); Table 1 provides details and information on complications).

Nyberg et al. (2017) have retrospectively analyzed their single-center cohort of patients with SVT and compared outcome data (mRS, 0–2 at 3 months) for patients treated with additional EVT ($n$ = 29) to those receiving anticoagulation only ($n$ = 37; 5-year time span (2011–2015)) [39]. The decision on whether to perform EVT was at the discretion of the treatment team and based on individual decision-making. The two treatment groups did not differ in outcome parameters (e.g., mRS, 0–2: 22% vs. 30%; mortality, $n$ = 6 vs. $n$ = 5; $p$ = 1.0).

Prospective case series, retrospective analyses and case series demonstrated the technical and procedural feasibility and safety of EVT in selected patients ($n$ = 19; details in Table 1) [19,40–57]. All reported patients were anticoagulated, and those with an expected poor prognosis (such as ICH or edema, neurological deterioration, coma (e.g., GCS < 9), progressive thrombus material observed on repeated imaging or signs of elevated intracranial pressure (e.g., papilledema)). Individual decision-making based on local experience and preferences was used to decide whether to perform EVT.

A total of 25 publications met the search criteria for COVID-19 and VITT-associated EVT in SVT. Of those, 14 records were excluded (because of lack of reported patient data, review articles and registry data without information on individual patients). Eleven records were eligible for analysis (Table 2) [61–71], comprising case reports and case series only. Of those, four case reports and case series presented data for four patients with COVID-19 and EVT [61–64]. The decision to perform EVT was made in cases with suspected poor prognosis, with criteria comparable to those described above. Aspiration in combination with local thrombolytic therapy was the preferred endovascular technique [61,62]. The overall outcome was poor [61–63].

The first reports of SVT caused by VITT emerged in 2021 [65–71]. As of 20 May 2022, seven records of EVT in 16 VITT patients were identified [65–71]. Most cases ($n$ = 15) were attributed to the ChAdOx1 nCoV-19 (AstraZeneca, Cambridge, UK) vaccine [65–67,69–71]. Only one case appeared to be associated with an mRNA vaccine (mRNA-1273 vaccine; Moderna, Cambridge, MA, USA) [68]. Excluding the latter, the time between vaccination and symptom onset was 4–27 days. Common features (except [68]) were thrombocytopenia, elevated D-dimer levels, and positivity for platelet factor 4 (PF4) antibodies (Table 2). Neurological deterioration potentially resulting in poor outcomes facilitated the use of EVT. The technical strategies described were aspiration plus stent retriever or balloon-guided thrombectomy in selected cases [65–67,69]. MRS of 0–1 was observed in seven patients during follow-up [65,66,69]. Three patients died [65,70].

**Table 1.** Summary of the 21 records included in this systematic review.

| Reference | | | | Treatment | | | | Outcome Assessment | | | | Localization | | | | Complications | | |
|---|---|---|---|---|---|---|---|---|---|---|---|---|---|---|---|---|---|---|---|
| Author (Year) | Study Type | Period | n (N) | Inclusion Criteria/Treatment Allocation | Pre-ICH | Endovascular Treatment | Control Group | FU (Month) | Outcome | Death | Recanal. | SSS | SS | Sig S | TS | DV | Catheter * | ICH ** | Other |
| Coutinho et al. (2020) [38] | RCT | 2011–2016 | 33 (67) | High probability of poor outcome, at least 1 of the following risk factors: mental status disorder, coma state (GCS <9), ICH, or thrombosis of the deep cerebral venous system (exclusion: duration from diagnosis of more than 10 days, pregnancy (women in the puerperium were eligible), thrombocytopenia (platelet count, <100 × 10^9/L), clinical and radiological signs of impending transtentorial herniation) | n = 22 | n = 33; LT (alteplase, urokinase; up to 72 h); n = 17 (52%); MT: n = 30 (91%) (Angiojet [n = 14], SR [n = 5], B [n = 3], aspiration (A) [n = 3; Penumbra], microcatheter [n = 3], other [n = 9]) | n = 34; standard care | 6, 12 | mRS 0–1 (12 months); n = 22 (67%) vs. n = 23 (68%); risk ratio 0.99 (95% CI 0.71–1.18) | 12 months; n = 4 (12%) [vs. n = 1 (3%)] | SSS (6–12 months); 79% vs. 52%; 1.52 (1.02–2.27); SS (6 months); 96% vs. 86%, 1.13 (0.95–1.33) | n = 23 (70%) | n = 17 (52%) | l: n = 12 r: n = 15 | l: n = 16 r: n = 22 | n = 14 (42%) | n = 3 (9%) | n = 6 (18%) (hem. compl.) | NA |
| Nyberg et al. (2017) [39] | retrosp | 2011–2015 | 29 (66) | SVT (anticoagulation), decision of treatment team | n = 17 (n = 10 in CC) | LT n = 29 (24–72 h); n = 21 additional MT (A, SR, B, Angiojet or combination; not specified) | n = 37; standard care | 3 | mRS 0–2: 22 vs. 30 (p = 1.0) | n = 6 (vs. n = 5) | n = 11; full (n = 8), partial (n = 3) | n = 25 | n = 0 | n = 21 | n = 25 | n = 7 | NN | n = 9 | NN |
| Siddiqui et al. (2014) [40] | retrosp | 1995–2012 | 63 (NN) | SVT (anticoagulation) and either coma (GCS < 9), ICH or deterioration | n = 29 | n = 63; n = 29 LT only; n = 34 MT (plus LT n = 27; Angiojet n = 28, A n = 3, SR n = 1, B n = 2) [LT bolus and continuously depending on recanalization] | NA | 3 | n = 53; mRS 0–1: n = 33 | n = 11 | full (n = 21), partial (n = 18) | NN | NN | NN | NN | NN | n = 5 | n = 3 | NN |
| Gao et al. (2020) [41] | retrosp | 2010–2019 | 56 (227 ss) | SVT under anticoagulation; ICH, lack of improvement or deterioration of symptoms | n = 56 | n = 56; LT only (n = 41); duration: 7 days]; additional MT (n = 15) [SR n = 5, A n = 3, B n = 3, combined n = 4] | NA | 6 | n = 54; mRS 0–2: n = 49 | n = 3 | (full and partial): LT n = 39; MT n = 14 | NN | NN | NN | NN | NN | n = 0 | LT n = 7, MT n = 1 | NN |
| Andersen et al. (2020) [42] | retrosp | 2007–2018 | 28 (NN) | SVT under anticoagulation; clinical deterioration and/or impaired consciousness | n = 18 | n = 28; LT (n = 26; 12–72 h), A combined (more than 2 techniques; n = 4) incl. PTA and stenting (n = 2) | NA | 6 | mRS 0–2: n = 20 | n = 5 | full (n = 15), partial (n = 11), no (n = 2) | n = 16 | n = 15 | n = 15 | n = 16 | n = 7 | n = 1 (retrsp. hem.) | n = 8 | NA |
| Yang et al. (2019) [43] | pros CS | 2014–2018 | 21 (22 ss) | SVT (anticoagulation) with: ICH (mental status impairment, coma (GCS < 9), DV thrombosis, cortical venous thrombosis, intracranial hypertension, or papilledema | NN | NN | NA | 12 | mRS 0–2: n = 21 | n = 0 | full (n = 5), partial (n = 9) | n = 16 | n = 0 | n = 17 | n = 19 | n = 14 | NN | NN | NN |

**Table 1.** *Cont.*

| Reference | | | | Treatment | | | Outcome Assessment | | | | Localization | | | | | Complications | | |
|---|---|---|---|---|---|---|---|---|---|---|---|---|---|---|---|---|---|---|
| Author (Year) | Study Type | Period | n (N) | Inclusion Criteria/Treatment Allocation | Pre-ICH | Endovascular Treatment | Control Group | FU (Month) | Outcome | Death | Recanal. | SSS | SS | Sig S | TS | DV | Catheter * | ICH ** | Other |
| Yang et al. (2021) [44] | retrosp | 2017–2019 | 23 (NN) | SVT (anticoagulation) with: deterioration after the initiation of anticoagulation, lethargy or coma, venous infarction with hemorrhagic transformation or ICH | n = 8 | n = 23; MT (B) plus LT (urokinase) | NA | 6 | n = 21; mRS 0-1: n = 21 | n = 0 | full (n = 9), partial (n = 13) | n = 20 | n = 11 | n = 21 | n = 21 | NN | n = 2 (failure) | n = 1 | NN |
| Stam et al. (2008) [45] | pros CS | NN | 20 (NN) | SVT (heparin) with assumed poor prognosis: altered mental status, coma, extensive edema, ICH, infarction | n = 14 | SVT (heparin), LT only (n = 15 additional MT [rheolytic catheter]) | NA | 3 (–6) | mRS 0-2: n = 12 | n = 6 | NN | NN | NN | NN | NN | n = 20 | NN | n = 1 (ICH progress) | NN |
| Lu et al. (2019) [46] | retrosp | 2015–2018 | 14 (NN) | SVT (best medical treatment); decision of treatment team | n = 1 | n = 14; MT (SR or A, combination), additional stenting in n = 5 (in case of failure of SR or A, re-occlusion) | NA | 2 (–16) | n = 5 (stenting); mRS 0-1: n = 4 | n = 0 | NN | n = 0 | n = 0 | n = 0 | n = 5 | NA | NN | n = 2 (increase) | NN |
| Qureshi et al. (2018) [47] | retrosp | 2006-2011/2016/2017 | 14 (NN) | SVT (anticoagulation), deterioration | n = 7 | n = 13 LT, MT: Angiojet n = 9, B n = 2, SR n = 2 (combined) [LT bolus up to 22 h after MT in case of incomplete recanalization] | NA | 1 (–3) | mRS 0-2: n = 10 | n = 1 | full (n = 3), partial (n = 4) | n = 10 | n = 1 | n = 10 | n = 13 | n = 0 | NN | n = 3 | NN |
| Styczen et al. (2019) [48] | retrosp | 2011–2018 | 13 (NN) | SVT (heparin) with assumed poor prognosis: altered mental status or coma, involvement of DV, ICH | n = 7 | n = 13; MT (A n = 4, A plus SR n = 9) | NA | 3 (median) | mRS 0-2: n = 12 | n = 1 | full (n = 4), partial (n = 7) | n = 9 | n = 5 | n = 7 | n = 10 | NN | n = 1 (perf) | n = 3 | NN |
| Mokin et al. (2015) [49] | retrosp | 2010–2013 | 13 (NN) | SVT (plus/minus anticoagulation), decision of treatment team | NN | n = 13 (LT n = 2 [sinus or ia]; A n = 2, LT plus A n = 3, A plus SR n = 2, Angiojet n = 2, combined n = 3) | NA | 3 | n = 11; mRS 0-2: n = 5 | n = 1 | full (n = 5), partial (n = 8) | n = 10 | n = 7 | n = 0 | n = 11 | n = 0 | NN | NN | NN |
| Dashti et al. (2011) [50] | retrosp | 2009/2010 | 13 (NN) | NA, decision of treatment team | NN | n = 13; Angiojet | NA | NN | n = 9; mRS 0-1: n = 7 | n = 2 | full (n = 6), partial (n = 7) | n = 9 | NN | NN | NN | NN | NN | NN | n = 1 (re-occl) |
| Lee et al. (2016) [51] | retrosp | 2008–2015 | 10 (NN) | SVT under anticoagulation, MT in case of ICH, deep venous thrombosis, deterioration | n = 9 | n = 10; MT (B plus A [combination]) plus LT (n = 3; before 2013; bolus) | NA | 3 | mRS 0-1: n = 8 | n = 1 | NN | n = 6 | n = 3 | n = 5 | n = 9 | NA | n = 0 | n = 1 | NN |
| Poulsen et al. (2013) [52] | retrosp | 2007–2011 | 9 (NN) | SVT (anticoagulation), deterioration | n = 4 | n = 6 MT (n = 5 prior LT [24–72 h]; not specified); n = 5 LT only | NA | 6 | mRS 0-2: n = 8 | n = 1 | full (n = 2), partial (n = 4) | n = 5 | n = 4 | n = 0 | n = 9 | n = 0 | n = 0 | n = 1 (SAH) | n = 3 (hem. eVOI) |

135

**Table 1.** Cont.

| Reference | | | | Treatment | | | | Outcome Assessment | | | Localization | | | | | Complications | | |
|---|---|---|---|---|---|---|---|---|---|---|---|---|---|---|---|---|---|---|
| Author (Year) | Study Type | Period | n (N) | Inclusion Criteria/Treatment Allocation | Pre-ICH | Endovascular Treatment | Control Group | FU (Month) | Outcome | Death | Recanal. | SSS | SS | Sig S | TS | DV | Catheter * | ICH ** | Other |
| Manninen et al. (2017) [53] | retrosp | (4 years) | 8 (243 sc) | SVT (anticoagulation), no response or deterioration | n = 1 | n = 8 (MT, A [Penumbra] plus additional B (n = 7) and LT (n = 3; bolus) | NA | 6 | mRS 0–2: n = 5 | n = 1 | full (n = 3), partial (n = 4) | n = 5 | n = 5 | n = 2 | n = 6 | n = 3 | n = 0 | n = 0 | n = 0 |
| Peng et al. (2021) [54] | retrosp | 2017–2020 | 7 (NN) | SVT (anticoagulation), one risk factor (poor outcome), coma (GCS < 9), ICH, DV thrombosis | n = 4 | n = 7 MT (SR; plus B plus A n = 4, plus heparin n = 4, plus LT n = 1 [bolus]) | NA | 3 | mRS 0–2: n = 6 | n = 0 | full (n = 4), partial (n = 3) | n = 7 | n = 0 | n = 4 | n = 5 | n = 0 | n = 0 | n = 0 | n = 0 |
| Mohdi et al. (2020) [55] | retrosp | 2018/2019 | 7 (NN) | SVT (anticoagulation), clinical and imaging deterioration (no signs of herniation) | n = 3 | n = 7 (MT, A) plus LT (n = 4, bolus 20 min) | NA | 1 (3, 6) | mRS 0–1: n = 5 | n = 0 | partial (n = 7) | n = 6 | n = 4 | n = 0 | n = 3 | n = 0 | n = 0 | n = 0 | n = 0 |
| Tsang et al. (2018) [56] | CS | 2014–2018 | 6 (NN) | SVT (anticoagulation) with deterioration or ICH | NN | n = 6; MT (A [Penumbra] plus LT (urokinase) | NA | 3 | mRS 0–1: n = 5 | n = 1 | NN | n = 5 | n = 2 | n = 3 | n = 4 | NN | n = 0 | n = 0 | n = 0 |
| Jankowitz et al. (2013) [19] | retrosp | 2009–2011 | 6 (27 sc) | SVT (best medical treatment); clinical (progressive deficits, coma) or radiological (hem., edema) deterioration | n = 4 | n = 6; MT (A (n = 6), additional LT n = 4 (bolus) | NA | 6 | mRS 0–2: n = 4 | n = 1 | n = 6 | n = 3 | n = 2 | n = 1 | n = 3 | NA | n = 0 | NN | n = 0 |
| Yue et al. (2010) [57] | retrosp | 2005–2008 | 6 (28 sc) | SVT (anticoagulation) with deterioration or assumed poor prognosis; coma, altered mental state, seizure, space-occupying lesions (edema or [hemorrhagic] infarct) | n = 2 | n = 6; MT (B) plus T (urokinase) | NA | 3 (–6) | mRS 0: n = 5 | n = 1 | full (n = 5) | n = 6 | n = 4 | n = 6 | n = 6 | n = 20 | n = 0 | n = 0 | n = 0 |

* catheter complications such as perforation; ** ICH: new hemorrhage or worsening of a pre-existing intracerebral hemorrhage; n, number of patients; N, total number of patients (patients screened: indicated by [sc]; ICH, intracerebral hemorrhage; FU, follow-up; Recanal., recanalization; SSS, sagittal superior sinus; SS, straight sinus; S Sig, sigmoid sinus; TS, transverse sinus; DV, deep cerebral veins; RCT, randomized controlled trial; restrosp, retrospective, pros, prospective; CS, case series; GCS, Glasgow Coma Scale; SVT, sinus or cerebral vein thrombosis; MT, mechanical thrombectomy; NN, unknown; NA, not applicable; LT, local (intrasinus) thrombolysis; A, aspiration thrombectomy; SR, stent retriever thrombectomy; B, balloon guided thrombectomy or angioplasty; PTA, percutaneous transluminal angioplasty; ia, intra-arterial; T, thrombolysis; mRS, modified Rankin Scale; hem, hemorrhagic or hemorrhage; retrop., retroperitoneal; compl, complication; perf, perforation; SAH, subarachnoid hemorrhage; occl, occlusion.

**Table 2.** Case reports of endovascular therapy in SVT due to COVID-19 or VITT.

| Reference | | | Etiology | Laboratory Findings | Treatment | | Outcome | | Location | Complications |
|---|---|---|---|---|---|---|---|---|---|---|
| Author (Year) | Study Type | n | COVID-19 (C-19), VITT | d (After Index) | Treatment Allocation | Endovascular Treatment | mRS | Recanalization | | |
| Ostovan et al. (2021) [62] | case series | 1 (of 9) | C-19 | TP (140 T/uL), elevated D-dimer levels (>10,000 ng/mL) 5 (?) | ICH | LT plus MT (A) | 6 | full | SSS, TS | NN |

**Table 2.** Cont.

| Reference | | | Etiology | | Laboratory Findings | Treatment | | | Outcome | | Location | Complications |
|---|---|---|---|---|---|---|---|---|---|---|---|---|
| Author (Year) | Study Type | n | COVID-19 (C-19), VITT | d (After Index) | | Treatment Allocation | Endovascular Treatment | mRS | Recanalization | | | |
| Cavalcanti et al. (2020) [63] | case series | 1 (of 3) | C-19 | 10 | TP (14 T/uL), elevated D-dimer levels (>55,000 ng/mL) | edema, rapid deterioration | MT (A) plus LT (microcatheter, cont.) | 6 | partial | | SSS, TS, SS, DV | NN |
| Omari et al. (2022) [64] | case report | 1 | C-19 | 30 | NN | visual deterioration, intracranial hypertension | NN | NN | NN | | TS, S Sig | blindness |
| Sajjad et al. (2021) [65] | case report | 1 | C-19 | 20 | TP (NN), PF4 antibodies (NN), elevated D-dimer levels (6.3 mg/L) | ICH plus edema, coma, deterioration | Fogarty catheter | 2 | full | | SSS | NN |
| Chew et al. (2021) [66] | case series | 6 | VITT (ChAdOx1 nCoV-19) * | 10 (−14) | TP (11 T–91 T/uL), PF4 antibodies and D-dimer levels NN | ICH (n = 5), progressive thrombus material, deterioration (coma) | Aspiration (Penumbra) | 0–1: n = 3; 6: n = 2 | satisf. (n = 5) | | NN | n = 1 (ICH-progression) |
| Wolf et al. (2021) [67] | case series | 3 | VITT (ChAdOx1 nCoV-19) | 4 (−17) | TP (60 T–92 T/uL), PF4 antibodies (positive), elevated D-dimer levels (2120–22,800 ng/mL) | SAH (1); ICH (2); coma due to bilateral thalamic edema (3) | MT (A [1, 3] plus B [2]) | 0 (1, 3); 1 (2) | full | | SSS, TS (1), SSS, TS, S Sig (2) | 2 MT sessions needed (2) |
| Cleaver et al. (2021) [68] | case series | 3 | VITT (ChAdOx1 nCoV-19) | 8 (−27) | TP (85 T/uL [1], 23 T/uL [2], 35 T/uL [3]); PF4-antibodies positive (all), elevated D-dimer levels (15.83–30.34 µg/mL) | progr. ICH/SAH, edema and deterioration (1); progr. ICH and thrombus material (2); new ICH, status epilepticus, intubation (3) | MT (A [1], A plus SR [2]) | 2 (all) | full (2), partial (1, 3) | | SSS (1), SS, S Sig, TS (2), SSS, S Sig, TS (3) | NN |
| Gurjar et al. (2022) [69] | case report | 1 | VITT (mRNA-1273 vaccine) ** | 3 months | TP (139 T/uL), PF4 antibodies (negative), elevated D-dimer levels (16.666 ng/mL) | coma, progressive symptoms | MT (not specified) | 3 | full | | SSS, TS, S Sig | NN |
| Mirandola et al. (2022) [70] | case report | 1 | VITT (ChAdOx1 nCoV-19) | 15 | TP (40 T/uL), PF4 antibodies (positive), elevated D-dimer levels (18 mcg/mL) | progressive thrombus material, edema, coma and seizure requiring intubation | MT (A plus SR) | 0 | partial (SS), full (rest) | | SSS, SS, TS, S Sig | NN |
| Choi et al. (2021) [71] | case report | 1 | VITT (ChAdOx1 nCoV-19) | 12 | TP (14 T/uL), PF4 antibodies (positive), elevated D-dimer levels (>32.5 mg/L [reference: < 0.5]) | progressive coma | MT (not specified) | 6 | full | | S Sig | NN |
| Waraich et al. (2021) [72] | case report | 1 | VITT (ChAdOx1 nCoV-19) | 13 | TP (14 T/uL), PF4 antibodies NN, elevated D-dimer levels 62.342 ng/mL) | deterioration, SAH, seizures requiring CPR | NN | NN (2 ***) | full | | SSS, TS, S Sig | NN |

* ChAdOx1 nCoV-19, AstraZeneca vaccine; ** mRNA-1273 vaccine, Moderna; *** not specified, mRS assumed by the authors depending on the symptom description provided; n, number; VITT, vaccine-induced thrombotic thrombocytopenia; d, days; mRS, modified Rankin Scale; TP, thrombocytopenia; PF4; platelet factor 4; T, thousand; ICH, intracerebral hemorrhage; SHA, subarachnoid hemorrhage; CPR, cardiopulmonary resuscitation; NN, unknown; SSS, sagittal superior sinus; SS, straight sinus; S Sig, sigmoid sinus; TS, transverse sinus; DV, deep cerebral veins; SVT, sinus or cerebral vein thrombosis; MT, mechanical thrombectomy; LT, local (intrasinus) thrombolysis; A, aspiration thrombectomy; SR, stent retriever thrombectomy; B, balloon guided thrombectomy or angioplasty; cont, continuous.

## 4. Discussion

The overall outcome after SVT can be unfavorable in terms of functional independence and survival [8,11,72]. A total of 75–84% of patients eventually become functionally independent, with excellent functional recovery (mRS, 0–1) [8,11,72]. However, a considerable number of patients remain functionally dependent or disabled (22.2%) or die (up to 14.6%) [11,72]. To identify patients prone to poor prognosis, several risk factors have been identified (independent of treatment strategies): GCS < 9, presence of ICH, involvement of the deep cerebral venous system, mental status disorder (not specified; additional conditions such as underlying malignancy, cerebral or systemic infection, and requirement for hemicraniectomy also apply) [11,72–74]. Neurological deterioration—as part of the natural course of the disease or due to factors such as heparin resistance—might necessitate an additional EVT approach to remove the thrombus load [75].

Retrospective and anecdotal data have demonstrated the safety and feasibility of EVT in selected patients, and have shown satisfying results [19,39–57]. Yet, because of their lack of a control group and their retrospective nature, those studies have been unable to demonstrate a treatment effect resulting in an outcome benefit. In addition, inconsistencies in the timing of the interventions, indications for surgical procedures such as decompressive hemicraniectomy, etiological considerations (e.g., malignancy or sepsis) and clinical complications interfering with outcomes (e.g., status epilepticus) make an interpretation difficult. To our knowledge, only one RCT (TO-ACT) has compared EVT to standard care in patients with SVT (again, with a suspected unfavorable prognosis, as described above). TO-ACT did not detect a modification of the treatment effect attributable to EVT (see Table 1 for inclusion criteria) [38]. The limitations of this trial include its small sample size (due to early termination recommended by the data and safety monitoring board because of futility), patient selection based on clinical presentations suspected to (and previously reported to) negatively influence outcomes and unrestricted use of available endovascular approaches and devices [38]. Therefore, non-significant but clinically relevant treatment effects as well as subgroups that might actually show considerable benefits remained undetected. In a meta-analysis using individual patient data (not including RCT data), EVT was associated with poor outcomes and mortality [76]. Because each treatment decision was made individually in each case (no clear indication; suspected poor prognosis), generalizability is limited. The baseline characteristics were poorer in EVT patients than in controls. Therefore, these retrospective results must be interpreted very cautiously. Important questions regarding patient selection (clinical versus imaging characteristics) and the timing of the intervention remain unanswered. Waiting until a patient is deteriorating might be too late.

Various treatment strategies have been investigated in EVT for SVT. Local thrombolytic therapy (urokinase or alteplase) was performed in most of the cases [19,38–42,44–49,51–57], with either a single periinterventional bolus or a continual infusion (locally, via a microcatheter) for up to 72 h (or longer, depending on the recanalization success). Yue et al. (2010) combined intraarterial thrombolysis with an endovascular thrombectomy approach (balloon-guided) [57]. Several thrombectomy procedures were discussed in the presented literature: aspiration thrombectomy [19,38–42,46,48,49,51,53–56], stent retriever thrombectomy [38–42,46–49,54], balloon-guided thrombectomy/angioplasty [19,38–41,44, 47,51,53,54,57], the (rheolytic) AngioJet device [38–40,47,49,50] as well as additional stenting [42,46]. The study by Dashti et al. was the only one performing thrombectomy without local thrombolysis (AngioJet) [50]. A meta-analysis published in 2019 did not detect differences in outcomes stratified by treatment approach [77]. Despite poor baseline characteristics, 70–80% of patients eventually achieved mRS scores of 0–2 in the follow-up [78]. Local thrombolysis in combination with EVT has not been associated with the development or worsening of an ICH (complication rate < 10%) [78]. Further complications observed were subarachnoid hemorrhage, vessel perforation, and treatment failure [38–42,50,52,54]. Experience and routine (i.e., adherence to a local protocol) might be important because centers following one specific approach showed higher recanalization rates (independently of the procedure or the combination of procedures chosen) than centers using various combinations of EVT strategies [77]. However, the described inconsistencies in device allocation and the small number of treated patients make comparisons regarding the superiority of any of the treatment strategies impossible. Thus, future trials are needed to make such a comparison. Endovascular trials in acute ischemic stroke have indicated that devices are crucial in facilitating treatment effects, recanalization rates, and good functional outcomes [79].

Both COVID-19 and COVID-19 vaccination have been reported to be associated with an increase in SVT incidence [5,6]. Patients with COVID-associated SVT (4.2% of all COVID-associated strokes) appear to be older, do not have specific risk factors and experience higher in-hospital mortality (up to 16.7%) [80,81]. In a New York cohort study, two of the 12 patients received endovascular local thrombolysis [5]. SVT associated with COVID-19 vaccination may be more severe and has higher reported mortality rates (39.2% as compared with approximately 2–5% in pre-pandemic SVT) [6]. The mechanism of pathogenesis (VITT; a prothrombotic state associated with an immunoglobin G reaction against PF4) predominantly occurs in adenovirus vector-type vaccinations (ChAdOx1 nCov-19 (AstraZeneca); recombinant adenovirus type 26 vector encoding S glycoprotein of SARS-CoV-2 (Johnson and Johnson/Janssen)) [6,82]. EVT might be reasonable in selected patients meeting the TO-ACT inclusion criteria (Table 1) [38,83]. Although observational data and case reports of EVT in those patients are scarce [65–71], these studies have indicated the feasibility and safety of EVT and have suggested that EVT can achieve good functional outcomes in a cohort with overall poor prognosis.

This systematic review is limited by the quality (and sample size) of the available data. The disadvantages of the TO-ACT trial have already been discussed. Because of the retrospective design of the remaining data, all the attributed limitations apply (e.g., selection bias or bias by indication) because the rationale for treatment allocation and the number of patients who were potentially eligible for treatment but were not considered are unknown. Therefore, the presented results and the conclusion require very cautious interpretation.

In conclusion, the available data do not support the routine use of EVT strategies in patients with SVT. In patients with a suspected poor outcome (meeting the TO-ACT inclusion criteria), EVT can be performed as part of individual healing attempts. EVT is feasible and safe and might possibly improve functional outcomes. No reasonable recommendation can be made regarding which endovascular technique to use (and in which cases). According to our own experience, patients with substantial thrombus material (without an early response to anticoagulation), those with ICH, those in need of intensive care, and those with VITT do benefit from EVT. Yet, whether patients with clinical and/or imaging risk factors might benefit from early treatment initiation (before deterioration occurs) remains unknown. Further RCTs are warranted to investigate treatment strategies, patient selection, and the timing of the intervention (using predefined therapeutic strategies and reproducible inclusion criteria).

**Author Contributions:** P.B. and H.H.: drafted the article and performed the primary literature research. P.B. wrote the manuscript. V.H.: expert in the endovascular treatment of intracranial venous sinus thrombosis, involved in the data collection and analysis of data concerning endovascular management. A.C.: expert in the endovascular treatment of intracranial venous sinus thrombosis, involved in the data collection and analysis of data concerning the outcome of different endovascular procedures. J.E.C.: endovascular neurosurgeon, contributed to aspects of endovascular and intensive care treatment concepts. T.H.: neurologist with significant stroke experience, analyzed the manuscript concerning the medicinal treatment of VST. O.G.: senior neurosurgeon with significant neurovascular experience, supervised the aspects of surgical treatment of VST. H.B.: senior neurologist with significant stroke experience, supervised the aspects of medicinal treatment of VST. All authors have read and agreed to the published version of the manuscript.

**Funding:** This research received no external funding.

**Institutional Review Board Statement:** Not applicable.

**Informed Consent Statement:** Not applicable.

**Data Availability Statement:** There are no data beyond the analyzed publications, which became the basis for this systematic review.

**Conflicts of Interest:** H.H. is coinventor of the Solitaire stent and the pRESET stent retriever and cofounder of phenox GmbH, femtos GmbH and CONTARA GmbH, which are medical device companies developing and/or selling products for the EVT of neurovascular disorders. All other authors declare no conflicts of interest in the context of this publication.

## References

1. Hopper, A.H.; Klein, J.P. Cerebral Venous Thrombosis. *N. Engl. J. Med.* **2021**, *385*, 59–64.
2. Bousser, M.; Ferro, J.M. Cerebral venous thrombosis: An update. *Lancet Neurol.* **2007**, *6*, 162–170. [CrossRef]
3. Coutinho, J.M.; Zuurbier, S.M.; Aramideh, M.; Stam, J. The Incidence of Cerebral Venous Thrombosis a Cross-Sectional Study. *Stroke* **2012**, *43*, 3375–3377. [CrossRef]
4. Stam, J. Thrombosis of the Cerebral Veins and Sinuses. *N. Engl. J. Med.* **2005**, *352*, 1791–1798. [CrossRef]
5. Al-Mufti, F.; Amuluru, K.; Sahni, R.; Bekelis, K.; Karimi, R.; Ogulnick, J.; Cooper, J.; Overby, P.; Nuoman, R.; Tiwari, A.; et al. Cerebral Venous Thrombosis in COVID-19: A New York Metropolitan Cohort Study. *AJNR Am. J. Neuroradiol.* **2021**, *42*, 1196–1200. [CrossRef]
6. Jaiswal, V.; Nepal, G.; Dijamco, P.; Ishak, A.; Dagar, M.; Sarfraz, Z.; Shama, N.; Sarfraz, A.; Lnu, K.; Mitra, S.; et al. Cerebral Venous Sinus Thrombosis Following COVID-19 Vaccination: A Systematic Review. *J. Prim. Care Community Health* **2022**, *13*, 1–10. [CrossRef]
7. Jung, S.; Mattle, H.; Horvath, T.; Seiffge, D.; Heldner, M.; Meinel, T.; Bühlmann, M.; Prange, U.; Salmen, S.; Humm, A.; et al. Stroke Guidelines of the Bern Stroke Network. Available online: http://www.neurologie.insel.ch/fileadmin/Neurologie/Dokumente/Stroke_Center/Stroke_Guidelines_2021_English.pdf (accessed on 26 May 2022).
8. Devianne, J.; Legris, N.; Crassard, I.; Bellesme, C.; Bejot, Y.; Guidoux, C.; Pico, F.; Germanaud, D.; Obadia, M.; Rodriguez, D.; et al. Epidemiology, Clinical Features, and Outcome in a Cohort of Adolescents with Cerebral Venous Thrombosis. *Neurology* **2021**, *97*, e1920–e1932. [CrossRef]
9. Einhäupl, K.M.; Villringer, A.; Meister, W.; Mehraein, S.; Garner, C.; Pellkofer, M.; Haberl, R.L.; Pfister, H.W.; Schmiedek, P. Heparin treatment in sinus venous thrombosis. *Lancet* **1991**, *338*, 597–600. [CrossRef]
10. De Bruijn, S.F.T.M.; Stam, J.; for the Cerebral Venous Sinus Thrombosis Study Group. Randomized, Placebo-Controlled Trial of Anticoagulant Treatment with Low-Molecular-Weight Heparin for Cerebral Sinus Thrombosis. *Stroke* **1999**, *30*, 484–488. [CrossRef]
11. Ferro, J.M.; Canhão, P.; Stam, J.; Bousser, M.; Barinagarrementeria, F.; ISCVT Investigators. Prognosis of Cerebral Vein and Dural Sinus Thrombosis Results of the International Study on Cerebral Vein and Dural Sinus Thrombosis (ISCVT). *Stroke* **2004**, *35*, 664–670.
12. Lee, S.-K.; Mokin, M.; Hetts, S.W.; Fifi, J.F.; Bousser, M.; Fraser, J.F.; Society of NeuroInterventional Surgery. Current endovascular strategies for cerebral venous thrombosis: Report of the SNIS Standards and Guidelines Committee. *NeuroInterv. Surg.* **2018**, *10*, 803–810. [CrossRef] [PubMed]
13. Coutinho, J.M.; Ferro, J.M.; Zuurbier, S.M.; Mink, M.S.; Canhão, P.; Crassard, I.; Majoie, J.B.; Reekers, J.A.; Houdart, E.; de Haan, R.J.; et al. Thrombolysis or anticoagulation for cerebral venous thrombosis: Rationale and design of the TO-ACT trial. *Int. J. Stroke* **2013**, *8*, 135–140. [CrossRef] [PubMed]
14. Simaan, N.; Molad, J.; Peretz, S.; Filioglo, A.; Auriel, E.; Hallevi, H.; Seyman, E.; Barnea, R.; Cohen, J.E.; Leker, R.R.; et al. Characteristics of Cerebral Sinus Venous Thrombosis Patients Presenting with Intracerebral Hemorrhage. *J. Clin. Med.* **2022**, *11*, 1040. [CrossRef]
15. Rahman, M.; Velat, G.J.; Hoh, B.L.; Mocco, J. Direct thrombolysis for cerebral venous sinus thrombosis. *Neurosurg. Focus* **2009**, *27*, E7. [CrossRef] [PubMed]
16. Baker, M.D.; Opatowsky, M.J.; Wilson, J.A.; Glazier, S.S.; Morris, P.P. Rheolytic catheter and thrombolysis of dural venous sinus thrombosis: A case series. *Neurosurgery* **2001**, *48*, 487–493. [CrossRef] [PubMed]
17. Canhao, P.; Falcao, F.; Ferro, J.M. Thrombolytics for cerebral sinus thrombosis: A systematic review. *Cereb. Dis* **2003**, *15*, 159–166. [CrossRef]
18. Choulakian, A.; Alexander, M.J. Mechanical thrombectomy with the penumbra system for treatment of venous sinus thrombosis. *J. Neurointerv. Surg.* **2010**, *2*, 153–156. [CrossRef]
19. Jankowitz, B.T.; Bodily, L.M.; Jumaa, M.; Syed, Z.F.; Jovin, T.G. Manual aspiration thrombectomy for cerebral venous sinus thrombosis. *J. Neurointerv. Surg.* **2013**, *5*, 534–538. [CrossRef]
20. Kirsch, J.; Rasmussen, P.A.; Masaryk, T.J.; Perl, J., II; Fiorella, D. Adjunctive rheolytic thrombectomy for central venous sinus thrombosis: Technical case report. *Neurosurgery* **2007**, *60*, E577–E578. [CrossRef]
21. La Barge, D.V.; Bishop, F.S.; Stevens, E.A.; Eskandari, R.; Schmidt, R.H.; Skalabrin, E.J.; Ng, P.P. Intrasinus catheter-directed heparin infusion the treatment of dural venous sinus thrombosis. *AJNR Am. J. Neuroradiol.* **2009**, *30*, 1672–1678. [CrossRef]
22. Zhang, A.; Collinson, R.L.; Hurst, R.W.; Weigele, J.B. Rheolytic thrombectomy for cerebral sinus thrombosis. *Neurocrit Care* **2008**, *9*, 17–26. [CrossRef] [PubMed]

3. Zhen, Y.; Zhang, N.; He, L.; Shen, L.; Yan, K. Mechanical thrombectomy combined with recombinant tissue plasminogen activator thrombolysis in the venous sinus for the treatment of severe tcerebral venous sinus thrombosis. *Exp. Ther. Med.* **2015**, *9*, 1080–1084. [CrossRef] [PubMed]
4. Shui, S.F.; Li, T.F.; Han, X.W.; Ma, J.; Guo, D. Balloon dilatation and thrombus extraction for the treatment of cerebral venous sinus thrombosis. *Neurol. India* **2014**, *62*, 371–375. [CrossRef] [PubMed]
5. Wasay, M.; Bakshi, R.; Kojan, S.; Bobustuc, G.; Dubey, N.; Unwin, D.H. Nonrandomized comparison of local urokinase thrombolysis versus systemic heparin anticoagulation for superior sagittal sinus thrombosis. *Stroke* **2001**, *32*, 2310–2317. [CrossRef] [PubMed]
6. Chow, K.Y.; Gobin, P.; Saver, J.; Kidwell, C.; Dong, P.; Viñuela, F. Endovascular Treatment of Dural Sinus Thrombosis with Rheolytic Thrombectomy and Intra-Arterial Thrombolysis. *Stroke* **2000**, *31*, 1420–1425. [CrossRef] [PubMed]
7. Najjar, A.A.; Rasheedi, J.K.; Kurdi, K.I.; Hasan, A.A.; Almekhlafi, M.A.; Baeesa, S.S. Endovascular suction thrombectomy for severe cerebral venous sinus thrombosis: A report of two cases. *J. Taibah Univ. Med. Sci.* **2018**, *13*, 87–92. [CrossRef]
8. Lee, D.J.; Ahmadpour, A.; Binyamin, T.; Dahlin, B.C.; Shahlaie, K.; Waldau, B. Management and outcome of spontaneous cerebral venous sinus thrombosis in a 5-year consecutive single-institution cohort. *J. NeuroInterv. Surg.* **2017**, *9*, 34–38. [CrossRef]
9. Adachi, H.; Mineharu, Y.; Ishikawa, T.; Imamura, H.; Yamamoto, S.; Todo, K.; Yamagami, H.; Sakai, N. Stenting for acute cerebral venous sinus thrombosis in the superior sagittal sinus. *Interv. Neuroradiol.* **2015**, *21*, 719–723. [CrossRef]
30. Liao, W.; Liu, Y.; Gu, W.; Yang, J.; Chen, C.; Liu, F.; Zeng, F.; Wang, X. Cerebral Venous Sinus Thrombosis: Successful Treatment of Two Patients Using the Penumbra System and Review of Endovascular Approaches. *Neuroradiol. J.* **2015**, *28*, 177–183. [CrossRef]
31. Philips, M.F.; Bagley, L.J.; Sinson, G.P.; Raps, E.C.; Galetta, S.L.; Zager, E.L.; Hurst, R.W. Endovascular thrombolysis for symptomatic cerebral venous thrombosis. *J. Neurosurg.* **1999**, *90*, 65–71. [CrossRef]
32. Dandapat, S.; Samaniego, E.A.; Szeder, V.; Siddiqui, F.M.; Duckwiler, G.R.; Kiddy, U.; Guerrero, W.R.; Zheng, B.; Hasan, D.; Derdeyn, C.; et al. Safety and efficacy of the use of large bore intermediate suction catheters alone or in combination for the treatment of acute cerebral venous sinus thrombosis: A multicenter experience. *Interv. Neuroradiol.* **2020**, *26*, 26–32. [CrossRef] [PubMed]
33. Siddiqui, F.; Weber, M.W.; Dandapat, S.; Scaife, S.; Buhnerkempe, M.; Ortega-Gutierrez, S.; Aksan, N.; Elias, A.; Coutinho, J.M. Endovascular Thrombolysis or Thrombectomy for Cerebral Venous Thrombosis: Study of Nationwide Inpatient Sample 2004–2014. *J. Stroke Cereb. Dis.* **2019**, *6*, 1440–1447. [CrossRef] [PubMed]
34. Ma, J.; Shui, S.; Han, X.; Guo, D.; Li, T.; Yan, L. Mechanical thrombectomy with Solitaire AB stents for the treatment of intracranial venous sinus thrombosis. *Acta Radiol.* **2016**, *57*, 1524–1530. [CrossRef] [PubMed]
35. Zhang, S.; Hu, Y.; Li, Z.; Huang, D.; Zhang, M.; Wang, C.; Wang, Z. Endovascular treatment for hemorrhagic cerebral venous sinus thrombosis: Experience with 9 cases for 3 years. *Am. J. Transl. Res.* **2018**, *10*, 1611–1619.
36. Liao, C.; Liao, N.; Chen, W.; Chen, H.; Shen, C.; Yang, S.; Tsuei, Y. Endovascular Mechanical Thrombectomy and On-Site Chemical Thrombolysis for Severe Cerebral Venous Sinus Thrombosis. *Sci. Rep.* **2020**, *10*, 4937. [CrossRef]
37. Li, X.; Li, T.; Fan, Y. Efficacy of intravascular mechanical thrombectomy combined with thrombolysis and anticoagulant therapy in the treatment of cerebral venous sinus thrombosis and its effect on neurological function and coagulation indices. *Am. J. Transl. Res.* **2021**, *13*, 6921–6928.
38. Coutinho, J.M.; Zuurbier, S.M.; Bousser, M.; Ji, X.; Canhão, P.; Boos, Y.B.; Crassard, I.; Nunes, A.P.; Uyttenboogaart, M.; Chen, J.; et al. Effect of Endovascular Treatment with Medical Management vs Standard Care on Severe Cerebral Venous Thrombosis: The TO-ACT Randomized Clinical Trial. *JAMA Neurol.* **2020**, *77*, 966–973. [CrossRef]
39. Nyberg, E.M.; Case, D.; Nagae, L.M.; Honce, J.M.; Reyenga, W.; Seinfeld, J.; Poisson, S.; Leppert, M.H. The addition of endovascular intervention for dural venous sinus thrombosis: Single-center experience and review of literature. *J. Stroke Cereb. Dis.* **2017**, *26*, 2240–2247. [CrossRef]
40. Siddiqui, F.M.; Banerjee, C.; Zuurbier, S.M.; Hao, Q.; Ahn, C.; Pride, G.L.; Wasay, M.; Majoie, C.B.; Liebeskind, D.; Johnsin, M.; et al. Mechanical thrombectomy versus intrasinus thrombolysis for cerebral venous sinus thrombosis: A non-randomized comparison. *Interv. Neuroradiol.* **2014**, *20*, 336–344. [CrossRef]
41. Guo, X.; Liu, S.; Guan, S. The clinical analysis and treatment strategy of endovascular treatment for cerebral venous sinus thrombosis combined with intracerebral hemorrhage. *Sci. Rep.* **2020**, *10*, 22300. [CrossRef]
42. Andersen, T.H.; Hansen, K.; Truelsen, T.; Cronqvist, M.; Stavngaard, T.; Cortsen, M.E.; Holtmannspötter, M.; Højgaard, J.L.S.; Stensballe, J.; Welling, K.L.; et al. Endovascular treatment for cerebral venous sinus thrombosis—A single center study. *Br. J. Neurosurg.* **2020**, *35*, 259–265. [CrossRef] [PubMed]
43. Yang, X.; Wu, F.; Liu, Y.; Duan, J.; Meng, R.; Chen, J.; Li, D.; Fan, Z.; Fisher, M.; Yang, Q.; et al. Predictors of successful endovascular treatment in severe cerebral venous sinus thrombosis. *Ann. Clin. Trans. Neur.* **2019**, *6*, 755–761. [CrossRef] [PubMed]
44. Yang, J.; Wang, H.; Chen, Y.; Qiu, M.; Zhang, B.; Chen, Z. Balloon-Assisted Thrombectomy and Intrasinus Urokinase Thrombolysis for Severe Cerebral Venous Sinus Thrombosis. *Front. Neurol.* **2021**, *12*, 735540. [CrossRef]
45. Stam, J.; Majoie, C.; Van Delden, O.M.; Van Lienden, K.P.; Reekers, J.A. Endovascular thrombectomy and thrombolysis for severe cerebral sinus thrombosis: A prospective study. *Stroke* **2008**, *39*, 1487–1490. [CrossRef] [PubMed]
46. Lu, G.; Shin, J.H.; Song, Y.; Lee, D.H. Stenting of symptomatic lateral sinus thrombosis refractory to mechanical thrombectomy. *Interv. Neuroradiol.* **2019**, *25*, 714–720. [CrossRef]

47. Qureshi, A.I.; Grigoryan, M.; Saleem, M.A.; Aytac, E.; Wallery, S.S.; Rodriguez, G.J.; Suri, M.F.K. Prolonged Microcatheter-Based Local Thrombolytic Infusion as a Salvage Treatment After Failed Endovascular Treatment for Cerebral Venous Thrombosis: A Multicenter Experience. *Neurocrit Care* **2018**, *29*, 54–61. [CrossRef]
48. Styczen, H.; Tsogkas, I.; Liman, J.; Maus, V.; Psychogios, M.N. Endovascular Mechanical Thrombectomy for Cerebral Venous Sinus Thrombosis: A Single-Center Experience. *World Neurosurg.* **2019**, *127*, e1097–e1103. [CrossRef]
49. Mokin, M.; Lopes, D.K.; Binning, M.J.; Veznedaroglu, E.; Liebman, K.M.; Arthur, A.S.; Doss, V.T.; Levy, E.I.; Siddiqui, A.H. Endovascular treatment of cerebral venous thrombosis: Contemporary multicenter experience. *Interv. Neuroradiol.* **2015**, *21*, 520–526. [CrossRef]
50. Dashti, S.H.; Hu, V.C.; Fiorella, D.; Mitha, A.P.; Abuquerque, F.C.; McDougall, C.G. Mechanical thrombectomy as first-line treatment for venous sinus thrombosis: Technical considerations and preliminary results using the AngioJet device. *J. Neurointerv. Surg.* **2011**, *5*, 49–53. [CrossRef]
51. Lee, C.; Liu, H.; Chen, Y.; Lin, Y.; Wang, J. Suction thrombectomy after balloon maceration for dural venous sinus thrombosis. *J. Neurol. Sci.* **2016**, *365*, 76–81. [CrossRef]
52. Poulsen, F.R.; Høgedal, L.; Stilling, M.V.; Birkeland, P.F.; Schultz, M.K.; Rasmussen, J.N. Good clinical outcome after combined endovascular and neurosurgical treatment of cerebral venous thrombosis. *Dan. Med. J.* **2013**, *60*, A4724. [PubMed]
53. Mammen, S.; Keshava, S.N.; Moses, V.; Aaron, S.; Ahmed, M.; Chiramel, G.K.; Mani, S.E.; Alexander, M. Role of penumbra mechanical thrombectomy device in acute dural sinus thrombosis. *Indian J. Radiol. Imaging* **2017**, *27*, 82–87. [CrossRef] [PubMed]
54. Peng, T.; Dan, B.; Zhang, Z.; Zhu, B.; Liu, J. Efficacy of Stent Thrombectomy Alone or Combined with Intermediate Catheter Aspiration for Severe Cerebral Venous Sinus Thrombosis: A Case-Series. *Front. Neurol.* **2021**, *12*, 783380. [CrossRef]
55. Medhi, G.; Parida, S.; Nicholson, P.; Senapati, S.B.; Padhy, B.P.; Medes Pareira, V. Mechanical Thrombectomy for Cerebral Venous Sinus Thrombosis: A Case Series. *World Neurosurg.* **2020**, *140*, 148–161. [CrossRef]
56. Tsang, A.C.O.; Hwang, A.C.; Chiu, R.H.Y.; Chan, D.Y.C.; Tsang, F.C.P.; Ho, W.S.; Lee, R.; Leung, G.K.K.; Lui, W.M. Combined aspiration thrombectomy and continuous intrasinus thrombolysis for cerebral venous sinus thrombosis: Technical note and case series. *Neuroradiology* **2018**, *60*, 1093–1096. [CrossRef] [PubMed]
57. Yue, X.; Xi, G.; Zhou, Z.H.; Xu, G.; Liu, X. Combined intraarterial and intravenous thrombolysis for severe cerebral venous sinus thrombosis. *J. Thromb. Thrombolysis* **2010**, *29*, 361–367. [CrossRef]
58. Saposnik, G.; Barinagarrementeria, F.; Brown, R.D., Jr.; Bushnell, C.D.; Cucchiara, B.; Cushman, M.; deVeber, G.; Ferro, J.M.; Tsai, F.Y. American Heart Association Stroke Council and the Council on Epidemiology and Prevention. Diagnosis and Management of Cerebral Venous Thrombosis A Statement for Healthcare Professionals from the American Heart Association/American Stroke Association. *Stroke* **2011**, *42*, 1158–1192. [CrossRef]
59. Ferro, J.M.; Bousser, M.; Canhão, P.; Coutinho, J.M.; Crassard, I.; Dentali, F.; Di Minno, M.; Maino, A.; Martinelli, I.; Masuhr, F.; et al. European Stroke Organization guideline for the diagnosis and treatment of cerebral venous thrombosis—Endorsed by the European Academy of Neurology. *Eur. J. Neurol.* **2017**, *24*, 1203–1213. [CrossRef]
60. Page, M.J.; McKenzie, J.E.; Bossuyt, P.M.; Boutron, I.; Hoffmann, T.C.; Mulrow, C.D.; Shamseer, L.; Tetzlaff, J.M.; Akl, E.A.; Brennan, S.E.; et al. The PRISMA 2020 statement: An updated guideline for reporting systematic reviews. *J. Clin. Epidemiol.* **2021**, *134*, 178–189. [CrossRef]
61. Ostovan, V.R.; Foroughi, R.; Rostami, M.; Almasi-Dooghaee, M.; Esmaili, M.; Akbar Bidaki, A.; Behzadi, Z.; Farzadfard, F.; Marbooti, H.; Rahimi-Jaberi, A.; et al. Cerebral venous sinus thrombosis associated with COVID-19: A case series and literature review. *J. Neurol.* **2021**, *268*, 3549–3560. [CrossRef]
62. Cavalcanti, D.D.; Raz, E.; Shapiro, M.; Dehkharghani, S.; Yaghi, S.; Lillemoe, K.; Nossek, E.; Torres, J.; Jain, R.; Riina, H.A.; et al. Cerebral Venous Thrombosis Associated with COVID-19. *AJNR Am. J. Neuroradiol.* **2020**, *41*, 1370–1376. [CrossRef] [PubMed]
63. Omari, A.; Kally, P.; Schimmel, O.; Kahana, A. Vision Loss Secondary to COVID-19 Associated Bilateral Cerebral Venous Sinus Thromboses. *Ophthalmic Plast. Reconstr. Surg.* **2022**, *38*, e65–e67. [CrossRef] [PubMed]
64. Sajjad, A.; Khan, A.F.; Jafri, L.; Kamal, A.K. Successful endovascular mechanical thrombectomy in anticoagulation-resistant COVID-19 associated cerebral venous sinus thrombosis. *BMJ Case Rep.* **2021**, *14*, e245405. [CrossRef]
65. Chew, H.S.; Al-Ali, S.; Butler, B.; Rajapakse, D.; Nader, S.K.; Chavda, S.; Lamin, S. Mechanical Thrombectomy for Treatment of Cerebral Venous Sinus Thrombosis in Vaccine-Induced Immune Thrombotic Thrombocytopenia. *AJNR Am. J. Neuroradiol.* **2022**, *43*, 98–101. [CrossRef] [PubMed]
66. Wolf, M.E.; Luz, B.; Niehaus, L.; Bhogal, P.; Bäzner, H.; Henkes, H. Thrombocytopenia and Intracranial Venous Sinus Thrombosis after "COVID-19 Vaccine AstraZeneca" Exposure. *J. Clin. Med.* **2021**, *10*, 1599. [CrossRef] [PubMed]
67. Cleaver, J.; Ibitoye, R.; Morrison, H.; Flood, R.; Crewdson, K.; Marsh, A.; Abhinav, K.; Bosnell, R.; Crossley, R.; Mortimer, A. Endovascular treatment for vaccine-induced cerebral venous sinus thrombosis and thrombocytopenia following ChAdOx1 nCoV-19 vaccination: A report of three cases. *J. NeuroInterv. Surg.* **2021**, 1–6. [CrossRef]
68. Gurjar, H.; Dhallu, M.; Lvovsky, D.; Sadullah, S.; Chilimuri, S. A Rare Case of Coronavirus Disease 2019 Vaccine-Associated Cerebral Venous Sinus Thrombosis Treated with Mechanical Thrombectomy. *Am. J. Case Rep* **2022**, *23*, e935355. [CrossRef]
69. Mirandola, L.; Arena, G.; Pagliaro, M.; Boghi, A.; Naldi, A.; Castellano, D.; Vaccarino, A.; Silengo, D.; Aprà, F.; Cavallo, R.; et al. Massive cerebral venous sinus thrombosis in vaccine-induced immune thrombotic thrombocytopenia after ChAdOx1 nCoV-19 serum: Case report of a successful multidisciplinary approach. *Neurol. Sci.* **2022**, *43*, 1499–1502. [CrossRef]

70. Chou, J.; Kim, S.; Kim, S.R.; Jin, J.Y.; Choi, S.W.; Kim, H.; Yoo, J.H.; Park, I.S.; Kim, S.R. Intracerebral Hemorrhage due to Thrombosis with Thrombocytopenia Syndrome after Vaccination against COVID-19: The First Fatal Case in Korea. *J. Korean Med. Sci.* **2021**, *36*, e223. [CrossRef]
71. Waraich, A.; Williams, G. Haematuria, a widespread petechial rash, and headaches following the Oxford AstraZeneca ChAdOx1 nCoV-19 Vaccination. *BMJ Case Rep.* **2021**, *14*, e245440. [CrossRef]
72. Karsy, M.; Harmer, J.R.; Guan, J.; Brock, A.A.; Ravindra, V.M.; Chung, L.S.; Tkach, A.; Majersik, J.J.; Park, M.S.; Schmidt, R.H. Outcomes in adults with cerebral venous sinus thrombosis: A retrospective cohort study. *J. Clin. Neurosci.* **2018**, *53*, 34–40. [CrossRef]
73. Yeo, L.L.L.; Lye, P.P.S.; Yee, K.W.; Cunli, Y.; Ming, T.T.; Ho, A.F.; Sharma, V.K.; Chan, B.P.; Tan, B.Y.; Gopinathan, A. Deep Cerebral Venous Thrombosis Treatment Endovascular Case using Aspiration and Review of the Various Treatment Modalities. *Clin. Neuroradiol.* **2020**, *30*, 661–670. [CrossRef] [PubMed]
74. Pfefferkorn, T.; Crassard, I.; Linn, J.; Dichgans, M.; Boukobza, M.; Bousser, M. Clinical features, course and outcome in deep cerebral venous system thrombosis: An analysis of 32 cases. *J. Neurol.* **2009**, *256*, 1839–1845. [CrossRef] [PubMed]
75. King, A.B.; O'Duffy, A.E.; Kumar, A.B. Heparin Resistance and Anticoagulation Failure in a Challenging Case of Cerebral Venous Sinus Thrombosis. *Neurohospitalist* **2015**, *6*, 118–121. [CrossRef]
76. Xu, Z.; Li, X.; Feng, D.; Wang, T.; Xu, X.; Deng, R.; Zhou, X.; Chen, G. Endovascular Therapy Versus Anticoagulation for Treatment of Cerebral Venous Sinus Thrombosis A Meta-Analysis. *Neurologist* **2022**, *27*, 69–73. [CrossRef]
77. Lewis, W.; Saber, H.; Sadeghi, M.; Rajah, G.; Narayanan, S. Transvenous Endovascular Recanalization for Cerebral Venous Thrombosis: A Systematic Review and Meta-Analysis. *World Neurosurg.* **2019**, *130*, 341–350. [CrossRef] [PubMed]
78. Ilyas, A.; Chen, C.H.-J.; Raper, D.M.; Ding, D.; Buell, T.; Mastorakos, P.; Liu, K.C. Endovascular mechanical thrombectomy for cerebral venous sinus thrombosis: A systematic review. *J. Neurointerv. Surg.* **2017**, *9*, 1086–1092. [CrossRef]
79. Boyle, K.; Joundi, R.A.; Aviv, R.I. An historical and contemporary review of endovascular therapy for acute ischemic stroke. *Neurovasc Imaging.* **2017**, *3*, 1. [CrossRef]
80. Shahjouei, S.; Tsivgoulis, G.; Farahmand, G.; Koza, E.; Mowla, A.; Sadr, A.V.; Kia, A.; Far, A.V.; Mondello, S.; Cernigliaro, A.; et al. SARS-CoV-2 and Stroke Characteristics A Report from the Multinational COVID-19 Stroke Study Group. *Stroke* **2021**, *52*, e117–e130. [CrossRef]
81. Mowla, A.; Shakibajahromi, B.; Shahjouei, S.; Borhani-Haghighi, A.; Rahimian, N.; Baharvahdat, H.; Naderi, S.; Khorvash, F.; Altafi, D.; Ebrahimzadeh, S.A.; et al. Cerebral venous sinus thrombosis associated with SARS-CoV-2; a multinational case series. *J. Neurol. Sci.* **2020**, *419*, 117183. [CrossRef]
82. McGonagle, D.; De Marco, G.; Bridgewood, C. Mechanisms of Immunothrombosis in Vaccine-Induced Thrombotic Thrombocytopenia (VITT) Compared to Natural SARS-CoV-2 Infection. *J. Autoimmun.* **2021**, *121*, 102662. [CrossRef] [PubMed]
83. Mahajan, A.; Hirsch, J.A. Cerebral venous thrombosis after COVID-19 vaccination: The role for endovascular treatment. *J. NeuroInterv. Surg.* **2022**, 1–2. [CrossRef] [PubMed]

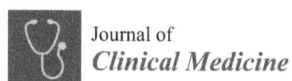

*Review*

# Blood Biomarkers for Triaging Patients for Suspected Stroke: Every Minute Counts

Radhika Kiritsinh Jadav [1], Reza Mortazavi [1,2,*] and Kwang Choon Yee [1]

[1] Faculty of Health, University of Canberra, Canberra, ACT 2617, Australia; radhikashah2529@gmail.com (R.K.J.); kwang_choon.yee@canberra.edu.au (K.C.Y.)
[2] Prehab Activity Cancer Exercise Survivorship Research Group, Faculty of Health, University of Canberra, Canberra, ACT 2617, Australia
* Correspondence: reza.mortazavi@canberra.edu.au

**Abstract:** Early stroke diagnosis remains a big challenge in healthcare partly due to the lack of reliable diagnostic blood biomarkers, which in turn leads to increased rates of mortality and disability. Current screening methods are optimised to identify patients with a high risk of cardio-vascular disease, especially among the elderly. However, in young adults and children, these methods suffer low sensitivity and specificity and contribute to further delays in their triage and diagnosis. Accordingly, there is an urgent need to develop reliable blood biomarkers for triaging patients suspected of stroke in all age groups, especially children and young adults. This review explores some of the existing blood biomarkers, as single biomarkers or biomarker panels, and examines their sensitivity and specificity for predicting stroke. A review was performed on PubMed and Web of Science for journal articles published in English during the period 2001 to 2021, which contained information regarding biomarkers of stroke. In this review article, we provide comparative information on the availability, clinical usefulness, and time-window periods of seven single blood biomarkers and five biomarker panels that have been used for predicting stroke in emergency situations. The outcomes of this review can be used in future research for developing more effective stroke biomarkers.

**Keywords:** stroke; CNS; ischaemic; haemorrhagic; biomarker; panel; young adults; children; triage; specificity; sensitivity; prediction values

## 1. Introduction

Stroke is the leading cause of disability and the second most common cause of death worldwide [1]. Early detection of stroke is essential for implementing timely diagnostic tests and radio-imaging, as well as subsequent intervention therapies such as thrombolysis (using tissue plasminogen activator), thrombectomy, or anti-platelet/anti-coagulant treatments [2–6]. However, early detection of stroke is still remaining elusive, and it has been reported that even in many advanced hospitals, only about one-third of the patients with ischaemic stroke (IS) are diagnosed early enough for a timely intervention [2].

Early screening tools, such as the Cincinnati Prehospital Stroke Scale (CPSS) or the Recognition of Stroke in the Emergency Room (ROSIER) scale, have demonstrated their values in high-risk patients, with a sensitivity between 80% and 85% [2,7]. However, these tools are less accurate in children and young adults, who account for 10–15% of all stroke cases [2,8]. Given there are approximately 12 million new cases of stroke diagnosed globally each year, it is estimated that there are around 1–2 million cases per year that are not detected appropriately using the current screening tools [9]. In addition, studies have found that current screening tools have poor performance in distinguishing stroke from stroke mimics such as migraine, epilepsy, central nervous system (CNS) infections, Bell's palsy, and conversion disorders, with a negative predictive value of approximately 20% [2,10].

The majority of the current screening tools for stroke are based on considering the patients' clinical signs and symptoms and demographic risk factors. The downside is that those patients who do not present with typical symptoms and those who are perceived as low risk (e.g., children and young adults) may not be consistently identified [8]. Therefore, we need alternative methods for detecting potential stroke cases which do not depend on the above-mentioned categorisations. Such screening tools would be a welcome addition to the diagnostic toolkit of clinicians at emergency departments, neurology departments, and regional hospitals, as well as paramedics.

The use of blood biomarkers plays an important role in the screening and diagnosis of some critical illnesses such as ischaemic heart disease. The inclusion of troponin into the screening/diagnostic protocols of ischaemic heart disease in the early 2000s significantly improved the clinical approach to this condition, and subsequently has contributed to remarkable improvements in patient outcomes [11]. Unfortunately, this is not the case with the screening and diagnosis of stroke.

The brain is a complex tissue comprising different unique cells, including various neurons and glial cells, as well as extracellular supportive matrices [12]. Therefore, in the event of a stroke where many neuronal tissues are damaged, a sudden release of CNS and/or vascular biomarkers into the peripheral blood would be expected. If such biomarkers are reliably measured in the peripheral blood specimens, then they could be used for screening or triaging purposes.

In this review, we have mentioned many currently available stroke biomarkers but have explained seven single blood biomarkers and five biomarker panels in more detail because of their potential usefulness for the detection or prediction of IS in suspected patients.

## 2. Materials and Methods

We performed a narrative review of the literature published in the English language from 2001 to 2021 using two online databases, PubMed and Web of Science. We used the search terms "stroke", "diagnosis", "biomarker", "humans", "sensitivity", and "specificity". We also screened the reference lists of the extracted articles to identify articles not computed from the original search.

## 3. Results and Discussion

The initial database search generated 170 results. Three articles were excluded as duplicates, and after screening the titles and abstracts of the remaining, we included 23 articles for this review (Figure 1 and Table 1).

**Table 1.** Included studies in this literature review.

| Author/s (Year), Reference Number | Type of Study, Country | Numbers of Participants and Controls, Mean or Median Age (Age Range When Available) | Type of Stroke | Biomarkers/Biomarker Panels Studied |
|---|---|---|---|---|
| Park S. Y., et al., (2013) [13] | Cohort study, Korea | Patients: n = 111, mean age 67; controls: n = 127, mean age 63 | IS | H-FABP and S100B |
| Dambinova S. A., et al., (2012) [14] | Cohort study, USA | Patients: n = 101, median age 62 (26–95); non-stroke patients (stroke mimics): n = 91, median age 61 (24–95); healthy controls: n = 52, median age 59 (29–92) | IS or TIA | NR2 peptide |

Table 1. Cont.

| Author/s (Year), Reference Number | Type of Study, Country | Numbers of Participants and Controls, Mean or Median Age (Age Range When Available) | Type of Stroke | Biomarkers/Biomarker Panels Studied |
|---|---|---|---|---|
| Allard L., et al., (2005) [15] | Cohort studies; one European (Switzerland) and two American (USA) cohorts. | European study: patients: n = 36, mean age 71.3 (25–92); controls: n = 35 mean age 71.1 (28–91); American study 1: patients: n = 53, controls: n = 30 (non-age or sex-matched); American study 2: patients: n = 533, controls: 100 (age matched with patients). | IS (most of the patients), TIA, HS | PARK7 and NDKA |
| Zhao X., et al., (2016) [16] | Cohort study, China | Patients: n = 94, mean age 61.8; controls: n = 37, mean age 47.1 | IS | APOA1-UP |
| Park K. Y., et al., (2018) [17] | Cohort study, USA | Patients: n = 172, mean age 68.8; controls: n = 133, mean age 71.0 | IS | GPBB |
| Zhou, S. et al., (2016) [18] | Single-centre pilot study, China | Patients: HS: n = 46, mean age 68.1; IS: n = 71, mean age 69.3; no control group | HS and IS | S100B |
| Losy, J. and Zaremba, J. (2001) [19] | Cohort study, Poland | Patients: n = 23, mean age 72.2; controls: n = 15 (age and sex-matched) | IS | MCP-1 |
| Sharma, R., et al., (2014) [20] | Cohort study, USA | Patients: IS: n = 56, mean age 66.9; HS: n = 32, mean age 64.7; TIA: n = 41, mean age 63.1; mimic: n = 37, mean age 61.8 | Mixed patient group (IS, HS, TIA, and mimics) | A 5-biomarker model was developed consisting of eotaxin, EGFR, metalloproteinase inhibitor-4, prolactin, and S100A12 |
| Supanc, V., et al., (2011) [21] | Cohort study, Croatia | Patients: n = 110; mean age 70.2 (36–86); controls: n = 93, median age 70 (47–86) | IS | ICAM-1 and VCAM-1 |
| Katan, M., Elkind, M. S. V. (2011) [22] | Review article, USA | N/A | IS | IL-1, IL-6, MM-9, TNF-alpha, TNF-a receptor, ICAM-1, VCAM, Lipoprotein-associated phospholipase A2, vWF; Fibrinogen; D-dimer, BNP, NT-proBNP, cortisol; PAI-1, and others |
| Kamtchum-Tatuene, J. and Jickling, G. C. (2019) [23] | Review article, Canada | N/A | IS and HS | S100B, GFAP, MBP, NSE, H-FABP, anti-NMDA receptors antibodies, vWF, D-dimer, fibrinogen, PAI, Fibronectin, MMP-9, caspase-3, thrombomodulin, and others |
| Abdel-Ghaffar, W. E. et al., (2019) [24] | Cohort study, Egypt | Patients: n = 40, age above 65 years old; no control group | IS and HS | S100B |
| Sen, J. and Belli, A. (2007) [25] | Review article, UK | N/A | N/A | S100B |

Table 1. *Cont.*

| Author/s (Year), Reference Number | Type of Study, Country | Numbers of Participants and Controls, Mean or Median Age (Age Range When Available) | Type of Stroke | Biomarkers/Biomarker Panels Studied |
|---|---|---|---|---|
| Kalev-Zylinska, M. L. et al., (2013) [26] | Cohort study, New Zealand | Patients: n = 48, Mean age 70; control group 1: health laboratory workers: n = 46, age range 30 years of age or younger; control group 2: healthy blood donors: n = 50, age range 50 years of age or older | IS | Anti-NMDAR antibodies |
| Lakhan S. E. et al., (2013) [27] | Review article, USA | N/A | IS | MMP-9 |
| Kelly, P. J. et al., (2008) [28] | Case–control study, Ireland | Patients: n = 52; mean age 70.1; controls: n = 27, mean age 68.2 | IS | MMP-9 and F2Ips |
| Castellanos, et al., (2007) [29] | Cohort study, Spain | Patients: n = 134, mean age 62; no control group | IS | MMP-9 |
| Eldeeb, M. A. et al., (2020) [30] | Case–control, Egypt | Patients: n = 60, mean age 60, age range 28–88; healthy controls: n = 30 (age and sex-matched) | IS | Apo-A1 |
| Kawata, K. et al., (2016) [31] | Review article, USA | N/A | IS and HS | S100B, NSE, MMP-9, sCD40L, TIMP-1, MDA, and others |
| Reynolds, M. A. (2003) [32] | Cohort study, USA | Patients: n = 223 (including 82 patients with IS), age not available; controls (healthy donors): n = 214, age not available | IS and HS (a mixed patient group) | A 5-biomarker panel was developed consisting of S100B, BNGF, vWF, MMP-9, MCP-1, |
| Lynch, J. R. et al., (2004) [33] | Cohort study, USA | Patients: n = 65, mean age 62; controls (non-stroke): n = 157, mean age 63.3 | IS | A 3-biomarker panel was developed consisting of vWF, MMP-9, and VCAM |
| Laskowitz, D. T. et al., (2005) [34] | Cohort study, USA | Patients: n = 130, age not available; controls: n = 10, age not available | IS | A 5-biomarker panel was developed using BNP, CRP, D-dimer, MMP-9, and S100B. |
| Moore, D. F. et al., (2005) [35] | Cohort study, Canada | Patients (IS): n= 20, mean age 75.5; controls (healthy): n = 20, mean age 66.0 | IS | A 22-gene expression panel was developed using peripheral blood mononuclear cells. |

H-FABP, heart-type fatty acid binding protein; S100B, S100 calcium-binding protein B; TIA, transient ischaemic attack; NR2 peptide, NMDA (N-methyl-d-aspartate) receptor 2 peptide; PARK7, Parkinson disease protein 7; NDKA, nucleoside diphosphate kinase A; APOA1-UP, apolipoprotein A1 unique peptide: GPBB, glycogen phosphorylase BB; IS, ischaemic stroke; HS, haemorrhagic stroke; MCP-1, monocyte chemoattractant protein-1; EGFR, epidermal growth factor receptor; S100A12, S100 calcium-binding protein A12; ICAM-1, inter-cellular adhesion molecule 1; VCAM-1, vascular cell adhesion molecule 1; IL-1, interleukin 1, IL-6, interleukin 6; MMP-9, matrix metalloproteinase-9; TNF: tumour necrosis factor; vWF, von Willebrand factor; BNP, brain natriuretic peptide; NT-pro BNP, N-terminal pro-brain natriuretic peptide; PAI-1, plasminogen activator inhibitor-1; GFAP, glial fibrillary acid protein; MBP, myelin basic protein; NSE, neuron-specific enolase; Anti-NMDAR, antibody against N-methyl-d-aspartate receptor; F2Ips, F2-isoprostanes; Apo-A1, apolipoprotein A1; NSE, neuron-specific enolase; sCD40L, soluble CD40 ligand; TIMP-1, tissue inhibitors of metalloproteinases-1; MDA, malondialdehyde; BNGF, B-type neurotrophic growth factor; MCP-1, monocyte chemotactic protein-1.

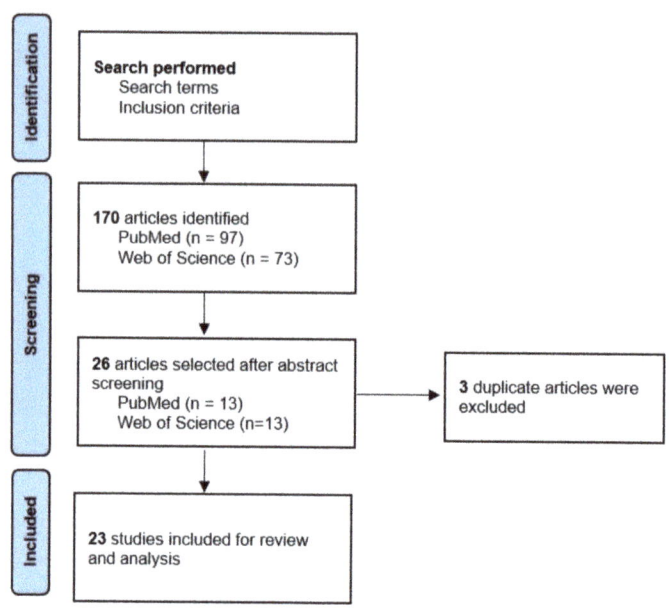

Figure 1. The literature search process.

### 3.1. Individual Biomarkers

Over the last 20 years, many biomarkers have been studied for stroke diagnosis; however, we still do not have a reliable biomarker that can detect stroke with a high accuracy compared to troponin in the diagnosis of ischaemic heart disease. Nonetheless, so far, many biomarkers have been identified whose blood levels increase following a stroke event, especially an acute IS. In general, those biomarkers can be divided into a few categories based on their origins, namely: (1) the neuronal injury markers (e.g., heart-type fatty acid binding protein (H-FABP), NR2 peptide (a degradation product of N-methyl-d-aspartate receptors found in plasma), Parkinson disease protein 7 (PARK7), nucleoside diphosphate kinase A (NDKA), apolipoprotein A1 unique peptide (APOA1-UP), matrix metalloproteinase-9 (MMP-9), glycogen phosphorylase isoenzyme BB (GPBB), and B-type neurotrophic growth factor (BNGF)) [13,15–17]; (2) the neuronal cell activation indicators (e.g., S100 calcium-binding protein B (S100B) and monocyte chemoattractant protein-1 (MCP-1)) [18,19]; (3) the neuroinflammation indicators (e.g., eotaxin and vascular cell adhesion molecule (VCAM)) [20,21]; (4) the endothelial dysfunction markers (e.g., D-dimer, von Willebrand factor (vWF); and (5) the neuro-endocrine markers such as B-type natriuretic peptide (BNP), and cortisol [22].

Despite the abundance of available biomarkers, only a few of them have demonstrated a sensitivity above 50% for stroke in clinical trials, which largely limits their clinical applicability [23]. In the process of this literature review, we focused on biomarkers that have undergone preliminary clinical evaluations. We selected seven individual biomarkers that have both sensitivity and specificity of more than 50% (Figure 2).

S100B is a member of the S100 protein superfamily. It is an intracellular protein found in glial cells and Schwann cells and is released into the blood circulation following cellular activation caused by tissue damage [24,25]. Zhou et al., (2016) reported a sensitivity of 95.7% and specificity of 70.4% for stroke for S100B, as well as an area under the curve (AUC) of 0.903 in differentiating between IS and intracranial haemorrhage (ICH) [18]. In another study, this biomarker was found useful in predicting the patient's short-term functional outcome after a stroke event [24]. However, the elevations of the plasma levels of this biomarker in other neurological and neuropsychological disorders such as Alzheimer's disease and schizophrenia means it would be of a reduced value in triaging the suspected patients for stroke [25].

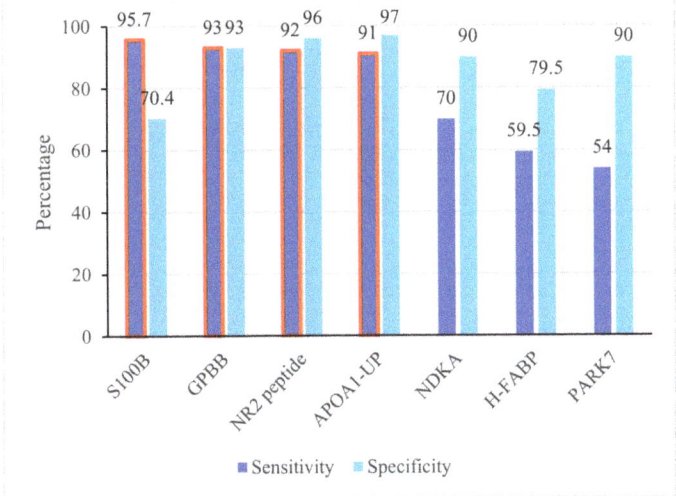

Figure 2. Single blood biomarkers for stroke. S100B, GPBB, NR2 peptide, and APOA1_UP all have sensitivities of >90% (highlighted in red). S100B, S100 calcium-binding protein B; GPBB, glycogen phosphorylase BB; NR2 peptide, a degradation product of N-methyl-d-aspartate receptors; APOA1-UP, apolipoprotein A1 unique peptide; NDKA, nucleoside diphosphate kinase A; H-FABP, heart-type fatty acid binding protein; PARK7, Parkinson disease protein 7.

GPBB is a glycogen phosphorylase isoenzyme found in the brain and heart tissues whose function is to make glucose-1-phosphate by breaking down glycogen, which helps restore the energy stores, which are depleted during a cerebral ischaemic event [17]. According to Park et al., (2018), increased plasma levels of GPBB have a sensitivity and a specificity of 93% for detecting stroke within 12 h from the onset of the symptoms [17]. However, this study did not find any correlation between GPBB levels and the severity of the stroke, infarct volume, or the clinical outcome, which suggests a less suitable position for this biomarker to be used for predicting the disease prognosis in patients with IS.

NR2 peptide is an N-terminal fragment of N-methyl-D-aspartate (NMDA) receptors, which can be measured in the plasma sample. Following cerebral ischaemia, NMDA receptors are released from endothelial cells of the brain's microvessels which are then cleaved by serine proteinases and are released into the blood stream as NR2 peptides [14]. In a study undertaken by Dambinova et al., in 2012, it was reported that NR2 peptide has a sensitivity of 92% and specificity of 96% for ischaemic stroke when measurable at 3 h post-stroke [14]. Also, it has been found that the plasma levels of anti-NMDA antibodies are predictive of stroke and a brain lesion size in high-risk patients [26].

MMP-9 is a $Zn^{2+}$-dependent proteolytic enzyme that is released from different cells such as neutrophils and has roles in the degradation of the extracellular matrix following IS and ICH [36]. Experimental studies have shown that systemic inflammation during stroke causes a neutrophil infiltration of the ischaemic area of the brain which eventually leads to increased plasma MMP-9 activity in patients with stroke [27]. The studies by Castellanos et al., (2007) and Kelly et al., (2008) showed that high levels of MMP-9 are predictive of blood–brain barrier disruption and haemorrhagic transformation after an IS [28,29]. Another benefit of measuring plasma MMP-9 has been reported to be its predictive value in detecting brain tissue haematoma following tissue plasminogen activator treatment in patients with IS (sensitivity of 92% and specificity of 74%) [29].

Apolipoprotein A1 (APOA1) is a major protein component of the high-density lipoprotein (HDL) and exhibits anti-inflammatory and antioxidant effects, hence playing an important role in the protection of the vascular system against oxidative stress. Studies have shown that the levels of APOA1 decrease in patients with stroke and/or infection [30]. Similarly, decreased levels of APOA1-UP, as a novel biomarker have been reported to have a high sensitivity (91%) and specificity (97%) for the prediction of IS, nominating it as a promising independent predictor of IS [16].

PARK7 and NDKA are released from the cerebrospinal fluid into the plasma after significant brain injury [15]. The study done by Allard et al., (2005) reported a sensitivity of 54% and a specificity of 90% for PARK7 at a cut-off level of 14.1 µg/L, when samples were taken at 3 h after the onset of the acute stroke. Accordingly, the reported sensitivity and specificity for NDKA, at a cut-off value of 22 µg/L were 70% and 90%, respectively [15].

H-FABP is a fatty acid binding protein that is released from CNS tissues after an ischaemic event into the blood. A study by Park et al., found that this protein had a sensitivity of 59.5%, specificity of 79.5%, and an AUC = 0.71 ($p < 0.001$) for identifying IS if the blood samples were collected after 24 h of the stroke onset [13]. Given the long timeframe and its low sensitivity, this protein might not be a good biomarker for stroke detection.

Although many of these biomarkers seem promising in the early screening of stroke, most of the findings are hardly generalisable to larger populations due to the small sample sizes of the original studies. In addition, because medical interventions need to be performed within a short timeframe to salvage the vulnerable neuronal tissues and minimise mortality or functional deficits, many of the suggested biomarkers do not seem to be very useful because of the relatively long time needed for the symptoms' onset until a reliably measurable change in the biomarkers' levels can be detected. Some biomarkers, such as PARK7, NDKA, and NR2 peptide, are released into the plasma and are detectable within the first three hours after the stroke onset, which makes them potentially promising biomarkers to be used in future studies in acute settings [15]. Unfortunately, many other biomarkers identified in this review have not yet been evaluated for their diagnostic reliability at the early stages of stroke. Table 2 summarises some of the key aspects of the clinical studies related to the biomarkers and biomarker panels reviewed in this article.

Table 2. Blood biomarkers for stroke diagnosis.

| Biomarker | Reference | Sample Size (n) | Cut-Off | Time from Symptoms Onset to Sample Collection (up to) |
|---|---|---|---|---|
| S100B | Zhou et al., (2016) [18] | 46 (ICH) 71 (IS) | 67 pg/mL | 6 h |
| GPBB | Park et al., (2018) [17] | 172 (IS) 133 (C) | 7.0 ng/mL | 4.5 h |
| NR2 peptide | Dambinova et al., (2012) [14] | 101 (IS) 91 (C) | 1.0 µg/L | 3 h |
| APOA1-UP | Zhao et al., (2016) [16] | 94 (IS) 37 (C) | APOA1-UP/LRP ratio 1.80 | 72 h |
| PARK-7 | Allard et al., (2005) [15] | 622 (S) 165 (C) | 9.33 µg/L | 3 h |
| NDKA | Allard et al., (2005) [15] | 622 (S) 165 (C) | 2 µg/L | 3 h |
| H-FABP | Park et al., (2013) [13] | 111 (IS) 127 (C) | 9.70 ng/ml | 24 h |
| Panel A | Reynolds et al., (2003) [32] | 223 (S) 214 (C) | - | 6 h |
| Panel B | Lynch et al., (2004) [33] | 65 (IS) 157 (C) | - | 6 h |
| Panel C | Sharma et al., (2014) [20] | 167 (S) | - | 24 h |
| Panel D | Laskowitz et al., (2005) [34] | 130 (IS) 10 (C) | - | 6 h |
| Panel E | Moore et al., 2005 [35] | 20 (IS) 20 (C) | - | <24 h (n = 7), 24–48 h (n = 10), >48 h (n = 3) |

Ischaemic stroke (IS), control (C), intracerebral haemorrhage (ICH), stroke (not specified or a mixed population) (S), labelled reference peptide (LRP).

As it can be seen from Figure 2, some of these biomarkers (e.g., S100B) have better sensitivity than others, but are less specific for stroke [37]. In addition, some comorbidities and other factors are also found to interfere with the accuracy of these biomarkers. However, when the biomarkers are combined in a panel, they may offer greater sensitivity and specificity values compared to individual biomarkers [37].

*3.2. Biomarker Panels*

Unavailability of single biomarkers with both high sensitivity and specificity has been a limiting factor in adopting blood biomarkers as stand-alone diagnostic tools in clinical situations such as stroke. To add to the complexity, patterns of biomarkers changes may differ depending on the type of stroke (e.g., IS versus ICH) or depending on the affected brain areas [31]. It has been suggested that by combining several biomarkers into a biomarker panel more useful information can be obtained particularly by including biomarkers specific to different areas of the brain [14,16,17,29]. In this review, we have identified five biomarker panels that have shown both a sensitivity and specificity above 50% (Figure 3). We have named these five biomarker panels as panels A through E in this review due to the lack of specific trade names for them in the original articles (Tables 2 and 3).

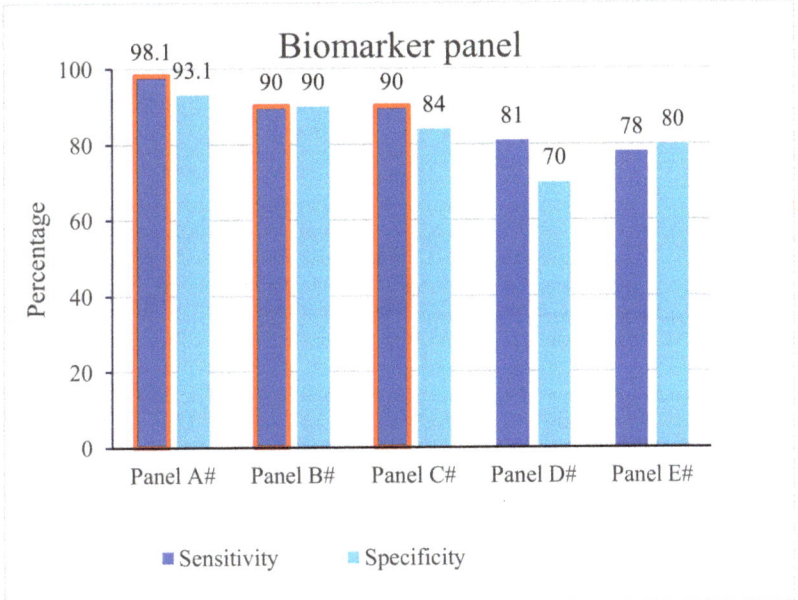

**Figure 3.** Panel biomarkers for stroke. Panels A, B and C have sensitivity of 90% or higher, which are highlighted in red. NB: The reported sensitivity and specificity for panels A, B, D, and E are related to ischaemic stroke only.

Most of these panels are composed of brain-specific biomarkers (neuronal cell activation and neuro-endocrine markers) and non-specific biomarkers (MMP-9, C-reactive protein (CRP), VCAM, vWF, and D-dimer), to represent different parts of the ischaemic cascade and provide complementary information for the diagnosis of stroke. Although the findings from those studies are not conclusive, the use of biomarker panels may have opened a new frontier in the development of highly sensitive and specific biomarkers. Therefore, the concept of diagnostic biomarker panels is a promising topic for future research.

Table 3. Panel biomarker composition.

| Biomarker Panel | Composition of Biomarkers |
|---|---|
| Panel A (5 proteins) | BNGF, MCP-1, MMP-9, S100B, vWF |
| Panel B (3 proteins) | vWF, MMP-9, VCAM |
| Panel C (5 proteins) | Eotaxin, EGFR, S100A12, Metalloproteinase inhibitor-4, Prolactin |
| Panel D (5 proteins) | S100B, MMP-9, D-dimer, BNP, CRP |
| Panel E (22 genes) | CD163; Hypothetical protein FLJ22662 Laminin A motif; Amyloid β(A4) precursor-like protein 2; N-acetylneuraminate pyruvate lyase; v-fos FBJ murine osteosarcoma viral oncogene homolog; Toll-like receptor 2; Ectonucleoside triphosphate diphosphohydrolase 1; Chondroitin sulfate proteoglycan 2 (versican); Interleukin 13 receptor, α1; CD14 antigen; Bone marrow stromal cell antigen 1/CD157; Complement component 1, q subcomponent, receptor 1; Paired immunoglobulin-like type 2 receptor α; Fc fragment of IgG, high-affinity Ia, receptor for (CD64); Adrenomedullin; Dual-specificity phosphatase 1; Cytochrome b-245, β polypeptide (chronic granulomatous disease); Leukotriene A4 hydrolase; v-ets Erythroblastosis virus E26 oncogene homolog 2 (avian); CD36 antigen (thrombospondin receptor); Baculoviral IAP repeat-containing protein 1 (Neuronal apoptosis inhibitory protein); and KIAA0146 protein |

BNGF, B-type neurotrophic growth factor; MCP-1, monocyte chemoattractant protein-1; MMP-9, matrix metalloproteinase-9; S100B, S100 calcium-binding protein B; vWF, von Willebrand factor; VCAM, vascular cell adhesion molecule; EGFR, epidermal growth factor receptor; S100A12, S100 calcium-binding protein A12; BNP, B-type natriuretic peptide; CRP, C-reactive protein.

Panel A is composed of five protein biomarkers that were studied by Reynolds et al., (Table 2) [32]. This panel has shown a sensitivity of approximately 98% and specificity of about 93% for prediction of IS for samples collected within 6 h from the appearance of symptoms. This is a significant improvement compared to many individual markers in previous studies [32]. Panel B includes three protein biomarkers based on a study by Lynch et al., in 2004. This panel had both 90% sensitivity and specificity where the samples were obtained within 6 h of the stroke onset [33]. Panel C comprises five protein biomarkers based on a study by Sharma et al., in which they reported a sensitivity of 90%, specificity of 84%, a positive predictive value (PPV) of 78%, and a negative predictive value (NPV) of 93% for stroke detection within 24 h of symptoms' onset [20]. Panel D, which was developed in a cohort of 130 patients with acute neurological symptoms, consists of five protein biomarkers. This panel showed a sensitivity of 81% and a specificity of 70% for the prediction of IS when the blood specimens were collected within 6 h of the stroke onset [35]. Given the above information, panels A, B, and D may be clinically useful for triaging purposes [32,33,35].

Panel E, made by Moore et al., in 2005 was created following a comparative study of gene expression profiles in confirmed stroke cases (IS; n = 20) versus matched healthy controls (n = 20) using microarray technology. Accordingly, and after the initial study of exhaustive gene expression patterns using the RNA samples extracted from peripheral blood mononuclear cells, they observed a significant change (mainly up-regulations) in the expression of 190 genes in patients with IS. Next, a panel of 22 genes was chosen for the derivation of a predictive model for the prediction of stroke using hierarchical cluster analysis (Table 3). The model was then prospectively validated in another cohort consisting of 9 stroke patients and 10 healthy individuals. This model showed a sensitivity of 78% and a specificity of 80% in the validation cohort [35]. These results are promising; however, the authors were unable to rule out the effects of non-stroke causes in the up-regulation of the genes. In addition, because of the small sample sizes both for the derivation and the validation studies, the results need to be validated in larger studies.

The above-mentioned biomarkers have not been approved for clinical diagnostic use yet due to several reasons, including the lack of large prospective trials, lack of the standards for measurement, unknown interference in certain population groups, or uncertainties in the time-concentration relationships. We believe that the available data are still limited, and explorative investigations such as in vitro studies on stroke biomarkers are still insufficient. We suggest that before starting large-scale clinical studies, we need to have a better understanding of the window periods of individual biomarkers for stroke detection (the time from symptoms' onset to a detectable change in the blood levels of a biomarker). As we know, the efficacy for current interventions for acute stroke is time-dependent, and most of the current guidelines recommend <4.5 h as a key target between the onset of symptoms and treatment intervention with fibrinolytic, and up to 6 h for mechanical thrombectomy [38,39]. Therefore, by taking into consideration the time required for radio-imaging to confirm the diagnosis prior to treatment (which is around 45 min in optimal settings and up to 1.5 h in average settings), any biomarker that can be reliably detected within 3 h of the onset of stroke could be a highly valuable diagnostic tool.

In this literature review, we did not allocate a great level of priority for exploring potential associations between blood levels of biomarkers and the size of brain lesions (extents of infarcts or bleedings) as our review was more of a diagnostic nature rather than prognostic. However, we found some limited, yet promising, evidence, which could be used in future research in those areas. For example, in terms of the IS, Kalev-Zylinska et. al. (2013) found that plasma levels of anti-NMDA antibodies were predictive of brain lesion's size in the patients and a high National Institutes of Health Stroke Scale score. However, they found this association only in 21 of the 48 patients (44%) studied. Accordingly, they identified this small sample size and the explanatory nature of their research as limiting factors for the applicability of their findings [26]. On the other hand, in a study by Park et al., (2018), the researchers did not find a correlation between GPBB levels and the clinical outcome or volume of the infarct in patients with IS [17]. In addition, in terms of the intracerebral haemorrhage, there is some promising evidence. For example, in 2007 Castellanos et al., in a multicentre prospective study reported high sensitivities and negative predictive values for the levels of serum cellular fibronectin and MMP-9 for the prediction of haemorrhagic transformation and parenchymal haematoma following thrombolytic therapy in patients with acute IS. However, they admitted that their small sample size (n = 134) and the smaller number of patients who developed parenchymal haemorrhage during the follow-up period were among the limiting factors for their findings. Having mentioned all the above, and despite the uncertainties in the usefulness of biomarkers in predicting the lesion size and clinical outcomes, this is a relatively less explored area of knowledge, and we believe that it is worth researching further.

## 4. Our Study Limitations

There are a few limitations to this paper. Firstly, we performed a narrative literature search using studies involving human only and excluded animal studies, which may have caused us to miss some of the current literature. Secondly, this was not a systematic review; therefore, we are not sure if we have identified and reported all the appropriate stroke biomarkers (hence we suggest a systematic review for this purpose). Thirdly, we only searched for articles published in English; as a result, we may have missed some important studies published in non-English languages. Lastly, because most of the patients in the included studies were middle-aged or older adults, some of the conclusions presented here might not be applicable to children and young adults because of age-related differences in the pathophysiology of stroke. Accordingly, we suggest that there is an urgent need for research into the role of blood biomarkers in the detection of stroke in different age groups, particularly children and young adults.

## 5. Conclusions

The results of this literature review indicate that there are potential biomarkers (both as individual biomarkers and as panels) with high-enough sensitivity and specificity that may serve as early detection tools for stroke diagnosis. However, most of the published studies had small sample sizes, which makes the clinical applicability of their findings challenging. Therefore, further research needs to be done in larger cohorts to confirm the clinical usefulness of the available data. In addition, most of the proposed biomarkers have not been examined in very acute patients within the first 3–5 h post-stroke, hence there is a need for further research in this area.

**Author Contributions:** Conceptualisation, R.K.J. and K.C.Y.; methodology, R.K.J.; literature search, R.K.J. and R.M.; data curation, R.K.J., R.M. and K.C.Y.; writing the original draft, R.K.J.; review, revision and editing R.K.J., R.M. and K.C.Y.; visualisation, R.K.J. and R.M.; supervision, R.M. and K.C.Y.; project administration, R.M. All authors have read and agreed to the published version of the manuscript.

**Funding:** This research was funded by the University of Canberra.

**Institutional Review Board Statement:** Not applicable.

**Informed Consent Statement:** Not applicable.

**Data Availability Statement:** No data were generated in this study.

**Conflicts of Interest:** The authors declare no conflict of interest.

## References

1. Donkor, E.S. Stroke in the 21(st) Century: A Snapshot of the Burden, Epidemiology, and Quality of Life. *Stroke Res. Treat.* **2018**, *2018*, 3238165. [PubMed]
2. Antipova, D.; Eadie, L.; Macaden, A.; Wilson, P. Diagnostic accuracy of clinical tools for assessment of acute stroke: A systematic review. *BMC Emerg. Med.* **2019**, *19*, 49. [CrossRef] [PubMed]
3. Falcione, S.; Kamtchum-Tatuene, J.; Sykes, G.; Jickling, G.C. RNA expression studies in stroke: What can they tell us about stroke mechanism? *Curr. Opin. Neurol.* **2020**, *33*, 24–29. [CrossRef] [PubMed]
4. Mokin, M.; Ansari, S.A.; McTaggart, R.A.; Bulsara, K.R.; Goyal, M.; Chen, M.; Fraser, J.F. Indications for thrombectomy in acute ischemic stroke from emergent large vessel occlusion (ELVO): Report of the SNIS Standards and Guidelines Committee. *J. Neurointerv. Surg.* **2019**, *11*, 215–220. [CrossRef]
5. Laskowitz, D.T.; Kasner, S.E.; Saver, J.; Remmel, K.S.; Jauch, E.C. Clinical usefulness of a biomarker-based diagnostic test for acute stroke: The Biomarker Rapid Assessment in Ischemic Injury (BRAIN) study. *Stroke* **2009**, *40*, 77–85. [CrossRef]
6. Yan, A.-R.; Naunton, M.; Peterson, G.M.; Fernandez-Cadenas, I.; Mortazavi, R. Effectiveness of Platelet Function Analysis-Guided Aspirin and/or Clopidogrel Therapy in Preventing Secondary Stroke: A Systematic Review and Meta-Analysis. *J. Clin. Med.* **2020**, *9*, 3907. [CrossRef]
7. Purrucker, J.C.; Hametner, C.; Engelbrecht, A.; Bruckner, T.; Popp, E.; Poli, S. Comparison of stroke recognition and stroke severity scores for stroke detection in a single cohort. *J. Neurol. Neurosurg. Psychiatr.* **2015**, *86*, 1021–1028. [CrossRef]
8. Smajlović, D. Strokes in young adults: Epidemiology and prevention. *Vasc. Health Risk Manag.* **2015**, *11*, 157–164. [CrossRef]
9. Feigin, V.L.; Stark, B.A.; Johnson, C.O.; Roth, G.A.; Bisignano, C.; Abady, G.G.; Abbasifard, M.; Abbasi-Kangevari, M.; Abd-Allah, F.; Abedi, V.; et al. Global, regional, and national burden of stroke and its risk factors, 1990–2013; 2019: A systematic analysis for the Global Burden of Disease Study 2019. *Lancet Neurol.* **2021**, *20*, 795–820. [CrossRef]
10. Mackay, M.T.; Churilov, L.; Donnan, G.A.; Babl, F.E.; Monagle, P. Performance of bedside stroke recognition tools in discriminating childhood stroke from mimics. *Neurology* **2016**, *86*, 2154–2161. [CrossRef]
11. Babuin, L.; Jaffe, A.S. Troponin: The biomarker of choice for the detection of cardiac injury. *CMAJ Can. Med. Assoc. J. J. L'assoc. Med. Can.* **2005**, *173*, 1191–1202. [CrossRef]
12. Viji Babu, P.K.; Radmacher, M. Mechanics of Brain Tissues Studied by Atomic Force Microscopy: A Perspective. *Front. Neurosci.* **2019**, *13*, 600. [CrossRef]
13. Park, S.Y.; Kim, M.H.; Kim, O.J.; Ahn, H.J.; Song, J.Y.; Jeong, J.Y.; Oh, S.-H. Plasma heart-type fatty acid binding protein level in acute ischemic stroke: Comparative analysis with plasma S100B level for diagnosis of stroke and prediction of long-term clinical outcome. *Clin. Neurol. Neurosurg.* **2013**, *115*, 405–410. [CrossRef]
14. Dambinova, S.A.; Bettermann, K.; Glynn, T.; Tews, M.; Olson, D.; Weissman, J.D.; Sowell, R.L. Diagnostic Potential of the NMDA Receptor Peptide Assay for Acute Ischemic Stroke. *PLoS ONE* **2012**, *7*, e42362. [CrossRef]
15. Allard, L.; Burkhard, P.R.; Lescuyer, P.; Burgess, J.A.; Walter, N.; Hochstrasser, D.F.; Sanchez, J.-C. PARK7 and Nucleoside Diphosphate Kinase A as Plasma Markers for the Early Diagnosis of Stroke. *Clin. Chem.* **2005**, *51*, 2043–2051. [CrossRef]
16. Zhao, X.; Yu, Y.; Xu, W.; Dong, L.; Wang, Y.; Gao, B.; Li, G.; Zhang, W. Apolipoprotein A1-Unique Peptide as a Diagnostic Biomarker for Acute Ischemic Stroke. *Int. J. Mol. Sci.* **2016**, *17*, 458. [CrossRef]
17. Park, K.Y.; Ay, I.; Avery, R.; Caceres, J.A.; Siket, M.S.; Pontes-Neto, O.M.; Zheng, H.; Rost, N.S.; Furie, K.L.; Sorensen, A.G.; et al. New biomarker for acute ischaemic stroke: Plasma glycogen phosphorylase isoenzyme BB. *J. Neurol. Neurosurg. Psychiatr.* **2018**, *89*, 404–409. [CrossRef]
18. Zhou, S.; Bao, J.; Wang, Y.; Pan, S. S100β as a biomarker for differential diagnosis of intracerebral hemorrhage and ischemic stroke. *Neurol. Res.* **2016**, *38*, 327–332. [CrossRef]

19. Losy, J.; Zaremba, J. Monocyte chemoattractant protein-1 is increased in the cerebrospinal fluid of patients with ischemic stroke. *Stroke* **2001**, *32*, 2695–2696. [CrossRef]
20. Sharma, R.; Macy, S.; Richardson, K.; Lokhnygina, Y.; Laskowitz, D.T. A blood-based biomarker panel to detect acute stroke. *J. Stroke Cereb. Dis.* **2014**, *23*, 910–918. [CrossRef]
21. Supanc, V.; Biloglav, Z.; Kes, V.B.; Demarin, V. Role of cell adhesion molecules in acute ischemic stroke. *Ann. Saudi. Med.* **2011**, *31*, 365–370. [CrossRef]
22. Katan, M.; Elkind, M.S. Inflammatory and neuroendocrine biomarkers of prognosis after ischemic stroke. *Expert. Rev. Neurother.* **2011**, *11*, 225–239. [CrossRef]
23. Kamtchum-Tatuene, J.; Jickling, G.C. Blood Biomarkers for Stroke Diagnosis and Management. *Neuromol. Med.* **2019**, *21*, 344–368. [CrossRef]
24. Abdel-Ghaffar, W.E.; Ahmed, S.; Mahmoud El reweny, E.; Elfatatry, A.; Elmesky, M.; Hashad, D. The role of s100b as a predictor of the functional outcome in geriatric patients with acute cerebrovascular stroke. *Egypt. J. Neurol. Psychiatr. Neurosurg.* **2019**, *55*, 75. [CrossRef]
25. Sen, J.; Belli, A. S100B in neuropathologic states: The CRP of the brain? *J. Neurosci. Res.* **2007**, *85*, 1373–1380. [CrossRef]
26. Kalev-Zylinska, M.L.; Symes, W.; Little, K.C.; Sun, P.; Wen, D.; Qiao, L.; Young, D.; During, M.J.; Barber, P.A. Stroke patients develop antibodies that react with components of N-methyl-D-aspartate receptor subunit 1 in proportion to lesion size. *Stroke* **2013**, *44*, 2212–2219. [CrossRef]
27. Lakhan, S.E.; Kirchgessner, A.; Tepper, D.; Leonard, A. Matrix metalloproteinases and blood-brain barrier disruption in acute ischemic stroke. *Front. Neurol.* **2013**, *4*, 32. [CrossRef]
28. Kelly, P.J.; Morrow, J.D.; Ning, M.; Koroshetz, W.; Lo, E.H.; Terry, E.; Ginger, L.M.; Hubbard, J.; Lee, H.; Stevenson, E.; et al. Oxidative stress and matrix metalloproteinase-9 in acute ischemic stroke: The Biomarker Evaluation for Antioxidant Therapies in Stroke (BEAT-Stroke) study. *Stroke* **2008**, *39*, 100–104. [CrossRef]
29. Castellanos, M.; Sobrino, T.; Millán, M.; García, M.; Arenillas, J.; Nombela, F.; Brea, D.; de la Ossa, N.P.; Serena, J.; Vivancos, J.; et al. Serum cellular fibronectin and matrix metalloproteinase-9 as screening biomarkers for the prediction of parenchymal hematoma after thrombolytic therapy in acute ischemic stroke: A multicenter confirmatory study. *Stroke* **2007**, *38*, 1855–1859. [CrossRef]
30. Eldeeb, M.A.; Zaki, A.S.; Ashour, S.; Abdel Nasser, A.; El Bassiouny, A.; Abdulghani, K.O. Serum apolipoprotein A1: A predictor and prognostic biomarker in acute ischemic stroke. *Egypt. J. Neurol. Psychiatr. Neurosurg.* **2020**, *56*, 3. [CrossRef]
31. Kawata, K.; Liu, C.Y.; Merkel, S.F.; Ramirez, S.H.; Tierney, R.T.; Langford, D. Blood biomarkers for brain injury: What are we measuring? *Neurosci. Biobehav. Rev.* **2016**, *68*, 460–473. [CrossRef] [PubMed]
32. Reynolds, M.A.; Kirchick, H.J.; Dahlen, J.R.; Anderberg, J.M.; McPherson, P.H.; Nakamura, K.K.; Laskowitz, D.T.; Valkirs, G.E.; Buechler, K.F. Early biomarkers of stroke. *Clin. Chem.* **2003**, *49*, 1733–1739. [CrossRef] [PubMed]
33. Lynch, J.R.; Blessing, R.; White, W.D.; Grocott, H.P.; Newman, M.F.; Laskowitz, D.T. Novel diagnostic test for acute stroke. *Stroke* **2004**, *35*, 57–63. [CrossRef] [PubMed]
34. Laskowitz, D.T.; Blessing, R.; Floyd, J.; White, W.D.; Lynch, J.R. Panel of biomarkers predicts stroke. *Ann. N. Y. Acad. Sci.* **2005**, *1053*, 30. [CrossRef]
35. Moore, D.F.; Li, H.; Jeffries, N.; Wright, V.; Cooper, R.A., Jr.; Elkahloun, A.; Gelderman, M.P.; Zudaire, E.; Blevins, G.; Yu, H.; et al. Using peripheral blood mononuclear cells to determine a gene expression profile of acute ischemic stroke: A pilot investigation. *Circulation* **2005**, *111*, 212–221. [CrossRef]
36. Rosell, A.; Ortega-Aznar, A.; Alvarez-Sabín, J.; Fernández-Cadenas, I.; Ribó, M.; Molina, C.A.; Lo, E.H.; Montaner, J. Increased brain expression of matrix metalloproteinase-9 after ischemic and hemorrhagic human stroke. *Stroke* **2006**, *37*, 1399–1406. [CrossRef]
37. Ishida, K.; Cucchiara, B. Blood Biomarkers for Stroke: Wolters Kluwer. 2014. Available online: https://www.uptodate.com/contents/blood-biomarkers-for-stroke (accessed on 27 April 2022).
38. Toyoda, K.; Koga, M.; Iguchi, Y.; Itabashi, R.; Inoue, M.; Okada, Y.; Ogasawara, K.; Tsujino, A.; Hasegawa, Y.; Hatano, H.; et al. Guidelines for Intravenous Thrombolysis (Recombinant Tissue-type Plasminogen Activator), the Third Edition, March 2019: A Guideline from the Japan Stroke Society. *Neurol. Med. Chir.* **2019**, *59*, 449–491. [CrossRef]
39. Powers, W.J.; Rabinstein, A.A.; Ackerson, T.; Adeoye, O.M.; Bambakidis, N.C.; Becker, K.; Biller, J.; Brown, M.; Demaerschalk, B.M.; Hoh, B.; et al. Guidelines for the early management of patients with acute ischemic stroke: 2019 update to the 2018 guidelines for the early management of acute ischemic stroke: A guideline for healthcare professionals from the American Heart Association/American Stroke Association. *Stroke* **2019**, *50*, e344–e418.

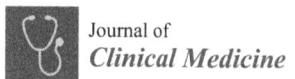 

Article

# Assessment of the Effect on Thromboprophylaxis with Multifaceted Quality Improvement Intervention based on Clinical Decision Support System in Hospitalized Patients: A Pilot Study

Qian Gao [1,2,3,†], Kaiyuan Zhen [1,2,3,4,†], Lei Xia [5], Wei Wang [6], Yaping Xu [6], Chaozeng Si [7], Zhu Zhang [1,2,3], Fen Dong [8], Jieping Lei [8], Peiran Yang [9], Jixiang Liu [1,2,3,10], Ziyi Sun [11,12], Tieshan Zhang [7], Jun Wan [13,14], Wanmu Xie [1,2,3], Peng Liu [15], Cunbo Jia [11,\*], Zhenguo Zhai [1,2,3,4,\*] and Chen Wang [1,2,3,4,10] on behalf of the Chinese Prevention Strategy for Venous Thromboembolism (CHIPS-VTE) Study Group

1. Department of Pulmonary and Critical Care Medicine, Center of Respiratory Medicine, China-Japan Friendship Hospital, Beijing 100029, China
2. Institute of Respiratory Medicine, Chinese Academy of Medical Sciences, Beijing 100029, China
3. National Clinical Research Center for Respiratory Diseases, Beijing 100029, China
4. Peking University China-Japan Friendship School of Clinical Medicine, Beijing 100029, China
5. Medical Affairs Department of China-Japan Friendship Hospital, Beijing 100029, China
6. Department of Nursing, China-Japan Friendship Hospital, Beijing 100029, China
7. Department of Information Management, China-Japan Friendship Hospital, Beijing 100029, China
8. Institute of Clinical Medical Sciences, China-Japan Friendship Hospital, Beijing 100029, China
9. Department of Physiology, Institute of Basic Medical Sciences, Chinese Academy of Medical Sciences, Peking Union Medical College, Beijing 100730, China
10. Chinese Academy of Medical Sciences and Peking Union Medical College, Beijing 100730, China
11. China-Japan Friendship Hospital, Beijing 100029, China
12. Department of Oncology, Beijing Electric Power Hospital, Capital Medical University, Beijing 100073, China
13. Department of Pulmonary and Critical Care Medicine, Beijing Anzhen Hospital, Capital Medical University, Beijing 100029, China
14. Beijing Institute of Heart, Lung and Blood Vessel Diseases, Beijing 100029, China
15. Department of Cardiovascular Surgery, China-Japan Friendship Hospital, Beijing 100029, China

\* Correspondence: jcb1973@163.com (C.J.); zhaizhenguo2011@126.com (Z.Z.)

† These authors contributed equally to this work.

**Abstract:** Background: To explore the feasibility and effectiveness of multifaceted quality improvement intervention based on the clinical decision support system (CDSS) in VTE prophylaxis in hospitalized patients. Methods: A randomized, department-based clinical trial was conducted in the department of respiratory and critical care medicine, orthopedic, and general surgery wards. Patients aged ≥18 years, without VTE in admission, were allocated to the intervention group and received regular care combined with multifaceted quality improvement intervention based on CDSS during hospitalization. VTE prophylaxis rate and the occurrence of hospital-associated VTE events were analyzed as primary and secondary outcomes. Results: A total of 3644 eligible residents were enrolled in this trial. With the implementation of the multifaceted quality improvement intervention based on the CDSS, the VTE prophylaxis rate of the intervention group increased from 22.93% to 34.56% ($p < 0.001$), and the incidence of HA-VTE events increased from 0.49% to 1.00% ($p = 0.366$). In the nonintervention group, the VTE prophylaxis rate increased from 24.49% to 27.90% ($p = 0.091$), and the incidence of HA-VTE events increased from 0.47% to 2.02% ($p = 0.001$). Conclusions: Multifaceted quality improvement intervention based on the CDSS strategy is feasible and expected to facilitate implementation of the recommended VTE prophylaxis strategies and reduce the incidence of HA-VTE in hospital. However, it is necessary to conduct more multicenter clinical trials in the future to provide more reliable real-world evidence.

**Keywords:** Venous thromboembolism; quality improvement; VTE prophylaxis

## 1. Introduction

Venous thromboembolism (VTE) includes pulmonary thromboembolism (PE) and deep vein thrombosis (DVT). The estimated incidence of VTE is 115–269 per 100,000 globally, and the mortality rate is 6.8–32.3 per 100,000 [1,2]. The majority (55–60%) of VTE events occur during hospitalization or 90 days after discharge, which are considered as hospital-associated VTE (HA-VTE) [3]. As a major preventable inpatient adverse event, the incidence of VTE can be effectively reduced by standardized preventive measures such as the prophylactic use of anticoagulants and mechanical prophylaxis [4–6].

VTE prophylaxis is the key measure in reducing VTE incidence and VTE-related mortality and morbidity in medical and surgical inpatients. The guidelines in China recommend that clinicians should adopt various individualized prophylaxis strategies based on adequate assessment of VTE risk and bleeding risk and adjust prophylaxis strategies based on dynamic assessment results [7,8]. The American College of Chest Physicians (ACCP) guidelines for thromboprophylaxis have clearly stated the importance of anticoagulant prophylaxis and mechanical prophylaxis [9]. Several academic institutions also have developed guidelines and recommendations on VTE prophylaxis [6,10–12].

Many initiatives have been taken in several countries to prevent VTE in hospitals with impressive results: In 2010, the National Health Service (NHS) launched the National Venous Thromboembolism Prophylaxis Programme. The National Institute for Health and Care Research published guidelines for inpatient VTE prophylaxis. Through the use of mandatory VTE risk assessment tools, the VTE risk assessment rate increased rapidly from 50% in 2010 to 90% at the beginning of Q4 2011 and has remained above 95% since 2013, achieving a 10.8% reduction in VTE-related mortality over the same period [11]. In 2008, the Agency for Healthcare Research and Quality Management (AHRQ) published guidelines for reducing HA-VTE, which were updated again in 2016 [6,13]. In 2012, the New Zealand Health Quality & Safety Commission also released a national policy document to prevent HA-VTE [14].

However, there remains a gap between the recommended preventive and measures clinical practice. Between 2007 and 2016, the incidence of VTE in Chinese inpatients increased from 3.2 to 17.5 per 100,000, while the in-hospital VTE-related mortality rate decreased from 4.7% to 2.1% [15]. At the same time, the DissolVE-2 study showed that VTE prophylaxis rates in China were severely underrepresented at only 19.0% and 9.3% among surgical and medical inpatients, respectively, with even lower rates of appropriate prophylaxis [16]. This result was much lower than the 40–60% VTE prophylaxis rates reported by a global multicenter study in 2008 [17]. The gap between the increasing incidence and the highly inadequate prophylaxis highlights the need to strengthen VTE prophylaxis, which has become an urgent clinical issue. Recent advances in machines learning and deep learning based on the increased availability of clinical data have stimulated new interest in a computerized clinical decision support system (CDSS) [18]. The CDSS shows great potential in improving health care, improving patient safety, and reducing medical costs. To facilitate implementation of appropriate thromboprophylaxis, the Chinese Prevention Strategy for Venous Thromboembolism (CHIPS-VTE) study network developed a system-wide multifaceted quality improvement strategy based on the CDSS [19]. This single-center study aims to explore the feasibility and effectiveness of multifaceted quality improvement intervention based on CDSS in VTE prophylaxis in hospitalized patients.

## 2. Methods

### 2.1. Study Design and Participants

In this pilot study, a single-center, department-based, cluster randomized trial was conducted at the China–Japan Friendship Hospital by comparing VTE prevention-related performance between departments applying multifaceted quality improvement intervention and those applying regular care. A total of ten medical or surgical units from the departments of Pulmonary and Critical Care Medicine, Orthopedics, and General Surgery participated in this study.

The study included two periods: the baseline period was from 1 October 2019 to 31 December 2019 and the intervention period from 1 April 2020 to 30 June 2020. Patient information was not collected from 1 January to 31 March 2020 due to the COVID-19 pandemic, during which the clinical care of inpatients was not representative of standard clinical practice.

Adult patients with a length-of-stay of more than 3 days or receiving surgery under anesthesia were considered to be included. Patients with hospitalization of less than 3 days without receiving surgery, diagnosed with VTE before admission or with community-acquired VTE after admission, with acute myocardial infarction (AMI), atrial fibrillation (AF), acute stroke (AS), mechanical heart valve replacement, extracorporeal membrane oxygenation (ECMO), or dialysis in admission were considered to be excluded.

*2.2. Cluster Randomization and Intervention*

We randomly divided medical or surgical units, based on the prophylaxis rates of each participating unit at the baseline period, into intervention groups and nonintervention groups, to reduce the contamination bias within the same clinical unit. Both groups were asked to include three different units of Orthopedic, Respiratory and Critical Care Medicine, and General Surgery.

The intervention group was subjected to multifaceted quality improvement intervention based on the CDSS, which included the application of the CDSS with electronic alertness assistance for VTE prophylaxis, dynamic VTE risk assessment, and prophylaxis. The CDSS has four fundamental functions: automatic, reminder, correction, and quality control analysis. The CDSS can automatically collect and analyze patients' information from various information platforms in-hospital such as electronic medical record (EMR), hospital information system (HIS), laboratory information system (LIS), picture archiving and communication system (PACS), etc. Through extract–transform–load (ETL), natural language processing (NLP), and other technologies, timely and accurate reminders and supporting decisions were automatically provided to clinicians according to clinical diagnosis and treatment guidelines (Figure 1). The CDSS could automatically analyze the patient medical records to assist medical staff in making decisions on VTE risk assessment and appropriate prophylaxis, with error correction and reminder features. Electronic alertness could automatically and actively remind medical staff to complete the VTE risk assessment and prophylaxis in a pop-up window in the electronic medical record system when they failed to complete the risk assessment or prophylaxis. If clinicians disagreed with the advice made by the CDSS, they could refuse the decisions with plausible explanations.

We established a multidisciplinary VTE prevention expert committee to formulate the VTE prevention process of the hospital. The units assigned to the nonintervention group implemented the hospital's current VTE prophylaxis measures which is according to the guidelines suggesting that doctors confirm the results of risk assessment conducted by nurses and make a prophylaxis order without additional interventions such as mandatory reminders and corrections.

*2.3. Statistical Analysis*

The primary outcome was the implementation of any VTE prophylaxis measurements in hospitalized patients. For patients at intermediate or high risk of VTE, VTE prophylaxis must be used if there were no other relevant contraindications; if there was a high risk of bleeding, mechanical prophylaxis should be applied; if there was no high risk of bleeding, pharmacological prophylaxis or pharmacological prophylaxis combined with mechanical prophylaxis should be applied.

The secondary outcome was HA-VTE events in hospitalization, which was determined by as follows: (1) admission diagnosis without VTE and discharge diagnosis of new-onset VTE, with manual verification; (2) patients who already had VTE or were already receiving anticoagulation for other diseases at admission were not included.

Normally distributed measurement data are presented as mean ± standard deviation, and an independent sample *t*-test was used for comparison between the two groups. Non-normally distributed measurement data are presented as median (upper and lower quartiles), and count data are expressed as absolute numbers (N) and percentages (%). For comparison of differences between groups, Wilcoxon rank sum test was used for non-normally distributed data, and chi-square test for qualitative data. A two-tailed $p < 0.05$ was regarded as statistically significant. SPSS 24.0 was used for statistical analysis in this study.

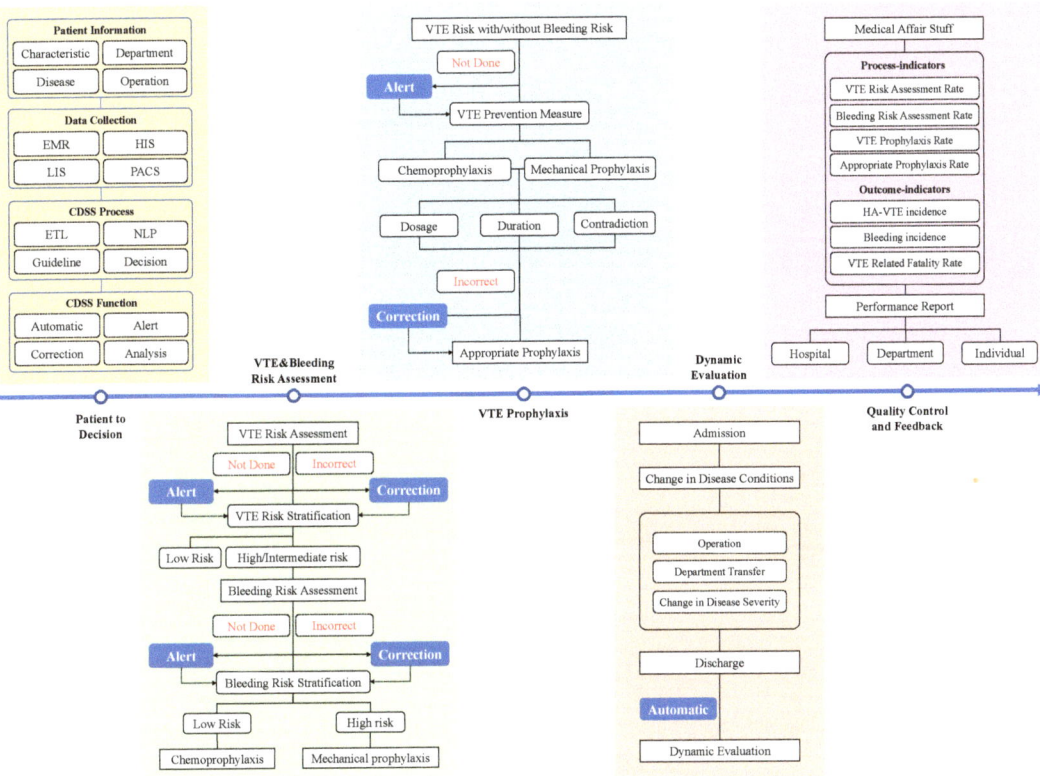

**Figure 1.** Process of multifaceted quality improvement intervention based on CDSS. EMR: electronic medical record; HIS: hospital information system; LIS: laboratory information system; PACS: picture archiving and communication system; ETL: extract–transform–load; NLP: natural language processing.

## 3. Results

### 3.1. Patient Characteristics

A total of 3644 eligible patients were enrolled in the study. Out of that total, 1624 cases were included in the intervention group, of which 1025 were in the baseline period, and 599 were in the intervention period; 2020 cases were included in the nonintervention group, of which 1278 were in the baseline period, and 742 were in the intervention period. The study flow is shown in Figure 2. There was no statistical difference between the two groups in terms of age more than 40 years and mean length-of-stay ($p > 0.05$). However, there were more male patients in the intervention group and a higher proportion of inpatients aged under 40 and between 61 and 74 in the nonintervention group. A comparison between patients in the two groups during each period is shown in Table 1.

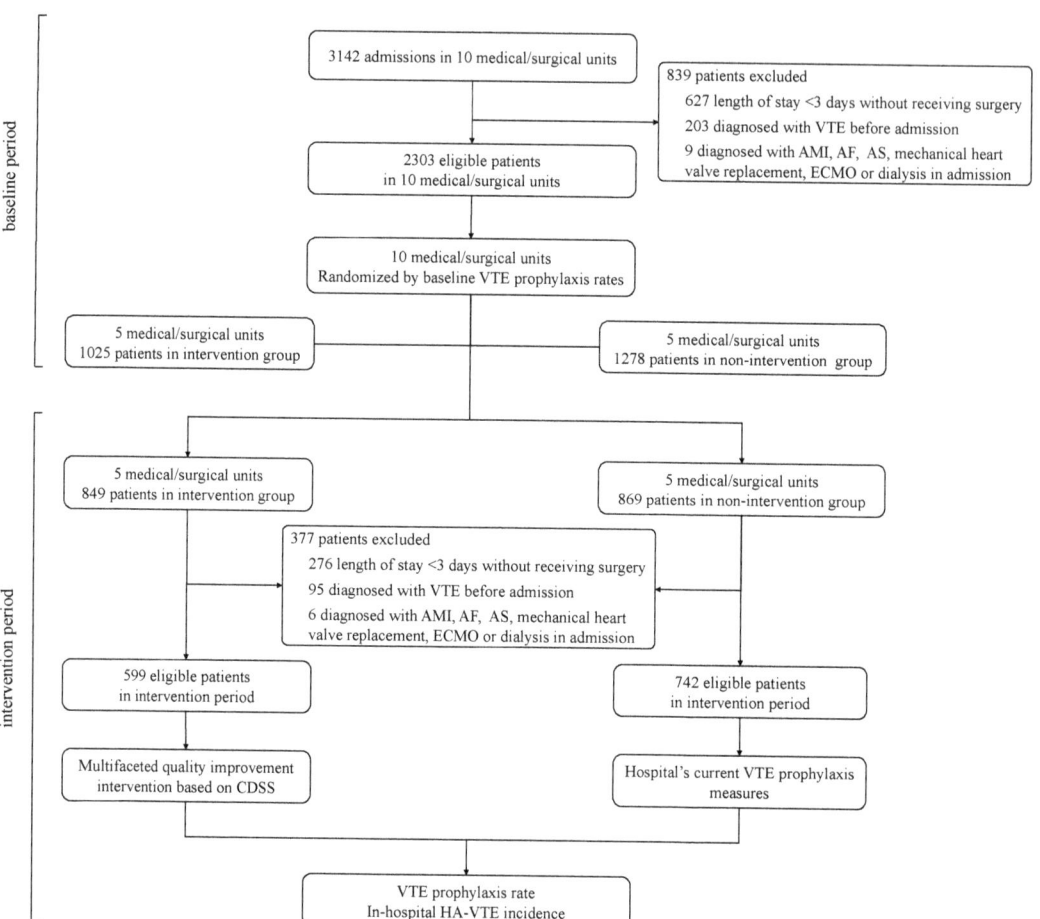

**Figure 2.** Recruitment process and flow through study. LOS: length of stay; AMI: acute myocardial infarction; AF: atrial fibrillation; AS: acute stroke; ECMO: extracorporeal membrane oxygenation.

**Table 1.** Characteristics of patients in baseline and intervention period.

|  | Baseline Period | Intervention Period [#] | |
|---|---|---|---|
|  |  | Intervention Group | Nonintervention Group |
|  | (n = 2303) | (n = 599) | (n = 742) |
| Male | 1088 (47.24%) | 349 (58.26%) | 339 (45.69%) |
| Age (Years) |  |  |  |
| ≤40 | 370 (16.07%) | 104 (17.36%) | 79 (10.65%) |
| 41–60 | 758 (32.91%) | 180 (30.05%) | 219 (29.51%) |
| 61–74 | 838 (36.39%) | 219 (36.56%) | 298 (40.16%) |
| ≥75 | 337 (14.63%) | 96 (16.03%) | 146 (19.68%) |
| Medical disease | 829 (36.00%) | 121 (20.20%) | 250 (33.69%) |
| Malignancy | 567 (24.62%) | 249 (41.57%) | 185 (24.93%) |
| Surgery | 1474 (64.00%) | 478 (79.80%) | 492 (66.31%) |
| VTE prophylaxis | 548 (23.80%) * | 207 (34.56%) | 207 (27.90%) |
| Length of stay (Days) | 8 | 8 | 8 |

[#]: Patients in each group were admitted in the same units in both periods. *: no statistical difference of VTE prophylaxis was found between the intervention group and nonintervention group during the baseline period (22.93% vs. 24.49%, $p = 0.091$).

## 3.2. Improvement in VTE Risk Assessment

A total of 3374 (92.59%) patients were given VTE risk assessment, including 2167 (94.09%) patients in the baseline period and 1207 (90.00%) in the intervention period.

For patients of the intervention group, the VTE risk assessment rates were slightly increased from 93.66% in the baseline period to 94.99% in the intervention period ($p = 0.269$). However, the VTE risk assessment rates were found decreased in the nonintervention group from 93.89% in the baseline period to 83.83% in the intervention period ($p < 0.001$), as shown in Figure 3. Among patients who received the VTE risk assessment, 1927 (57.11%) patients were stratified into intermediate or high risk of VTE.

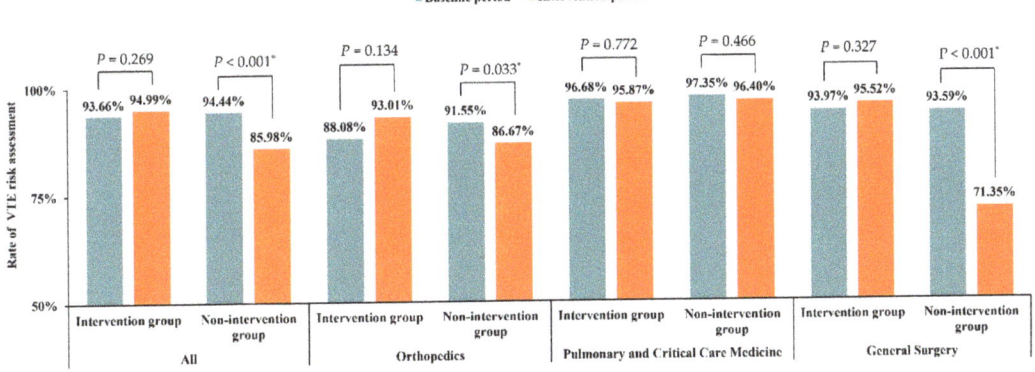

**Figure 3.** Improvement in VTE risk assessment in different departments. * $p < 0.05$.

The rate of VTE risk assessment remained stable in the intervention group in the departments of Orthopedics, Pulmonary and Critical Care Medicine, and General Surgery across the study (Figure 3). However, significant decreases were found in nonintervention group in the departments of Orthopedics and General Surgery ($p < 0.001$ for both).

## 3.3. Improvement in VTE Prophylaxis

As for VTE prophylaxis, 962 (26.40%) patients were given VTE prophylaxis in the study. No statistical differences between intervention and nonintervention groups were found in the baseline period (22.93% vs. 24.49%, $p = 0.091$) (Table 1). Although patients in both groups showed a poor rate of VTE prophylaxis, a significant increase was found in the intervention group from the baseline period to the intervention period (22.93% to 34.56%, $p < 0.001$). In contrast, in the nonintervention group, the VTE prophylaxis rate changed from 21.65% in the baseline period to 27.16% in the intervention period ($p = 0.269$), as shown in Figure 4. There was also a statistically significant difference between the two groups in the intervention period (27.90% vs. 34.56%, $p = 0.009$).

In the intervention group, significant improvements of VTE prophylaxis were observed in the departments of Orthopedics, Pulmonary and Critical Care Medicine, and General Surgery. The corresponding $p$ values were 0.032, 0.003, and 0.005, respectively. No statistical differences were found in nonintervention group in any department. The corresponding $p$ values were 0.790, 0.174, and 0.202, respectively (Figure 4).

Among patients receiving VTE prophylaxis, 952 (98.96%) patients had pharmacological prophylaxis, and 132 (13.72%) patients received mechanical prophylaxis. Low molecular weight heparin (LMWH) was used the most for pharmacological prophylaxis. However, both graduated compression stockings (GCS) ($n = 33$, 25.00%) and intermittent pneumatic compression (IPC) ($n = 31$, 23.48%) were used for mechanical prophylaxis.

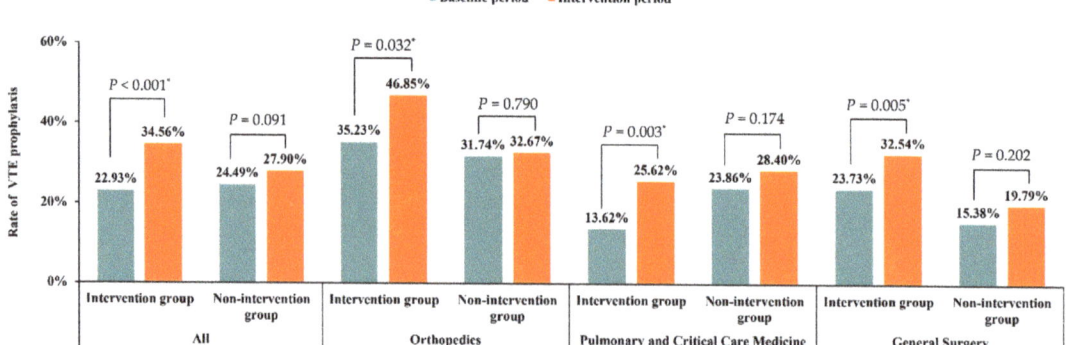

**Figure 4.** Improvement of VTE prophylaxis in different departments. * $p < 0.05$.

### 3.4. Change in In-Hospital HA-VTE Incidents

During the baseline period, the intervention group had a total of five hospital-associated VTE events, with an HA-VTE incidence of 0.49%. During the intervention period, a total of six in-hospital HA-VTE events were reported in the intervention group, with an HA-VTE incidence of 1.00%. There was no significant difference in the change in HA-VTE incidence before and after the intervention ($p = 0.366$). The nonintervention group registered a total of 6 HA-VTE events at baseline, with an HA-VTE incidence of 0.47%, and a total of 15 HA-VTE events in the intervention period, with an HA-VTE incidence of 2.02%. For the nonintervention group, HA-VTE incidence increased significantly between the two periods ($p = 0.001$). Figure 5 shows the change of in-hospital HA-VTE events from baseline to the end of intervention.

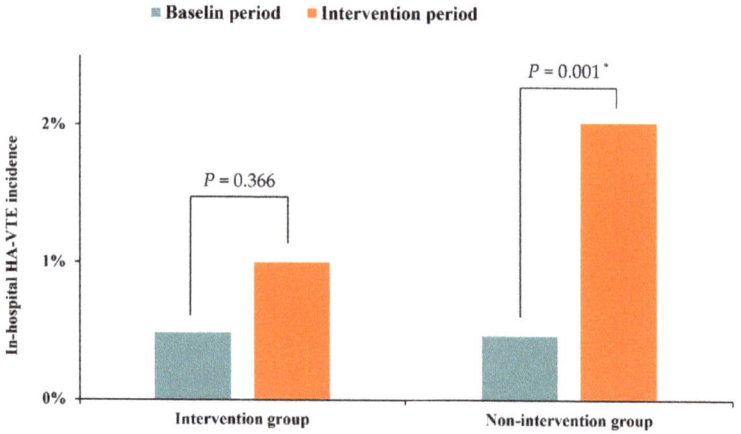

**Figure 5.** Change in in-hospital HA-VTE Event from baseline to the end of intervention. * $p < 0.05$.

## 4. Discussion

Multifaceted quality improvement intervention based on the CDSS is a multidisciplinary collaborative strategy that integrates a series of effective measures. We conducted a pilot study to explore the effect of multifaceted quality improvement intervention on VTE prophylaxis for inpatients. The results of the single-center, department-based, cluster randomized trial showed feasibility for implementation and positive effect on the improvement of VTE prophylaxis with multifaceted quality improvement intervention based on the CDSS, which may provide real-world evidence of multifaceted quality improvement intervention for further development.

The adoption of the CDSS will help improve quality of healthcare and patient safety, reduce waste in the healthcare system, and reduce the risk of an overwhelming overload for clinicians [18]. Current VTE prophylaxis strategies focus on assessing patients' VTE risk and bleeding risk and proactively taking the appropriate prophylactic measures based on these risks [8]. Currently, clinically available VTE risk scoring models are generally developed based on European and American evidence. Since the risk factors for acquired VTE in Asian populations are similar to those in European and American populations among hospitalized patients, these models have also been partially validated in Asian populations and are gradually being used in clinical practice in China. In our study, the VTE risk assessment for inpatients was initially performed by the nurses and then confirmed by the physicians. The assessment results were recorded in the nursing system and then automatically sent to the attending physicians' electronic medical record system for confirmation. The collaboration between nurses and doctors has resulted in a stable and high rate of VTE risk assessment among inpatients.

The VTE risk assessment rate in the intervention group in our study remained largely stable from the baseline period (93.66%) to the intervention period (94.99%). There was a decrease in the VTE risk assessment rate in the general surgery department of the nonintervention group, which could be due to the COVID-19 pandemic (Figure 1). A study analyzing inpatient data before and after the implementation of a VTE risk assessment model (with Padua and IMPROVE risk scales) in hospitals found no significant difference in the incidence of PE and major bleeding among 413 patients, and only 43.3% of patients received pharmacological prophylaxis after the use of the VTE risk assessment scale, compared to 56.7% before [20]. Thus, VTE risk assessment may reduce the medical costs of VTE prophylaxis while keeping patients safe.

In our study, the VTE prophylaxis rate was approximately the same in the intervention and nonintervention groups at baseline. After intervention, the VTE prophylaxis rate increased by 12% in the intervention group with a statistically significant difference, while in the nonintervention group the rate only increased by 5% with no statistically significant difference. Several studies have been conducted to investigate the effectiveness and safety of multiple interventions in VTE prophylaxis. A Cochrane review included 13 RCT studies with a total of 35,997 subjects for analysis, and the results support the conclusion that systematic intervention strategies with proactive reminders can help improve VTE prophylaxis [21]. Kucher et al. included 2506 patients at high risk for VTE and randomized them into two groups with or without electronic alerts. The study found that a significantly greater proportion of patients in the intervention group received mechanical (10.0% vs. 1.5%; $p < 0.001$) or pharmacological prophylaxis (23.6% vs. 13.0%; $p < 0.001$) compared with those in the nonintervention group, and patients in the intervention group had a 41% lower rate of VTE events within 90 days (HR 0.59 [95% CI 0.43–0.81]; $p = 0.001$) [22].

Although our study found no decrease in HA-VTE incidence in the intervention group, a significant increase in the incidence of HA-VTE was found in nonintervention group, revealing an important role of the intervention in limiting the occurrence of HA-VTE. We considered the increase in HA-VTE incidence was mainly due to the limitation of patient activity during the COVID-19 pandemic. Researchers from Johns Hopkins Hospital introduced a mandatory decision support system to facilitate VTE prophylaxis implementation in their hospital information system and enrolled 1599 patients undergoing trauma surgery into their analysis. The study showed that implementation of the mandatory decision support system significantly increased VTE prophylaxis rates in clinical practice (66.2% vs. 84.4%; $p < 0.001$). Moreover, the incidence of HA-VTE decreased significantly after the implementation (1.0% vs. 0.17%; $p = 0.04$) [23]. The University of Virginia Hospital adopted the scheme of Johns Hopkins Hospital and introduced a mandatory CDSS in the implementation of VTE prophylaxis in general surgery patients. The hospital's 30-day VTE incidence dropped significantly after implementing (1.25% vs. 0.64%; $p = 0.033$), which helped the hospital improve its ranking to the top 10% of 760 hospitals in the National Surgical Quality Improvement Program (NSQIP) in the United States [24]. After participating in the NSQIP, Boston University Hospital also implemented mandatory VTE risk assessment and stratification, and the CDSS automatically recommended the appropriate prophylaxis measures and duration based on the Caprini scores. The result was a significant reduction in the incidence of DVT (from 1.9% to 0.3%) and PE (from 1.1% to 0.5%) in the hospital, highlighting the contribution of the mandatory alert system to the promotion of VTE prophylaxis [25].

We acknowledge that the limited number of participating departments in our study may hinder extrapolation and applicability of the findings, and further validation is needed in studies with larger populations. The department-based cluster randomization in this study can reduce intergroup contamination. The quality control approach of real-time monitoring and reminding through a CDSS enables timely implementation of VTE prophylaxis among multidisciplinary medical staff. Besides the use of different anticoagulant prophylaxis, other efficacy outcomes such as fatal events and VTE events after discharge should also be taken into consideration in evaluating the effect of the VTE prophylaxis in future study [26]. This study forms a pilot study to provide evidence for the feasibility of future trials of multifaceted quality improvement intervention strategies for VTE prophylaxis in multiple centers.

## 5. Conclusions

The multifaceted quality improvement intervention strategies in clinical practice could help improve VTE prevention and reduce the VTE-related safety events in hospitalized patients at risk of VTE. Further study to validation and broader generalization were needed to solve the insufficient VTE prevention in Chinese inpatients.

**Author Contributions:** Conceptualization, C.J., Z.Z. (Zhenguo Zhai) and C.W.; methodology, C.J., Z.Z. (Zhenguo Zhai) and C.W.; software, C.S. and T.Z.; validation, J.W., W.X. and P.L.; formal analysis, Q.G. and K.Z.; investigation, Z.Z. (Zhu Zhang), L.X., W.W., Y.X.; resources, T.Z., J.W., W.X. and P.L.; data curation, F.D. and J.L. (Jieping Lei); writing—original draft preparation, Q.G. and K.Z.; writing—review and editing, Q.G., K.Z. and P.Y.; visualization, J.L. (Jixiang Liu) and Z.S.; supervision, C.W.; project administration, C.J.; funding acquisition, Z.Z. (Zhenguo Zhai). All authors have read and agreed to the published version of the manuscript.

**Funding:** This study is funded by the CAMS Innovation Fund for Medical Sciences (CIFMS) (2020-I2M-A-022) and the National Key Research and Development Program of China (No. 2016YFC0905600).

**Institutional Review Board Statement:** This study is approved by the ethics committee in China-Japan Friendship Hospital (approval number 2016-SSW-7).

**Informed Consent Statement:** Participants were given informed consent to participate in the study before taking part.

**Data Availability Statement:** Data are available upon reasonable request.

**Acknowledgments:** We appreciate all members within CHIPS-VTE network. Doctors, nurses, health administrators, researchers, and patients' engagement in the study will be appreciated.

**Conflicts of Interest:** The authors declare no conflict of interest.

## References

1. Barco, S.; Mahmoudpour, S.H.; Valerio, L.; Klok, E.; Münzel, T.; Middeldorp, S.; Ageno, W.; Cohen, A.T.; Hunt, B.J.; Konstantinides, S. Trends in Mortality Related to Pulmonary Embolism in the European Region, 2000–2015: Analysis of Vital Registration Data from the WHO Mortality Database. *Lancet Respir. Med.* **2020**, *8*, 277–287. [CrossRef]
2. Wendelboe, A.M.; Raskob, G.E. Global Burden of Thrombosis: Epidemiologic Aspects. *Circ. Res.* **2016**, *118*, 1340–1347. [CrossRef] [PubMed]
3. Hunt, B.J. Preventing Hospital Associated Venous Thromboembolism. *BMJ* **2019**, *365*, l4239. [CrossRef] [PubMed]
4. Gould, M.K.; Garcia, D.A.; Wren, S.M.; Karanicolas, P.J.; Arcelus, J.I.; Heit, J.A.; Samama, C.M. Prevention of VTE in Nonorthopedic Surgical Patients. Antithrombotic Therapy and Prevention of Thrombosis, 9th ed: American College of Chest Physicians Evidence-Based Clinical Practice Guidelines. *Chest* **2012**, *141* (Suppl. S2), e227S–e277S. [CrossRef] [PubMed]

1. Geerts, W.H.; Bergqvist, D.; Pineo, G.F.; Heit, J.A.; Samama, C.M.; Lassen, M.R.; Colwell, C.W. Prevention of Venous Thromboembolism: American College of Chest Physicians Evidence-Based Clinical Practice Guidelines (8th Edition). *Chest* **2008**, *133* (Suppl. S6), 381S–453S. [CrossRef]
2. Maynard, G. *Preventing Hospital-Acquired Venous Thromboembolism: A Guide for Effective Quality Improvement*, 2nd ed.; Agency for Healthcare Research and Quality: Rockville, MA, USA, 2016.
3. Expert Committee on the Special Fund for Thrombosis and Blood Vessels of China Health Promotion Foundation; Pulmonary Embolism and Pulmonary Vascular Diseases Group of Respiratory Disease Branch of Chinese Medical Association. Pulmonary embolism and Pulmonary Vascular Disease Working Committee of Chinese Association of Chest Physicians. Prophylaxis and Management of Venous Thromboembolism in Hospital. *Chin. Med. J.* **2018**, *98*, 1383–1388.
4. Pulmonary Embolism and Pulmonary Vascular Diseases Group of Chinese Thoracic Society; Pulmonary Embolism and Pulmonary Vascular Disease Working Committee of Chinese Association of Chest Physicians. National Collaborative group on Prevention and Treatment of Pulmonary Embolism and Pulmonary Vascular Disease. Guidelines for the Diagnosis, Treatment and Prevention of Pulmonary Thromboembolism. *Chin. Med. J.* **2018**, *98*, 1060–1087.
5. Cesarman-Maus, G.; Ruiz-Argüelles, G.J. News in the Indications of Direct Oral Anticoagulants According to the American College of Chest Physicians 2016 Guidelines. *Curr. Drug Metab.* **2017**, *18*, 651–656. [CrossRef]
6. Hill, J.; Treasure, T. Reducing the Risk of Venous Thromboembolism (Deep Vein Thrombosis and Pulmonary Embolism) in Patients Admitted to Hospital: Summary of the NICE Guideline. *Heart* **2010**, *96*, 879–882. [CrossRef]
7. Roberts, L.N.; Durkin, M.; Arya, R. Annotation: Developing a National Programme for VTE Prevention. *Br. J. Haematol.* **2017**, *178*, 162–170. [CrossRef]
8. Henke, P.K.; Kahn, S.R.; Pannucci, C.J.; Secemksy, E.A.; Evans, N.S.; Khorana, A.A.; Creager, M.A.; Pradhan, A.D.; On behalf of the American Heart Association Advocacy Coordinating Committee. Call to Action to Prevent Venous Thromboembolism in Hospitalized Patients: A Policy Statement From the American Heart Association. *Circulation* **2020**, *2010*, 297–298. [CrossRef] [PubMed]
9. Maynard, G.; Stein, J. *Preventing Hospital-Acquired Venous Thromboembolism: A Guide for Effective Quality Improvement*; AHRQ Publ. No. 08-0075; Society of Hospital Medicine: Philadelphia, PA, USA, 2008.
10. Blumgart A, Merriman E G, Jackson S; Singh, V. ; Royle, G. National Policy Framework: VTE Prevention in Adult Hospitalised Patients in NZ; Health Quality & Safety Commission: Wellington, New Zealand, 2012.
11. Zhang, Z.; Lei, J.; Shao, X.; Dong, F.; Wang, J.; Wang, D.; Wu, S.; Xie, W.; Wan, J.; Chen, H.; et al. Trends in Hospitalization and In-Hospital Mortality From VTE, 2007 to 2016, in China. *Chest* **2019**, *155*, 342–353. [CrossRef] [PubMed]
12. Zhai, Z.; Kan, Q.; Li, W.; Qin, X.; Qu, J.; Shi, Y.; Xu, R.; Xu, Y.; Zhang, Z.; Wang, C.; et al. VTE Risk Profiles and Prophylaxis in Medical and Surgical Inpatients: The Identification of Chinese Hospitalized Patients' Risk Profile for Venous Thromboembolism (DissolVE-2)—A Cross-Sectional Study. *Chest* **2019**, *155*, 114–122. [CrossRef] [PubMed]
13. Cohen, A.T.; Tapson, V.F.; Bergmann, J.-F.; Goldhaber, S.Z.; Kakkar, A.K.; Deslandes, B.; Huang, W.; Zayaruzny, M.; Emery, L.; A Anderson, F. Venous Thromboembolism Risk and Prophylaxis in the Acute Hospital Care Setting (ENDORSE Study): A Multinational Cross-Sectional Study. *Lancet* **2008**, *371*, 387–394. [CrossRef]
14. Mahadevaiah, G.; Rv, P.; Bermejo, I.; Jaffray, D.; Dekker, A.; Wee, L. Artificial Intelligence-Based Clinical Decision Support in Modern Medical Physics: Selection, Acceptance, Commissioning, and Quality Assurance. *Med. Phys.* **2020**, *47*, e228–e235. [CrossRef]
15. Dong, F.; Zhen, K.; Zhang, Z.; Si, C.; Xia, J.; Zhang, T.; Xia, L.; Wang, W.; Jia, C.; Shan, G.; et al. Effect on Thromboprophylaxis among Hospitalized Patients Using a System-Wide Multifaceted Quality Improvement Intervention: Rationale and Design for a Multicenter Cluster Randomized Clinical Trial in China. *Am. Heart J.* **2020**, *225*, 44–54. [CrossRef]
16. Depietri, L.; Marietta, M.; Scarlini, S.; Marcacci, M.; Corradini, E.; Pietrangelo, A.; Ventura, P. Clinical Impact of Application of Risk Assessment Models (Padua Prediction Score and Improve Bleeding Score) on Venous Thromboembolism, Major Hemorrhage and Health Expenditure Associated with Pharmacologic VTE Prophylaxis: A "Real Life" Prospective and Re. *Intern. Emerg. Med.* **2018**, *13*, 527–534. [CrossRef]
17. Kahn, S.R.; Morrison, D.R.; Diendéré, G.; Piché, A.; Filion, K.B.; Klil-Drori, A.J.; Douketis, J.D.; Emed, J.; Roussin, A.; Tagalakis, V.; et al. Interventions for Implementation of Thromboprophylaxis in Hospitalized Patients at Risk for Venous Thromboembolism. *Cochrane Database Syst. Rev.* **2018**, *2018*, CD008201. [CrossRef]
18. Kucher, N.; Tapson, V.F.; Goldhaber, S.Z. Risk Factors Associated with Symptomatic Pulmonary Embolism in a Large Cohort of Deep Vein Thrombosis Patients. *Thromb. Haemost.* **2005**, *93*, 494–498. [CrossRef]
19. Haut, E.R.; Lau, B.D.; Kraenzlin, F.S.; Hobson, D.B.; Kraus, P.S.; Carolan, H.T.; Haider, A.H.; Holzmueller, C.G.; Efron, D.T.; Pronovost, P.J.; et al. Improved Prophylaxis and Decreased Rates of Preventable Harm with the Use of a Mandatory Computerized Clinical Decision Support Tool for Prophylaxis for Venous Thromboembolism in Trauma. *Arch. Surg.* **2012**, *147*, 901–907. [CrossRef]
20. Turrentine, F.E.; Sohn, M.-W.; Wilson, S.L.; Stanley, C.; Novicoff, W.; Sawyer, R.G.; Williams, M.D. Fewer Thromboembolic Events after Implementation of a Venous Thromboembolism Risk Stratification Tool. *J. Surg. Res.* **2018**, *225*, 148–156. [CrossRef] [PubMed]

25. Cassidy, M.R.; Rosenkranz, P.; McAneny, D. Reducing Postoperative Venous Thromboembolism Complications with a Standardized Risk-Stratified Prophylaxis Protocol and Mobilization Program. *J. Am. Coll. Surg.* **2014**, *218*, 1095–1104. [CrossRef] [PubMed]
26. Spyropoulos, A.C.; Ageno, W.; Albers, G.W.; Elliott, C.G.; Halperin, J.L.; Hiatt, W.R.; Maynard, G.A.; Steg, P.G.; Weitz, J.I.; Suh, E.; et al. Rivaroxaban for Thromboprophylaxis after Hospitalization for Medical Illness. *N. Engl. J. Med.* **2018**, *379*, 1118–1127. [CrossRef] [PubMed]

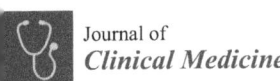 

Article

# Exploring the Complex Network of Heme-Triggered Effects on the Blood Coagulation System

Sarah Mubeen [1], Daniel Domingo-Fernández [1,2], Sara Díaz del Ser [1,3], Dhwani M. Solanki [4], Alpha T. Kodamullil [1,5], Martin Hofmann-Apitius [1], Marie-T. Hopp [4,*] and Diana Imhof [4,*]

1. Department of Bioinformatics, Fraunhofer Institute for Algorithms and Scientific Computing (SCAI), Schloss Birlinghoven, D-53757 Sankt Augustin, Germany
2. Enveda Biosciences, Inc., San Francisco, CA 94080, USA
3. Polytechnic University of Madrid, E-28040 Madrid, Spain
4. Pharmaceutical Biochemistry and Bioanalytics, Pharmaceutical Institute, University of Bonn, An der Immenburg 4, D-53121 Bonn, Germany
5. Causality Biomodels, Kinfra Hi-Tech Park, Kalamassery, Cochin 683503, Kerala, India
* Correspondence: mhopp@uni-bonn.de (M.-T.H.); dimhof@uni-bonn.de (D.I.); Tel.: +49-228-73-5231 (M.-T.H.); +49-228-73-5254 (D.I.)

**Abstract:** Excess labile heme, occurring under hemolytic conditions, displays a versatile modulator in the blood coagulation system. As such, heme provokes prothrombotic states, either by binding to plasma proteins or through interaction with participating cell types. However, despite several independent reports on these effects, apparently contradictory observations and significant knowledge gaps characterize this relationship, which hampers a complete understanding of heme-driven coagulopathies and the development of suitable and specific treatment options. Thus, the computational exploration of the complex network of heme-triggered effects in the blood coagulation system is presented herein. Combining hemostasis- and heme-specific terminology, the knowledge available thus far was curated and modeled in a mechanistic interactome. Further, these data were incorporated in the earlier established heme knowledge graph, "HemeKG", to better comprehend the knowledge surrounding heme biology. Finally, a pathway enrichment analysis of these data provided deep insights into so far unknown links and novel experimental targets within the blood coagulation cascade and platelet activation pathways for further investigation of the prothrombotic nature of heme. In summary, this study allows, for the first time, a detailed network analysis of the effects of heme in the blood coagulation system.

**Keywords:** blood coagulation cascade; data mining; heme; hemolysis; knowledge graph; platelet activation; thrombosis

## 1. Introduction

Hemolysis-associated thrombosis is a common complication observed in diseases, such as sickle cell disease (SCD) and paroxysmal nocturnal hemoglobinuria (PNH), or as a side effect of transfusions [1–3]. The cumulative incidence for thrombosis with ~11–27% in autoimmune hemolytic anemia, ~17% in SCD, and ~29–44% in PNH is as high as in inherited thrombophilias, such as protein C deficiency (~21%) [4–6]. Thereby, predominantly venous thrombotic events occur, encompassing deep vein thrombosis and pulmonary embolism, which can even lead to death in the most severe cases [4,6,7]. Among other disorder-specific factors, such as glycosylphosphatidylinositol anchor deficiency in PNH or vessel obstruction by sickle-shaped red blood cells in SCD, the major pathophysiological event underlying these hypercoagulopathies is intravascular hemolysis, which is characterized by an excessive, premature rupture of red blood cells that ultimately leads to a massive release and accumulation of hemoglobin and heme into the bloodstream [8,9]. Both are rapidly scavenged and cleared by the respective plasma proteins, involving haptoglobin,

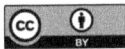

albumin, and hemopexin [10–14]. However, overwhelming of the heme-binding capacity of the plasma (~1.2–1.8 mM [15,16]) provokes the accumulation of labile heme. Labile heme, in turn, has been shown to be capable of binding and functionally affecting a wide range of plasma proteins, thereby causing most of the observed clinical outcomes in hemolytic disorders [9]. The underlying signaling pathways were recently contextualized in the Heme Knowledge Graph (HemeKG), which provided novel mechanistic insights at the molecular level [17]. Specifically, Toll-like receptor 4 (TLR4) signaling was identified as the main route for heme-driven proinflammatory action [17–19]. The exact mechanism of the pathway activation has not yet been unraveled; however, evidence for heme-mediated TLR4 activation has been associated with increased excretion of proinflammatory cytokines, elevated complement deposits on endothelial cells, and vasoocclusion [18,20,21]. Furthermore, the main driver of the complement system, component 3 (C3), binds, among other proteins, heme, which results in the deposition of activation fragments on endothelial cells and, thus, complement overactivation, as has been monitored in hemolytic diseases [21–25]. The versatile effects of heme as a modulator in the blood coagulation system have also been extensively described, -either as a matter of side effects during heme injection for the treatment of acute intermittent porphyria (AIP) or because of excessive heme release in hemolytic disorders, such as SCD and PNH [4,26,27]. Thus, initial efforts were made to investigate the molecular basis of the interference of heme in the coagulation system, identifying a few proteins that are affected by heme [26]. However, the currently available data are partially contradictory with respect to the pathophysiological outcome (bleeding vs. thrombosis) and exhibit conspicuous knowledge gaps with respect to the broad spectrum and complexity of the blood coagulation system with its primary (platelet adhesion, activation, and aggregation) and secondary (enzymatic clotting cascade) pathways.

The present study aimed at mapping and contextualizing the current knowledge on heme-driven thrombosis. We therefore established a novel knowledge graph, called "HemeThrombKG", focusing on heme-driven effects in the blood coagulation system. A pathway analysis, which includes information from three pathway databases, sheds light on important effector proteins that were not analyzed in the context of heme so far, revealing future targets for further exploration of the molecular basis of heme-driven thrombosis. Finally, the extension of the earlier established HemeKG by the novel heme-thrombosis knowledge graph provides a large network on heme-driven effects under hemolytic conditions, comprising a total of more than 800 nodes and 3000 relations, which is freely accessible and will enable researchers and physicians to independently explore the heme biology network for future study development.

## 2. Materials and Methods

### 2.1. Knowledge Modeling and Inclusion of the Knowledge Graph into HemeKG

An earlier published review article concerning the link between heme and thrombosis [26], which presented knowledge from over 200 articles, formed the basis for the present study. Therein, knowledge on (1) the side effects observed after heme injection, (2) the impact of heme intoxication on cells participating in blood coagulation, and (3) the effect of heme on proteins acting in blood coagulation is depicted in three supplementary tables [26]. This information was used to construct a knowledge graph, specifically focusing on the relations between heme and the development of coagulation disorders. As previously described [17], the detailed knowledge was extracted and manually coded into biological expression language (BEL; Figure 1), incorporating information about the experimental setting (e.g., dose of heme, type of injection, and cell type) as well as binding affinity data if applicable. While "heme", "hemin", and "hematin" were consistently curated as "heme", formulations of heme (e.g., heme arginate and heme-albumin formulations) were excluded, since these were established to prevent from heme-driven side effects in the treatment of porphyrias (heme deficiency diseases). The BEL statements were then used to generate a knowledge graph, designated as "HemeThrombKG" in the following, which models the different effects caused by heme in the context of thrombosis and/or bleeding and thus, was subjected to further analysis. Furthermore, we enriched the earlier established HemeKG with these coagulation-related data by merging the HemeKG with the novel HemeThrombKG (Figure 1).

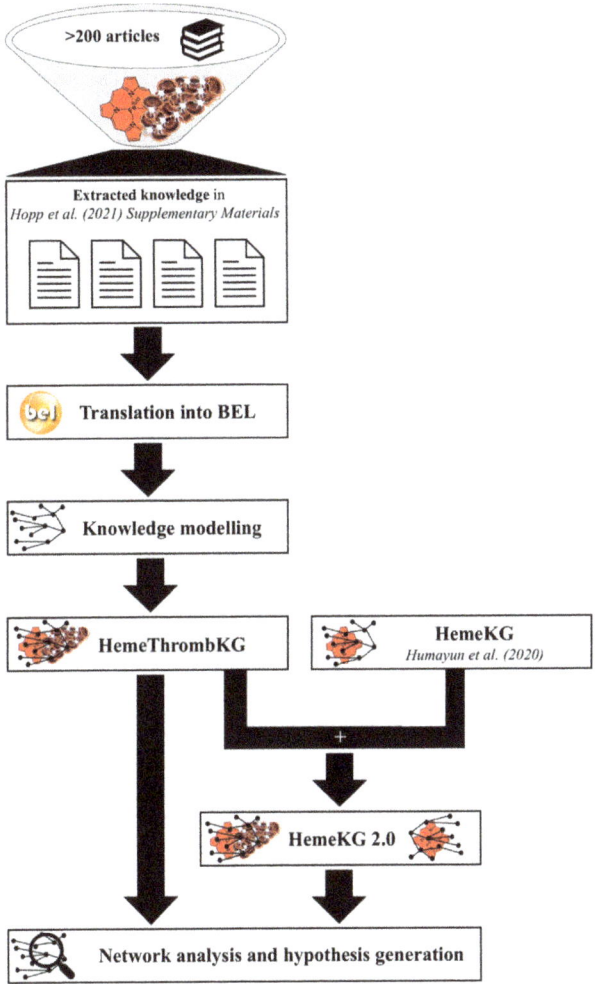

**Figure 1.** Workflow for the generation, progression, and analysis of HemeThrombKG. Using the knowledge comprehensively collected in a recent review article by the authors [26], the current information about heme's interference in the blood coagulation system was extracted and translated into BEL to generate the novel knowledge graph "HemeThrombKG". Furthermore, this new network of heme effects was included in the earlier established knowledge graph "HemeKG" [17], resulting in the expanded knowledge graph on heme biology "HemeKG 2.0". Both computational networks can be used for pathway and causality analysis, which can be applied for e.g., basic research on the effects of heme but also for the development of suitable drugs for the treatment of hemolysis-driven pathophysiology, such as thrombosis.

*2.2. Analysis of the Crosstalk of Heme with the Blood Coagulation System*

First, the relevant pathways for blood coagulation at the molecular level were selected and extracted from three pathway databases KEGG [28], Reactome [29], and WikiPathways [30], comprising the platelet activation pathway (KEGG, HSA04611), the extrinsic pathway of fibrin clot formation (Reactome, R-HSA-140834), the intrinsic pathway of fibrin clot formation (Reactome, R-HSA-140837), the common pathway of fibrin clot formation (Reactome, R-HSA-140875), the platelet aggregation/plug formation (Reactome, R-HSA-76009), and the blood clotting cascade (WikiPathways, WP272).

The data from these pathways were combined and explored by using the web application PathMe [31], resulting in a network with more than 400 edges (Figure S1). Subsequently, this network was used to enrich the generated HemeThrombKG by integrating this knowledge into the original knowledge graph, as described earlier [17,32]. The enrichment led to a network consisting of 848 nodes (including 246 proteins) and 3430 edges. Due to the size of the graph, the investigation of common components was split into the analysis of common extracellular plasma proteins and effects on the cellular level with respect to common membrane-associated and intracellular proteins. For that purpose, the list of 246 proteins was screened for their location (extracellular vs. intracellular and transmembrane proteins) using annotations available from QuickGO [33]. Subsequently, the extracellular and the intracellular/membrane-associated proteins from the database network were independently overlaid with the protein network extracted from HemeThrombKG. In total, 22 extracellular proteins, 10 transmembrane and membrane-associated proteins (incl. adhesion proteins, channels, and receptors), and 18 intracellular proteins were found in the HemeThrombKG, whereas the network extracted from the databases encompassed 54 extracellular proteins, 24 transmembrane and membrane-associated proteins, and 101 intracellular proteins. For clarity, the analysis of the extracellular pathway (i.e., the blood coagulation cascade) was split into the intrinsic, the extrinsic, and the common pathway, as provided by Reactome (R-HSA-140834, R-HSA-140837, and R-HSA-140875 [29]). In the case of membrane-associated proteins and intracellular proteins, a pathway-level analysis was performed by using HemeKG 2.0 in order to include a greater number of relevant proteins. Due to the highest overlap, the pathway-level analysis was performed by focusing on the platelet activation signaling pathways as provided by KEGG (HSA04611 [28]). Common nodes were highlighted, and the node size automatically arranged according to the abundance in the underlying BEL relations.

## 3. Results

*3.1. HemeThrombKG Illustrates the Knowledge about Heme's Interference in the Blood Coagulation System*

After the establishment of the first knowledge graph on heme biology ("HemeKG") in 2020 [17], in which data regarding heme-driven thrombosis were underrepresented, the herein introduced knowledge graph "HemeThrombKG" specifically focuses on the effects of heme on the blood coagulation system. HemeThrombKG is based on extracted and filtered knowledge from over 200 publications over the last 110 years, which was comprehensively combined in a recent review [26]. HemeThrombKG contains 151 nodes and 426 edges with 47 proteins involved (Figure 2A). In addition, contextual information, such as cell type and heme-binding kinetics, is deposited where applicable. In particular, lodging of the heme-binding affinity data will allow to rank the proteins for mechanistic analysis of heme-driven coagulation disorders in the future. Since administered heme for the treatment of AIP was reported to cause prothrombotic effects (e.g., thrombophlebitis), clinical symptoms that occur upon heme injection were incorporated in the network as well.

To further extend and network the knowledge contained in the earlier established HemeKG [17], the relations from HemeThrombKG were incorporated into HemeKG. In the following, the combined knowledge graph is designated as "HemeKG 2.0" and consists of 868 nodes (incl. 246 proteins) and 3430 edges (Figure 2B).

Finally, to allow researchers global access to the network, the BEL documents of the curated content have been made publicly available (https://github.com/HemeThrombKG/HemeThrombKG).

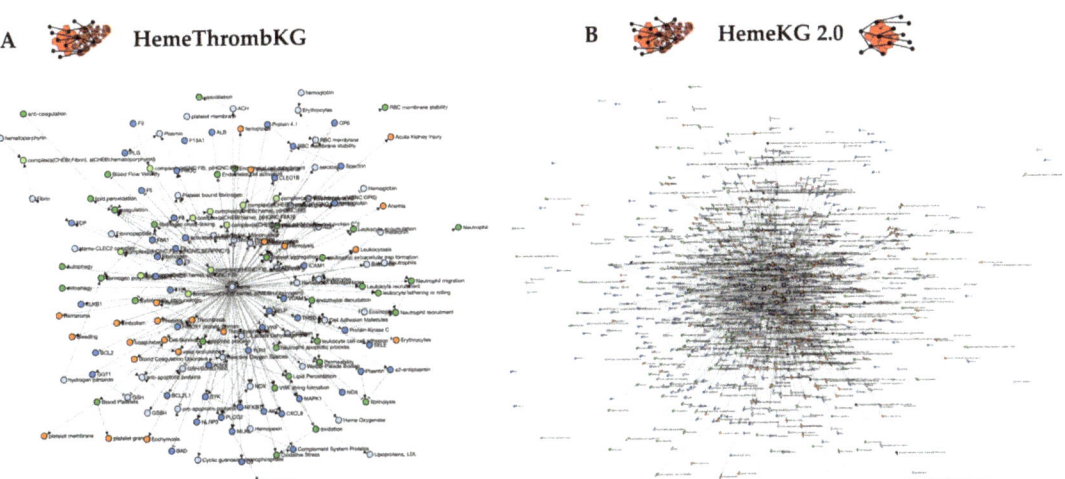

**Figure 2.** (**A**) The novel HemeThrombKG, consisting of 151 nodes and 426 edges, comprises the current knowledge of heme's interferences in the blood coagulation system. (**B**) HemeKG 2.0 displays the extended knowledge graph of the earlier established HemeKG [17] by inclusion of the relations of HemeThrombKG. The network combines 868 nodes and 3430 edges. Nodes are colored according to their different functions in BEL (blue: protein, orange: pathology, green: biological process, red: miRNA, light green: complex, black: reaction, light orange: gene, light blue: abundance, pink: RNA).

*3.2. HemeThrombKG and HemeKG 2.0 Enable the Detailed Analysis of Heme-Triggered Thrombosis at the Molecular Level*

As described earlier [17,34], a knowledge graph is highly conducive to study the crosstalk of the effects that are driven by heme under hemolytic conditions with pathways or pathophysiologies of interest. To explore the pathway crosstalk of heme with the underlying pathways of the blood coagulation system, HemeThrombKG was enriched with the relevant pathways from the three databases KEGG [28], Reactome [29], and WikiPathways [30], which showed the greatest overlap with the process of fibrin clot formation (blood coagulation cascade) with respect to plasma proteins and platelet activation signaling in the case of membrane-associated and intracellular proteins (Figures 3 and 4). Thus, the crosstalk analysis focused on these pathways, which is described in detail in the following subsections.

3.2.1. Crosstalk of Heme and the Plasma Proteins of the Blood Coagulation System

To study the crosstalk of heme-driven signaling with the blood coagulation cascade, the network of HemeThrombKG was separately superimposed with each of the three parts (i.e., intrinsic, extrinsic, and common pathway) of the cascade (Figure 3A–C). The blood coagulation cascade can be initiated by the activation of the coagulation factor XII (intrinsic pathway) on the one hand and cellular exposure of tissue factor to the bloodstream (extrinsic pathway) on the other hand. Both pathways culminate in the common pathway, which finally leads to the formation of a fibrin clot.

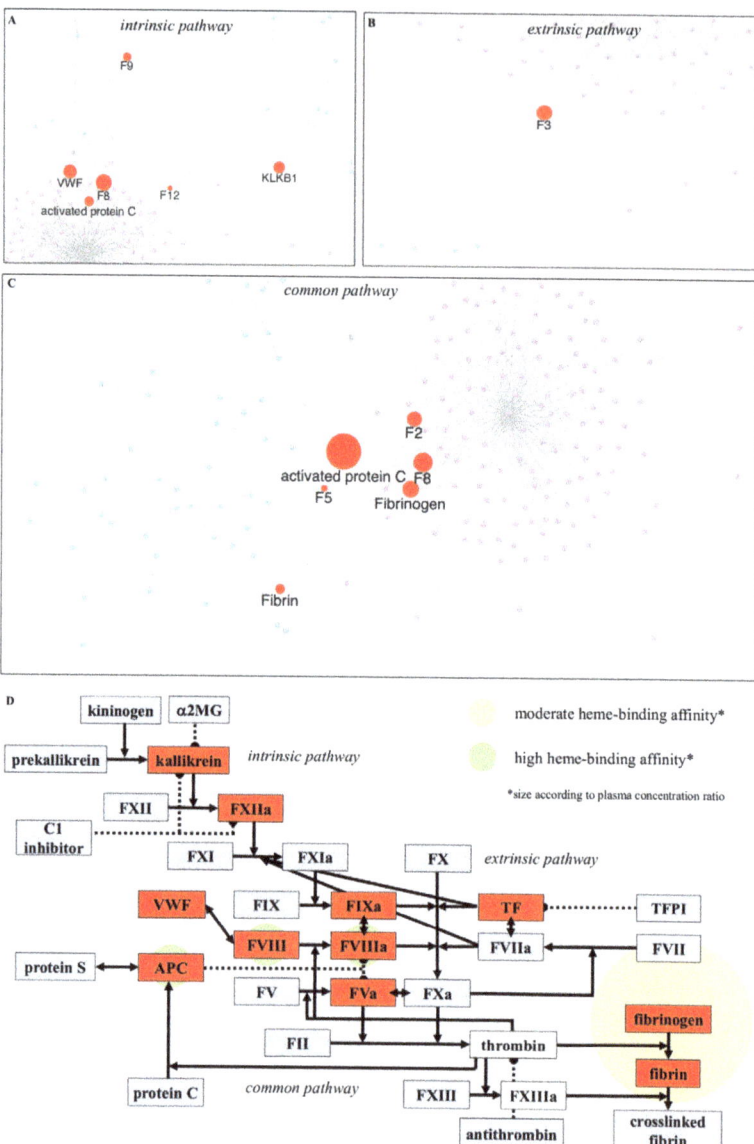

**Figure 3.** Crosstalk analysis of the blood coagulation cascade and HemeThrombKG. (**A**) The overlay of HemeThrombKG (light purple) and the intrinsic pathway (light blue) of the blood coagulation cascade (Reactome, R-HSA-140837) revealed plasma kallikrein, the coagulation factors VIII, IX, and XII, as well as APC and VWF as common nodes. (**B**) When superimposed with the extrinsic pathway (Reactome, R-HSA-140834; light blue), only TF appeared as a protein affected by heme. (**C**) In the common pathway (light blue), crosstalk analysis demonstrated thrombin, APC, coagulation factors V and VIII, as well as fibrinogen and fibrin as common proteins that are affected in the usual coagulation process as well as in heme-triggered thrombosis. (**D**) The superimposition of the complete blood coagulation cascade (Reactome, R-HSA-140877) with HemeThrombKG demonstrated that heme is capable of affecting the intrinsic, the extrinsic, and the common pathway of the cascade. Common effector proteins as found in the crosstalk analysis are highlighted (dark red). Recently, it was shown that the enzymatic function of thrombin and FXIIIa is not influenced by heme (white). Direct heme

binding was only demonstrated for APC, FVIII/FVIIIa, and fibrinogen (circles depict the relation of their plasma concentration and heme-binding affinity; see legend in the figure on the right). Further search for a correlation of the remaining participating proteins and heme in the literature did not reveal any further relations, which highlights these effector proteins as interesting future targets. F2: thrombin, F3: tissue factor, F5: coagulation factor Va, F8: coagulation factor VIII(a), F9: coagulation factor IXa, F12: coagulation factor XIIa, KLKB1: plasma kallikrein.

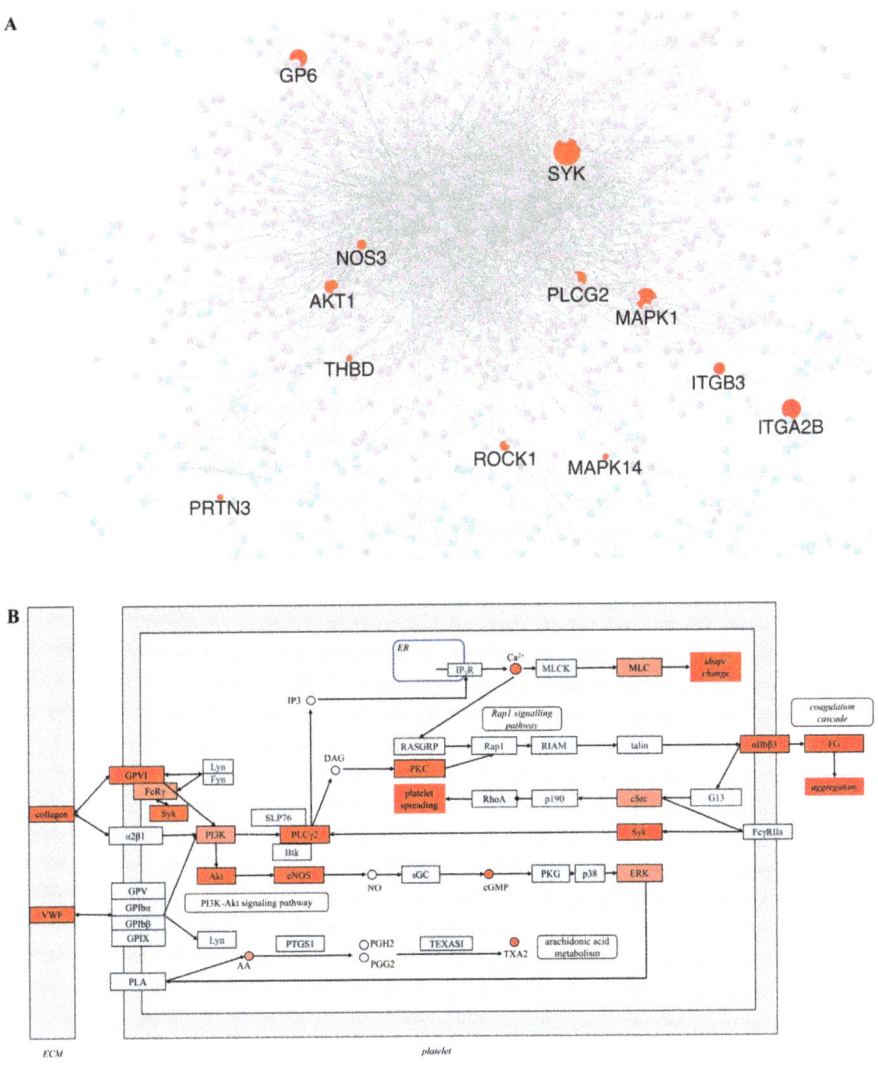

**Figure 4.** Heme-affected membrane-associated and intracellular proteins in clotting processes. (**A**) The overlay of HemeThrombKG (light purple nodes) and the clotting pathways extracted from databases (light blue nodes) reveals several membrane-associated (i.e., receptors and integrins) and intracellular proteins as common nodes (red). (**B**) HemeKG 2.0 shares distinct proteins with the platelet activation signaling pathways (HSA04611, KEGG [28]). The pathways with the highest level of overlap are depicted, with the common proteins highlighted in red. Relevant small molecules, i.e., IP3, DAG, PGH2, PGG2, TXA2, NO, and cGMP, $Ca^{2+}$ ions, as well as essential platelet activation

processes (e.g., spreading, aggregation) are included. Effector proteins that are not included in HemeKG 2.0 but reported in the context of heme signaling are marked in light red, whereas molecules that were not yet described in relation with heme are shown in light blue. AKT: AKT serine/threonine kinase, Btk: Bruton's tyrosine kinase, DAG: diacylglycerol, ECM: extracellular matrix, ER: endoplasmatic reticulum, ERK: extracellular-signal regulated kinase, FCγRIIa: FCγ receptor IIa, FcRγ: Fc receptor γ, FG: fibrinogen, GPV/Ibα/Ibβ/IX: glycoproteins V/Ibα/Ibβ/IX, GP6/GPVI: platelet glycoprotein VI, IP3: inositol trisphosphate, IP3R: inositol trisphosphate receptor, ITGA2B + ITGB3: integrin αIIbβ3, MAPK: mitogen-activated protein kinase, MLC: myosin light chain, MLCK: myosin light chain kinase, NOS: nitric oxide synthase, PI3K: phosphoinositide 3 kinase, PIP2: phosphatidylinositol-4,5-bisphosphate, PKC: protein kinase C, PKG: cGMP-dependent protein kinase or protein kinase G, PLA: phospholipase A, PLCG2/PLCγ2: phospholipase C γ2, PRTN3: proteinase 3, PTGS1: cyclooxygenase 1, RASGRP: RAS guanyl releasing protein 1, RhoA: Ras homolog family member A, RIAM: amyloid beta precursor protein binding family B member 1 interacting protein, ROCK1: Rho kinase 1, sGC: soluble guanylate cyclase, SLP76: SH2 domain-containing leukocyte protein of 76 kDa; SYK: spleen-associated tyrosine kinase, TEXAS1: thromboxane A synthase, VWF: von Willebrand factor.

Superimposition of the HemeThrombKG network and the intrinsic pathway (Reactome, R-HSA-140837) revealed the coagulation factors VIII, IX, and XII, the coagulation inhibitor activated protein C (APC), the adhesive protein von Willebrand factor (VWF), and plasma kallikrein as common nodes, which were described in the past to bind and/or to be affected by heme in vitro and partially in vivo [20,35–39] (Figure 3A).

One of the initial intrinsic pathway serine proteases, plasma kallikrein is activated in the presence of heme (up to 24 nmol), leading to the procoagulant induction of the intrinsic pathway in plasma samples [35]. In the same context, heme-triggered autoactivation of FXII has been suggested [35]. However, upon retroorbital injection (up to 35 μmol/kg) into mice, immunoblockage of FXII did not reduce the heme-triggered coagulation activation, which is why a role of the proposed FXII-heme interaction in vivo appears questionable [40].

Apart from potential procoagulant effects on these proteins of the intrinsic pathway, high-affinity heme binding [$K_D$ ~1.9 nM (FVIII) and $K_D$ ~12.7 nM (FVIIIa)] to FVIII(a) abolishes its interaction with FIX, which ultimately leads to the inhibition of the clotting process in vitro [37]. In contrast, persistent FVIII-VWF complex formation and increased binding of this complex to human platelets in the presence of heme directs again towards procoagulant signaling [38]. VWF itself has been found to show higher expression levels, string formation, and secretion from Weibel–Palade bodies upon incubation of endothelial cells with heme (up to 100 μM; in vitro) and/or heme injection (3.2 μmol/kg) into mice (in vivo) [20,23]. In vitro, VWF was also capable of the protection of FVIII(a) from its heme-driven inhibition [37]. Furthermore, heme upregulates proteases (e.g., MMP9), which regulate VWF digestion, as has been observed in plasma from SCD patients and with heme (up to 60 μM) incubated endothelial cells [39]. In line with these procoagulant effects on FVIII and VWF, the function of the natural inactivator of FVIIIa, APC, is completely abrogated upon direct heme binding ($K_D$ ~400 nM) to the serine protease in vitro (up to 100 μM heme), tending towards prothrombotic consequences of heme excess as well [36].

The superimposition of HemeThrombKG with the extrinsic clotting pathway (Reactome, R-HSA-140834) revealed tissue factor (TF) as a common component and, thus, as the only so far known heme-affected factor in the extrinsic pathway (Figure 3B). Thereby, heme initiates the extrinsic pathway by induction of TF expression and thus provision of an increased level of functionally active TF [40–42]. This was observed in different cell types (i.e., endothelial cells and leukocytes; up to 100 μM heme), ex vivo in blood (30 μM heme), as well as upon intravenous (100 μmol/kg) or (35 μmol/kg) retroorbital injection in mice (in vivo) [40–43]. Subsequent steps on the molecular level that are explicitly induced by heme-driven TF upregulation were so far not analyzed.

Regarding the common pathway (Reactome, R-HSA-140875), the two networks share the following proteins: APC, FV, thrombin, fibrin, and fibrinogen (Figure 3C). The inhibitory effect of heme on APC has been described above. Whether heme prevents APC-mediated inactivation of the two cofactors, FV and FVIII, from both the intrinsic and the common pathway, has not yet been explored. In contrast, it is already known that heme can abolish the prothrombinase ([FXa + FVa])-catalyzed reaction, which was attributed to direct inhibition of the involved cofactor FVa in vivo (4 mg/kg heme injection in an AIP patient) [44]. The central enzyme of the common pathway, i.e., thrombin, has been suggested to be affected by strong heme binding in vitro as well, but the earlier reported decrease in its amidolytic activity in the presence of heme could not be reproduced in a recent study [36,45]. Although FXIIIa, the fibrin stabilizing factor, has been disproven as a heme-regulated protein [36], it is well known that fibrinogen itself binds heme in vitro, which results in fibrinogen binding to platelets as well as crosslinking and polymer formation in plasma and/or blood samples (up to 500 µM heme applied), ultimately leading to clot formation [46–48].

As such, direct heme binding has only been described for FVIII(a), fibrinogen, and APC so far, all possessing heme-binding affinities in the nano- to micromolar range (Figure 3D) [36,37,48]. In addition, several components of the blood coagulation cascade, which are present in the three databases, were not found in the herein established HemeThrombKG, e.g., FX(a), FX(a), and several coagulation inhibitors. Therefore, a specific screening for literature reports of these proteins in the context of heme signaling was conducted by entering the respective queries in PubMed, as this knowledge might not be covered in HemeThrombKG. However, no further relations were identified, proving the quality of the new knowledge graph and revealing novel targets for studying the effect of heme on the blood coagulation cascade (Figure 3D).

### 3.2.2. Crosstalk of Heme within the Pathways of Platelet Activation

The crosstalk of heme with intracellular signaling pathways of the blood coagulation system was analyzed by superimposition of HemeKG 2.0 with the membrane-associated and intracellular proteins involved in the selected pathways from the databases KEGG [28], Reactome [29], and WikiPathways [30], revealing two receptors (Glycoprotein VI and thrombomodulin), one integrin ($\alpha$IIb$\beta$3), and eight intracellular proteins as common nodes (Figure 4A). The greatest overlap occurred between the HemeKG 2.0 network and a part of the platelet activation signaling pathways as extracted from KEGG (HSA04611, [28]; Figure 4B).

Initiation of platelet adhesion and activation is mediated either by adhesion proteins of the extracellular matrix (e.g., collagen and VWF) through interaction with integrins, glycoproteins on the platelet surface and/or by stimulation of receptors through agonists (e.g., ADP and thromboxane A2) [49–51]. As a result of intracellular signaling, the cytosolic level of $Ca^{2+}$ ions increases and finally induces the change in platelet shape, secretion of granule content, and activation of the integrin $\alpha$IIb$\beta$3, which enables "communication" with plasma proteins, such as fibrinogen [51]. This, in turn, potentiates platelet adhesion, activation, aggregation, and spreading with the result of clot formation and retraction [51].

Superimposition of the HemeKG 2.0 network and the underlying pathways of these platelet activation mechanisms revealed that the two proteins of the extracellular matrix, collagen and VWF, as well as the glycoprotein VI, the integrin, $\alpha$IIb$\beta$3 and the intracellular proteins spleen-associated tyrosine kinase (Syk), AKT serine/threonine kinase (Akt), nitric oxide synthase (NOS), phospholipase C $\gamma$2 (PLC$\gamma$2), and protein kinase C (PKC) were common (Figure 4B). In contrast, several other effector proteins, which were found in the respective pathways in the KEGG database (part of HSA04611; [28]), were not found in HemeKG 2.0 (e.g., glycoprotein V, cGMP-dependent protein kinase or protein kinase G, or the extracellular-signal regulated kinase (ERK); Figure 4B). Thus, specific literature screening for reports of these effector proteins in the context of heme signaling was performed in the same way as described for the plasma proteins above (see Section 3.2.1).

As a result, Fc receptor $\gamma$ (FcR$\gamma$), phosphoinositide 3 kinase (PI3K), myosin, cSrc, and ERK were additionally found and highlighted in the network as well (Figure 4B; Table S1).

In the initial phase of heme-induced platelet activation, collagen and VWF seem to play a crucial role (Figure 4B). As already described herein (Section 3.2.1), heme excess (up to 100 µM tested) causes elevated VWF expression and string formation in vitro and in vivo, which might coordinate platelet adhesion to the vessel wall [20,23]. In an ex vivo model (mouse aorta), heme (1 mM)-triggered endothelial collagen expression was associated with increased platelet aggregation [52]. Until now, however, only the relevance of these proteins for platelet adhesion to the extracellular matrix and platelet aggregation caused by heme-driven upregulation of their expression has been described. Our analysis revealed that there is an indication for their contribution to heme-triggered platelet activation pathways as well (Figure 4B). In case of the pathway that follows platelet adhesion to collagen, its counterpart protein, GPVI, has been already described to bind heme with a rather low affinity ($K_D$ ~29.4 µM), which induces platelet aggregation upon heme exposure in vitro (up to ~115 µM) [53]. The participation of FcRγ, which is intracellularly associated with GPVI, has also been suggested to participate in this process [54]. Usually, GPVI crosslinking or platelet adhesion to collagen induces phosphorylation of FcRγ, leading to recruitment and activation of intracellular signaling proteins, such as Syk, PI3K, and PLCγ2 [50,53]. Since heme seems to be capable of inducing platelet activation by targeting both collagen and GPVI, this might account for a direct and indirect activation of this pathway (Figure 4B) and, thus, an amplification of the observed effects. Syk and PLCγ2 phosphorylation in platelets was associated with heme (up to 50–115 µM) exposure as well [53,55]. This has been attributed to GPVI and C-type lectin-like receptor 2 (CLEC2) activation by heme [53,55]. CLEC2 itself is found in HemeThrombKG in relation to heme as well but did not occur as a common node in the crosstalk analysis since it is not yet curated into the database platelet activation signaling pathways.

In contrast to Syk and PLCγ2, the intermediary effector protein PI3K did neither occur in HemeThrombKG nor in HemeKG 2.0, because it has not yet been found in the context of heme and coagulation processes. Literature screening revealed that PI3K was identified as a mediator of heme-induced PLC phosphorylation in neutrophils (up to 30 µM heme tested) [56], which may apply for heme-driven intracellular platelet signaling as well. Activated PLCγ2 usually catalyzes phosphatidylinositol-4,5-bisphosphate ($PIP_2$) hydrolysis to inositol trisphosphate ($IP_3$) and diacylglycerol (DAG), leading to calcium mobilization and protein kinase C (PKC) activation [51]. A heme-induced increase in IP3 and DAG levels has not yet been described; however, elevated intracellular calcium levels and mobilization in platelets as well as PKC activation in neutrophils has already been monitored (in the presence of up to 20 µM heme) [46,57,58]. In general, calcium mobilization enables contractile activity through myosin, which leads to the characteristic shape change of activated platelets [50]. The calcium–myosin axis has not been highlighted in the context of heme signaling, but heme-induced oxidation of myosin in human skeletal muscle fiber segments and platelet shape change has been shown in vitro (up to 300 µM heme applied) [46,59]. Several of the other involved effector proteins (e.g., $IP_3$ receptor, myosin light chain kinase, and RAS guanyl releasing protein 1) were not recognized and/or reported in the context of heme signaling (Figure 4B) and, thus, display suitable targets for future investigation of the underlying pathways of heme-triggered platelet activation.

Under conditions of heme excess, platelet aggregation through fibrinogen binding to platelets was observed (~11 µM heme applied) [46], proposing a heme-induced αIIbβ3-fibrinogen "communication", since both components evolved in our crosstalk analysis as common nodes (Figure 4B). Furthermore, this integrin is capable of intracellular signaling induction. This, in turn, promotes platelet spreading, which also occurred as a node in HemeThrombKG. From the involved effector proteins, only the tyrosine kinase Src was already described to be activated by heme, but only in epithelial cells so far and not in platelets [60]. Src, in turn, can phosphorylate the FCγ receptor IIa (FCγRIIa) and induce Syk signaling (Figure 4B) [51]. This indicates that this pathway may be affected by heme as well, although FCγRIIa has not yet been reported in the context of heme signaling.

Apart from PLC activation (see above), PI3K can catalyze Akt phosphorylation, explaining its activation in platelets upon incubation with heme (2.5 µM) [57]. Heme-triggered platelet activation along with Akt phosphorylation was demonstrated to be dependent on TLR4 [57]. Although the TLR4 signaling pathway is highly pronounced in the HemeThrombKG network, it did not emerge during crosstalk analysis, since it is not yet recognized for its contribution to procoagulant processes in the databases. This pathway has been previously highlighted in the context of heme-driven inflammation and suitable future targets from this signaling were already pointed out [17].

Akt phosphorylation can further lead to eNOS activation in platelets, a hemoprotein, whose production has been reported to be influenced by heme [61,62]. Many of the subsequent effector proteins of this pathway have not yet been described in relation to heme signaling, but ERK has been found to contribute to heme signaling in other cell types (e.g., neutrophils) (Table S1) [43,57,63]. Furthermore, an interrelation of heme with the messenger molecules cyclic guanosine monophosphate (cGMP; in vivo), arachidonic acid, and thromboxane A2 (in vitro) in platelets has already been reported [46,64–66], suggesting the induction and progression of the respective pathways in the presence of heme.

In contrast to the collagen/GPVI-mediated platelet activation signaling, the pathway induced by platelet adhesion to VWF is largely unexplored as a potential route for heme signaling. None of the proteins of the GPIb-IX-V complex were mentioned in context with heme-mediated platelet activation. However, the pathway shares several effector proteins with the collagen/GPVI-initiated signaling, which could be activated by heme as part of the VWF-associated signaling pathway as well.

## 4. Discussion

The high prevalence of thrombosis in hemolytic disorders and the associated harmful complications emphasize the importance of the in-depth investigation of the molecular basis of heme-driven prothrombotic effects.

Thus, a mechanistic model of heme signaling in the context of blood coagulation is presented herein. "HemeThrombKG" represents the contextualization of the current knowledge about the interference of heme in the blood coagulation system. Furthermore, the analysis of the complex interrelations by enrichment and superimposition with information available from databases provides novel insights into underlying pathways with a focus on the enzymatic coagulation cascade and platelet activation signaling. In addition, crucial knowledge gaps were identified and highlighted that need to be targeted in future research.

In the past, several components of the blood coagulation cascade were reported to be affected by heme with contradictory outcome (anticoagulant (e.g., FV and FVIII) vs. procoagulant (e.g., APC and fibrinogen) signaling) but to date only three proteins (i.e., APC, fibrinogen, and FVIII(a)) out of this complex network were shown to bind heme in vitro. The heme-binding affinities along with the plasma levels of the coagulation factors (Figure 3D) could enable a temporal and heme concentration-dependent ranking of the processes in the blood coagulation system. The highest heme-binding affinity of the so far known heme-binding coagulation proteins exhibit FVIII (12.7 nM)/FVIIIa (1.9 nM) and APC (~400 nM), whereas fibrinogen possesses a moderate heme-binding affinity (~3.3 µM) [36,37,47]. However, while FVIII/FVIIIa and APC occur only in very low amounts in the plasma (subnano- to nanomolar range), fibrinogen is the clotting factor with the highest plasma concentration (micromolar range). Thus, it is highly probable that fibrinogen will be in the first line affected by heme, whereas APC and FVIII might only be regulated under conditions of heme excess. Still, several participating proteins have not yet been analyzed for these heme-binding characteristics, which were outlined in this study (e.g., FX, FXI, and various coagulation inhibitors). These should be analyzed for their potential heme-binding capacity in the future to enable a complete understanding of the temporal and spatial hierarchy of heme-triggered effects in the blood coagulation cascade and, thus, evaluation of the progression of hemolysis-driven thrombotic complications.

Beyond the effects on the coagulation cascade, heme has been associated with cellular events, including platelet adhesion, activation, and aggregation [46,53,55,57,67]. However, the underlying intracellular signaling pathways and, in particular, the interrelations of the already described effector proteins, are largely unexplored. To enable a more comprehensive analysis of potential intracellular signaling pathways, HemeKG 2.0, a combination of the previous (HemeKG [17]) and the novel (HemeThrombKG) heme knowledge graph, were used for the analysis of cellular signaling pathways. Thereby, the platelet activation signaling pathways were highly pronounced, emphasizing the importance of the collagen/GPVI signaling route for heme-driven platelet activation. As pointed out in this study, several effector proteins of this signaling pathway (e.g., Btk, SLP76, $IP_3R$, MLCK, RASGRP, and Rap1) have not yet been described in the context of heme biology and should thus be experimentally investigated as potential heme-induced signaling proteins. The same applies for the VWF/GPIb-XI-V signaling route, where only VWF and messenger molecules were reported to be influenced under conditions of heme excess. However, it should be noted that a few of the herein included effector proteins (e.g., PLC$\gamma$2) have not yet been reported to be activated and/or induced by heme in platelets but only in other cell types, such as endothelial cells and leukocytes, which thus requires future experimental investigation in platelets. Beside the different cell types, the different heme concentrations that were used for the studies impede a direct comparison of the results. Furthermore, our analysis emphasizes the need for suitable and comparable in vivo studies that support the in vitro results and observations.

Beyond the herein described components of the blood coagulation system, other proteins occurred in the HemeThrombKG network that participate in the prothrombotic reactions, including receptors (TLR4, CLEC2 and thrombomodulin), adhesion proteins (selectin E, selectin P, ICAM1, and VCAM1), and several intracellular proteins (e.g., MAPK1, NLRP3, GGT1, and actin). Future analysis should include these proteins to generate a more complete picture of the procoagulant effects of heme.

The high complexity of the actions of heme as a modulator in the blood coagulation system is further evident by indirectly triggered prothrombotic mechanisms, such as LDL oxidation by heme or heme-released iron followed by endothelial cell damage [68]. These links were not analyzed in the present study but are already (at least partially) included in HemeKG 2.0 and are, thus, also available for further exploration.

Finally, HemeThrombKG as well as the combined HemeKG 2.0 were curated with standard vocabularies (e.g., from ChEBI [69] and MeSH [70]) using BEL, which makes it linkable to public databases. The networks and analyses performed on these networks have been made available at https://github.com/HemeThrombKG/HemeThrombKG, to allow the public to interactively explore the knowledge graphs and gain additional mechanistic insights [71]. Thus, researchers can easily inspect further relations and dependencies in the herein provided networks on their own. As such, the networks can be used to predict suitable drugs and their response in hemolytic disorders (e.g., SCD and PNH) in the future, supporting the selection of suitable drug candidates for the targeted treatment of hemolysis-associated thrombosis.

## 5. Conclusions

In conclusion, this study emphasizes the importance and relevance of the blood coagulation cascade and platelet activation signaling pathways for the reported prothrombotic effects of heme as occurring in hemolytic disorders. Furthermore, several effector proteins are highlighted for future studies, which will allow for a more detailed characterization of the pathophysiological outcome on the molecular level and, thus, establishment of novel perspectives for targeted treatment options of prothrombotic complications in patients with hemolytic disorders.

**Supplementary Materials:** The following supporting information can be downloaded at: https://www.mdpi.com/article/10.3390/jcm11195975/s1, Figure S1: Overview of the extracted knowledge from the common pathway databases; Table S1: Evidence for heme relations in the platelet activation signaling pathways from additional literature screening.

**Author Contributions:** Conceptualization, D.I. and M.-T.H.; methodology, S.M., S.D.d.S. and D.D.-F.; validation, D.D.-F., D.M.S. and M.-T.H.; resources, M.H.-A.; data curation, S.M., S.D.d.S., D.M.S. and M.-T.H.; writing—original draft preparation, S.M. and M.-T.H.; writing—review and editing, all authors; visualization, S.M. and M.-T.H.; supervision, D.D.-F., A.T.K., M.-T.H. and D.I. All authors have read and agreed to the published version of the manuscript.

**Funding:** This work was funded by the Deutsche Forschungsgemeinschaft (DFG, German Research Foundation) under the project number: 507218303 (to M.-T.H.) and the STEP4 program of the University of Bonn (to D.I.).

**Institutional Review Board Statement:** Not applicable.

**Informed Consent Statement:** Not applicable.

**Data Availability Statement:** The herein established knowledge graph (HemeThrombKG) and its inclusion into HemeKG (HemeKG 2.0) are publicly accessible at https://github.com/HemeThrombKG/HemeThrombKG.

**Acknowledgments:** Financial support by the University of Bonn (to M.-T.H. and D.I.) is acknowledged.

**Conflicts of Interest:** D.D.-F. received salary from Enveda Biosciences and the company has no competing interests with the published results. The rest of the authors declare that they have no conflict of interest.

# References

1. Shet, A.S.; Lizarralde-Iragorri, M.A.; Naik, R.P. The Molecular Basis for the Prothrombotic State in Sickle Cell Disease. *Haematologica* **2020**, *105*, 2368–2379. [CrossRef] [PubMed]
2. van Bijnen, S.T.A.; van Heerde, W.L.; Muus, P. Mechanisms and Clinical Implications of Thrombosis in Paroxysmal Nocturnal Hemoglobinuria. *J. Thromb. Haemost.* **2012**, *10*, 1–10. [CrossRef] [PubMed]
3. Panch, S.R.; Montemayor-Garcia, C.; Klein, H.G. Hemolytic Transfusion Reactions. *New Engl. J. Med.* **2019**, *381*, 150–162. [CrossRef] [PubMed]
4. Delvasto-Nuñez, L.; Jongerius, I.; Zeerleder, S. It Takes Two to Thrombosis: Hemolysis and Complement. *Blood Rev.* **2021**, *50*, 100834. [CrossRef]
5. Srisuwananukorn, A.; Raslan, R.; Zhang, X.; Shah, B.N.; Han, J.; Gowhari, M.; Molokie, R.E.; Gordeuk, V.R.; Saraf, S.L. Clinical, Laboratory, and Genetic Risk Factors for Thrombosis in Sickle Cell Disease. *Blood Adv.* **2020**, *4*, 1978–1986. [CrossRef]
6. Naik, R.P.; Streiff, M.B.; Haywood, C.; Nelson, J.A.; Lanzkron, S. Venous Thromboembolism in Adults with Sickle Cell Disease: A Serious and under-Recognized Complication. *Am. J. Med.* **2013**, *126*, 443–449. [CrossRef]
7. Nouraie, M.; Lee, J.S.; Zhang, Y.; Kanias, T.; Zhao, X.; Xiong, Z.; Oriss, T.B.; Zeng, Q.; Kato, G.J.; Gibbs, J.S.R.; et al. The Relationship between the Severity of Hemolysis, Clinical Manifestations and Risk of Death in 415 Patients with Sickle Cell Anemia in the US and Europe. *Haematologica* **2013**, *98*, 464–472. [CrossRef]
8. Roumenina, L.T.; Rayes, J.; Lacroix-Desmazes, S.; Dimitrov, J.D. Heme: Modulator of Plasma Systems in Hemolytic Diseases. *Trends Mol. Med.* **2016**, *22*, 200–213. [CrossRef]
9. Rother, R.P.; Bell, L.; Hillmen, P.; Gladwin, M.T. The Clinical Sequelae of Intravascular Hemolysis and Extracellular Plasma Hemoglobin. *J. Am. Med Assoc.* **2005**, *293*, 1653. [CrossRef]
10. Samuel, P.P.; White, M.A.; Ou, W.C.; Case, D.A.; Phillips, G.N.; Olson, J.S. The Interplay between Molten Globules and Heme Disassociation Defines Human Hemoglobin Disassembly. *Biophys. J.* **2020**, *118*, 1381–1400. [CrossRef]
11. Andersen, C.B.F.; Stødkilde, K.; Sæderup, K.L.; Kuhlee, A.; Raunser, S.; Graversen, J.H.; Moestrup, S.K. Haptoglobin. *Antioxid. Redox Signal.* **2017**, *26*, 814–831. [CrossRef] [PubMed]
12. Alayash, A.I.; Andersen, C.B.F.; Moestrup, S.K.; Bülow, L. Haptoglobin: The Hemoglobin Detoxifier in Plasma. *Trends Biotechnol.* **2013**, *31*, 2–3. [CrossRef]
13. Kumar, S.; Bandyopadhyay, U. Free Heme Toxicity and Its Detoxification Systems in Human. *Toxicol. Lett.* **2005**, *157*, 175–188. [CrossRef] [PubMed]
14. Soares, M.P.; Bozza, M.T. Red Alert: Labile Heme Is an Alarmin. *Curr. Opin. Immunol.* **2016**, *38*, 94–100. [CrossRef]
15. Noé, R.; Bozinovic, N.; Lecerf, M.; Lacroix-Desmazes, S.; Dimitrov, J.D. Use of Cysteine as a Spectroscopic Probe for Determination of Heme-Scavenging Capacity of Serum Proteins and Whole Human Serum. *J. Pharm. Biomed. Anal.* **2019**, *172*, 311–319. [CrossRef] [PubMed]

16. Pires, I.S.; Govender, K.; Munoz, C.J.; Williams, A.T.; O'Boyle, Q.T.; Savla, C.; Cabrales, P.; Palmer, A.F. Purification and Analysis of a Protein Cocktail Capable of Scavenging Cell-free Hemoglobin, Heme, and Iron. *Transfusion* **2021**, *61*, 1894–1907. [CrossRef] [PubMed]
17. Humayun, F.; Domingo-Fernández, D.; Paul George, A.A.; Hopp, M.-T.; Syllwasschy, B.F.; Detzel, M.S.; Hoyt, C.T.; Hofmann-Apitius, M.; Imhof, D. A Computational Approach for Mapping Heme Biology in the Context of Hemolytic Disorders. *Front. Bioeng. Biotechnol.* **2020**, *8*, 74. [CrossRef]
18. Figueiredo, R.T.; Fernandez, P.L.; Mourao-Sa, D.S.; Porto, B.N.; Dutra, F.F.; Alves, L.S.; Oliveira, M.F.; Oliveira, P.L.; Graça-Souza, A.V.; Bozza, M.T. Characterization of Heme as Activator of Toll-like Receptor 4. *J. Biol. Chem.* **2007**, *282*, 20221–20229. [CrossRef]
19. Janciauskiene, S.; Vijayan, V.; Immenschuh, S. TLR4 Signaling by Heme and the Role of Heme-Binding Blood Proteins. *Front. Immunol.* **2020**, *11*, 1964. [CrossRef]
20. Belcher, J.D.; Chen, C.; Nguyen, J.; Milbauer, L.; Abdulla, F.; Alayash, A.I.; Smith, A.; Nath, K.A.; Hebbel, R.P.; Vercellotti, G.M.; et al. Heme Triggers TLR4 Signaling Leading to Endothelial Cell Activation and Vaso-Occlusion in Murine Sickle Cell Disease. *Blood* **2014**, *123*, 377–390. [CrossRef]
21. Merle, N.S.; Paule, R.; Leon, J.; Daugan, M.; Robe-Rybkine, T.; Poillerat, V.; Torset, C.; Frémeaux-Bacchi, V.; Dimitrov, J.D.; Roumenina, L.T. P-Selectin Drives Complement Attack on Endothelium during Intravascular Hemolysis in TLR-4/Heme-dependent Manner. *Proc. Natl. Acad. Sci. USA* **2019**, *116*, 6280–6285. [CrossRef] [PubMed]
22. Roumenina, L.T.; Chadebech, P.; Bodivit, G.; Vieira-Martins, P.; Grunenwald, A.; Boudhabhay, I.; Poillerat, V.; Pakdaman, S.; Kiger, L.; Jouard, A.; et al. Complement Activation in Sickle Cell Disease: Dependence on Cell Density, Hemolysis and Modulation by Hydroxyurea Therapy. *Am. J. Hematol.* **2020**, *95*, 456–464. [CrossRef] [PubMed]
23. Frimat, M.; Tabarin, F.; Dimitrov, J.D.; Poitou, C.; Halbwachs-Mecarelli, L.; Fremeaux-Bacchi, V.; Roumenina, L.T. Complement Activation by Heme as a Secondary Hit for Atypical Hemolytic Uremic Syndrome. *Blood* **2013**, *122*, 282–292. [CrossRef]
24. Pawluczkowycz, A.W.; Lindorfer, M.A.; Waitumbi, J.N.; Taylor, R.P. Hematin Promotes Complement Alternative Pathway-Mediated Deposition of C3 Activation Fragments on Human Erythrocytes: Potential Implications for the Pathogenesis of Anemia in Malaria. *J. Immunol.* **2007**, *179*, 5543–5552. [CrossRef] [PubMed]
25. Frimat, M.; Boudhabhay, I.; Roumenina, L.T. Hemolysis Derived Products Toxicity and Endothelium: Model of the Second Hit. *Toxins* **2019**, *11*, 660. [CrossRef]
26. Hopp, M.-T.; Imhof, D. Linking Labile Heme with Thrombosis. *J. Clin. Med.* **2021**, *10*, 427. [CrossRef]
27. Conran, N.; De Paula, E.V. Thromboinflammatory Mechanisms in Sickle Cell Disease—Challenging the Hemostatic Balance. *Haematologica* **2020**, *105*, 2380. [CrossRef]
28. Kanehisa, M.; Furumichi, M.; Tanabe, M.; Sato, Y.; Morishima, K. KEGG: New Perspectives on Genomes, Pathways, Diseases and Drugs. *Nucleic Acids Res.* **2017**, *45*, D353–D361. [CrossRef]
29. Fabregat, A.; Jupe, S.; Matthews, L.; Sidiropoulos, K.; Gillespie, M.; Garapati, P.; Haw, R.; Jassal, B.; Korninger, F.; May, B.; et al. The Reactome Pathway Knowledgebase. *Nucleic Acids Res.* **2018**, *46*, D649–D655. [CrossRef]
30. Slenter, D.N.; Kutmon, M.; Hanspers, K.; Riutta, A.; Windsor, J.; Nunes, N.; Mélius, J.; Cirillo, E.; Coort, S.L.; Digles, D.; et al. WikiPathways: A Multifaceted Pathway Database Bridging Metabolomics to Other Omics Research. *Nucleic Acids Res.* **2018**, *46*, D661–D667. [CrossRef]
31. Domingo-Fernández, D.; Mubeen, S.; Marín-Lló, J.; Hoyt, C.T.; Hofmann-Apitius, M. PathMe: Merging and Exploring Mechanistic Pathway Knowledge. *BMC Bioinform.* **2019**, *20*, 243. [CrossRef] [PubMed]
32. Hoyt, C.T.; Domingo-Fernández, D.; Aldisi, R.; Xu, L.; Kolpeja, K.; Spalek, S.; Wollert, E.; Bachman, J.; Gyori, B.M.; Greene, P.; et al. Re-Curation and Rational Enrichment of Knowledge Graphs in Biological Expression Language. *Database* **2019**, *2019*, baz068. [CrossRef] [PubMed]
33. Huntley, R.P.; Binns, D.; Dimmer, E.; Barrell, D.; O'Donovan, C.; Apweiler, R. QuickGO: A User Tutorial for the Web-Based Gene Ontology Browser. *Database* **2009**, *2009*, bap010. [CrossRef] [PubMed]
34. Hopp, M.T.; Domingo-Fernández, D.; Gadiya, Y.; Detzel, M.S.; Graf, R.; Schmalohr, B.F.; Kodamullil, A.T.; Imhof, D.; Hofmann-Apitius, M. Linking COVID-19 and Heme-Driven Pathophysiologies: A Combined Computational–Experimental Approach. *Biomolecules* **2021**, *11*, 644. [CrossRef]
35. Becker, C.G.; Wagner, M.; Kaplan, A.P.; Silverberg, M.; Grady, R.W.; Liem, H.; Muller-Eberhard, U. Activation of Factor XII-Dependent Pathways in Human Plasma by Hematin and Protoporphyrin. *J. Clin. Investig.* **1985**, *76*, 413–419. [CrossRef]
36. Hopp, M.-T.; Alhanafi, N.; Paul George, A.A.; Hamedani, N.S.; Biswas, A.; Oldenburg, J.; Pötzsch, B.; Imhof, D. Molecular Insights and Functional Consequences of the Interaction of Heme with Activated Protein, C. *Antioxid. Redox Signal.* **2021**, *34*, 32–48. [CrossRef]
37. Repessé, Y.; Dimitrov, J.D.; Peyron, I.; Moshai, E.F.; Kiger, L.; Dasgupta, S.; Delignat, S.; Marden, M.C.; Kaveri, S.V.; Lacroix-Desmazes, S. Heme Binds to Factor VIII and Inhibits Its Interaction with Activated Factor IX. *J. Thromb. Haemost.* **2012**, *10*, 1062–1071. [CrossRef] [PubMed]
38. Green, D.; Furby, F.H.; Berndt, M.C. The Interaction of the VIII/von Willebrand Factor Complex with Hematin. *Thromb. Haemost.* **1986**, *56*, 277–282.
39. Hunt, R.C.; Katneni, U.; Yalamanoglu, A.; Indig, F.E.; Ibla, J.C.; Kimchi-Sarfaty, C. Contribution of ADAMTS13-independent VWF Regulation in Sickle Cell Disease. *J. Thromb. Haemost.* **2022**, *20*, 2098–2108. [CrossRef]

40. Sparkenbaugh, E.M.; Chantrathammachart, P.; Wang, S.; Jonas, W.; Kirchhofer, D.; Gailani, D.; Gruber, A.; Kasthuri, R.; Key, N.S.; Mackman, N.; et al. Excess of Heme Induces Tissue Factor-Dependent Activation of Coagulation in Mice. *Haematologica* **2015**, *100*, 308–313. [CrossRef]
41. Setty, B.N.Y.; Betal, S.G.; Zhang, J.; Stuart, M.J. Heme Induces Endothelial Tissue Factor Expression: Potential Role in Hemostatic Activation in Patients with Hemolytic Anemia. *J. Thromb. Haemost.* **2008**, *6*, 2202–2209. [CrossRef] [PubMed]
42. Souza, G.R.; Fiusa, M.M.L.; Lanaro, C.; Colella, M.P.; Montalvao, S.A.L.; Saad, S.T.O.; Costa, F.F.; Traina, F.; Annichino-Bizzacchi, J.M.; de Paula, E.V. Coagulation Activation by Heme: Evidence from Global Hemostasis Assays. *Blood* **2014**, *124*, 455. [CrossRef]
43. May, O.; Yatime, L.; Merle, N.S.; Delguste, F.; Howsam, M.; Daugan, M.V.; Paul-Constant, C.; Billamboz, M.; Ghinet, A.; Lancel, S.; et al. The Receptor for Advanced Glycation End Products Is a Sensor for Cell-free Heme. *FEBS J.* **2021**, *288*, 3448–3464. [CrossRef] [PubMed]
44. Glueck, R.; Green, D.; Cohen, I.; Ts'ao, C. Hematin: Unique Effects on Hemostasis. *Blood* **1983**, *61*, 243–249. [CrossRef] [PubMed]
45. Green, D.; Reynolds, N.; Klein, J.; Kohl, H.; Ts'ao, C.H. The Inactivation of Hemostatic Factors by Hematin. *J. Lab. Clin. Med.* **1983**, *102*, 361–369. [PubMed]
46. Neely, S.M.; Gardner, D.V.; Reynolds, N.; Green, D.; Ts'ao, C. Mechanism and Characteristics of Platelet Activation by Haematin. *Br. J. Haematol.* **1984**, *58*, 305–316. [CrossRef]
47. Ke, Z.; Huang, Q. Haem-Assisted Dityrosine-Cross-Linking of Fibrinogen under Non-Thermal Plasma Exposure: One Important Mechanism of Facilitated Blood Coagulation. *Sci. Rep.* **2016**, *6*, 26982. [CrossRef]
48. Hou, T.; Zhang, Y.; Wu, T.; Wang, M.; Zhang, Y.; Li, R.; Wang, L.; Xue, Q.; Wang, S. Label-Free Detection of Fibrinogen Based on Fibrinogen-Enhanced Peroxidase Activity of Fibrinogen-Hemin Composite. *Analyst* **2018**, *143*, 725–730. [CrossRef]
49. Bergmeier, W.; Hynes, R.O. Extracellular Matrix Proteins in Hemostasis and Thrombosis. *Cold Spring Harb. Perspect. Biol.* **2012**, *4*, a005132. [CrossRef]
50. Nieswandt, B.; Pleines, I.; Bender, M. Platelet Adhesion and Activation Mechanisms in Arterial Thrombosis and Ischaemic Stroke. *J. Thromb. Haemost.* **2011**, *9*, 92–104. [CrossRef]
51. Li, Z.; Delaney, M.K.; O'Brien, K.A.; Du, X. Signaling During Platelet Adhesion and Activation. *Arterioscler. Thromb. Vasc. Biol.* **2010**, *30*, 2341–2349. [CrossRef] [PubMed]
52. Woollard, K.J.; Sturgeon, S.; Chin-Dusting, J.P.F.; Salem, H.H.; Jackson, S.P. Erythrocyte Hemolysis and Hemoglobin Oxidation Promote Ferric Chloride-Induced Vascular Injury. *J. Biol. Chem.* **2009**, *284*, 13110–13118. [CrossRef] [PubMed]
53. Oishi, S.; Tsukiji, N.; Otake, S.; Oishi, N.; Sasaki, T.; Shirai, T.; Yoshikawa, Y.; Takano, K.; Shinmori, H.; Inukai, T.; et al. Heme Activates Platelets and Exacerbates Rhabdomyolysis-Induced Acute Kidney Injury via CLEC-2 and GPVI/FcRγ. *Blood Adv.* **2021**, *5*, 2017–2026. [CrossRef] [PubMed]
54. Tsuji, M.; Ezumi, Y.; Arai, M.; Takayama, H. A Novel Association of Fc Receptor γ-Chain with Glycoprotein VI and Their Co-Expression as a Collagen Receptor in Human Platelets. *J. Biol. Chem.* **1997**, *272*, 23528–23531. [CrossRef]
55. Bourne, J.H.; Colicchia, M.; Di, Y.; Martin, E.; Slater, A.; Roumenina, L.T.; Dimitrov, J.D.; Watson, S.P.; Rayes, J. Heme Induces Human and Mouse Platelet Activation through C-Type-Lectin-like Receptor-2. *Haematologica* **2020**, *106*, 626–629. [CrossRef]
56. Porto, B.N.; Alves, L.S.; Fernández, P.L.; Dutra, T.P.; Figueiredo, R.T.; Graça-Souza, A.V.; Bozza, M.T. Heme Induces Neutrophil Migration and Reactive Oxygen Species Generation through Signaling Pathways Characteristic of Chemotactic Receptors. *J. Biol. Chem.* **2007**, *282*, 24430–24436. [CrossRef]
57. Annarapu, G.K.; Nolfi-Donegan, D.; Reynolds, M.; Wang, Y.; Kohut, L.; Zuckerbraun, B.; Shiva, S. Heme Stimulates Platelet Mitochondrial Oxidant Production to Induce Targeted Granule Secretion. *Redox Biol.* **2021**, *48*, 102205. [CrossRef]
58. Graça-Souza, A.V.; Arruda, M.A.B.; de Freitas, M.S.; Barja-Fidalgo, C.; Oliveira, P.L. Neutrophil Activation by Heme: Implications for Inflammatory Processes. *Blood* **2002**, *99*, 4160–4165. [CrossRef]
59. Alvarado, G.; Tóth, A.; Csősz, É.; Kalló, G.; Dankó, K.; Csernátony, Z.; Smith, A.; Gram, M.; Akerström, B.; Édes, I.; et al. Heme-Induced Oxidation of Cysteine Groups of Myofilament Proteins Leads to Contractile Dysfunction of Permeabilized Human Skeletal Muscle Fibres. *Int. J. Mol. Sci.* **2020**, *21*, 8172. [CrossRef]
60. Yao, X.; Balamurugan, P.; Arvey, A.; Leslie, C.; Zhang, L. Heme Controls the Regulation of Protein Tyrosine Kinases Jak2 and Src. *Biochem. Biophys. Res. Commun.* **2010**, *403*, 30–35. [CrossRef]
61. da Guarda, C.C.; Santiago, R.P.; Pitanga, T.N.; Santana, S.S.; Zanette, D.L.; Borges, V.M.; Goncalves, M.S. Heme Changes HIF-α, ENOS and Nitrite Production in HUVECs after Simvastatin, HU, and Ascorbic Acid Therapies. *Microvasc. Res.* **2016**, *106*, 128–136. [CrossRef] [PubMed]
62. Chen, P.F.; Tsai, A.L.; Wu, K.K. Cysteine 184 of Endothelial Nitric Oxide Synthase Is Involved in Heme Coordination and Catalytic Activity. *J. Biol. Chem.* **1994**, *269*, 25062–25066. [CrossRef]
63. Arruda, M.A.; Rossi, A.G.; de Freitas, M.S.; Barja-Fidalgo, C.; Graça-Souza, A.V. Heme Inhibits Human Neutrophil Apoptosis: Involvement of Phosphoinositide 3-Kinase, MAPK, and NF-KB. *J. Immunol.* **2004**, *173*, 2023–2030. [CrossRef]
64. Peng, L.; Mundada, L.; Stomel, J.M.; Liu, J.J.; Sun, J.; Yet, S.-F.; Fay, W.P. Induction of Heme Oxygenase-1 Expression Inhibits Platelet-Dependent Thrombosis. *Antioxid. Redox Signal.* **2004**, *6*, 729–735. [CrossRef] [PubMed]
65. Peterson, D.A.; Gerrard, J.M.; Rao, G.H.; Mills, E.L.; White, J.G. Interaction of Arachidonic Acid and Heme Iron in the Synthesis of Prostaglandins. *Adv. Prostaglandin Thromboxane Res.* **1980**, *6*, 157–161.
66. Green, D.; Ts'ao, C. Hematin: Effects on Hemostasis. *J. Lab. Clin. Med.* **1990**, *115*, 144–147.

67. NaveenKumar, S.K.; SharathBabu, B.N.; Hemshekhar, M.; Kemparaju, K.; Girish, K.S.; Mugesh, G. The Role of Reactive Oxygen Species and Ferroptosis in Heme-Mediated Activation of Human Platelets. *ACS Chem. Biol.* **2018**, *13*, 1996–2002. [CrossRef]
68. Nagy, E.; Eaton, J.W.; Jeney, V.; Soares, M.P.; Varga, Z.; Galajda, Z.; Szentmiklósi, J.; Méhes, G.; Csonka, T.; Smith, A.; et al. Red Cells, Hemoglobin, Heme, Iron, and Atherogenesis. *Arterioscler. Thromb. Vasc. Biol.* **2010**, *30*, 1347–1353. [CrossRef]
69. Hastings, J.; de Matos, P.; Dekker, A.; Ennis, M.; Harsha, B.; Kale, N.; Muthukrishnan, V.; Owen, G.; Turner, S.; Williams, M.; et al. The ChEBI Reference Database and Ontology for Biologically Relevant Chemistry: Enhancements for 2013. *Nucleic Acids Res.* **2012**, *41*, D456–D463. [CrossRef]
70. Lipscomb, C.E. Medical Subject Headings (MeSH). *Bull. Med Libr. Assoc.* **2000**, *88*, 265–266.
71. Hoyt, C.T.; Domingo-Fernández, D.; Hofmann-Apitius, M. BEL Commons: An Environment for Exploration and Analysis of Networks Encoded in Biological Expression Language. *Database* **2018**, *2018*, bay126. [CrossRef] [PubMed]

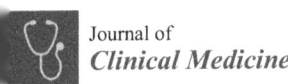 

*Review*

# Patients with Bicuspid Aortopathy and Aortic Dilatation

Francesco Nappi [1,*,†], Omar Giacinto [2,†], Mario Lusini [2], Marialuisa Garo [2], Claudio Caponio [2], Antonio Nenna [2], Pierluigi Nappi [3], Juliette Rousseau [1], Cristiano Spadaccio [4] and Massimo Chello [2]

1. Department of Cardiac Surgery, Centre Cardiologique du Nord, 93200 Saint-Denis, France
2. Department of Cardiovascular Surgery, Università Campus Bio-Medico di Roma, 00128 Rome, Italy
3. Department of Clinical and Experimental Medicine, University of Messina, 98122 Messina, Italy
4. Department of Cardiac Surgery, Massachusetts General Hospital & Harvard Medical School, Boston, MA 02115, USA
* Correspondence: francesconappi2@gmail.com; Tel.: +33-1-4933-4104; Fax: +33-1-4933-4119
† These authors contributed equally to this work.

**Abstract:** (1) Background: Bicuspid aortic valve (BAV) is the most frequent congenital cardiac disease. Alteration of ascending aorta diameter is a consequence of shear stress alterations due to haemodynamic abnormalities developed from inadequate valve cusp coaptation. (2) Objective: This narrative review aims to discuss anatomical, pathophysiological, genetical, ultrasound, and radiological aspects of BAV disease, focusing on BAV classification related to imaging patterns and flux models involved in the onset and developing vessel dilatation. (3) Methods: A comprehensive search strategy was implemented in PubMed from January to May 2022. English language articles were selected independently by two authors and screened according to the following criteria. (4) Key Contents and Findings: Ultrasound scan is the primary step in the diagnostic flowchart identifying structural and doppler patterns of the valve. Computed tomography determines aortic vessel dimensions according to the anatomo-pathology of the valve. Magnetic resonance identifies hemodynamic alterations. New classifications and surgical indications derive from these diagnostic features. Currently, indications correlate morphological results, dissection risk factors, and genetic alterations. Surgical options vary from aortic valve and aortic vessel substitution to aortic valve repair according to the morphology of the valve. In selected patients, transcatheter aortic valve replacement has an even more impact on the treatment choice. (5) Conclusions: Different imaging approaches are an essential part of BAV diagnosis. Morphological classifications influence the surgical outcome.

**Keywords:** bicuspid aortic valve; aortopathy; classification; diagnosis; treatment

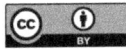

## 1. Introduction

Bicuspid aortic valve (BAV) is the most frequent congenital cardiac pathology; has a prevalence of 1–2% [1], a high incidence of adverse outcomes, especially aortic stenosis (AS) and aortic regurgitation (MR) [2]; and is at least three times more common in males than females [3].

Bicuspid aortopathy, reported in 50% of BAV patients, consists of the aorta enlargement starting from the aortic root and involving the aortic arch and depends on blood flux turbulences characterized by power vectors directed against the aortic toot and the convexity of the vessel [4–7]. Recently, micro-RNA (miRNA) has been studied regarding post-transcriptional regulation of genes in aortopathy manifestation. [8,9]. This paper aims to discuss the current knowledge about anatomical, pathophysiological, genetical, ultrasound, and radiological aspects of BAV disease, focusing on BAV classification related to imaging patterns and flux models involved in the onset of aortic dilatation and its developed process. We present the following article in accordance with the narrative review reporting checklist.

## 2. Methods

This narrative review was carried out from January 2022 to May 2022. The following search strategy was implemented on PubMed: (BAV OR bicuspid aortopathy OR bicuspid aortic valve) AND (ultrasound OR computed tomography OR magnetic resonance OR US OR CT or MR). Published articles were evaluated from database inception up to search date. Only articles in the English language were included. Details are reported in Table 1.

Table 1. Narrative review searching strategies.

| Items | Specification |
|---|---|
| Date of Search (specified to date, month and year) | From January 2022 to May 2022 |
| Databases and other sources searched | PubMed |
| Search terms used (including MeSH and free text search terms and filters) | (BAV OR bicuspid aortopathy OR bicuspid aortic valve) AND (ultrasound OR computed tomography OR magnetic resonance OR US OR CT or MR) |
| Time frame | Up to May 2022 |
| Inclusion and exclusion criteria (study type, language restrictions, etc.) | English language |
| Selection process | Two authors independently selected articles after screening for duplicates. |

## 3. Genetics and Molecular Biology

Estimating mutation genes and their inheritance patterns is challenging [7] because locus 9q34.3 alteration causes mutations in regulators NOTCH1 with secondary pathological aortic valve development [10,11]; gene damages on 18q, 5q, and 13q induces BAV [12]; and finally, damages to the smooth muscle alfa actine (ACTA 2) gene produce BAV and aortic aneurysms [13].

There is a tight linkage between BAV expression and other congenital pathologies such as the coarctation of the aorta. Concerning BAV phenotype, Shone's syndrome with a left-sided lesion that can cause inflow and outflow obstruction, Turner's syndrome with aortic coarctation, and William's syndrome involving supravalvular stenosis may be observed. Moreover, ventricular septal defect, atrial septal defect, patent ductus arteriosus, and coronary vessels, which may mainly involve single coronary and reversal coronary dominance, have been reported [14–16].

Micro-RNAs (MiRNAs) need to be considered in biochemical and molecular changes in BAV and aortopathy (Table 2). MiRNAs are small, single-stranded, noncoding RNA molecules that determine the post-transcriptional regulation of gene expression. The effects of miRNAs are the result of base pairing with complementary sequences within mRNA molecules that are silenced by cleavage of the mRNA strand, destabilization of the mRNA by shortening its tail, and less efficient translation into proteins by ribosomes [17]. MiRNA expression profiling studies show that the expression levels of certain miRNAs change in diseased human hearts, suggesting their involvement in cardiomyopathies. MiR-712 is a potential predictor of atherosclerosis, has blood flow-dependent expression, and miR-712 is also upregulated in endothelial cells exposed to naturally occurring d-flow in the greater curvature of the aortic arch [18]. Several studies have investigated the cooperation of miRNA, metalloproteinases (MMP), and tissue inhibitor of matrix metalloproteinases (TIMP) in aortopathy secondary to morphological alteration of the aortic valve. miRNAs related to dilation of the thoracic aorta (TA) are upregulated in transcriptional and epigenetic ways: different levels of MMP-2, MMP-9, TIMP-1, and TIMP-9 were observed [19]. A high level of MMP-2 and increased levels of miR-17 and miRNAs with the same genetic features as miR-17 were found in a comparative study involving patients with mild and severe aorta dilation, with a decreased level of TIMP -1, TIMP-2, and TIMP-3, thus hypothesizing a continuous development of TA influenced by BAV [20]. A recent study showed a relationship between miR-133a and TIMP-1 and TIMP-2 without reporting a statistically significant association between miR-143 and MMP-2 [21].

**Table 2.** Gene expression involved in valve and aortic diseases. ACTA 2: alfa actine 2, AXIN: gene encodes a cytoplasmic protein that contains a regulation of G-protein signaling (RGS) domain and a disheveled and axin (DIX) domain, BAV: bicuspid aortic valve, ENG: Endoglin, FBN1: fibrillin 1, GATA (sequence for transcription factors for zinc proteins' binding DNA sequence), NOS3: nitric oxide synthase 3, NOTCH1 (gene encoding transmembrane proteins), PDIA2: protein disulfide isomerase family A member 2, PECAM-1: platelet endothelial cell adhesion molecule-1, TGF: transforming growth factor, TIMP: tissue inhibitor of matrix metalloproteinases.

| Gene Expression | Pathology |
| --- | --- |
| miR-146-5p | BAV, aortic aneuurysm (convex region) |
| miR-21-5p | BAV, aortic aneuurysm (convex region) |
| miR-17 | Aoritc anurysm |
| miR 21 | Aortic aneurysm |
| miR-34 a | Aortic aneurysm |
| miR-122 | BAV |
| miR 130 a | BAV |
| miR-133a | TIMP1,TIMP2, aortic aneurysm |
| mi-R 143 | Aortic aneurysm |
| mi-R 145 | Aortic aneurysm |
| miR 146-5p | Aortic aneurysm |
| miR-200 | Endothelial-mesenchimal/epithelial mesenchimal |
| miR-423-5p | BAV, aortic aneurysm |
| miR-424-3p downregulation | Cell proliferation, apoptosis, endothelial cells alterations, aortic anuerysm |
| miR-486 | BAV |
| miR-494 | PECAM |
| miR-712 | Atherosclerosis, aortic aneurysm |
| miR-718 | Aortic aneurysm |
| ACTA2 | BAV. Aortic aneurysm |
| AXIN1-PDIA2 | BAV |
| ENG | BAV |
| FBN 1 | BAV |
| GATA4/GATA5/GATA6 | BAV |
| NOS3 | BAV |
| NOTCH1 (9q34.3) | BAV, outflow tract malformation |
| TGFb1/TGFb2 | Sporadic BAV, Loeys-Dietz syndrome |
| 18q | BAV |
| 5q | BAV |
| 13q | BAV |

Plasma exosomal miR-423-5p regulates TGF-β signaling by targeting "similar mothers against decapentaplegic Drosophila gene" 2 (SMAD2), exerting functions in the initiation and development of BAV disease and its complication, bicuspid aortopathy [22,23]. Circulating miRNAs may reflect remodeling processes in the proximal aorta in patients with bicuspid aortopathy, and a recent study found a significant association between miRNA expression in peripheral blood and aortic tissue, as levels of miR-21, miR-133a, miR-143, and miR-145 were associated with dilated aorta [24].

Since abnormalities in vascular smooth muscle cells (VSMCs) may influence the development of TA dilation, primarily when contractile function converts to secretory function, this molecular situation causes cell apoptosis, in which the role of miRNA regulation may play a crucial role. Specifically, the convex part of ascending thoracic aorta (ATA) in BAV has increased miR-146-5p and miR-21-5p and reduced miR-133a-3p levels [25]; miR-424-3p and miR-3688-3p are downregulated in Hippo, ErbB, and TGF-beta signalling pathways, an epiphenomenon of cell proliferation and apoptosis [26]; and, finally, endothelial cells may have alterations due to abnormal flux patterns and genetic factors. This last alteration results in a less resistant vessel wall and can start a process of aortic dilation. Moreover, miR-494 is associated with platelet endothelial cell adhesion molecule (PECAM) and microparticles derived from endothelial cells [26], and the decreased expression of the miR-200 group can determine the involvement of the miR-200 family in endothelial–mesenchymal/epithelial–mesenchymal transition (EndMT/EMT) [27].

Observing the role of miRNAs as aortopathy biomarker of aortic dilation and increasing aortic dilation, it has been observed that miR-133a has a special linkage with the aneurysms' incidence [28]; miR-122, miR-130a, and miR-486 are expressed in BAV; and miR-718 is used to predict aneurysms [29] similar to miR-34a [30].

Fibrillin 1 (FBN1) mutations have been found in BAV and aortic dilation. This gene encodes a glycoprotein of extracellular matrix (ECM), which manteins elastic fibers, and is also involved in the linkage of epithelial cells to interstitial matrix. A downregualtion of this gene has been associated with BAV [31]. GATA (sequence for transcription factors for zinc proteins' binding DNA sequence) variations are involved in BAV: a missense p. Arg202Gln in GATA5 and three synonymous variants—p. Cys274 and p. His302 in GATA4, and p. Asn458 in GATA6 [32]. Alterations in nitric oxide synthase 3 (NOS3) are also associated with BAV. A single nucleotide polymorphism (SNP) is present in aneurysmal and non-aneurysmal BAV [33]. A haplotype within the AXIN-1-protein disulfide isomerase family A member 2 (AXIN1-PDIA2) locus and in the Endoglin (ENG) gene has been found to be linked to BAV [34]. Cilia and excyst have a main role in regulate mitogen-activated protein kinase (MAPK) signaling. An alteration of this mechanism is the cause of an activation of MAPK and the formation of BAV and calcified aortic stenosis [35].

## 4. Classification and Nomenclature

Since 1970, several classifications of BAV, derived from pathology, US scan, CT scan, and MR patterns (Table 3), have been proposed [36]. Recently, an international consensus statement developed a classification based on the progression of cusps fusion and geometry of commissurae [37], with particular attention to surgical indications and techniques.

**Table 3.** BAV classifications (adapted from Michelena HI et al./European Journal of cardio-thoracic surgery). Abbreviations; BAV, bicuspid aortic valve; BAVCon, bicuspid aortic valve consortium; LN, left non-coronary fusion; RL, right–left fusion; RN, right non-coronary fusion.

| Author | Nomenclature |
|---|---|
| Roberts [36] 1970 | Anterior–posterior cusps<br>Right–left cusps<br>Presence of raphe |
| Brandenburg et al. [38] 1983 | Clock-face nomenclature:<br>Commissures at 4–10 o'clock with raphe at 2 o'clock (R-L)<br>Commissures at 1–6 o'clock with raphe at 10 o'clock (RN)<br>Commissures at 3–9 o'clock without raphe (L-N) |
| Angelini et al. [39] 1989 | Anterior–posterior cusps<br>Right–left cusps<br>Presence of raphe |
| Sabet et al. [40] 1999 | RL<br>RN<br>LN<br>Presence of raphe |
| Sievers and Schmidtke [41] 2007 | Type 0 (no raphe): anteroposterior or lateral cusps (true BAV)<br>Type 1 (1 raphe): R-L, RN, L-N<br>Type 2 (2 raphes): L-R, RN |

Table 3. Cont.

| Author | Nomenclature |
|---|---|
| Schaefer et al. [42] 2008 | Type 1: RL<br>Type 2: RN<br>Type 3: LN<br>Presence of raphe<br>Aorta:<br>Type N: normal shape<br>Type E: sinus effacement<br>Type A: ascending aorta dilatation |
| Kang et al. [43] 2013 | Anteroposterior orientation:<br>type 1: R-L with raphe type; 2: R-L without raphe<br>Right–left orientation:<br>Type 3: RN with raphe<br>Type 4: L-N with raphe<br>Type 5: symmetrical cusps with 1 coronary artery originating from each cusp<br>Aorta:<br>Type 0: normal<br>Type 1: dilated root<br>Type 2: dilated ascending aorta<br>Type 3: diffuse involvement of the ascending aorta and arch |
| Michelena et al. [44] 2014 | BAVCon nomenclature:<br>Type 1: R-L<br>Type 2: RN<br>Type 3: L-N<br>Presence of raphe |
| Jilaihawi et al. [45] 2016 | Tricommissural: functional or acquired bicuspidity of a trileaflet valve<br>Bicommissural with raphe<br>Bicommissural without raphe |
| Sun et al. [46] 2017 | Dichotomous nomenclature:<br>R-L<br>Mixed: (RN or L-N) |
| Murphy et al. [47] 2017 | Clock-face nomenclature:<br>Type 0: partial fusion/eccentric leaflet?<br>Type 1: RN, RL, LN partial fusion/eccentric leaflet?<br>Type 2: RL and RN, RL and LN, RN and LN partial fusion/eccentric leaflet? |

From this consensus statement, three BAV patterns related to the fusion of cusps and the number of sinuses may be observed. Every pattern should be considered like a schematic-based US short-axis scan at the base of the heart; the ideal circumference of the aortic valve is subdivided into parts like the face of a clock, in which the points over the watch are the coordinates of the anatomical features of the BAV.

In normal cardiogenesis, endothelium-derived nitric oxide syntethase (eNOS) expression is related to endocardial cells and is dependent upon the shear stress [48,49]. Nitric oxide is the promotor of podokinesis. In this way, cardiac jelly is populated by endocardil cells to make endocardil cushions [50]. In a study on mice, eNOS deficency may cause an alteration of cell migration with impairment in the development of valvular cushions, and an alteration of the function of cardiac neural crest cells has a role in this pathogenetic pattern [7,51].

The first pattern related to embryological events is defined as the fused bicuspid aortic valve (Figure 1) and diagnosed in 90–95% of cases [44] and presents three subtypes defined according to the cusps involved.

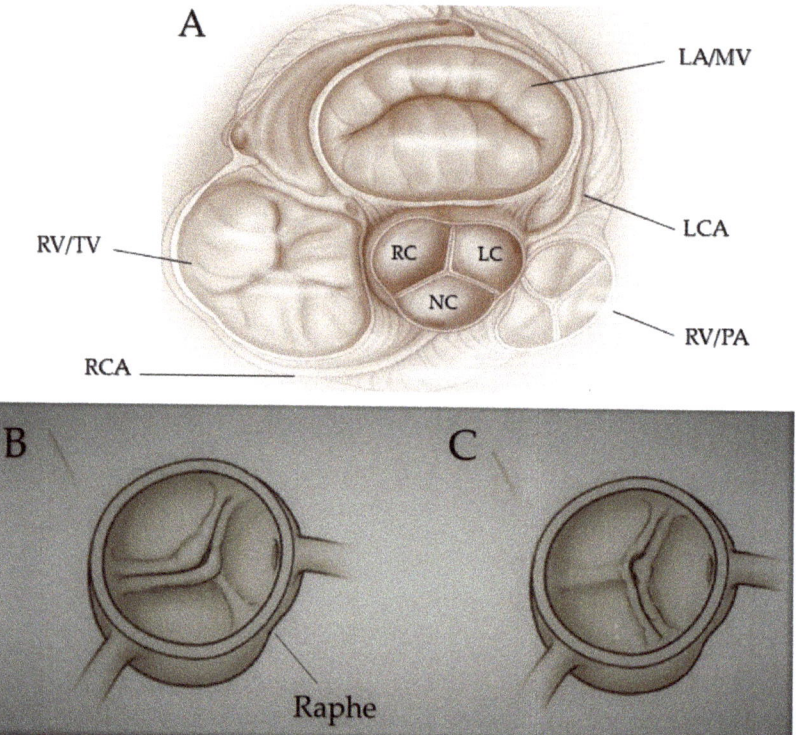

**Figure 1.** Fused bicuspid aortic valve. (**A**) Represents short-axis normal tricuspidal aortic pattern with anatomical proximities. Cusps' fusion patterns seen in short heart axis: right-left coronary fusion (**B**), right-non coronary fusion (**C**). All BAVs have three sinuses. Raphe structure is between the fused cusps. Non-fused cusp is prominent in respect to the fused ones. The commissure angle of the non-fused cusp has a degree < 180°. Abbreviations: LA, left atrium; LC, left cusp; LCA, left coronary artery; MV, mitral valve; NC, non-coronary cusp; PA, pulmonary artery; RA, right atrium; RC, right cusp; RCA, right coronary artery; RV, right ventricule; TV, tricuspidalic valve. Licenses Centre Cardiologique du Nord; order date 8 September 2022; order number 5384080341542; publication NEJM; Title: Mitral valve Repair for Mitral valve prolapse.

In normal conditions, valve cushions are modelled by an excavation process resulting in fusion of the cusps in case of process alteration [51–55]. It is possible to distinguish three sinuses and the fusion of two of the three cusps. In contrast, the non-fused cusp commissure has an angle of different degrees and generally is more prominent than the fused cusps, as occurs for its sinus compared to the other two sinuses. A fibrous raphe, a predictor of further development of AS [56] between the two fused cusps, has been frequently observed [40,57]. The right–left cusp fusion, observed in 70–80% of patients [58] and often associated with AS and aortic regurgitation (AR) [44], is derived from a mild alteration in the outflow tract septation during embryogenesis and is linked to the formation of aneurysms in every section of the aorta (aortic root, ascending aorta, aortic arch) and frequently characterized by root dilation. An association has also been observed between right–left cusp fusion and aortic coarctation. The right–left cusp fusion is common in genetic syndromes, such as Turner's one and Shone's complex and people with Down syndrome [59]. In 20–30% of BAV cases, a proper non-coronary cusp fusion is present, more common among the Asian population [60] and frequently associated with AS in adults [56].

Moreover, it may be observed combined with an alteration of the process involved in the formation of the endocardial cushion, an independent predictor of AR [61]. In children, this phenotype may induce a more rapid development of AS and AR [62,63]. Left non-coronary cusp fusion is only present in 3–6% of patients [37].

The second type of BAV is referred to as the two sinuses BAV type (Figure 2).

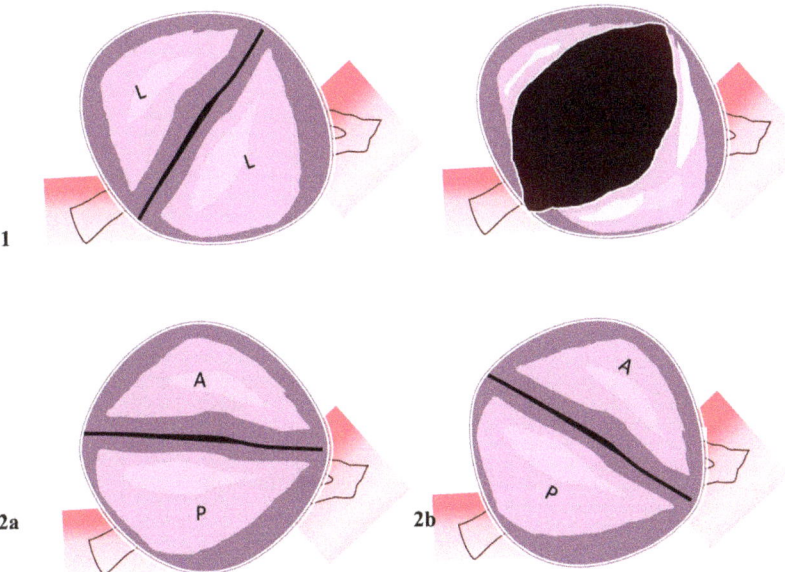

**Figure 2.** Two-sinus bicuspid aortic valve. Figure represents two cusps' non-fusion patterns seen in the short heart axis. Aortic valves have two sinuses with two leaflets non-derived from fusion mechanisms. (**1**) Coronary arteries originate from the two sinuses with two lateral leaflets. The opened valve in systole phase has the oval-ball image. (**2a**) In this position, coronary arteries originate from the anterior sinus (right coronary artery) and posterior sinus (common left stem). (**2b**) Right coronary artery and common left stem both originate from anterior sinus. Abbreviations; A, anterior; L, lateral P, posterior.

Its incidence ranges between 5 and 7% of cases [40,44,64]. In this pattern, it is possible to identify two cusps corresponding to homologous sinuses, not depending upon fusion but upon the abnormal embryological constitution. Typically, the cusps are the same in size, a raphe is not present, and the aortic orifice is divided into two portions: laterolateral (Figure 2(1)) and anteroposterior (Figure 2(2a,2b)). In the laterolateral pattern, coronary setup is from each sinus; in the anteroposterior type, coronaries may originate from each sinus or the anterior one. Embryological alteration involved in the laterolateral pattern is secondary to abnormal endocardial cushion formation and positioning. The aetiology of the anteroposterior model is due to abnormal outflow tract septation. The same mechanism in the fused aortic bicuspid valve type is present in this second morphological pattern, but the two-sinus valve may constitute a more severe embryological development alteration [37].

The third BAV type is a partial fusion bicuspid aortic valve (Figure 3), with an unknown prevalence [65].

Morphological features are similar to a tricuspid valve with symmetry of the cusps, and the aortic orifice area is less comprehensive than the normal surface. A raphe is localized at the base of each commissure, causing a fixed portion of the cusp to the artic wall. For this reason, this phenotype is also called form fruste aortic valve [66–68]. An alteration of normal embryological processes may be identified. Therefore, it is assumed that a mild defect in outflow tract septation and remodelling of aortic valve cushions are present.

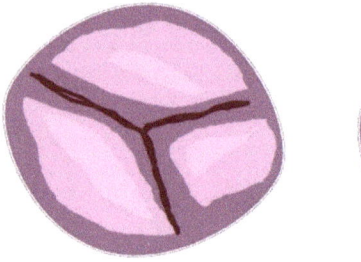
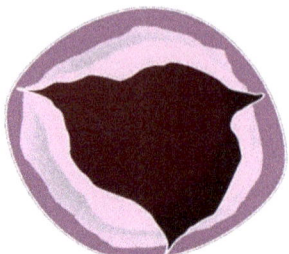

**Figure 3.** Partial fusion aortic valve. Figure represents three cusps with partial leaflets fusion seen in the short heart axis (**left**). In this case, the opened (**right**) aortic valve is similar to the normal valve but with a more narrow area.

The above classifications (Table 3) have implications for daily clinical practice. Siever's classification is still the most important for diagnosis and surgical indication. The classifications with the determination of the leaflets and the fusion patterns of the commissures are crucial for the development of aortic dilatation [69]. Even aortic valve morphology, flow changes, and prognostic evaluation are well determined by models derived from fusion pattern classification.

## 5. BAV Geometry Types and Surgical Implications

In every subtype of the previous classification, we can identify the BAV geometrical pattern by evaluating the position of commissures related to the aortic orifice, their angle in the coaptation zone, the presence of raphe, and the morphology and the area of the cusps. In the fused BAV type, it is relevant to establish the relationships between the fused cusps and non-fused cusp and the angle of the commissures of the non-fused cusps (Figure 4).

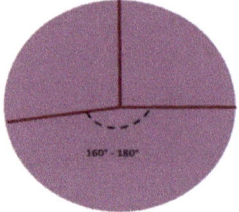
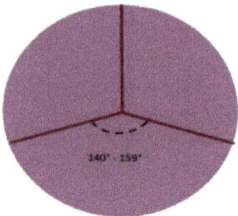
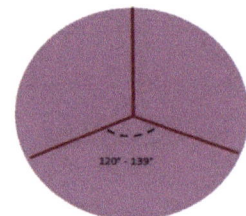

**Figure 4.** Symmetry of fused bicuspid aortic valve (adapted from Michelena HI et al./European Journal of cardio-thoracic surgery). Figure represents the angles determined by aortic valve leaflets fusion patterns. The length of raphe causes the retraction of fused leaflets and the non-physiological coaptation of the non-fused leaflet with fused leaflets. The geometry of the three patterns can be summarized as symmetrical, asymmetrical, and very asymmetrical The degree of the angle is important for surgical technique.

When the two fused cusps are retracted over the raphe, AR may develop. Therefore, the coaptation line and angle must be described mainly for surgical indications and practice. The coaptation angle may vary from 180° to less than 150°; to ensure a higher probability of valve repair, the ideal angle should range between 180° and 160°. When the angle approximates 140°, valve sparing and repairing is more complex [70]. Pre-cardiopulmonary bypass transoesophageal echocardiography establishes the coaptation model and commissural angle.

The two-cusp fusion model, more frequent in AS, has the two cusps/two sinuses feature, and the commissural angle is nearly close to 180° [37]. In partial fusion, the commissural angle resembles the one present in the normal aortic valve.

Surgical valve-preserving techniques are indicated by the commissural geometry of the aortic valve, as mentioned by a recent paper that also considers the relationship of the aortic root from the virtual basal ring (VBR) to the sinitubular junction [71].

## 6. Pathophysiology

Histological and hemodynamic features have a critical role in understanding BAV development. Histological changes in the aortic wall structure may be ascribed to cystic medial necrosis. The process involved in smooth muscle cells' regulatory pathways is well known. Extracellular matrix fibrillin 1, abnormally processed by smooth muscle cells, causes the separation of smooth muscle cells from the extracellular matrix layer. After that, MMPs are activated with consequences on the fragmentation of elastin and cellular apoptosis, and the media tunica becomes less prone to flexibility than normal aortic wall [72–74].

Hemodynamic implications cooperate with histological patterns in developing aortopathy in BAV. Biophysics may significantly confirm pathological evidence, given the relationship between hemodynamic and histological patterns. Analysis of the flux, especially in fused bicuspid valves, helps understand the way of aortic dilation, remembering that even a normofunctioning bicuspid valve may cause a flux alteration. A notable contribution to these aspects is due to cineMR of the heart and ascending thoracic aorta [75]: assessing the development of aortic dilation and its complications, such as the dissection, allows for considering flux modification rather than the normal one. For this purpose, the Wall Shear Stress (WSS), peak velocity, normalized flow displacement, and in-plane rotational flow (IPRF) should be observed (Figure 5).

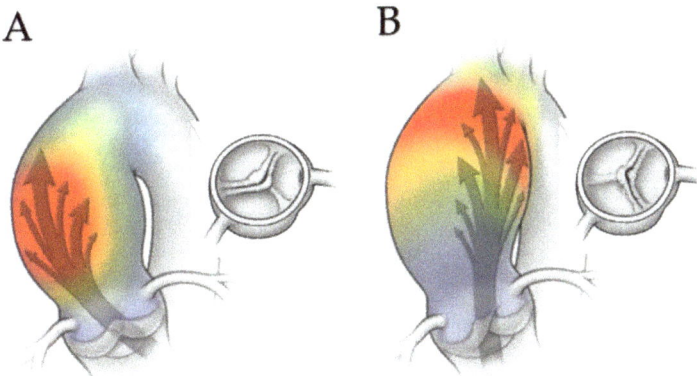

**Figure 5.** (**A**,**B**). Representation of morphologic chacteristic of the bicuspid aortic valve influencing the pattern of aortopathy. The fusion pattern of the aortic valve cusps is responsible for changes due to shear stress on the aortic wall and in the resulting flow pattern. (**A**) In the right–left fusion model, the jet is directed towards the right anterior wall of the ascending aorta, where it moves in a right-hand helical direction to promote dilation predominantly of the ascending aorta. (**B**) In contrast, in the model characterized by a fusion of the right and non-coronary cusps, the jet is directed towards the posterior wall of the aorta, so the model of shear stress of the wall it causes can favor aortic expansion at the internal proximal arch. Licenses Centre Cardiologique du Nord; order date 27 July 2022; order number 5357160571198; publication NEJM; Title: Aortic Dilatation in Patients with Bicuspid Aortic Valve.

Given that the morphology of BAV influences WSS, this should be evaluated considering its two main axial and circumferential components. Especially in fused patterns and a particular portion of the aorta, WSS may be incidental in aortic dilation (Figure 5). In this case, two distinct models of aortic dilation may be identified: the tubular aortic dilation and the root dilation. The R-L fusion type (Figure 5A) causes more WSS to the root and the outer curvature of the proximal part of the ascending aorta with a lower influence upon the upper tubular portion of the aorta itself; instead, R non-cusp fusion (Figure 5B) exerts a stronger WSS on the convexity of ascending aorta with involvement of the aortic arch [76,77]. Moreover, WSS is also dependent on the degree of AS, given its contribution to a more abnormal flux pattern and the consequent possibility of developing hybrid forms of aortic dilation.

Root aneurysms may be associated with tubular aortic and arch enlargement. This type of aortic dilation is called root phenotype extended [37,78]. Root phenotype is more frequently associated with aortic dissection, especially in patients who have previously undergone aortic valve replacement (AVR). This is determined by WSS and genetic factors [79]. The ascending phenotype is determined from WSS and the significant curvature of the tubular portion, which can determine a more substantial power of WSS [80,81]. In this context, Sigovan et al. described how the flow jet angle (FJA) and normalized flow displacement (NFD) might act upon the aortic wall, causing dilation [82]. In-plane rotational flow (IPRF), determined in MR imaging, is valuable for measuring rotation flow through a surface. In this sense, the vorticity ($\omega$) and circulation ($\Gamma$) are calculated by the integral of vorticity related to a sectional area [83]. Flow volumes are registered as the time integral of forward and backward flow measurements through the aortic surface, thus allowing for the calculation of the systolic flow reversal ratio (SFRR) [84]. Together with biophysical considerations, these parameters are instrumental for a deep CT and RM imaging reading. They may be used during patients' follow-up, especially in those for whom stratifying the risk of developing and increasing an abnormal aortic diameter is needed. Combining these features with risk factors control and pharmacological approach may be helpful in primary and secondary prophylaxis of aortic dilation.

## 7. Imaging Diagnostic

### 7.1. Echocardiographic Imaging

The role of transesophageal echocardiography (TTE) in diagnosing BAV and its sequelae is well known [38,85–87] and mandatory in particular conditions such as AS. It has been estimated that TTE has a sensitivity of 78%, a specificity of 96%, and an accuracy of 93% [38]. In patients with AS, ECG-gated CT is recommended.

TTE determines the morphology of the valve, the connected hemorheology, the anatomical features of the root system, the diameter and the wall alteration of ascending aorta, and conditions like the aortic coarctation associated with BAV. In aortic root determination, TTE allows for measuring the sinotubular junction (STJ), especially in some aortopathy related to BAV (Figure 6).

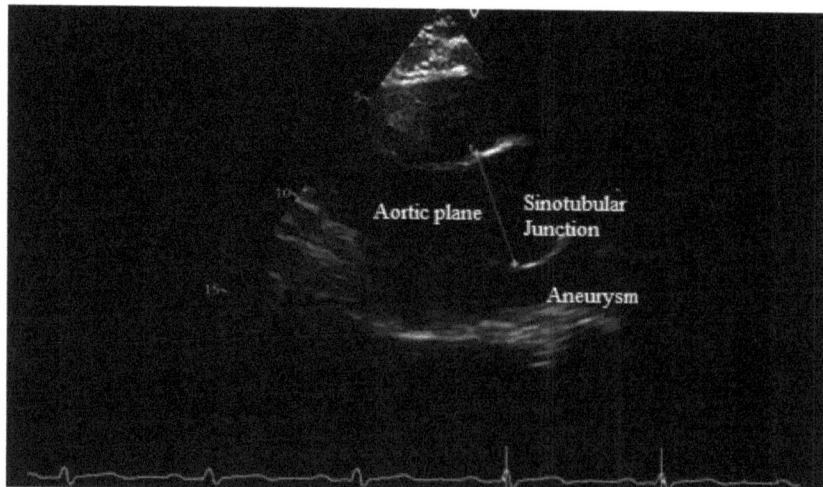

**Figure 6.** TTE shows enlargement of the sinotubular junction related to R-L cusp fusion.

It is performed using a parasternal short-axis and subcostal short-axis 2D scan, in which the first parameter helps detect two aortic valve cusps. A long axis may be used to investigate the doming in the systolic phase of the fused cusps.

To describe patterns in BAV classification, a short-axis 2D scan is the best US view because it allows for detecting all the aortic orifices and characterizing cusps fusion and position. It is helpful to determine the presence of raphe and the calcification of the structures related to the components of the aortic valve. Furthermore, TTE, combined with a TC scan, supports determining the relations between cusps, or the angle of commissures, which is important for surgical methods and the width of the sinuses (Figure 7).

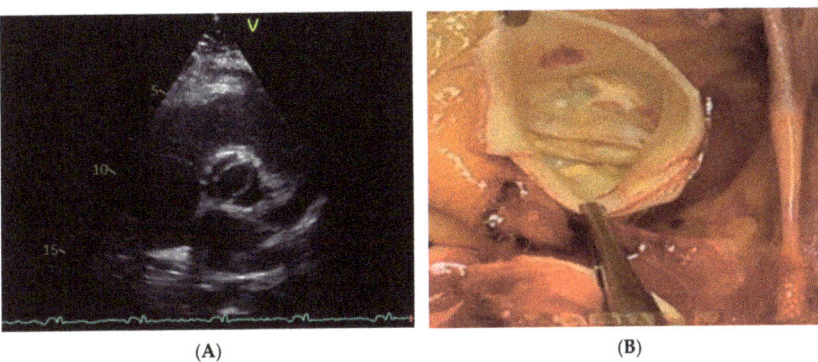

**Figure 7.** (**A**) TTE. Right non-coronary cusps fusion. (**B**) In the picture from operation theater, it is possible to appreciate the fusion between the right cusp and the non-coronary cusp. Three sinuses are still viewed. Commissural geometrical juxtaposition forms a 180-degree angle.

Deeping the role of the US in determining BAV features, the evaluation of the symmetry of the fused cusps related to non-fused cusps is fundamental. Generally, the fused cusps form a new structure that is greater and asymmetrical than the non-fused cusp, while the sinus corresponding to the non-fused cusp is larger than the other two sinuses [88].

The valvular function should be well established since flux alterations are present in BAV patterns. Normal functioning valves have to be studied, considering that many of them may evolve into stenosis or regurgitation. Recognizing valves with systolic relevant bending strain, systolic flow models [89], and transaortic fluximetry (peak velocity Doppler) is mandatory. The left ventricular outflow tract (LVOT) is studied with a continuous equation and generally has a larger surface than normal valves. Guidelines recommend employing the peak systolic velocity and mean gradient where the normal ejection fraction is registered [90].

In AR, every part of the aortic valve and STJ may be investigated. Prolapse of one or both cusps may be observed, usually associated with dilation of the annulus and root system [91]. TTE may contribute to determining the mechanism of regurgitation and establishing if the valve may be repaired or not; in case of positive indication, TTE supports the identification of repair measurements. To obtain a coaptation zone without residual insufficiency, the commissure angle should reach not less than 160°. It is also relevant to determine the presence of calcification and the mobility of the cusps [86].

Furthermore, through the parasternal long-axis and short-axis images derived by TTE, it is possible to measure the diameter of the ascending aorta segments. In particular, the parasternal long axis may not represent the actual diameter of the aorta correctly [92], but, since aortic diameters are orthogonal to blood flow and X-rays form a 90° angle with vectors of blood flow, the CT scan is valuable in determining every single diameter in aortic segments. Furthermore, TTE registers aortic wall measurements at the end-diastolic phase, taking them from the leading edge to the leading edge. This technique allows for identifying aortic enlargement related to the single patterns of BAV.

Since there is an agreement of no greater than 2 mm between echocardiography and CT or MR measurements (difference not more than 2 mm), TTE has a primary role during follow-up. It may be performed every 3–5 years if the diameter is normal, every 12 months if the diameter is 40–49 mm, and every 24 months if the stability should be assessed. In the presence of a diameter ranging from 50 to 54 mm, TTE must be repeated every 12 months. The function of the aortic valve should be considered for indication of surgery [93].

*7.2. Cardiac Computed Tomography*

Cardiac computed tomography (CCT) complements US scans in BAV diagnosis. It is relevant in determining aortic dilation, the anatomical edges and correlation with closer structures, and discovering other pathologies correlated with BAV, such as aortic coarctation. Therefore, the radiological protocol is scheduled to determine those features useful for surgeons in the act of choosing traditional surgical approach or transcatheter aortic valve replacement (TAVR) [94] (Figure 8).

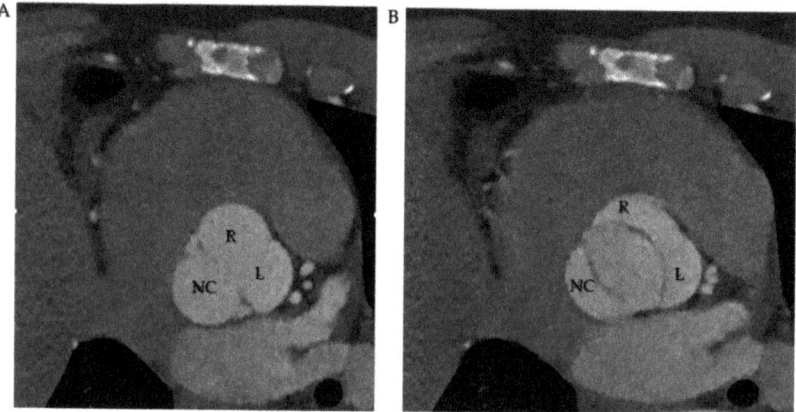

**Figure 8.** (**A**,**B**). CT scan in R-L cusp fusion. (**A**) Three sinuses are represented. (**B**). Opening mechanism in fusion pattern. Abbreviations; R, right coronary cusp; L, left coronary cusp; NC, non-coronary cusp.

In order to diagnose BAV, a 64-slice CT with a venous infusion of 50–100 mL of iodine contrast medium is usually performed. It is helpful to evaluate both systolic and diastolic ECG gating phases, and in the case of BAV, a true commissure or a raphe should be determined [95]. The systolic phase shows the opening pattern of the valve and helps to register the size of the annulus and the leaflets. In the diastolic phase, the edges of the leaflets, their hinge to the aortic wall, the way they close the left ventricle outflow, and the presence of calcifications on their surfaces may be evaluated; coronaries' imaging should also be evaluated keeping a strict monitoring of heart rate. The role of CCT in determining coronary origin in BAV deserves special mention. Eccentricity of the ostium of the right coronary artery is more frequent (> 20°) than the origin of the left coronary artery. In 95.5% of BAV patients, the obstruction of the right coronary artery is located at the border between the right cusp and the non-coronary cusp. It is also possible to assess the right and left cusps and the right and left coronary midlines. In 97% of BAV patients, the right and left cusps are slightly displaced from the commissure. In 93% of BAV patients, a displacement of less than 20° was noted between the right and left coronary cusps and between the right and left coronary arteries as centered lines [96].

Virtual Basal Ring (VBR) software estimates the size and anatomical features [95], especially the anatomical region between the plane passing across the ventricle outflow where this muscular structure encounters leaflets nadir and STJ. The cylindrical geometrical figure can be developed into a rectangular shape, where it is possible to identify hinge regions, sines, and interleaflet triangles. This multiplanar reconstruction (MPR) is particularly significant for surgical technical choices. To have a correct profile of the entire valve, aortic wall measurements should be taken by tracing curved lines in the inner surface of the aorta.

Every BAV pattern may be localized through a CT scan given the capacity to determine the exact anatomical coordinates as in the echocardiography. The valve orifice may be divided into parts like a clock face, while coronary cusps and non-coronary cusps have the same place as in the TTE.

Fusion patterns, the presence of raphe, leaflets coaptation, and commissure angles may be identified according to the general classification [37].

A recent radiological classification considering a morphological and geometrical approach derived from the valve, commissural orientation, and the aortic annulus shape was developed with the help of a CT scan [97]. The elliptical index of the annulus is measured related to the angle formed by commissure coaptation. Using this approach, three pattern types can be identified. The first type has a low elliptical index (more circular than the others) with a coaptation angle of 160°–180°. The second pattern has a moderate ellipse eccentricity with a coaptation angle estimated between 140° and 159°. Finally, the third type has a very elliptical annulus and a commissural orientation angle of 120°–139°.

According to the BAV classification, aneurysm phenotypes may be identified on CCT. The RL cusps' fusion pattern is better linked to root dilation and the initial portion of the tubular thoracic ascending aorta. RN cusp fusion is involved in the dilation of ascending aorta and aortic arch. CCT enables to measure the diameter of the thoracic aorta at different levels, the structure of the aortic wall, the presence of other aortic pathologies, and aortic wall destabilization/intramural hematomas/dissections. The diameter should be measured from the inner wall to the inner wall in the diastolic phase to correctly estimate the magnitude of ascending aorta.

*7.3. Magnetic Resonance*

The contribution of the MR is relevant in those cases in which the echocardiography cannot estimate the morphology of the aortic valve and root and the diameter of ascending aorta and arch (Figure 9). It also has a complementary role in determining the aortic wall structure and the viability of myocardial muscle. It has a main role in determining scarry zones inside a healthy myocardium and the efficiency of cardiac chambers. EF may be estimate with this technique. These features should be matched with other decision elements derived from other imaging techniques to identify the proper surgical indication and forecast the patients' prognosis. These factors make MR more useful in clinical practice than CT scan regarding functional evaluation [98] (Figure 9).

For hemorheological aspects secondary to BAV, MR is crucial. Time-resolved three-dimensional phase-contrast cardiovascular magnetic resonance (CMR 4D-flow) is necessary for optimal investigation. It allows us to study peak velocity, jet angle, normalized flow displacement, and in-plane rotational flow [75].

Velocity measured through the plane passing along the aortic valve may be associated with its vector figure. Ideally, the angle between the velocity vector and the valve plane is approximately equal to 90°. However, in the presence of BAV, this condition is altered. Therefore, it is necessary to investigate how the velocity vector and the power vector determined by the left ventricular ejection effort influence the blood flux and, consequently, the impact on the aortic wall. This biophysical model considers two particular BAV patterns: The R-L fusion causes a displacement of power against the root portion and to the convex line of the aorta. In contrast, the R-non cusp model shows vector forces directed in the posterior part of the ascending aorta. Interestingly, these power lines are modified in pathological patterns relating to the normal aortic valve, assuming a wider spectrum of action in the CMR 4D flow phase.

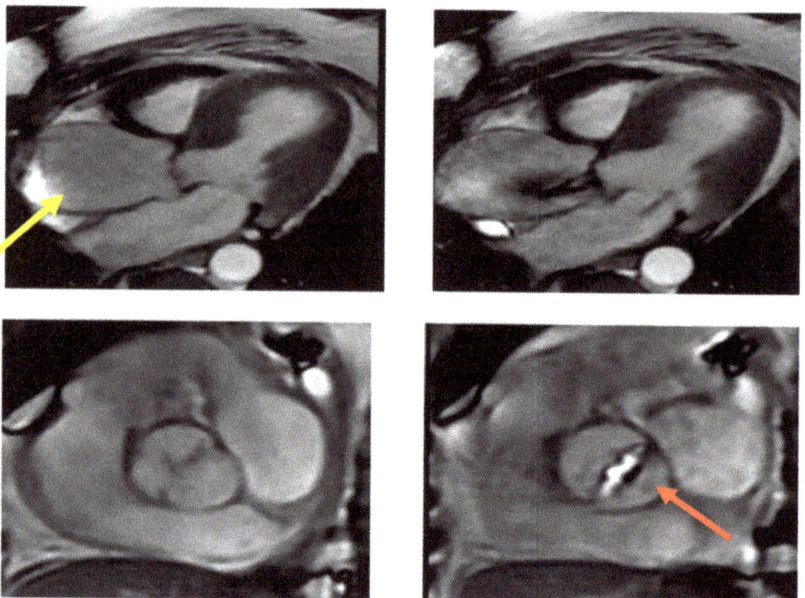

**Figure 9.** Calcific bicuspid aorta Sievert Type 2 with fusion of the two coronary cusps for a raphe (red arrow). The patient had a transvalvular gradient of 40 mmHg. The ascending thoracic aorta is dilated above the Valsalva sinuses with a maximum diameter of 53 mm measured at the intersection with the right pulmonary artery (yellow arrow).

MR also contributes to evaluating IPRF and SFRR [75] through a right-handed circular model that describes the geometry of the flux in BAV. IPRF seems higher in R-N-cusp than in the R-L pattern in mid and distal sections of ascending aorta [75,99–102] and has a higher value even in BAV with the dilated aorta. Higher IPRF values in ascending aortic aneurysm pattern than in the root pattern have also been observed. Rotational flux impacts the circular WSS because it may be possible, in this case, for the conjunction of powers with power vectors effort in double action on the aortic wall. SFRR has higher values in the BAV pattern than healthy persons without no difference between R-L and RN cusp patterns. SFRR levels are higher in ascending thoracic aorta than in the root pattern. In IPRF and SFRR, alterations of effort vectors with alteration of WSS may be observed.

MR imaging helps determine the geometrical and biophysical ascending aorta (AA) features. So far, the morphology of AA is connected to the diameter measure. A retrospective study [103] presented an AA segmentation from the aortic annulus to the emerging of the brachio-cephalic vessel-specific using a 3D segmentation MR software platform to relate the aortic vessel to an idealized cylinder. MR values in every segment were added to reproduce a volume pattern, and the volumetric growth index was determined by comparing baseline and follow-up measurements.

Interestingly results highlighted a difference between diameter measure and volume calculation. In this latter case, the growth index of the aorta was greater than diameter enhancement. Volume representation is more helpful in achieving information from every segment of the aorta than diameter measure, giving a synchronic vision of the idealized cylinder.

AA segmentation by 4D flow MR is a unique technique employed to investigate biophysical aortic features, such as flow rate, distensibility, local strain, and stiffness [104]. Pulse wave velocity (PWV) is determined in aortic regions from Valsalva's sinuses to the descending aorta (DA). The flow rate is obtained by multiplying the average velocity by the area of a single aortic section. PWV is influenced by diameter expansion, Young's elastic module, and reduced elasticity (E). PWV decreases when the diameter is larger than a normal aorta diameter and changes when stiffness is greater in pathological patterns than in normal situations.

## 8. Assessment and Treatment

The patterns of aortic involvement guide the surgical choice, and it can be classified into three types (Figure 10).

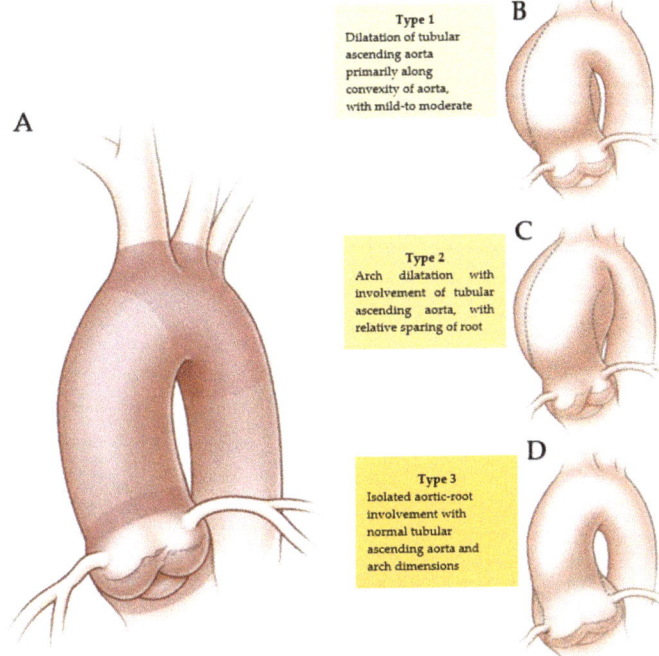

**Figure 10.** (A–D). Depict patterns of bicuspid aortopathy revealing the biologic features of the aorta and the three types of bicuspid aortopathy. The three morphological types reported provide a substantial contribution to the best surgical procedure to be used for the treatment of the bicuspid aortopathy. Licenses Centre Cardiologique du Nord; order date 27 July 2022; order number 5357160571198; publication NEJM; title: Aortic Dilatation in Patients with Bicuspid Aortic Valve.

Type 1 (B) is the most common type involving dilatation of the tubular ascending aorta with particular regard along its convexity, associated by varying degrees of aortic-root dilatation. Patients who develop this type of morphology have an older age at diagnosis (>50 years). Valvular stenosis and a preferentially RL fusion pattern are disclosed [6,90–92]. Type 2 (C) offers as typical feature an isolated involvement of the tubular ascending aorta associated to a relative sparing of the aortic root. Frequently, the morphological type 2 can be extended into the transverse aortic arch, and it has been associated with the presence of the RN fusion pattern [6,63,90–92]. Finally, type 3, due to its substantial characteristics, is called the root phenotype, and involves an isolated dilation of the aortic root (D). Its rarity is to be underlined as well as the frequent manifestation in a younger age at diagnosis (<40 years), in the male sex, and the occurrence of aortic regurgitation. Morphological type 3 has been referred to as the form of bicuspid aortopathy that is most likely to be associated with a genetic cause [6,58,64].

An early diagnosis of bicuspid aortopathy is likely offered by the use of TTE [42,105–108]. Although TTE is substantially a method for assessing the morphology of the aortic root and proximal ascending aorta, it is known that the correct visualization of the mid-distal portion of ascending aorta and the arch may present some difficulty in adults. In these cases, both computed tomographic (CT) and MR investigation may be offered a better visualization with a global evaluation of the ascending aorta. In patients who have contraindications to CT or MR, a TTE is suitable for reaching the diagnosis [43,105,109,110]. Likewise, in scheduling serial surveillance, it is more convenient to use MR than CT since it avoids extensive radiation exposure. (Figure 11)

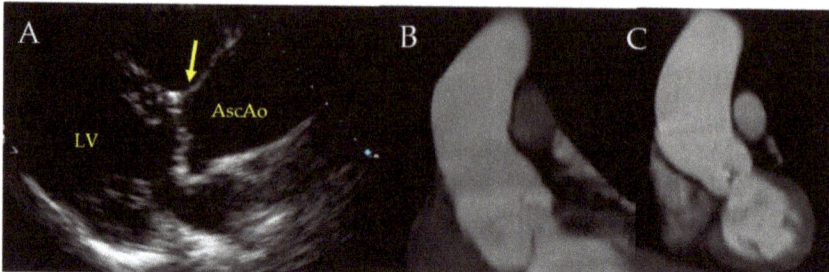

**Figure 11.** (**A**–**C**). Depicts representative findings on echocardiography and computed tomography (CT). In (**A**), the transthoracic echocardiogram shows normal dimensions of the sinuses of Valsalva (arrow) and a dilated ascending aorta. Ascending aorta denotes proximal ascending aorta, and LV denotes left ventricle. In (**B**,**C**), the CT images reveal dilatation of the aortic root and dilatation of the ascending aorta and proximal arch, respectively. Licenses Centre Cardiologique du Nord; order date 27 July 2022; order number 5357160571198; publication NEJM; Title: Aortic Dilatation in Patients with Bicuspid Aortic Valve.

*8.1. Decision-Making Algorithm for Treatment Option*

In patients suffering from bicuspid aortopathy, some risk factors, such as smoking and hypertension, require crucial attention. From a pharmacological point of view, the recent ACC/AHA guidelines recommend using antihypertensive drugs such as beta-adrenergic blockers, angiotensin-converting enzyme inhibitors, and angiotensin-receptor blockers. The use of beta-adrenergic blockers may offer the theoretical advantage of reducing the shear stress phenomenon of the aortic wall, thus avoiding the risk of rupture [111]. Conversely, angiotensin-receptor blockers favor decreasing the aortic growth rate in patients with Marfan syndrome [112].

Scheduling a continuous evaluation of the aorta diameter may be indicated in patients with bicuspid aortopathy. If the size of the aortic or ascending root aorta reaches a diameter between 45 and 48 mm, a CT or an MR scan is recommended [43,105,108]. It is important to emphasize that if concomitant indications exist to perform aortic valve correction or associated CABG surgery, a personalized surgical approach is evaluated considering rigorous parameters such as the pattern of aortopathy, the perioperative risk, the skill of the surgeon, and the experience of the referral center [109,113]. In patients in whom the lesion assumes the main characteristic of dilation of the tubular ascending aorta, the various surgical options are directed towards a more or less aggressive approach. The surgeon may choose between isolated supracoronary replacement of the ascending aorta or, in patients with a substantial aortic valve dysfunction associated with aortic root dilation, a replacement of the aortic valve, aortic root, or ascending aorta [114–122]. The surgical approach differs substantially in those patients who exhibit bicuspid aortopathy involving dilation of the ascending aorta in association with an aortic arch expansion. The treatment option may be the replacement of the aortic valve combined with the supracoronary replacement of the ascending aorta and with the involvement of the aortic hemiarch. Again, in case of the involvement of this distal part of the aorta, surgical treatment requires more or less deep hypothermia with the circulatory arrest that may be associated with the use of an anterograde or retrograde cerebral perfusion approach [114–122].

In patients with isolated aortic root involvement, the surgical option is directed towards the Bentall procedure, which includes aortic valve and aortic root replacement using a mechanical or biological composite valve conduit. A conservative surgical repair revealed excellent results in cases that present an ideal patho-anatomy of bicuspid aortopathy, although patients must be addressed to expert referral centers [120,121,123–125]. Indication of the combined aortic valve and ascending aorta replacement surgery should consider nonsurgical factors integrated into the final decision-making process. Therefore, the patient's lifestyle, the need for long-term anticoagulants, and future reproductive plans in the case of female patients should be considered. A Ross procedure may represent the ideal option for special populations because it uses the pulmonary autograft, which constitutes a living tissue [111,126–130].

Patients with no indication for valve replacement and who reveal dimensions of the aortic root or ascending aorta with a diameter ranging from 45 to 50 mm should be referred for surgery only if they have substantial high-risk characteristics such as a family history of aortic dissection, evidence of sudden rupture, and evidence-based imaging of an aortic growth rate greater than 5 mm per year [115,117–119,122,131]. On the other hand, the ratio of aortic area to body height greater than 10 $cm^2$ per meter is also effective for patients with short body stature [109,110,132]. If these conditions are insufficient to establish a correct clinical evaluation, an annual reassessment of risk stratification using CT or MR should be reconsidered.

Current ACC/AHA guidelines and the position papers of professional societies recommend a threshold of 5.5 cm and a more individualized approach. COR I and LOE A of ACC/AHA state that in asymptomatic or symptomatic BAV patients with a diameter of the aortic sinuses or ascending aorta higher than 5.5 cm, operative intervention to replace the aortic sinuses, and/or the ascending aorta is recommended. In asymptomatic patients with an aortic root or ascending aorta with a diameter ranging between 5.0 and 5.5 cm and an additional risk factor for dissection (COR 2a, LOE B-NR), surgery is recommended [111,113,133].

In other specific clinical conditions, different approaches may be adopted. For asymptomatic BAV patients with low surgical risk and a diameter of the aortic sinuses or ascending ranging from 5.0 to 5.5 cm without additional risk factors for dissection, surgery to replace the aortic sinuses and/or the ascending aorta may be considered if the surgery is performed at a comprehensive valve center (COR 2b, LOE B-NR) [115,117–120,122,131,133,134]. BAV patients who meet the criteria for replacement of the aortic sinuses may be considered for valve-sparing surgery when the surgery is performed at a comprehensive valve center (COR 2b LOE C-LD) [114]. European guidelines recommend the aortic replacement in patients who experience a diameter of the aortic root or ascending aorta at 5.0 cm or more and when patients have associated risk factors that include coarctation of the aorta, systemic hypertension, family history of dissection, or an increase in the aortic diameter of more than 2 mm per year [93]. International guidelines recommend ascending aortic replacement surgery in patients with a lower threshold (aortic diameter: 45 mm) for whom there is an indication for aortic valve surgery and when valve repair can be performed in an expert center [93,111]. As for patients who received an AVR related to BAV disease and presented with an aortic sinus or ascending aortic diameter greater than 4.0 cm, serial surveillance with lifelong aortic imaging is advisable [135,136].

Finally, the Canadian guidelines recommend the surgical option for an aortic diameter threshold that ranges between 5 and 5.5 cm, also considering the body surface and specific patient risk factors as fundamental criteria, such as the time when the procedure is performed and the nature of the elective aortic replacement [137,138]. Prophylactic surgery is recommended for patients with a lower threshold limit of 50 mm and substantial risk factors for developing an aortic complication, such as rapid aortic growth, concomitant aortic valve disease, and disorders related to connective tissue or genetic syndromes. However, the prophylactic surgery option is not recommended in patients with an increased risk of complications during surgery. Canadian guidelines assume that, since the aortic complications represent a long-term risk that increases with time, they may be prevented if patients undergo elective aortic valve replacement and when aortic surgery is executed in centers with a mortality rate less than 1% [137] (Figure 12).

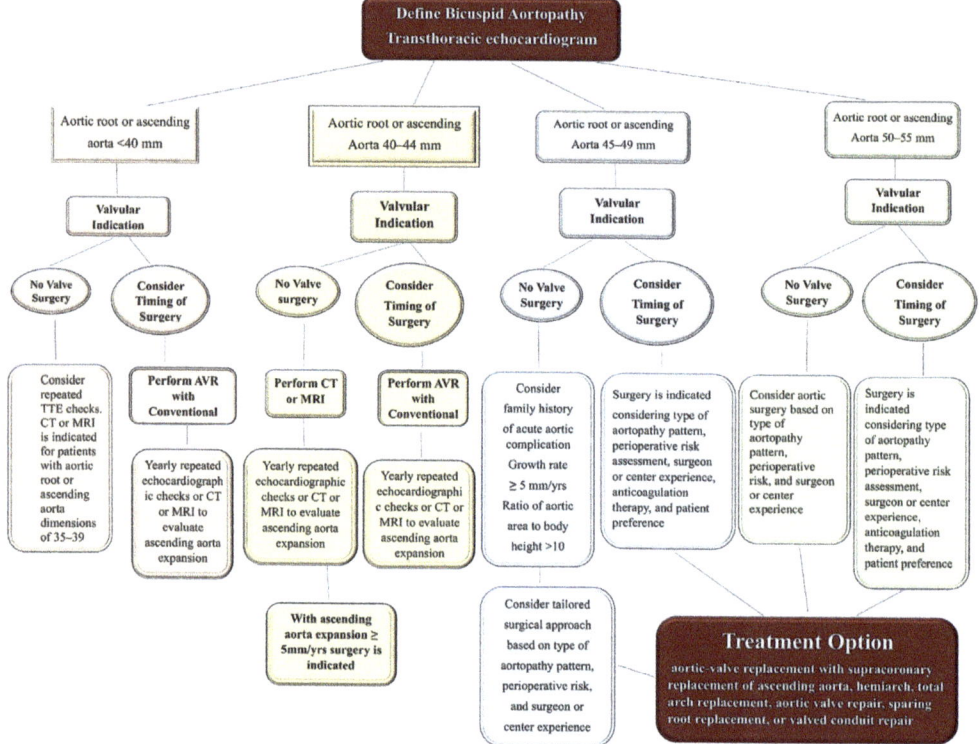

**Figure 12.** Decision-making algorithm for the management of the bicuspid aortopathy. Abbreviations; AVR, aortic valve replacement; CT, computed tomography; MRI, magnetic resonance imaging; TTE, transthoracic echocardiography.

*8.2. Special Populations*

During pregnancy, women who experience a bicuspid aortic valve with concomitant aortic dilatation may record changes in hemodynamics and the level of the tunica media of the aorta leading to an increased risk of complications. In women who reveal a bicuspid aortic valve associated with an aortic diameter greater than 4.5 cm, general guidelines recommend discontinuing pregnancy. For athletes with aortic root or ascending aortic dilatation greater than 45 mm diameter, regardless of valve dysfunction, guidelines recommend participating in low-intensity events.

For patients who experience symptomatic BAV with severe AS, the transthoracic aortic valve replacement (TAVR) procedure may be considered a valid alternative to AVR after evaluation of patient-specific procedural risks, values, trade-offs, and if executed in a comprehensive valve center (ACC/AHA; COR 2b, B-NR) [139–141]. Finally, the familiarity with bicuspid aortic disease, such as that which occurs in the first degree of kinship, should involve marked surveillance for early detection of an asymptomatic bicuspid aortic valve and aortic disease [93,111,142].

*8.3. Surgery in Special Population*

The Ross procedure with Pulmonary Autograft (PA) is a valuable option for treating bicuspid aortopathy in young or middle-aged patients. PA implanted in an aortic position offers a lasting solution, especially in pregnant women [123,130,143–152]. Patients who underwent the Ross operation disclosed a retrieval of normal life expectancy, reaching an excellent quality of life with a low number of valve-related complications [127–130]. The Ross procedure is particularly recommended for women who plan pregnancy because prolonged administration of anticoagulant drugs is not necessary [153–156]. Consequently, the use of PA as a substitute for the diseased aortic valve has a reduced risk of developing valve thrombosis, thromboembolism, and bleeding compared to the use of mechanical valve prosthesis [157,158]. Furthermore, several studies revealed the superiority of the Ross procedure over other surgical options for AVR in the long term [123,143–151,159,160]; nevertheless, ESC/ESCTS does not consider the Ross procedure as a recommendation among surgical options (Class IIb) [93]. Conversely, AHA/ACC guidelines (COR IIb LOE C) recommend using the Ross procedure in patients who require a replacement of the aortic valve [66]. The guidelines support the use of PA in aortic valve and/or aortic root surgery in specific conditions, such as patients no older than 50 years, with non-disabling comorbidity and an aortic stenosis anatomical pattern, and with a small or normal-sized aortic ring. Finally, an experienced surgeon should be involved in the use of pulmonary autograft in young patients with bicuspid aortopathy when AVK anticoagulation is contraindicated or undesirable. We are unaware of any randomized studies comparing the use of Ross operation with cryopreserved aortic homograft for infectious BAV and it is unlikely that such a study will be conducted. Therefore, the current recommendation for the treatment of endocarditis in patients with BAV is based on observational data. Again, evidence from RCTs is lacking for patients who are suitable to receive surgical treatment for a BAV and asymptomatic for a functional or degenerative disorder of mitral valve but who have severe mitral regurgita-tion without a left ventricular dysfunction or dilation, atrial fibrillation, or pulmonary hy-pertension. These patients should undergo early combined mitro-aortic surgery [160–164] (Figure 13).

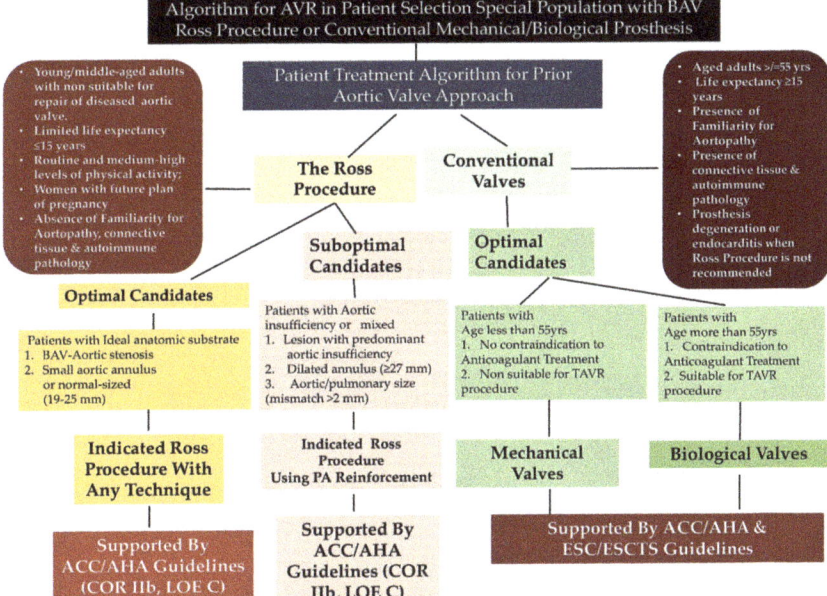

Figure 13. Algorithm for patient special population selection for aortic valve replacement. Ross procedure or conventional mechanical/biological prosthesis may be used according with international guidelines. Abbreviations; ACC, American College of Cardiology; AHA, American Heart Association; BAV, bicuspid aortic valve; COR, class of recommendation; ESCTS, European Society of Cardiothoracic Surgery; ESC, European Society of Cardiology; LOE, level of evidence; TAVR, transthoracic aortic valve replacement.

## 9. Conclusions

BAV remains challenging in everyday clinics. Since patients may present a broad spectrum of anatomy, pathophysiological, clinical, and surgical features, disease classification is complex. A synthetic classification should help elucidate fusion patterns and the geometry of the valve commissures to distinguish valves considered for reparation from valves needing a classical substitution. In the diagnostic field, biophysics may be integrated into regular clinical activity, especially for patients who have no surgical indications but need monitoring to predict the developing enlargement and control risk factors related to dilation velocity.

In the surgical approach, international guidelines focus on the coexistence of the structural pathology and risk factors for aortic dissection and rupture. Therefore, in the new clinical procedures, the alteration of valve structure and aortic enlargement should be considered two aspects of the same disease.

**Author Contributions:** Conceptualization, F.N.; methodology, F.N., O.G., M.L. and M.G.; software, M.G., C.C., A.N. and P.N.; validation, F.N. and O.G.; formal analysis, F.N., O.G., M.L. and M.G.; investigation, F.N, O.G., C.C., A.N. and P.N.; data curation, F.N., O.G., M.L., A.N. and J.R.; writing—original draft preparation, F.N.; writing—review and editing, F.N., O.G., M.G. and A.N.; visualization, F.N., J.R., C.S. and M.C.; supervision, F.N., J.R., C.S. and M.C. All authors have read and agreed to the published version of the manuscript.

**Funding:** This research received no external funding.

**Institutional Review Board Statement:** Not applicable.

**Informed Consent Statement:** Not applicable.

**Data Availability Statement:** Not applicable.

**Conflicts of Interest:** The authors declare no conflict of interest.

## Abbreviations

| | |
|---|---|
| ATA | Ascending thoracic aorta |
| ACTA | Alfa actine |
| AS | Aortic stenosis |
| AR | Aortic regurgitation |
| AV | Aortic valve |
| AVK | Anti-vitamin K |
| AVR | Aortic valve replacement |
| AXIN | gene encodes a cytoplasmic protein, which contains a regulation of G-protein signaling (RGS) domain and a disheveled and axin (DIX) domain |
| BAV | Bicuspid aortic valve |
| CABG | Coronary artery bypass grafting |
| CCT | Cardiac computed tomography |
| CineMR | Cine magnetic resonance |
| CMR 4D-flow | Time-resolved three-dimensional phase-contrast cardiovascular magnetic resonance |
| COR | Class of recommendation |
| CT | Computed tomography |
| DA | Descending aorta |
| E | Young's elastic module |
| EMT | Epithelial–mesenchymal transition |
| EndMT | Endothelial–mesenchymal transition |
| ENG | Endoglin |
| eNOS | Endothelium-derived nitric oxide synthetase |
| Erb | Tyrosine kinase receptor |
| FBN 1 | Fibrillin 1 |

| | |
|---|---|
| FJA | flow jet angle |
| GATA | sequence for transcription factors for zinc proteins' binding DNA sequence |
| IPRF | In-plane rotational flow |
| LOE | Level of evidence |
| LVOT | Left ventricular outflow tract |
| MAPK | Mitogen-activated protein kinase |
| miRNA | Micro-RNA |
| MMP | Metalloproteinases |
| MR | Magnetic resonance |
| MRI | Magnetic resonance Imaging |
| NFD | normalized flow displacement |
| NOTCH1 | gene encoding transmembrane proteins |
| NOS3 | nitric oxide synthase 3 |
| PA | pulmonary autograft |
| PDIA2 | Protein disulfide isomerase family A member 2 |
| PECAM | Platelet endothelial cell adhesion molecule |
| PWV | Pulse wave velocity |
| SFRR | systolic flow reversal ratio |
| SMAD 2 | similar mothers against decapentaplegic Drosophila gene 2 |
| SNP | single nucleotide polymorphism |
| STJ | Sinotubular junction |
| TA | Thoracic aorta |
| TAVR | Transcatheter aortic valve replacement |
| TEE | transesophageal echocardiography |
| TGF | Transforming growth factor |
| TIMP | Tissue inhibitor of matrix metalloproteinases |
| TTE | Transthoracic Echocardiography |
| VSMCs | Vascular smooth muscle cells |
| VBR | Virtual Basal Ring |
| WSS | Wall Shear Stress |
| $\Gamma$ | circulation |
| $\omega$ | vorticity |

## References

1. Ward, C. Clinical significance of the bicuspid aortic valve. *Heart* **2000**, *83*, 81–85. [CrossRef]
2. Tzemos, N.; Therrien, J.; Yip, J.; Thanassoulis, G.; Tremblay, S.; Jamorski, M.T.; Webb, G.D.; Siu, S.C. Outcomes in adults with bicuspid aortic valves. *JAMA* **2008**, *300*, 1317–1325. [CrossRef] [PubMed]
3. Tutar, E.; Ekici, F.; Atalay, S.; Nacar, N. The prevalence of bicuspid aortic valve in newborns by echocardiographic screening. *Am. Heart J.* **2005**, *150*, 513–515. [CrossRef] [PubMed]
4. Carro, A.; Teixido-Tura, G.; Evangelista, A. Aortic Dilatation in Bicuspid Aortic Valve Disease. *Rev. Esp. Cardiol.* **2012**, *65*, 977–981. [CrossRef] [PubMed]
5. Fedak, P.; Verma, S.; David, T.E.; Leask, R.; Weisel, R.D.; Butany, J. Clinical and Pathophysiological Implications of a Bicuspid Aortic Valve. *Circulation* **2002**, *106*, 900–904. [CrossRef] [PubMed]
6. Girdauskas, E.; Borger, M.; Secknus, M.-A.; Girdauskas, G.; Kuntze, T. Is aortopathy in bicuspid aortic valve disease a congenital defect or a result of abnormal hemodynamics? A critical reappraisal of a one-sided argument. *Eur. J. Cardio-Thorac. Surg.* **2011**, *39*, 809–814. [CrossRef] [PubMed]
7. Siu, S.C.; Silversides, C.K. Bicuspid aortic valve disease. *J. Am. Coll. Cardiol.* **2010**, *55*, 2789–2800. [CrossRef]
8. Jia, H.; Kang, L.; Ma, Z.; Lu, S.; Huang, B.; Wang, C.; Zou, Y.; Sun, Y. MicroRNAs involve in bicuspid aortic aneurysm: Pathogenesis and biomarkers. *J. Cardiothorac. Surg.* **2021**, *16*, 230. [CrossRef]
9. Nappi, F.; Iervolino, A.; Singh, S.S.A.; Chello, M. MicroRNAs in Valvular Heart Diseases: Biological Regulators, Prognostic Markers and Therapeutical Targets. *Int. J. Mol. Sci.* **2021**, *22*, 12132. [CrossRef]
10. Garg, V.; Muth, A.N.; Ransom, J.F.; Schluterman, M.K.; Barnes, R.; King, I.N.; Grossfeld, P.D.; Srivastava, D. Mutations in NOTCH1 cause aortic valve disease. *Nature* **2005**, *437*, 270–274. [CrossRef]
11. Mohamed, S.A.; Aherrahrou, Z.; Liptau, H.; Erasmi, A.W.; Hagemann, C.; Wrobel, S.; Borzym, K.; Schunkert, H.; Sievers, H.H.; Erdmann, J. Novel missense mutations (p. T596M and p. P1797H) in NOTCH1 in patients with bicuspid aortic valve. *Biochem. Biophys. Res. Commun.* **2006**, *345*, 1460–1465. [CrossRef]
12. Martin, L.; Ramachandran, V.; Cripe, L.H.; Hinton, R.B.; Andelfinger, G.; Tabangin, M.; Shooner, K.; Keddache, M.; Benson, D.W. Evidence in favor of linkage to human chromosomal regions 18q, 5q and 13q for bicuspid aortic valve and associated cardiovascular malformations. *Hum. Genet.* **2007**, *121*, 275–284. [CrossRef]

13. Guo, D.-C.; Pannu, H.; Tran-Fadulu, V.; Papke, C.L.; Yu, R.K.; Avidan, N.; Bourgeois, S.; Estrera, A.L.; Safi, H.J.; Sparks, E.; et al. Mutations in smooth muscle α-actin (ACTA2) lead to thoracic aortic aneurysms and dissections. *Nat. Genet.* **2007**, *39*, 1488–1493. [CrossRef]
14. Higgins, C.B.; Wexler, L. Reversal of dominance of the coronary arterial system in isolated aortic stenosis and bicuspid aortic valve. *Circulation* **1975**, *52*, 292–296. [CrossRef]
15. Hutchins, G.M.; Nazarian, I.H.; Bulkley, B.H. Association of left dominant coronary arterial system with congenital bicuspid aortic valve. *Am. J. Cardiol.* **1978**, *42*, 57–59. [CrossRef]
16. Rashid, A.; Saucedo, J.F.; Hennebry, T.A. Association of Single Coronary Artery and Congenital Bicuspid Aortic Valve with Review of Literature. *J. Interv. Cardiol.* **2005**, *18*, 389–391. [CrossRef]
17. Bartel, D.P. MicroRNAs: Target Recognition and Regulatory Functions. *Cell* **2009**, *136*, 215–233. [CrossRef]
18. Insull, W., Jr. The Pathology of Atherosclerosis: Plaque Development and Plaque Responses to Medical Treatment. *Am. J. Med.* **2009**, *122*, S3–S14. [CrossRef]
19. LeMaire, S.A.; Wang, X.; Wilks, J.A.; Carter, S.A.; Wen, S.; Won, T.; Leonardelli, D.; Anand, G.; Conklin, L.D.; Wang, X.L.; et al. Matrix metalloproteinases in ascending aortic aneurysms: Bicuspid versus trileaflet aortic valves1. *J. Surg. Res.* **2005**, *123*, 40–48. [CrossRef]
20. Wu, J.; Song, H.-F.; Li, S.-H.; Guo, J.; Tsang, K.; Tumiati, L.; Butany, J.; Yau, T.M.; Ouzounian, M.; Fu, S.; et al. Progressive Aortic Dilation Is Regulated by miR-17–Associated miRNAs. *J. Am. Coll. Cardiol.* **2016**, *67*, 2965–2977. [CrossRef]
21. Naito, S.; Petersen, J.; Sequeira-Gross, T.; Neumann, N.; Escobar, J.D.; Zeller, T.; Reichenspurner, H.; Girdauskas, E. Bicuspid aortopathy—Molecular involvement of microRNAs and MMP-TIMP. *Biomarkers* **2020**, *25*, 711–718. [CrossRef] [PubMed]
22. Zhang, H.; Liu, D.; Zhu, S.; Wang, F.; Sun, X.; Yang, S.; Wang, C. Plasma Exosomal Mir-423-5p Is Involved in the Occurrence and Development of Bicuspid Aortopathy via TGF-beta/SMAD2 Pathway. *Front. Physiol.* **2021**, *12*, 759035. [CrossRef] [PubMed]
23. Zheng, R.; Zhu, P.; Gu, J.; Ni, B.; Sun, H.; He, K.; Bian, J.; Shao, Y.; Du, J. Transcription factor Sp2 promotes TGFB-mediated interstitial cell osteogenic differentiation in bicuspid aortic valves through a SMAD-dependent pathway. *Exp. Cell Res.* **2022**, *411*, 112972. [CrossRef] [PubMed]
24. Naito, S.; Sequeira-Gross, T.; Petersen, J.; Detlef, I.; Sachse, M.; Zeller, T.; Reichenspurner, H.; Girdauskas, E. Circulating microRNAs in the prediction of BAV aortopathy: Do the expression patterns correlate between blood and aortic tissue? *Rev. Cardiovasc. Med.* **2022**, *23*, 47. [CrossRef]
25. Albinsson, S.; Della Corte, A.; Alajbegovic, A.; Krawczyk, K.K.; Bancone, C.; Galderisi, U.; Cipollaro, M.; De Feo, M.; Forte, A. Patients with bicuspid and tricuspid aortic valve exhibit distinct regional microrna signatures in mildly dilated ascending aorta. *Heart Vessel.* **2017**, *32*, 750–767. [CrossRef]
26. Borghini, A.; Foffa, I.; Pulignani, S.; Vecoli, C.; Ait-Ali, L.; Andreassi, M.G. miRNome Profiling in Bicuspid Aortic Valve-Associated Aortopathy by Next-Generation Sequencing. *Int. J. Mol. Sci.* **2017**, *18*, 2498. [CrossRef]
27. Martínez-Micaelo, N.; Beltrán-Debón, R.; Aragonès, G.; Faiges, M.; Alegret, J.M. MicroRNAs Clustered within the 14q32 Locus Are Associated with Endothelial Damage and Microparticle Secretion in Bicuspid Aortic Valve Disease. *Front. Physiol.* **2017**, *8*, 648. [CrossRef]
28. Maleki, S.; Cottrill, K.A.; Poujade, F.-A.; Bhattachariya, A.; Bergman, O.; Gådin, J.R.; Simon, N.; Lundströmer, K.; Franco-Cereceda, A.; Björck, H.M.; et al. The mir-200 family regulates key pathogenic events in ascending aortas of individuals with bicuspid aortic valves. *J. Intern. Med.* **2019**, *285*, 102–114. [CrossRef]
29. Martínez-Micaelo, N.; Beltrán-Debón, R.; Baiges, I.; Faiges, M.; Alegret, J.M. Specific circulating microRNA signature of bicuspid aortic valve disease. *J. Transl. Med.* **2017**, *15*, 76. [CrossRef]
30. Gallo, A.; Agnese, V.; Coronnello, C.; Raffa, G.M.; Bellavia, D.; Conaldi, P.G.; Pilato, M.; Pasta, S. On the prospect of serum exosomal miRNA profiling and protein biomarkers for the diagnosis of ascending aortic dilatation in patients with bicuspid and tricuspid aortic valve. *Int. J. Cardiol.* **2018**, *273*, 230–236. [CrossRef]
31. Giusti, B.; Sticchi, E.; De Cario, R.; Magi, A.; Nistri, S.; Pepe, G. Genetic Bases of Bicuspid Aortic Valve: The Contribution of Traditional and High-Throughput Sequencing Approaches on Research and Diagnosis. *Front. Physiol.* **2017**, *8*, 612. [CrossRef]
32. Alonso-Montes, C.; Martín, M.; Martínez-Arias, L.; Coto, E.; Naves-Díaz, M.; Morís, C.; Cannata-Andía, J.B.; Rodríguez, I. Variants in cardiac GATA genes associated with bicuspid aortic valve. *Eur. J. Clin. Investig.* **2018**, *48*, e13027. [CrossRef]
33. Hill, J.C.; Billaud, M.; Richards, T.D.; Kotlarczyk, M.P.; Shiva, S.; Phillippi, J.A.; Gleason, T.G. Layer-specific Nos3 expression and genotypic distribution in bicuspid aortic valve aortopathy. *Eur. J. Cardio-Thorac. Surg.* **2022**, ezac237. [CrossRef]
34. Wooten, E.C.; Iyer, L.K.; Montefusco, M.C.; Hedgepeth, A.K.; Payne, D.D.; Kapur, N.K.; Housman, D.E.; Mendelsohn, M.E.; Huggins, G.S. Application of gene network analysis techniques identifies AXIN1/PDIA2 and endoglin haplotypes associated with bicuspid aortic valve. *PLoS ONE* **2010**, *5*, e8830. [CrossRef]
35. Fulmer, D.; Toomer, K.; Guo, L.; Moore, K.; Glover, J.; Moore, R.; Stairley, R.; Lobo, G.; Zuo, X.; Dang, Y.; et al. Defects in the Exocyst-Cilia Machinery Cause Bicuspid Aortic Valve Disease and Aortic Stenosis. *Circulation* **2019**, *140*, 1331–1341. [CrossRef]
36. Roberts, W.C. The congenitally bicuspid aortic valve. A study of 85 autopsy cases. *Am. J. Cardiol.* **1970**, *26*, 72–83. [CrossRef]
37. Michelena, H.I.; Della Corte, A.; Evangelista, A.; Maleszewski, J.J.; Edwards, W.D.; Roman, M.J.; Devereux, R.B.; Fernández, B.; Asch, F.M.; Barker, A.J.; et al. International consensus statement on nomenclature and classification of the congenital bicuspid aortic valve and its aortopathy, for clinical, surgical, interventional and research purposes. *Eur. J. Cardiothorac. Surg.* **2021**, *60*, 448–476. [CrossRef]

48. Brandenburg, R.O.; Tajik, A.J.; Edwards, W.D.; Reeder, G.S.; Shub, C.; Seward, J.B. Accuracy of 2-dimensional echocardiographic diagnosis of congenitally bicuspid aortic valve: Echocardiographic-anatomic correlation in 115 patients. *Am. J. Cardiol.* **1983**, *51*, 1469–1473. [CrossRef]
49. Angelini, A.; Ho, S.Y.; Anderson, R.H.; Devine, W.A.; Zuberbuhler, J.R.; Becker, A.E.; Davies, M.J. The morphology of the normal aortic valve as compared with the aortic valve having two leaflets. *J. Thorac. Cardiovasc. Surg.* **1989**, *98*, 362–367. [CrossRef]
50. Sabet, H.Y.; Edwards, W.D.; Tazelaar, H.D.; Daly, R.C. Congenitally Bicuspid Aortic Valves: A Surgical Pathology Study of 542 Cases (1991 Through 1996) and a Literature Review of 2,715 Additional Cases. *Mayo Clin. Proc.* **1999**, *74*, 14–26. [CrossRef]
51. Sievers, H.-H.; Schmidtke, C. A classification system for the bicuspid aortic valve from 304 surgical specimens. *J. Thorac. Cardiovasc. Surg.* **2007**, *133*, 1226–1233. [CrossRef]
52. Schaefer, B.M.; Lewin, M.B.; Stout, K.K.; Gill, E.; Prueitt, A.; Byers, P.H.; Otto, C.M. The bicuspid aortic valve: An integrated phenotypic classification of leaflet morphology and aortic root shape. *Heart* **2008**, *94*, 1634–1638. [CrossRef]
53. Kang, J.-W.; Song, H.G.; Yang, D.H.; Baek, S.; Kim, D.-H.; Song, J.-M.; Kang, D.-H.; Lim, T.-H.; Song, J.-K. Association Between Bicuspid Aortic Valve Phenotype and Patterns of Valvular Dysfunction and Bicuspid Aortopathy: Comprehensive Evaluation Using MDCT and Echocardiography. *JACC Cardiovasc. Imaging* **2013**, *6*, 150–161. [CrossRef]
54. Michelena, H.I.; Prakash, S.K.; Della Corte, A.; Bissell, M.M.; Anavekar, N.; Mathieu, P.; Bossé, Y.; Limongelli, G.; Bossone, E.; Benson, D.W.; et al. Bicuspid aortic valve: Identifying knowledge gaps and rising to the challenge from the International Bicuspid Aortic Valve Consortium (BAVCon). *Circulation* **2014**, *129*, 2691–2704. [CrossRef]
55. Jilaihawi, H.; Chen, M.; Webb, J.; Himbert, D.; Ruiz, C.E.; Rodés-Cabau, J.; Pache, G.; Colombo, A.; Nickenig, G.; Lee, M.; et al. A Bicuspid Aortic Valve Imaging Classification for the TAVR Era. *JACC Cardiovasc. Imaging* **2016**, *9*, 1145–1158. [CrossRef]
56. Sun, B.J.; Lee, S.; Jang, J.Y.; Kwon, O.; Bae, J.S.; Lee, J.H.; Kim, D.-H.; Jung, S.-H.; Song, J.-M.; Kang, D.-H.; et al. Performance of a Simplified Dichotomous Phenotypic Classification of Bicuspid Aortic Valve to Predict Type of Valvulopathy and Combined Aortopathy. *J. Am. Soc. Echocardiogr.* **2017**, *30*, 1152–1161. [CrossRef]
57. Murphy, I.G.; Collins, J.; Powell, A.; Markl, M.; McCarthy, P.; Malaisrie, S.C.; Carr, J.C.; Barker, A.J. Comprehensive 4-stage categorization of bicuspid aortic valve leaflet morphology by cardiac MRI in 386 patients. *Int. J. Cardiovasc. Imaging* **2017**, *33*, 1213–1221. [CrossRef]
58. Bernard, C.; Morgant, M.C.; Guillier, D.; Cheynel, N.; Bouchot, O. Point on the Aortic Bicuspid Valve. *Life* **2022**, *12*, 518. [CrossRef]
59. Groenendijk, B.C.; Hierck, B.P.; Gittenberger-De Groot, A.C.; Poelmann, R.E. Development-related changes in the expression of shear stress responsive genes KLF-2, ET-1, and NOS-3 in the developing cardiovascular system of chicken embryos. *Dev. Dyn.* **2004**, *230*, 57–68. [CrossRef]
60. Noiri, E.; Lee, E.; Testa, J.; Quigley, J.; Colflesh, D.; Keese, C.R.; Giaever, I.; Goligorsky, M.S. Podokinesis in endothelial cell migration: Role of nitric oxide. *Am. J. Physiol. Physiol.* **1998**, *274*, C236–C244. [CrossRef]
61. Fernández, B.; Durán, A.C.; Fernández-Gallego, T.; Fernández, M.C.; Such, M.; Arqué, J.M.; Sans-Coma, V. Bicuspid Aortic Valves with Different Spatial Orientations of the Leaflets Are Distinct Etiological Entities. *J. Am. Coll. Cardiol.* **2009**, *54*, 2312–2318. [CrossRef]
62. Fernández, B.; Soto-Navarrete, M.T.; López-García, A.; López-Unzu, M.; Durán, A.C.; Fernández, M.C. Bicuspid Aortic Valve in 2 Model Species and Review of the Literature. *Veter. Pathol.* **2020**, *57*, 321–331. [CrossRef] [PubMed]
63. Phillips, H.M.; Mahendran, P.; Singh, E.; Anderson, R.H.; Chaudhry, B.; Henderson, D.J. Neural crest cells are required for correct positioning of the developing outflow cushions and pattern the arterial valve leaflets. *Cardiovasc. Res.* **2013**, *99*, 452–460. [CrossRef] [PubMed]
64. Sans-Coma, V.; Fernández, B.; Durán, A.C.; Thiene, G.; Arqué, J.M.; Muñoz-Chápuli, R.; Cardo, M. Fusion of valve cushions as a key factor in the formation of congenital bicuspid aortic valves in Syrian hamsters. *Anat. Rec.* **1996**, *244*, 490–498. [CrossRef]
65. Soto-Navarrete, M.T.; López-Unzu, M.; Durán, A.C.; Fernández, B. Embryonic development of bicuspid aortic valves. *Prog. Cardiovasc. Dis.* **2020**, *63*, 407–418. [CrossRef]
66. Evangelista, A.; Gallego, P.; Calvo-Iglesias, F.; Bermejo, J.; Robledo-Carmona, J.; Sánchez, V.; Saura, D.; Arnold, R.; Carro, A.; Maldonado, G.; et al. Anatomical and clinical predictors of valve dysfunction and aortic dilation in bicuspid aortic valve disease. *Heart* **2018**, *104*, 566–573. [CrossRef]
67. Kong, W.K.F.; Delgado, V.; Poh, K.K.; Regeer, M.V.; Ng, A.C.; McCormack, L.; Yeo, T.C.; Shanks, M.; Parent, S.; Enache, R.; et al. Prognostic Implications of Raphe in Bicuspid Aortic Valve Anatomy. *JAMA Cardiol.* **2017**, *2*, 285–292. [CrossRef]
68. Kong, W.K.F.; Regeer, M.V.; Poh, K.K.; Yip, J.W.; van Rosendael, P.; Yeo, T.C.; Tay, E.; Kamperidis, V.; Van Der Velde, E.T.; Mertens, B.; et al. Inter-ethnic differences in valve morphology, valvular dysfunction, and aortopathy between Asian and European patients with bicuspid aortic valve. *Eur. Heart J.* **2018**, *39*, 1308–1313. [CrossRef]
69. Niaz, T.; Poterucha, J.T.; Olson, T.M.; Johnson, J.N.; Craviari, C.; Nienaber, T.; Palfreeman, J.; Cetta, F.; Hagler, D.J. Characteristic Morphologies of the Bicuspid Aortic Valve in Patients with Genetic Syndromes. *J. Am. Soc. Echocardiogr.* **2018**, *31*, 194–200. [CrossRef]
70. Sun, B.J.; Jin, X.; Song, J.-K.; Lee, S.; Lee, J.H.; Park, J.-B.; Lee, S.-P.; Kim, D.-H.; Park, S.-J.; Kim, Y.-J.; et al. Clinical Characteristics of Korean Patients with Bicuspid Aortic Valve Who Underwent Aortic Valve Surgery. *Korean Circ. J.* **2018**, *48*, 48–58. [CrossRef]
71. Yang, L.T.; Pellikka, P.A.; Enriquez-Sarano, M.; Maalouf, J.F.; Scott, C.G.; Michelena, H.I. Stage B Aortic Regurgitation in Bicuspid Aortic Valve: New Observations on Progression Rate and Predictors. *JACC Cardiovasc. Imaging* **2020**, *13*, 1442–1445. [CrossRef]

62. Fernandes, S.M.; Khairy, P.; Sanders, S.P.; Colan, S.D. Bicuspid Aortic Valve Morphology and Interventions in the Young. *J. Am. Coll. Cardiol.* **2007**, *49*, 2211–2214. [CrossRef]
63. Fernandes, S.M.; Sanders, S.P.; Khairy, P.; Jenkins, K.J.; Gauvreau, K.; Lang, P.; Simonds, H.; Colan, S.D. Morphology of bicuspid aortic valve in children and adolescents. *J. Am. Coll. Cardiol.* **2004**, *44*, 1648–1651. [CrossRef]
64. Michelena, H.I.; Della Corte, A.; Evangelista, A.; Maleszewski, J.J.; Enriquez-Sarano, M.; Bax, J.J.; Otto, C.M.; Schäfers, H.-J Speaking a common language: Introduction to a standard terminology for the bicuspid aortic valve and its aortopathy. *Prog. Cardiovasc. Dis.* **2020**, *63*, 419–424. [CrossRef]
65. Sperling, J.S.; Lubat, E. Forme fruste or 'Incomplete' bicuspid aortic valves with very small raphes: The prevalence of bicuspid valve and its significance may be underestimated. *Int. J. Cardiol.* **2015**, *184*, 1–5. [CrossRef]
66. American College of Cardiology Foundation Appropriate Use Criteria Task Force; American Society of Echocardiography; American Heart Association; American Society of Nuclear Cardiology; Heart Failure Society of America; Heart Rhythm Society; Society for Cardiovascular Angiography and Interventions; Society of Critical Care Medicine; Society of Cardiovascular Computed Tomography; Society for Cardiovascular Magnetic Resonance; et al. ACCF/ASE/AHA/ASNC/HFSA/HRS/SCAI/SCCM/SCCT/SCMR 2011 Appropriate Use Criteria for Echocardiography. A Report of the American College of Cardiology Foundation Appropriate Use Criteria Task Force, American Society of Echocardiography, American Heart Association, American Society of Nuclear Cardiology, Heart Failure Society of America, Heart Rhythm Society, Society for Cardiovascular Angiography and Interventions, Society of Critical Care Medicine, Society of Cardiovascular Computed Tomography, Society for Cardiovascular Magnetic Resonance American College of Chest Physicians. *J. Am. Soc. Echocardiogr.* **2011**, *24*, 229–267.
67. Guala, A.; Rodriguez-Palomares, J.; Galian-Gay, L.; Teixido-Tura, G.; Johnson, K.M.; Wieben, O.; Avilés, A.S.; Evangelista, A. Partial Aortic Valve Leaflet Fusion Is Related to Deleterious Alteration of Proximal Aorta Hemodynamics. *Circulation* **2019**, *139*, 2707–2709. [CrossRef]
68. Michelena, H.I.; Yang, L.-T.; Enriquez-Sarano, M.; Pochettino, A. The elusive 'forme fruste' bicuspid aortic valve: 3D transoesophageal echocardiography to the rescue. *Eur. Heart J. Cardiovasc. Imaging* **2020**, *21*, 1169. [CrossRef]
69. Borger, M.A.; Fedak, P.W.; Stephens, E.H.; Gleason, T.G.; Girdauskas, E.; Ikonomidis, J.S.; Khoynezhad, A.; Siu, S.C.; Verma, S.; Hope, M.D.; et al. The American Association for Thoracic Surgery consensus guidelines on bicuspid aortic valve–related aortopathy: Full online-only version. *J. Thorac. Cardiovasc. Surg.* **2018**, *156*, e41–e74. [CrossRef]
70. Aicher, D.; Kunihara, T.; Issa, O.A.; Brittner, B.; Gräber, S.; Schäfers, H.-J. Valve Configuration Determines Long-Term Results After Repair of the Bicuspid Aortic Valve. *Circulation* **2011**, *123*, 178–185. [CrossRef]
71. Jahanyar, J.; de Kerchove, L.; El Khoury, G. Bicuspid aortic valve repair: The 180 degrees -Reimplantation technique. *Ann. Cardiothorac. Surg.* **2022**, *11*, 473–481. [CrossRef]
72. Ikonomidis, J.S.; Ruddy, J.M.; Benton, S.M.; Arroyo, J.; Brinsa, T.A.; Stroud, R.E.; Zeeshan, A.; Bavaria, J.E.; Gorman, J.H.; Gorman, R.C.; et al. Aortic Dilatation with Bicuspid Aortic Valves: Cusp Fusion Correlates to Matrix Metalloproteinases and Inhibitors. *Ann. Thorac. Surg.* **2012**, *93*, 457–463. [CrossRef] [PubMed]
73. Tadros, T.M.; Klein, M.D.; Shapira, O.M. Ascending aortic dilatation associated with bicuspid aortic valve: Pathophysiology, molecular biology, and clinical implications. *Circulation* **2009**, *119*, 880–890. [CrossRef] [PubMed]
74. Verma, S.; Siu, S.C. Aortic Dilatation in Patients with Bicuspid Aortic Valve. *New Engl. J. Med.* **2014**, *370*, 1920–1929. [CrossRef] [PubMed]
75. Rodríguez-Palomares, J.F.; Dux-Santoy, L.; Guala, A.; Kale, R.; Maldonado, G.; Teixidó-Turà, G.; Galian, L.; Huguet, M.; Valente, F.; Gutiérrez, L.; et al. Aortic flow patterns and wall shear stress maps by 4D-flow cardiovascular magnetic resonance in the assessment of aortic dilatation in bicuspid aortic valve disease. *J. Cardiovasc. Magn. Reson.* **2018**, *20*, 28. [CrossRef] [PubMed]
76. Barker, A.J.; Markl, M.; Bürk, J.; Lorenz, R.; Bock, J.; Bauer, S.; Schulz-Menger, J.; von Knobelsdorff-Brenkenhoff, F. Bicuspid Aortic Valve Is Associated with Altered Wall Shear Stress in the Ascending Aorta. *Circ. Cardiovasc. Imaging* **2012**, *5*, 457–466. [CrossRef] [PubMed]
77. Pepe, G.; Nistri, S.; Giusti, B.; Sticchi, E.; Attanasio, M.; Porciani, C.; Abbate, R.; Bonow, R.O.; Yacoub, M.; Gensini, G.F. Identification of fibrillin 1 gene mutations in patients with bicuspid aortic valve (BAV) without Marfan syndrome. *BMC Med. Genet.* **2014**, *15*, 23. [CrossRef] [PubMed]
78. Fazel, S.S.; Mallidi, H.R.; Lee, R.S.; Sheehan, M.P.; Liang, D.; Fleischmann, D.; Herfkens, R.; Mitchell, R.S.; Miller, D.C. The aortopathy of bicuspid aortic valve disease has distinctive patterns and usually involves the transverse aortic arch. *J. Thorac. Cardiovasc. Surg.* **2008**, *135*, 901–907.e2. [CrossRef]
79. Girdauskas, E.; Disha, K.; Rouman, M.; Espinoza, A.; Borger, M.; Kuntze, T. Aortic events after isolated aortic valve replacement for bicuspid aortic valve root phenotype: Echocardiographic follow-up study. *Eur. J. Cardio-Thorac. Surg.* **2015**, *48*, e71–e76. [CrossRef]
80. Forte, A.; Yin, X.; Fava, M.; Bancone, C.; Cipollaro, M.; De Feo, M.; Mayr, M.; Jahangiri, M.; Della Corte, A. Locally different proteome in aortas from patients with stenotic tricuspid and bicuspid aortic valvesdagger. *Eur. J. Cardiothorac. Surg.* **2019**, *56*, 458–469. [CrossRef]
81. Guzzardi, D.G.; Barker, A.J.; Van Ooij, P.; Malaisrie, S.C.; Puthumana, J.J.; Belke, D.D.; Mewhort, H.E.; Svystonyuk, D.A.; Kang, S.; Verma, S.; et al. Valve-Related Hemodynamics Mediate Human Bicuspid Aortopathy: Insights from Wall Shear Stress Mapping. *J. Am. Coll. Cardiol.* **2015**, *66*, 892–900. [CrossRef]

82. Sigovan, M.; Hope, M.D.; Dyverfeldt, P.; Saloner, D. Comparison of four-dimensional flow parameters for quantification of flow eccentricity in the ascending aorta. *J. Magn. Reson. Imaging* **2011**, *34*, 1226–1230. [CrossRef]
83. Hess, A.T.; Bissell, M.M.; Glaze, S.J.; Pitcher, A.; Myerson, S.; Neubauer, S.; Robson, M.D. Evaluation of Circulation, Γ, as a quantifying metric in 4D flow MRI. *J. Cardiovasc. Magn. Reson.* **2013**, *15*, E36. [CrossRef]
84. Bensalah, M.Z.; Bollache, E.; Kachenoura, N.; Giron, A.; De Cesare, A.; Macron, L.; Lefort, M.; Redheuill, A.; Mousseaux, E. Geometry is a major determinant of flow reversal in proximal aorta. *Am. J. Physiol. Circ. Physiol.* **2014**, *306*, H1408–H1416. [CrossRef]
85. Ayad, R.F.; Grayburn, P.A.; Ko, J.M.; Filardo, G.; Roberts, W.C. Accuracy of Two-Dimensional Echocardiography in Determining Aortic Valve Structure in Patients > 50 Years of Age Having Aortic Valve Replacement for Aortic Stenosis. *Am. J. Cardiol.* **2011**, *108*, 1589–1599. [CrossRef]
86. Michelena, H.I.; Chandrasekaran, K.; Topilsky, Y.; Messika-Zeitoun, D.; Della Corte, A.; Evangelista, A.; Schäfers, H.-J.; Enriquez-Sarano, M. The Bicuspid Aortic Valve Condition: The Critical Role of Echocardiography and the Case for a Standard Nomenclature Consensus. *Prog. Cardiovasc. Dis.* **2018**, *61*, 404–415. [CrossRef]
87. Michelena, H.I.; Khanna, A.D.; Mahoney, D.; Margaryan, E.; Topilsky, Y.; Suri, R.M.; Eidem, B.; Edwards, W.D.; Sundt, T.M.; Enriquez-Sarano, M. Incidence of Aortic Complications in Patients with Bicuspid Aortic Valves. *JAMA* **2011**, *306*, 1104–1112. [CrossRef]
88. Ugur, M.; Schaff, H.V.; Suri, R.M.; Dearani, J.A.; Joyce, L.D.; Greason, K.L.; Connolly, H.M. Late Outcome of Noncoronary Sinus Replacement in Patients with Bicuspid Aortic Valves and Aortopathy. *Ann. Thorac. Surg.* **2014**, *97*, 1242–1246. [CrossRef]
89. Robicsek, F.; Thubrikar, M.J.; Cook, J.W.; Fowler, B. The congenitally bicuspid aortic valve: How does it function? Why does it fail? *Ann. Thorac. Surg.* **2004**, *77*, 177–185. [CrossRef]
90. Nishimura, R.A.; Otto, C.M.; Bonow, R.O.; Carabello, B.A.; Erwin, J.P., 3rd; Fleisher, L.A.; Jneid, H.; Mack, M.J.; McLeod, C.J.; O'Gara, P.T.; et al. 2017 AHA/ACC Focused Update of the 2014 AHA/ACC Guideline for the Management of Patients with Valvular Heart Disease: A Report of the American College of Cardiology/American Heart Association Task Force on Clinical Practice Guidelines. *Circulation* **2017**, *135*, e1159–e1195. [CrossRef]
91. Niaz, T.; Poterucha, J.T.; Johnson, J.N.; Craviari, C.; Nienaber, T.; Palfreeman, J.; Cetta, F.; Hagler, D.J. Incidence, morphology, and progression of bicuspid aortic valve in pediatric and young adult subjects with coexisting congenital heart defects. *Congenit. Heart Dis.* **2017**, *12*, 261–269. [CrossRef]
92. Park, J.Y.; Foley, T.A.; Bonnichsen, C.R.; Maurer, M.J.; Goergen, K.M.; Nkomo, V.T.; Enriquez-Sarano, M.; Williamson, E.E.; Michelena, H.I. Transthoracic Echocardiography versus Computed Tomography for Ascending Aortic Measurements in Patients with Bicuspid Aortic Valve. *J. Am. Soc. Echocardiogr.* **2017**, *30*, 625–635. [CrossRef] [PubMed]
93. Beyersdorf, F.; Vahanian, A.; Milojevic, M.; Praz, F.; Baldus, S.; Bauersachs, J.; Capodanno, D.; Conradi, L.; De Bonis, M.; De Paulis, R.; et al. 2021 ESC/EACTS Guidelines for the management of valvular heart disease. *Eur. J. Cardio-Thorac. Surg.* **2021**, *60*, 727–800. [CrossRef] [PubMed]
94. Francone, M.; Budde, R.P.; Bremerich, J.; Dacher, J.N.; Loewe, C.; Wolf, F.; Natale, L.; Pontone, G.; Redheuil, A.; Vliegenthart, R.; et al. CT and MR imaging prior to transcatheter aortic valve implantation: Standardisation of scanning protocols, measurements and reporting-a consensus document by the European Society of Cardiovascular Radiology (ESCR). *Eur. Radiol.* **2020**, *30*, 2627–2650. [CrossRef] [PubMed]
95. Amoretti, F.; Cerillo, A.G.; Mariani, M.; Stefano, P. A simple method to visualize the bicuspid aortic valve pathology by cardiac computed tomography. *J. Cardiovasc. Comput. Tomogr.* **2020**, *14*, 195–198. [CrossRef] [PubMed]
96. Wang, X.; De Backer, O.; Bieliauskas, G.; Wong, I.; Bajoras, V.; Xiong, T.-Y.; Zhang, Y.; Kofoed, K.F.; Chen, M.; Sondergaard, L. Cusp Symmetry and Coronary Ostial Eccentricity and its Impact on Coronary Access Following TAVR. *JACC Cardiovasc. Interv.* **2022**, *15*, 123–134. [CrossRef]
97. Chirichilli, I.; Irace, F.G.; Weltert, L.P.; Salica, A.; Wolf, L.G.; Fusca, S.; Ricci, A.; De Paulis, R. A direct correlation between commissural orientation and annular shape in bicuspid aortic valves: A new anatomical and computed tomography classification. *Interact. Cardiovasc. Thorac. Surg.* **2020**, *30*, 666–670. [CrossRef] [PubMed]
98. Spath, N.B.; Singh, T.; Papanastasiou, G.; Baker, A.; Janiczek, R.J.; McCann, G.P.; Dweck, M.R.; Kershaw, L.; Newby, D.E.; Semple, S. Assessment of stunned and viable myocardium using manganese-enhanced MRI. *Open Heart* **2021**, *8*, e001646. [CrossRef]
99. Bissell, M.; Hess, A.T.; Biasiolli, L.; Glaze, S.J.; Loudon, M.; Pitcher, A.; Davis, A.; Prendergast, B.; Markl, M.; Barker, A.J.; et al. Aortic dilation in bicuspid aortic valve disease: Flow pattern is a major contributor and differs with valve fusion type. *Circ. Cardiovasc. Imaging* **2013**, *6*, 499–507. [CrossRef]
100. Hope, M.D.; Hope, T.A.; Crook, S.E.; Ordovas, K.G.; Urbania, T.H.; Alley, M.T.; Higgins, C.B. 4D Flow CMR in Assessment of Valve-Related Ascending Aortic Disease. *JACC Cardiovasc. Imaging* **2011**, *4*, 781–787. [CrossRef]
101. Lorenz, R.; Bock, J.; Barker, A.J.; von Knobelsdorff-Brenkenhoff, F.; Wallis, W.; Korvink, J.G.; Bissell, M.M.; Schulz-Menger, J.; Markl, M. 4D flow magnetic resonance imaging in bicuspid aortic valve disease demonstrates altered distribution of aortic blood flow helicity. *Magn. Reson. Med.* **2014**, *71*, 1542–1553. [CrossRef]
102. Meierhofer, C.; Schneider, E.P.; Lyko, C.; Hutter, A.; Martinoff, S.; Markl, M.; Hager, A.; Hess, J.; Stern, H.; Fratz, S. Wall shear stress and flow patterns in the ascending aorta in patients with bicuspid aortic valves differ significantly from tricuspid aortic valves: A prospective study. *Eur. Heart J. Cardiovasc. Imaging* **2013**, *14*, 797–804. [CrossRef]

103. Trinh, B.; Dubin, I.; Rahman, O.; Botelho, M.P.; Naro, N.; Carr, J.C.; Collins, J.D.; Barker, A.J. Aortic Volumetry at Contrast-Enhanced Magnetic Resonance Angiography: Feasibility as a Sensitive Method for Monitoring Bicuspid Aortic Valve Aortopathy. *Investig. Radiol.* **2017**, *52*, 216–222. [CrossRef]
104. Pascaner, A.F.; Houriez–Gombaud-Saintonge, S.; Craiem, D.; Gencer, U.; Casciaro, M.E.; Charpentier, E.; Bouaou, K.; De Cesare, A.; Dietenbeck, T.; Chenoune, Y.; et al. Comprehensive assessment of local and regional aortic stiffness in patients with tricuspid or bicuspid aortic valve aortopathy using magnetic resonance imaging. *Int. J. Cardiol.* **2021**, *326*, 206–212. [CrossRef]
105. Goldstein, S.A.; Evangelista, A.; Abbara, S.; Arai, A.; Asch, F.M.; Badano, L.P.; Bolen, M.A.; Connolly, H.M.; Cuéllar-Calàbria, H.; Czerny, M.; et al. Multimodality imaging of diseases of the thoracic aorta in adults: From the American Society of Echocardiography and the European Association of Cardiovascular Imaging: Endorsed by the Society of Cardiovascular Computed Tomography and Society for Cardiovascular Magnetic Resonance. *J. Am. Soc. Echocardiogr.* **2015**, *28*, 119–182.
106. Keane, M.G.; Wiegers, S.E.; Plappert, T.; Pochettino, A.; Bavaria, J.E.; Sutton, M.G. Bicuspid aortic valves are associated with aortic dilatation out of proportion to coexistent valvular lesions. *Circulation* **2000**, *102*, III35–III39. [CrossRef]
107. Kerstjens-Frederikse, W.S.; Sarvaas, G.J.; Ruiter, J.S.; Van Den Akker, P.C.; Temmerman, A.M.; Van Melle, J.P.; Hofstra, R.M.; Berger, R.M. Left ventricular outflow tract obstruction: Should cardiac screening be offered to first-degree relatives? *Heart* **2011**, *97*, 1228–1232. [CrossRef]
108. Masri, A.; Svensson, L.G.; Griffin, B.P.; Desai, M.Y. Contemporary natural history of bicuspid aortic valve disease: A systematic review. *Heart* **2017**, *103*, 1323–1330. [CrossRef]
109. Hiratzka, L.F.; Bakris, G.L.; Beckman, J.A.; Bersin, R.M.; Carr, V.F.; Casey, D.E., Jr.; Eagle, K.A.; Hermann, L.K.; Isselbacher, E.M.; Kazerooni, E.A.; et al. 2010 ACCF/AHA/AATS/ACR/ASA/SCA/SCAI/SIR/STS/SVM guidelines for the diagnosis and management of patients with thoracic aortic disease: Executive summary. A report of the American College of Cardiology Foundation/American Heart Association Task Force on Practice Guidelines, American Association for Thoracic Surgery, American College of Radiology, American Stroke Association, Society of Cardiovascular Anesthesiologists, Society for Cardiovascular Angiography and Interventions, Society of Interventional Radiology, Society of Thoracic Surgeons, and Society for Vascular Medicine. *Catheter. Cardiovasc. Interv.* **2010**, *76*, E43–E86.
110. MacKay, E.J.; Zhang, B.; Augoustides, J.G.; Groeneveld, P.W.; Desai, N.D. Association of Intraoperative Transesophageal Echocardiography and Clinical Outcomes After Open Cardiac Valve or Proximal Aortic Surgery. *JAMA Netw. Open* **2022**, *5*, e2147820. [CrossRef]
111. Otto, C.M.; Nishimura, R.A.; Bonow, R.O.; Carabello, B.A.; Erwin, J.P., III; Gentile, F.; Jneid, H.; Krieger, E.V.; Mack, M.; McLeod, C.; et al. 2020 ACC/AHA Guideline for the Management of Patients with Valvular Heart Disease: Executive Summary: A Report of the American College of Cardiology/American Heart Association Joint Committee on Clinical Practice Guidelines. *J. Am. Coll. Cardiol.* **2021**, *77*, 450–500. [CrossRef]
112. Van Andel, M.M.; Indrakusuma, R.; Jalalzadeh, H.; Balm, R.; Timmermans, J.; Scholte, A.J.; van den Berg, M.P.; Zwinderman, A.H.; Mulder, B.J.; de Waard, V.; et al. Long-term clinical outcomes of losartan in patients with Marfan syndrome: Follow-up of the multicentre randomized controlled COMPARE trial. *Eur. Heart J.* **2020**, *41*, 4181–4187. [CrossRef] [PubMed]
113. Elefteriades, J.A. Natural history of thoracic aortic aneurysms: Indications for surgery, and surgical versus nonsurgical risks. *Ann. Thorac. Surg.* **2002**, *74*, S1877–S1880. [CrossRef]
114. Beckerman, Z.; Kayatta, M.O.; McPherson, L.; Binongo, J.N.; Lasanajak, Y.; Leshnower, B.G.; Chen, E.P. Bicuspid aortic valve repair in the setting of severe aortic insufficiency. *J. Vis. Surg.* **2018**, *4*, 101. [CrossRef] [PubMed]
115. Borger, M.A.; Preston, M.; Ivanov, J.; Fedak, P.W.; Davierwala, P.; Armstrong, S.; David, T.E. Should the ascending aorta be replaced more frequently in patients with bicuspid aortic valve disease? *J. Thorac. Cardiovasc. Surg.* **2004**, *128*, 677–683. [CrossRef]
116. David, T.E.; Feindel, C.M.; David, C.M.; Manlhiot, C. A quarter of a century of experience with aortic valve-sparing operations. *J. Thorac. Cardiovasc. Surg.* **2014**, *148*, 872–880. [CrossRef]
117. Davies, R.; Kaple, R.K.; Mandapati, D.; Gallo, A.; Botta, D.M.; Elefteriades, J.A.; Coady, M.A. Natural History of Ascending Aortic Aneurysms in the Setting of an Unreplaced Bicuspid Aortic Valve. *Ann. Thorac. Surg.* **2007**, *83*, 1338–1344. [CrossRef]
118. Ergin, M.A.; Spielvogel, D.; Apaydin, A.; Lansman, S.L.; McCullough, J.N.; Galla, J.D.; Griepp, R.B. Surgical treatment of the dilated ascending aorta: When and how? *Ann. Thorac. Surg.* **1999**, *67*, 1834–1839. [CrossRef]
119. Svensson, L.G.; Kim, K.-H.; Lytle, B.W.; Cosgrove, D.M. Relationship of aortic cross-sectional area to height ratio and the risk of aortic dissection in patients with bicuspid aortic valves. *J. Thorac. Cardiovasc. Surg.* **2003**, *126*, 892–893. [CrossRef]
120. Park, C.B.; Greason, K.L.; Suri, R.M.; Michelena, H.I.; Schaff, H.V.; Sundt, T.M. Fate of nonreplaced sinuses of Valsalva in bicuspid aortic valve disease. *J. Thorac. Cardiovasc. Surg.* **2011**, *142*, 278–284. [CrossRef]
121. Schneider, U.; Feldner, S.K.; Hofmann, C.; Schöpe, J.; Wagenpfeil, S.; Giebels, C.; Schäfers, H.-J. Two decades of experience with root remodeling and valve repair for bicuspid aortic valves. *J. Thorac. Cardiovasc. Surg.* **2017**, *153*, S65–S71. [CrossRef]
122. Yasuda, H.; Nakatani, S.; Stugaard, M.; Tsujita-Kuroda, Y.; Bando, K.; Kobayashi, J.; Yamagishi, M.; Kitakaze, M.; Kitamura, S.; Miyatake, K. Failure to Prevent Progressive Dilation of Ascending Aorta by Aortic Valve Replacement in Patients with Bicuspid Aortic Valve: Comparison with Tricuspid Aortic Valve. *Circulation* **2003**, *108* (Suppl. S1), II291–II294. [CrossRef]
123. Mastrobuoni, S.; de Kerchove, L.; Solari, S.; Astarci, P.; Poncelet, A.; Noirhomme, P.; Rubay, J.; El Khoury, G. The Ross procedure in young adults: Over 20 years of experience in our Institution. *Eur. J. Cardio-Thorac. Surg.* **2015**, *49*, 507–513. [CrossRef]

24. De Meester, C.; Vanovershelde, J.L.; Jahanyar, J.; Tamer, S.; Mastrobuoni, S.; Van Dyck, M.; Navarra, E.; Poncelet, A.; Astarci, P.; El Khoury, G.; et al. Long-term durability of bicuspid aortic valve repair: A comparison of 2 annuloplasty techniques. *Eur. J. Cardiothorac. Surg.* **2021**, *60*, 286–294. [CrossRef]
25. Nazer, R.I.; Elhenawy, A.M.; Fazel, S.S.; Garrido-Olivares, L.E.; Armstrong, S.; David, T.E. The Influence of Operative Techniques on the Outcomes of Bicuspid Aortic Valve Disease and Aortic Dilatation. *Ann. Thorac. Surg.* **2010**, *89*, 1918–1924. [CrossRef]
26. Mazine, A.; El-Hamamsy, I.; Verma, S.; Peterson, M.D.; Bonow, R.O.; Yacoub, M.H.; David, T.E.; Bhatt, D.L. Ross Procedure in Adults for Cardiologists and Cardiac Surgeons: JACC State-of-the-Art Review. *J. Am. Coll. Cardiol.* **2018**, *72*, 2761–2777. [CrossRef]
27. Nappi, F.; Nenna, A.; Spadaccio, C.; Chello, M. Pulmonary autograft in aortic position: Is everything known? *Transl. Pediatr.* **2017**, *6*, 11–17. [CrossRef]
28. Nappi, F.; Singh, S.S.A.; Bellomo, F.; Nappi, P.; Iervolino, A.; Acar, C. The Choice of Pulmonary Autograft in Aortic Valve Surgery: A State-of-the-Art Primer. *BioMed. Res. Int.* **2021**, *2021*, 5547342. [CrossRef]
29. Nappi, F.; Spadaccio, C.; Acar, C.; El-Hamamsy, I. Lights and Shadows on the Ross Procedure: Biological Solutions for Biological Problems. *Semin. Thorac. Cardiovasc. Surg.* **2020**, *32*, 815–822. [CrossRef]
30. Nappi, F.; Spadaccio, C.; Chello, M.; Acar, C. The Ross procedure: Underuse or under-comprehension? *J. Thorac. Cardiovasc. Surg.* **2015**, *149*, 1463–1464. [CrossRef]
31. Svensson, L.G.; Kim, K.H.; Blackstone, E.H.; Rajeswaran, J.; Gillinov, A.M.; Mihaljevic, T.; Griffin, B.P.; Grimm, R.; Stewart, W.J.; Hammer, D.F.; et al. Bicuspid aortic valve surgery with proactive ascending aorta repair. *J. Thorac. Cardiovasc. Surg.* **2011**, *142*, 622–629. [CrossRef]
32. Wang, Y.; Yang, J.; Lu, Y.; Fan, W.; Bai, L.; Nie, Z.; Wang, R.; Yu, J.; Liu, L.; Liu, Y.; et al. Thoracic Aorta Diameter Calculation by Artificial Intelligence Can Predict the Degree of Arterial Stiffness. *Front. Cardiovasc. Med.* **2021**, *8*, 737161. [CrossRef]
33. Davies, R.R.; Goldstein, L.J.; Coady, M.A.; Tittle, S.L.; Rizzo, J.A.; Kopf, G.S.; Elefteriades, J.A. Yearly rupture or dissection rates for thoracic aortic aneurysms: Simple prediction based on size. *Ann. Thorac. Surg.* **2002**, *73*, 17–28. [CrossRef]
34. Russo, C.F.; Mazzetti, S.; Garatti, A.; Ribera, E.; Milazzo, A.; Bruschi, G.; Lanfranconi, M.; Colombo, T.; Vitali, E. Aortic complications after bicuspid aortic valve replacement: Long-term results. *Ann. Thorac. Surg.* **2002**, *74*, S1773–S1776. [CrossRef]
35. Girdauskas, E.; Disha, K.; Borger, M.; Kuntze, T. Long-term prognosis of ascending aortic aneurysm after aortic valve replacement for bicuspid versus tricuspid aortic valve stenosis. *J. Thorac. Cardiovasc. Surg.* **2014**, *147*, 276–282. [CrossRef]
36. McKellar, S.H.; Michelena, H.I.; Li, Z.; Schaff, H.V.; Sundt, T.M. Long-Term Risk of Aortic Events Following Aortic Valve Replacement in Patients with Bicuspid Aortic Valves. *Am. J. Cardiol.* **2010**, *106*, 1626–1633. [CrossRef]
37. Boodhwani, M.; Andelfinger, G.; Leipsic, J.; Lindsay, T.; McMurtry, M.S.; Therrien, J.; Siu, S.C. Canadian Cardiovascular Society Position Statement on the Management of Thoracic Aortic Disease. *Can. J. Cardiol.* **2014**, *30*, 577–589. [CrossRef]
38. Pacheco, C.; Mullen, K.A.; Coutinho, T.; Jaffer, S.; Parry, M.; van Spall, H.G.C.; Clavel, M.-A.; Clavel Ma Edwards, J.D.; Sedlak, T.; Norris, C.M.; et al. The Canadian Women's Heart Health Alliance Atlas on the Epidemiology, Diagnosis, and Management of Cardiovascular Disease in Women—Chapter 5: Sex- and Gender-Unique Manifestations of Cardiovascular Disease. *CJC Open* **2022**, *4*, 243–262. [CrossRef]
39. Kanjanahattakij, N.; Horn, B.; Vutthikraivit, W.; Biso, S.M.; Ziccardi, M.R.; Lu, M.L.R.; Rattanawong, P. Comparing outcomes after transcatheter aortic valve replacement in patients with stenotic bicuspid and tricuspid aortic valve: A systematic review and meta-analysis. *Clin. Cardiol.* **2018**, *41*, 896–902. [CrossRef]
40. Makkar, R.R.; Yoon, S.-H.; Leon, M.B.; Chakravarty, T.; Rinaldi, M.; Shah, P.B.; Skipper, E.R.; Thourani, V.H.; Babaliaros, V.; Cheng, W.; et al. Association Between Transcatheter Aortic Valve Replacement for Bicuspid vs Tricuspid Aortic Stenosis and Mortality or Stroke. *JAMA* **2019**, *321*, 2193–2202. [CrossRef]
41. Takagi, H.; Hari, Y.; Kawai, N.; Kuno, T.; Ando, T. Meta-analysis of transcatheter aortic valve implantation for bicuspid versus tricuspid aortic valves. *J. Cardiol.* **2019**, *74*, 40–48. [CrossRef]
42. Biner, S.; Rafique, A.M.; Ray, I.; Cuk, O.; Siegel, R.J.; Tolstrup, K. Aortopathy Is Prevalent in Relatives of Bicuspid Aortic Valve Patients. *J. Am. Coll. Cardiol.* **2009**, *53*, 2288–2295. [CrossRef] [PubMed]
43. David, T.E.; Woo, A.; Armstrong, S.; Maganti, M. When is the Ross operation a good option to treat aortic valve disease? *J. Thorac. Cardiovasc. Surg.* **2010**, *139*, 68–75. [CrossRef] [PubMed]
44. Nappi, F.; Nenna, A.; Larobina, D.; Carotenuto, A.R.; Jarraya, M.; Spadaccio, C.; Fraldi, M.; Chello, M.; Acar, C.; Carrel, T. Simulating the ideal geometrical and biomechanical parameters of the pulmonary autograft to prevent failure in the Ross operation. *Interact. Cardiovasc. Thorac. Surg.* **2018**, *27*, 269–276. [CrossRef] [PubMed]
45. Sievers, H.H.; Stierle, U.; Charitos, E.I.; Takkenberg, J.J.; Hoerer, J.; Lange, R.; Franke, U.; Albert, M.; Gorski, A.; Leyh, R.G.; et al. A multicentre evaluation of the autograft procedure for young patients undergoing aortic valve replacement: Update on the German Ross Registrydagger. *Eur. J. Cardiothorac. Surg.* **2016**, *49*, 212–218. [CrossRef]
46. Sievers, H.-H.; Stierle, U.; Petersen, M.; Klotz, S.; Richardt, D.; Diwoky, M.; Charitos, E.I. Valve performance classification in 630 subcoronary Ross patients over 22 years. *J. Thorac. Cardiovasc. Surg.* **2018**, *156*, 79–86.e2. [CrossRef]
47. Andreas, M.; Seebacher, G.; Reida, E.; Wiedemann, D.; Pees, C.; Rosenhek, R.; Heinze, G.; Moritz, A.; Kocher, A.; Laufer, G. A Single-Center Experience with the Ross Procedure Over 20 Years. *Ann. Thorac. Surg.* **2014**, *97*, 182–188. [CrossRef]
48. Da Costa, F.D.; Takkenberg, J.J.; Fornazari, D.; Balbi Filho, E.M.; Colatusso, C.; Mokhles, M.M.; da Costa, A.B.; Sagrado, A.G.; Ferreira, A.D.; Fernandes, T.; et al. Long-term results of the Ross operation: An 18-year single institutional experience. *Eur. J. Cardiothorac. Surg.* **2014**, *46*, 415–422. [CrossRef]

149. David, T.E.; David, C.; Woo, A.; Manlhiot, C. The Ross procedure: Outcomes at 20 years. *J. Thorac. Cardiovasc. Surg.* **2014**, *147*, 85–94. [CrossRef]
150. Martin, E.; Mohammadi, S.; Jacques, F.; Kalavrouziotis, D.; Voisine, P.; Doyle, D.; Perron, J. Clinical Outcomes Following the Ross Procedure in Adults: A 25-Year Longitudinal Study. *J. Am. Coll. Cardiol.* **2017**, *70*, 1890–1899. [CrossRef]
151. Skillington, P.D.; Mokhles, M.M.; Takkenberg, J.; Larobina, M.; O'Keefe, M.; Wynne, R.; Tatoulis, J. The Ross procedure using autologous support of the pulmonary autograft: Techniques and late results. *J. Thorac. Cardiovasc. Surg.* **2015**, *149*, S46–S52 [CrossRef]
152. Spadaccio, C.; Montagnani, S.; Acar, C.; Nappi, F. Introducing bioresorbable scaffolds into the show. A potential adjunct to resuscitate Ross procedure. *Int. J. Cardiol.* **2015**, *190*, 50–52. [CrossRef]
153. Bouhout, I.; Poirier, N.; Mazine, A.; Dore, A.; Mercier, L.-A.; Leduc, L.; El-Hamamsy, I. Cardiac, Obstetric, and Fetal Outcomes During Pregnancy After Biological or Mechanical Aortic Valve Replacement. *Can. J. Cardiol.* **2014**, *30*, 801–807. [CrossRef]
154. Buratto, E.; Shi, W.Y.; Wynne, R.; Poh, C.L.; Larobina, M.; O'Keefe, M.; Goldblatt, J.; Tatoulis, J.; Skillington, P.D. Improved Survival After the Ross Procedure Compared with Mechanical Aortic Valve Replacement. *J. Am. Coll. Cardiol.* **2018**, *71*, 1337–1344 [CrossRef]
155. Mazine, A.; David, T.; Rao, V.; Hickey, E.; Christie, S.; Manlhiot, C.; Ouzounian, M. Long-term outcomes of the ross procedure versus mechanical aortic valve replacement: A propensity-matched cohort study. *Can. J. Cardiol.* **2016**, *32*, S234–S235. [CrossRef]
156. Steinberg, Z.L.; Dominguez-Islas, C.P.; Otto, C.M.; Stout, K.K.; Krieger, E.V. Maternal and Fetal Outcomes of Anticoagulation in Pregnant Women with Mechanical Heart Valves. *J. Am. Coll. Cardiol.* **2017**, *69*, 2681–2691. [CrossRef]
157. Ikonomidis, J.S.; Kratz, J.M.; Crumbley, A.J., III; Stroud, M.R.; Bradley, S.M.; Sade, R.M.; Crawford, F.A., Jr. Twenty-year experience with the St Jude Medical mechanical valve prosthesis. *J. Thorac. Cardiovasc. Surg.* **2003**, *126*, 2022–2031. [CrossRef]
158. Van Nooten, G.J.; Caes, F.; Francois, K.; Van Bellleghem, Y.; Bové, T.; Vandenplas, G.; Taeymans, Y. Twenty years' single-center experience with mechanical heart valves: A critical review of anticoagulation policy. *J. Heart Valve Dis.* **2012**, *21*, 88–98.
159. Takkenberg, J.J.; Klieverik, L.M.; Schoof, P.H.; van Suylen, R.J.; van Herwerden, L.A.; Zondervan, P.E.; Roos-Hesselink, J.W.; Eijkemans, M.J.; Yacoub, M.H.; Bogers, A.J. The Ross procedure: A systematic review and meta-analysis. *Circulation* **2009**, *119*, 222–228. [CrossRef]
160. El-Hamamsy, I.; Eryigit, Z.; Stevens, L.-M.; Sarang, Z.; George, R.; Clark, L.; Melina, G.; Takkenberg, J.J.; Yacoub, M.H. Long-term outcomes after autograft versus homograft aortic root replacement in adults with aortic valve disease: A randomised controlled trial. *Lancet* **2010**, *376*, 524–531. [CrossRef]
161. Charitos, E.I.; Takkenberg, J.J.; Hanke, T.; Gorski, A.; Botha, C.; Franke, U.; Dodge-Khatami, A.; Hoerer, J.; Lange, R.; Moritz, A.; et al. Reoperations on the pulmonary autograft and pulmonary homograft after the Ross procedure: An update on the German Dutch Ross Registry. *J. Thorac. Cardiovasc. Surg.* **2012**, *144*, 813–823. [CrossRef]
162. Mokhles, M.M.; Rizopoulos, D.; Andrinopoulou, E.R.; Bekkers, J.A.; Roos-Hesselink, J.W.; Lesaffre, E.; Bogers, A.J.; Takkenberg, J.J. Autograft and pulmonary allograft performance in the second post-operative decade after the Ross procedure: Insights from the Rotterdam Prospective Cohort Study. *Eur. Heart J.* **2012**, *33*, 2213–2224. [CrossRef]
163. Nappi, F.; Spadaccio, C.; Fraldi, M. Reply: Papillary Muscle Approximation Is an Anatomically Correct Repair for Ischemic Mitral Regurgitation. *J. Am. Coll. Cardiol.* **2016**, *68*, 1147–1148. [CrossRef]
164. Nappi, F.; Nenna, A.; Petitti, T.; Spadaccio, C.; Gambardella, I.; Lusini, M.; Chello, M.; Acar, C. Long-term outcome of cryopreserved allograft for aortic valve replacement. *J. Thorac. Cardiovasc. Surg.* **2018**, *156*, 1357–1365. [CrossRef]

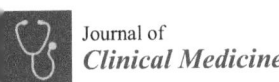 

*Review*

# Tailored Direct Oral Anticoagulation in Patients with Atrial Fibrillation: The Future of Oral Anticoagulation?

Matej Samoš [1,*], Tomáš Bolek [1], Lucia Stančiaková [2], Martin Jozef Péč [1], Kristína Brisudová [1], Ingrid Škorňová [2], Ján Staško [2], Marián Mokáň [1] and Peter Kubisz [2]

1 Department of Internal Medicine I, Jessenius Faculty of Medicine in Martin, Comenius University in Bratislava, 03659 Martin, Slovakia
2 National Centre of Hemostasis and Thrombosis, Department of Hematology and Blood, Transfusion, Jessenius Faculty of Medicine in Martin, Comenius University in Bratislava, 03601 Martin, Slovakia
* Correspondence: matej.samos@gmail.com; Tel.: +421-907-612-943 or +421-43-4203-820

**Abstract:** Direct oral anticoagulants (DOAC) are currently the drug of choice for drug prevention of stroke or systemic embolism in patients with atrial fibrillation (AF). However, repeated ischemic stroke or systemic embolism and bleeding while on DOAC is still a challenging clinical phenomenon in the management of future long-term anticoagulation. It is not known whether tailoring the DOAC therapy to achieve optimal therapeutic drug levels could improve the clinical course of DOAC therapy. To be able to tailor the therapy, it is necessary to have a valid laboratory method for DOAC level assessment, to be aware of factors influencing DOAC levels and to have clinical options to tailor the treatment. Furthermore, the data regarding clinical efficacy/safety of tailored DOAC regimes are still lacking. This article reviews the current data on tailored direct oral anticoagulation in patients with AF.

**Keywords:** direct oral anticoagulants; tailored medicine; DOAC laboratory monitoring; atrial fibrillation; adverse thrombotic and hemorrhagic events

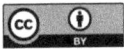

## 1. Introduction

Direct oral anticoagulants (DOAC) (Table 1), drugs directly inhibiting thrombin (dabigatran) or activated coagulation factor X (apixaban, edoxaban and rivaroxaban), are currently the drugs of choice for the pharmacological prevention of stroke or systemic embolism [1] in patients with atrial fibrillation (AF). Thrombosis (ischemic stroke or systemic embolism) and bleeding while on DOAC is still a challenging clinical phenomenon in the management of future long-term anticoagulation. Patients with ischemic stroke on DOAC have a high 90-day mortality (35.1% reported in previous study), with the majority of deaths due to the stroke itself [2]. The unfavorable clinical course can also be seen in DOAC-treated patients who suffer from adverse bleeding. For example, adjusted one-year mortality is significantly higher in patients who suffered from gastric bleeding on DOAC therapy compared with those who did not [3]. In addition, previous studies have demonstrated that these adverse events correlate with in-optimal plasma levels of DOAC [4–6]. The question is whether tailoring the DOAC therapy to achieve optimal therapeutic drug levels could improve the clinical course of DOAC therapy. The aim of this article is to review the current data about tailored direct oral anticoagulation in patients with AF.

**Table 1.** Direct oral anticoagulants: targets, indications, and pharmacology.

| Parameter | Apixaban | Dabigatran | Edoxaban | Rivaroxaban |
|---|---|---|---|---|
| Target | Factor Xa | Thrombin (Factor IIa) | Factor Xa | Factor Xa |
| FDA-approved indications | Nonvalvular AF, VTE (treatment *, secondary prevention, prophylaxis ‡) | Nonvalvular AF, VTE (treatment ‖, secondary prevention, prophylaxis) | Nonvalvular AF, VTE (treatment §) | Nonvalvular AF, VTE (treatment *, secondary prevention, prophylaxis ‡) |
| Safety in nonvalvular AF | Lower risk of major bleeding than with warfarin | Higher risk of GI bleeding than with warfarin | Lower risk of major bleeding than with warfarin; higher risk of GI bleeding (60 mg dose) than with warfarin | Higher risk of GI bleeding than with warfarin |
| Specific reversal agent | Andexanet alpha (specific for all factor Xa inhibitors) | Idarucizumab | Andexanet alpha (specific for all factor Xa inhibitors) | Andexanet alpha (specific for all factor Xa inhibitors) |
| Half-life (hours) | 12 | 8–15 | 10–14 | 7–11 |
| Renal clearance (%) | 25 | 80 | 50 | 33 |
| Dialyzable | No | Yes | No | No |
| Prodrug | No | Yes | No | No |
| Bioavailability (%) | 60 | 6 | 62 | 60–80 |
| Time to peak effect (hours) | 1–2 | 1–3 | 1–2 | 2–4 |
| Gene polymorphism studied | ABCB1 | CES1, ABCB1 | ABCB1, SLCO1B1 | ABCB1 |
| Non-pharmacologic interactions | Age, reduced body weight, reduced GFR (only if two conditions are simultaneously present), probably severe liver damage | Age, reduced GFR (do not use if eGFR < 30 mL/min/1.73 m$^2$) | Reduced GFR (do not use if eGFR < 15 mL/min/1.73 m$^2$), probably severe liver damage | Age (although dose reduction is not recommended), reduced GFR (do not use if eGFR < 15 mL/min/1.73 m$^2$), probably severe liver damage |
| Drug interactions | Avoid apixaban with concomitant use of dual P-gp and moderate CYP 3A4 inhibitors | Dose reduces dabigatran with concomitant P-gp inhibitor, be cautious when gastric acidity reducing drugs are administered | Avoid concomitant use of rifampin; No adjustments for concomitant P-gp inhibitors | Avoid rivaroxaban with concomitant use of dual P-gp and moderate CYP 3A4 inhibitors |

AF—atrial fibrillation; CYP—cytochrome P450; eGFR/GFR—(estimated) glomerular filtration rate, FDA—food and drugs administration; GI—gastrointestinal; P-gp—glycoprotein P; VTE—venous thromboembolism. * Twice daily for the first 21 days of VTE treatment; once daily for other indications for rivaroxaban or twice daily for apixaban. ‡ Approved for VTE prophylaxis after knee or hip surgery only. § Prophylaxis of VTE in adult patients hospitalized for an acute medical illness and for extended use. ‖ After 5–10 days of parental anticoagulant treatment only.

## 2. In-Optimal DOAC Levels and the Risk of Future Adverse Events

As mentioned, currently there are quite convincing data regarding the association between the risk of future adverse events and in-optimal (too low or too high) plasma levels of DOAC in AF patients on long-term DOAC therapy. First, a sub-analysis of the RE–LY trial showed that, in this trial, the occurrence of stroke and adverse bleeding correlated with dabigatran plasma levels. In this trial, on average, individuals who had a major hemorrhagic event had higher trough and post-dose dabigatran levels than individuals who did not experience a bleeding event. In the multivariate analysis of ischemic stroke/systemic embolism, there was an inverse relation between dabigatran trough levels and the probability of an event. Second, Testa et al. reported in their studies [5,6] that bleeding during DOAC therapy was more frequent in AF patients with high peak drug levels [5] and thrombotic events developed in individuals who had low baseline trough drug levels [6]. Third, looking at the drug levels at the time of the bleeding or ischemic event [7,8], patients with a DOAC therapy-related bleeding had significantly higher and patients with a stroke despite taking DOAC had significantly lower DOAC levels at the time of this event compared to individuals tolerating the DOAC therapy without any adverse events. Finally, in a recent observational study performed by Siedler et al. [9] patients who suffered from early ischemic stroke recurrence despite the use of DOAC had low DOAC plasma levels (this was demonstrated for apixaban and dabigatran after propensity score matching). In summary, the current evidence suggests an association between DOAC plasma levels and the risk of future adverse events, and that monitoring the DOAC levels may help to identify patients with increased risk for these events. The following questions should be answered: what method should be used for DOAC laboratory assessment and what are the optimal therapeutic levels for effective and safe DOAC therapy?

## 3. How to Measure DOAC Levels in AF Patients on Long-Term DOAC Therapy?

Although liquid chromatography-mass spectrometry (LC-MS) is still honored as a standard laboratory method for DOAC levels quantification [10–12], especially in the settings of preclinical/clinical research, there is a general consensus that the method is not very useful for the assessment of DOAC levels in routine clinical practice [13], mostly due to its limitations, such as bad availability, the need for specially equipped laboratory with specially skilled staff and time demands. Furthermore, standard coagulation test (prothrombin time, activated partial thromboplastin time, thrombin time) do not have sufficient sensitivity for DOAC levels assessment, especially when low DOAC levels are expected [10,13], and this could probably also be applied to standard reagents of novel viscoelastic hemostatic assays [14]. Therefore, DOAC-specific coagulation assays (ecarin clotting time assay or diluted thrombin time assays for dabigatran, and drug-specific chromogenic anti-Xa assays for apixaban, edoxaban and rivaroxaban) are arguably the most appropriate tests from the currently available laboratory methods for routine DOAC levels assessment (Table 2), as the assays demonstrated good correlation with LC-MS [11,12] and good clinical utility in previous post-marketing studies [15–17]. Nevertheless, the assays could be inaccurate at very low DOAC levels [10], and clinicians should always be aware of the limitations of DOAC laboratory testing when interpreting the results and choosing future strategies [13]. Although preliminary experience with novel thrombin generation assays [18] or novel automated thromboelastography [19] are promising, there is currently no sufficient evidence to recommend the use of these assays to guide clinical decisions in DOAC-treated patients [13].

The next, clinically important but yet not fully answered point is the question of the optimal timing of blood sampling for DOAC levels testing. As the majority of the published studies to date have reported an association between trough (pre-drug dose) and/or peak (post-drug-dose) drug levels with the risk of adverse events, it is quite reasonable to assess both drug levels. Trough drug level should definitely be measured in individuals with severe renal function impairment, with extremely high body weight (body mass index > 40 kg/m$^2$), in those with advanced age (elderly ones), and if a new DOAC-levels-modifying drug interaction is expected [13]. As all commercially available DOAC reach their drug steady-state within the first two days after starting therapy, it is probably reasonable to test DOAC levels on the forth to fifth day after the drug initiation (after five or more intakes), and to repeat the measurement whenever needed (new adverse bleeding or thrombosis, new decrease in renal/hepatic function, new possible drug interaction, questionable patient drug compliance, etc.). However, this recommendation is only based on the data from pharmacokinetic studies and on expert opinion [13], and more research in this area is still warranted.

Table 2. Specific assays for determination of DOAC levels/activity.

| Test | Dabigatran | Rivaroxaban | Apixaban | Edoxaban | Note |
|---|---|---|---|---|---|
| Liquid chromatography-mass spectrometry (LC-MS) | ↑↑↑ | ↑↑↑ | ↑↑↑ | ↑↑↑ | Standard method for preclinical/clinical research, the most accurate method (especially when low levels are expected); limited usefulness in clinical practice |
| Diluted thrombin time assay | ↑↑ | x | x | x | Good correlation with LC-MS, lower accuracy if drug levels are low; good usefulness in clinical research/practice |
| Ecarin clotting time assay | ↑↑ | x | x | x | Good correlation with LC-MS, lower accuracy if drug levels are low; good usefulness in clinical research/practice |
| Drug-specific chromogenic anti-Xa assays | x | ↑↑ | ↑↑ | ↑↑ | Good correlation with LC-MS, lower accuracy if drug levels are low; good usefulness in clinical research/practice |
| Thrombin generation assays | ↑↑ | ↑↑ | ↑↑ | ↑↑ | Promising method, but not validated; usefulness in clinical research |
| Automated thromboelastography with drug-specific reagents | ↑↑ | ↑↑ | ↑↑ | not known/not examined | Promising method, but not validated; usefulness in clinical research |

↑—sensitivity (↑↑—good, ↑↑↑—excellent), x—not sensitive.

## 4. Optimal DOAC Plasma Levels for Long-Term Anticoagulation

Another issue which should be reslved prior to recommending a tailored DOAC strategy is the issue of optimal therapeutic DOAC plasma levels for long-term anticoagulation. Therapeutic drug levels can probably be established, in part, for dabigatran. In the aforementioned sub-analysis of the RE–LY trial [4] which showed a correlation between dabigatran plasma levels and the risk of adverse events, patients with trough dabigatran levels > 210 ng/mL had a two-fold higher risk of dabigatran-related bleeding. Thus, dabigatran plasma level 210 ng/mL can likely be used as the upper limit for safe anticoagulation. Going further, patients with dabigatran trough levels < 28 ng/mL had a two-fold higher risk of adverse thrombosis; therefore, dabigatran plasma levels of at least 28 ng/mL appear to be necessary for efficient anticoagulation. Nevertheless, these levels were established based on the results of a sub-analysis of a single phase III clinical trial, as no other study dealing with this issue is currently available. Testa et al. were not able to establish cut-off limits for the risk of adverse ischemic [6] or bleeding [5] events due to the low patient sample and low rate of adverse events. In our previous studies, which aimed to establish DOAC plasma levels at the time of an adverse event, in dabigatran-treated patients with bleeding, dabigatran levels of 261.4 ± 163.7 ng/mL were determined on average [7]. In patients with embolic stroke, average dabigatran plasma levels of 40.7 ± 36.9 ng/mL were found [8]. This observation probably supports the upper reference range of 210 ng/mL in terms of safety, but questions the lower reference range of 28 ng/mL in terms of efficacy.

This issue remains unexplained for apixaban, edoxaban and rivaroxaban at present. Sakaguchi et al. [20] showed, in their analysis of Japanese rivaroxaban-treated patients with bleeding complications, higher peak rivaroxaban levels (anti-Xa activity), and peak rivaroxaban levels independently predicted bleeding. In another interesting retrospective study, rivaroxaban trough deficiency (defined as trough rivaroxaban levels < 12 ng/mL) was associated with an increased risk of thrombotic events (but not bleeding) in Chinese patients with AF [21]. Additionally, Sin et al. [17] showed, in their prospective study enrolling rivaroxaban-treated AF patients with different stages of chronic kidney disease (Stage 1–3), that rivaroxaban trough levels in those with hemorrhage were higher (59.9 ± 35.6 ng/mL) than in those who were free from a bleeding episode (41.1 ± 29.2 ng/mL; $p < 0.05$). This study enrolled only 92 patients. In our previous analyses [7,8], there were significantly higher rivaroxaban levels at the time of bleeding compared to the trough levels of patients who did not have complications during rivaroxaban administration (245.9 ± 150.2 ng/mL versus 52.5 ± 36.4 ng/mL; $p < 0.001$), and rivaroxaban levels tended to be lower in those experiencing embolic stroke (42.7 ± 31.9 ng/mL); however, the variability in drug plasma levels was the highest in rivaroxaban-treated patients. For apixaban, Limcharoen et al. [22] reported an association between apixaban trough levels and the risk of bleeding. In apixaban-treated patients with bleeding, apixaban trough levels of 139.15 ng/mL were reported. These levels are lower than our previous observation of apixaban levels of 311.8 ± 142.5 ng/mL at the time of a bleeding event [7]. It is interesting that, in the study performed by Limcharoen et al., almost all the patients presented apixaban plasma levels within the expected range, which was defined as a range of 34.0–230.0 ng/mL for trough and 69.0–321.0 ng/mL for peak drug levels [22]. The ranges were derived from a pharmacokinetic study with apixaban [23]. Unfortunately, there is no other study dedicated to the relationship between apixaban plasma levels and the risk of adverse ischemic or bleeding events (except for the previously mentioned ones performed by Testa et al. [5,6]), and no such study for edoxaban.

Summarizing this issue, the determination of optimal DOAC plasma levels for long-term anticoagulation still needs further research (especially for rivaroxaban, apixaban and edoxaban); nevertheless, levels derived from pharmacokinetic studies should probably not be used, as these data report only the expected drug level when a defined dose of the drug is taken, but do not correlate with the risk of bleeding or thrombosis during long-term therapy.

## 5. Factors Influencing DOAC Plasma Levels

When deciding on a tailored DOAC strategy (Figure 1), one should be aware of clinical features/factors that could possibly influence DOAC plasma levels (Table 1). Looking at the currently available data [24], DOAC levels could be changed (increased) in patients with a reduced glomerular filtration rate (to a lesser extent in case of apixaban administration), in elderly individuals (increased, especially when dabigatran is used) [25–27], and there are several relevant drug interactions [28] leading either to a change in gastric pH, which is important for the absorption of dabigatran [29], or to changed P-glycoprotein (P-gp) or cytochrome P450 (CYP) activity, which could, in theory, affect the pharmacokinetics of all the available DOAC (P-gp) or the pharmacokinetics of oral factor Xa inhibitors (CYP) [28]. At present, it is not entirely clear whether extreme body weight (extremely high or extremely low) affects DOAC plasma levels. In their retrospective analysis, Piran et al. [30] reported that most of the patients with body weight over 120 kg had peak plasma levels higher than the median trough level for each of the three DOAC (apixaban, dabigatran, rivaroxaban); but 21% of patients had a peak plasma concentration that was below the usual on-therapy range. On the other side, the authors of another prospective study showed that patients with extreme obesity (mean body mass index 44.4 kg/m$^2$) and AF who were receiving DOAC therapy had DOAC plasma levels, within the expected range [31]. Obesity did not affect the plasma levels of apixaban and rivaroxaban in another prospective study (in patients with venous thromboembolism) [32], and plasma levels of apixaban in a previously published case of morbidly obese patient treated for AF [33]. Data from post-marketing studies regarding the DOAC levels in patients with extremely low body weight are still lacking. In addition, several studies suggested a possible role of genetic polymorphism in several candidate genes (CES1 gene encoding plasmatic esterase for dabigatran; ABCB1 gene encoding P-gp for apixaban, dabigatran, rivaroxaban and edoxaban; and SLCO1B1 gene encoding organic anion transporter protein 1B1 for edoxaban); however, the results of the studies published to date are controversial [34–38].

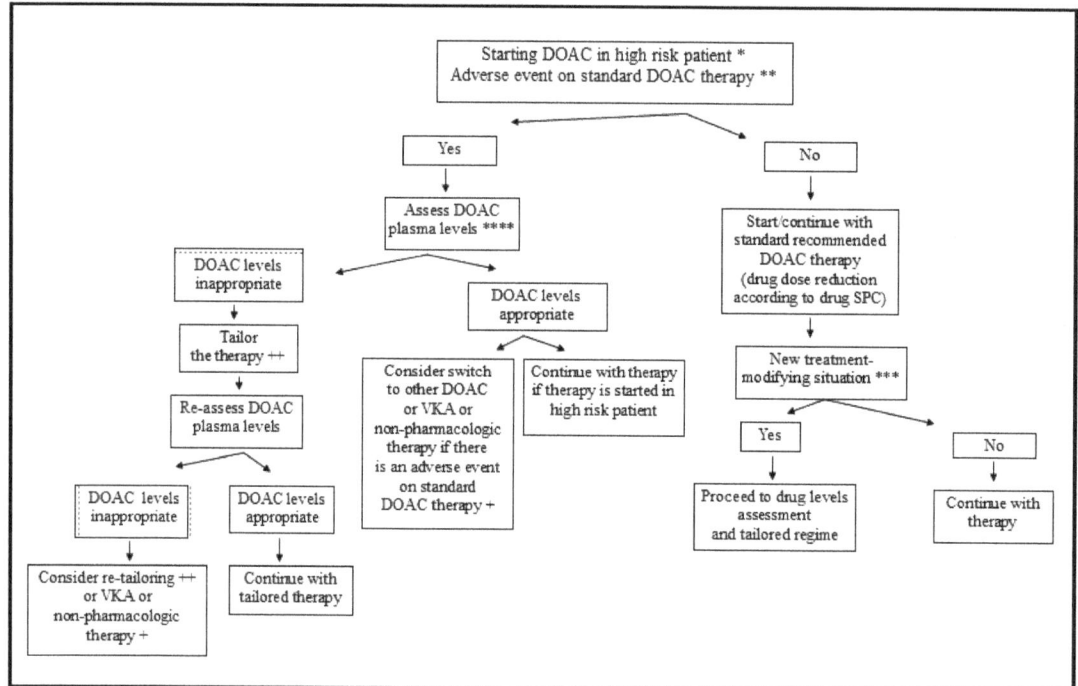

**Figure 1.** A proposed scheme for tailored direct oral anticoagulation. DOAC—direct oral anticoagulants; INR—international normalized ratio; LC-MS—liquid chromatography-mass spectrometry; SPC—summary of product characteristics; VKA—vitamin K antagonists. * severe renal/hepatic function impairment, extremely high body weight, advanced age, drug interactions. ** embolic stroke/systemic embolism or bleeding on labeled DOAC therapy. *** new adverse bleeding or thrombosis, new decrease in renal/hepatic function, new possible drug interaction, questionable patient drug compliance. **** LC-MS (if available) or drug-specific coagulation assays; test for trough (pre-drug dose) and peak (post-drug dose) levels. + VKA with target INR 2-3 or left atrial appendage (surgical/transcatheter) occlusion. ++ by optimizing drug dose or switch strategy or by modification of (modifiable) factors influencing DOAC drug levels.

## 6. How to Tailor DOAC Therapy

Another issue is the question of optimal approach for tailoring the DOAC therapy. In theory, DOAC therapy might be tailored by optimizing the drug dose (increasing/decreasing) or by switching the drug. None of these approaches have been validated in clinical trials. The strategy of tailoring the drug dose has a possible disadvantage in the use of a drug dose that is higher than the dose tested in clinical trials (for example if there is a need to increase the dose in a patient already taking dabigatran 150 mg twice daily or apixaban 5 mg twice daily). Similarly, if there is a need to reduce the dose in a patient already taking a reduced drug dose (for example, the need to reduce drug dose in a patient taking 15 mg of rivaroxaban or 30 mg of edoxaban daily), the second reduction will lead to a drug dosing thatwas not previously tested in the settings of prevention of stroke or systemic embolism related to AF. Therefore, the second strategy (switch strategy) seems to be more favorable, as it does not have the disadvantage of off-label drug dosing. On the other hand, in a recent study performed by Suwa et al. [39], a laboratory monitoring based an off-label underdosing of rivaroxaban and apixaban in selected patients did not lead to an increased risk of bleeding or thromboembolic events during follow up, and achieved acceptable peak drug levels (155–400 ng/mL for rivaroxaban, 90–386.4 ng/mL for apixaban, respectively). Nevertheless, only 73 patients used off-label underdosed rivaroxaban and only 46 patients used off-label underdosed apixaban, and there is a strong risk of selection bias. All these disadvantages should be taken into account when interpreting the results of this study. Another possible way of tailoring DOAC therapy is to try to modify the modifiable factors influencing DOAC drug levels. For example, DOAC levels could be optimized by the reduction of possible food and drug interactions. In addition, non-pharmacologic procedures, such as left atrial appendage occlusion, could be further use to reduce the risk of stroke if pharmacological prophylaxis is difficult to manage [1].

## 7. Is It Possible to Improve DOAC Therapy by a Tailored Strategy?

To answer this question, it is important to validate the hypothesis that tailoring the DOAC therapy according to DOAC plasma levels detected by a laboratory monitoring would lead to reduced incidence of future thromboembolic and bleeding events in a randomized clinical trial. That trial should randomize AF patients with the need for long-term anticoagulation, fulfilling criteria for DOAC administration to either standard treatment regimen (fixed dosing according to drug summary of product characteristics, without any laboratory assessment of drug levels) or to a tailored treatment regimen (with laboratory assessment of DOAC dosing and either modifying the drug dose or switching to other DOAC if in-optimal DOAC levels are detected). The primary outcome of the trial should be the incidence of stroke or systemic embolism and bleeding during the follow- up period. To date, no study with this design is on-going or planned. Therefore, there is no direct evidence that a tailored DOAC strategy would lead to improved clinical outcomes of long-term DOAC therapy, and the question: "Is it possible to improve DOAC therapy by a tailored strategy?" remains unanswered. However, as several factors that may significantly affect DOAC plasma levels have been identified, the tailored regime can be considered in selected risk patients, such as those experiencing stroke despite labeled DOAC anticoagulation, those with repeated bleeding while on DOAC therapy, those with a need for combined antiplatelet and anticoagulant therapy and those with multiple risk factors for in-optimal DOAC drug levels [24,40]. However, the risk/benefit ratio should be carefully evaluated before making the decision to use a tailored DOAC strategy.

## 8. Conclusions

Considering the aforementioned data, unanswered issues and possible limitations, at present, tailored DOAC therapy should not be recommended as a routine strategy in clinical practice. The tailored regime should be used with caution, only in selected patients, and after an appropriate evaluation of the risk/benefit ratio. However, further research of tailored DOAC strategy should definitely be advocated.

**Author Contributions:** M.S., T.B. and L.S. designed the study; M.S. and T.B. drafted the manuscript; M.J.P., K.B. and I.Š. performed the search of the literature, analyzed and interpreted the data; L.S., I.Š., J.S., M.M. and P.K. revised the manuscript critically. All authors have read and agreed to the published version of the manuscript (except of P.K. who, unfortunately, died before the submission of the final version of the manuscript).

**Funding:** This study was supported by project APVV (Slovak Research and Development Agency) 16-0020, and by Projects of Research Agency of Slovak Ministry of Education, Science and Sports (VEGA) 1/0549/19 and 1/0090/20.

**Institutional Review Board Statement:** The research was conducted according to ethical standards. There is no need for a Formal Consent for this type of study.

**Informed Consent Statement:** Not applicable.

**Data Availability Statement:** All the source data are available at the Corresponding Author uppon a request.

**Acknowledgments:** The authors would like to thank Jurica, J. and McCullough, P. for revision of English language.

**Conflicts of Interest:** Matej Samoš, Tomáš Bolek, Lucia Stančiaková, Martin Jozef Péč, Kristína Brisudová, Ingrid Škorňová, Ján Staško, Marián Mokáň and Peter Kubisz have no conflict of interest to declare.

## References

1. Hindricks, G.; Potpara, T.; Dagres, N.; Arbelo, E.; Bax, J.J.; Blomström-Lundqvist, C.; Boriani, G.; Castella, M.; Dan, G.A.; Dilaveris, P.E.; et al. 2020 ESC Guidelines for the diagnosis and management of atrial fibrillation developed in collaboration with the European Association for Cardio-Thoracic Surgery (EACTS): The Task Force for the diagnosis and management of atrial fibrillation of the European Society of Cardiology (ESC) Developed with the special contribution of the European Heart Rhythm Association (EHRA) of the ESC. *Eur. Heart J.* **2021**, *42*, 373–498.
2. Basso, C.; Goldstein, E.; Dai, X.; Rana, M.; Shu, L.; Chen, C.; Sweeney, J.; Stretz, C.; Smith, E.E.; Gurol, M.E.; et al. Acute ischemic stroke on anti-Xa inhibitors: Pharmacokinetics and outcomes. *J. Stroke Cerebrovasc. Dis.* **2022**, *31*, 106612. [CrossRef] [PubMed]
3. Verso, M.; Giustozzi, M.; Vinci, A.; Franco, L.; Vedovati, M.C.; Marchesini, E.; Becattini, C.; Agnelli, G. Risk factors and one-year mortality in patients with direct oral anticoagulant-associated gastrointestinal bleeding. *Thromb. Res.* **2021**, *208*, 138–144. [CrossRef]
4. Reilly, P.A.; Lehr, T.; Haertter, S.; Connolly, S.J.; Yusuf, S.; Eikelboom, J.W.; Ezekowitz, M.D.; Nehmiz, G.; Wang, S.; Wallentin, L.; et al. The effect of dabigatran plasma concentrations and patient characteristics on the frequency of ischemic stroke and major bleeding in atrial fibrillation patients: The RE-LY Trial (Randomized Evaluation of Long-Term Anticoagulation Therapy). *J. Am. Coll. Cardiol.* **2014**, *63*, 321–328. [CrossRef] [PubMed]
5. Testa, S.; Legnani, C.; Antonucci, E.; Paoletti, O.; Dellanoce, C.; Cosmi, B.; Pengo, V.; Poli, D.; Morandini, R.; Testa, R.; et al. Drug levels and bleeding complications in atrial fibrillation patients treated with direct oral anticoagulants. *J. Thromb. Haemost.* **2019**, *17*, 1064–1072. [CrossRef]
6. Testa, S.; Paoletti, O.; Legnani, C.; Dellanoce, C.; Antonucci, E.; Cosmi, B.; Pengo, V.; Poli, D.; Morandini, R.; Testa, R.; et al. Low drug levels and thrombotic complications in high-risk atrial fibrillation patients treated with direct oral anticoagulants. *J. Thromb. Haemost.* **2018**, *16*, 842–848. [CrossRef] [PubMed]
7. Škorňová, I.; Samoš, M.; Bolek, T.; Kameništʼáková, A.; Stančiaková, L.; Galajda, P.; Staško, J.; Kubisz, P.; Mokáň, M. Direct Oral Anticoagulants Plasma Levels in Patients with Atrial Fibrillation at the Time of Bleeding: A Pilot Prospective Study. *J. Cardiovasc. Pharmacol.* **2021**, *78*, e122–e127. [CrossRef]
8. Nosáľ, V.; Petrovičová, A.; Škorňová, I.; Bolek, T.; Dluhá, J.; Stančiaková, L.; Sivák, Š.; Babálová, L.; Hajaš, G.; Staško, J.; et al. Plasma levels of direct oral anticoagulants in atrial fibrillation patients at the time of embolic stroke: A pilot prospective multicenter study. *Eur. J. Clin. Pharmacol.* **2022**, *78*, 557–564. [CrossRef] [PubMed]
9. Siedler, G.; Macha, K.; Stoll, S.; Plechschmidt, J.; Wang, R.; Gerner, S.T.; Strasser, E.; Schwab, S.; Kallmünzer, B. Monitoring of direct oral anticoagulants plasma levels for secondary stroke prevention. *J. Thromb. Haemost.* **2022**, *20*, 1138–1145. [CrossRef]
10. Favaloro, E.J.; Pasalic, L.; Curnow, J.; Lippi, G. Laboratory Monitoring or Measurement of Direct Oral Anticoagulants (DOACs): Advantages, Limitations and Future Challenges. *Curr. Drug Metab.* **2017**, *18*, 598–608. [CrossRef] [PubMed]
11. Maier, V.; Slavík, L.; Ondra, P. A synergy of liquid chromatography with high-resolution mass spectrometry and coagulation test for determination of direct oral anticoagulants for clinical and toxicological purposes. *Biomed. Chromatogr.* **2021**, *35*, e5195. [CrossRef] [PubMed]
12. Slavik, L.; Lukes, J.; Friedecky, D.; Zhanelova, M.; Nemcova, M.; Ulehlova, J.; Prochazkova, J.; Hlusi, A.; Palova, M.; Vaclavik, J. Multianalyte Determination of NOACs Using LC-MS/MS and Comparison with Functional Coagulation Assays. *Clin. Lab.* **2018**, *64*, 1611–1621. [CrossRef] [PubMed]
13. Douxfils, J.; Adcock, D.M.; Bates, S.M.; Favaloro, E.J.; Gouin-Thibault, I.; Guillermo, C.; Kawai, Y.; Lindhoff-Last, E.; Kitchen, S.; Gosselin, R.C. 2021 Update of the International Council for Standardization in Haematology Recommendations for Laboratory Measurement of Direct Oral Anticoagulants. *Thromb. Haemost.* **2021**, *121*, 1008–1020. [CrossRef] [PubMed]
14. Korpallová, B.; Samoš, M.; Bolek, T.; Kühnelová, L.; Škorňová, I.; Kubisz, P.; Staško, J.; Mokáň, M. ROTEM Testing for Direct Oral Anticoagulants. *Semin. Thromb. Hemost.* **2021**, *47*, 815–823. [CrossRef] [PubMed]
15. Samoš, M.; Stančiaková, L.; Ivanková, J.; Staško, J.; Kovář, F.; Dobrotová, M.; Galajda, P.; Kubisz, P.; Mokáň, M. Monitoring of dabigatran therapy using Hemoclot® Thrombin Inhibitor assay in patients with atrial fibrillation. *J. Thromb. Thrombolysis* **2015**, *39*, 95–100. [CrossRef]
16. Samoš, M.; Bolek, T.; Stančiaková, L.; Škorňová, I.; Bánovčin, P., Jr.; Kovář, F.; Staško, J.; Galajda, P.; Kubisz, P.; Mokáň, M. Anti-Xa activity in oral factor Xa inhibitor-treated patients with atrial fibrillation and a higher risk of bleeding: A pilot study. *Blood Coagul. Fibrinolysis* **2018**, *29*, 369–373. [CrossRef] [PubMed]
17. Sin, C.F.; Wong, K.P.; Wong, H.M.; Siu, C.W.; Yap, D.Y.H. Plasma Rivaroxaban Level in Patients With Early Stages of Chronic Kidney Disease-Relationships With Renal Function and Clinical Events. *Front. Pharmacol.* **2022**, *13*, 888660. [CrossRef] [PubMed]
18. Sairaku, A.; Nakano, Y.; Onohara, Y.; Hironobe, N.; Matsumura, H.; Shimizu, W.; Kihara, Y. Residual anticoagulation activity in atrial fibrillation patients with temporary interrupted direct oral anticoagulants: Comparisons across 4 drugs. *Thromb. Res.* **2019**, *183*, 119–123. [CrossRef] [PubMed]

19. Artang, R.; Dias, J.D.; Walsh, M.; Bliden, K.; Nielsen, J.D.; Anderson, M.; Thurston, B.C.; Tantry, U.S.; Hartmann, J.; Gurbel, P.A. Measurement of Anticoagulation in Patients on Dabigatran, Rivaroxaban, and Apixaban Therapy by Novel Automated Thrombelastography. *TH Open* **2021**, *5*, e570–e576. [CrossRef]
20. Sakaguchi, T.; Osanai, H.; Murase, Y.; Ishii, H.; Nakashima, Y.; Asano, H.; Suzuki, S.; Takefuji, M.; Inden, Y.; Sakai, K.; et al. Monitoring of anti-Xa activity and factors related to bleeding events: A study in Japanese patients with nonvalvular atrial fibrillation receiving rivaroxaban. *J. Cardiol.* **2017**, *70*, 244–249. [CrossRef]
21. Gao, H.; Li, Y.; Sun, Y.; Huang, X.; Chen, H.; Lin, W.; Chen, M. Trough Concentration Deficiency of Rivaroxaban in Patients with Nonvalvular Atrial Fibrillation Leading to Thromboembolism Events. *J. Cardiovasc. Pharmacol.* **2022**, *13*, 888660. [CrossRef] [PubMed]
22. Limcharoen, S.; Pongchaidecha, M.; Pimsi, P.; Limprasert, S.; Suphanklang, J.; Saelim, W.; Santimaleeworagun, W.; Boonmuang, P. Do Apixaban Plasma Levels Relate to Bleeding? The Clinical Outcomes and Predictive Factors for Bleeding in Patients with Non-Valvular Atrial Fibrillation. *Biomedicines* **2022**, *10*, 2001. [CrossRef] [PubMed]
23. Cirincione, B.; Kowalski, K.; Nielsen, J.; Roy, A.; Thanneer, N.; Byon, W.; Boyd, R.; Wang, X.; Leil, T.; LaCreta, F.; et al. Population Pharmacokinetics of Apixaban in Subjects With Nonvalvular Atrial Fibrillation. *CPT Pharmacomet. Syst. Pharmacol.* **2018**, *7*, 728–738. [CrossRef] [PubMed]
24. Steffel, J.; Collins, R.; Antz, M.; Cornu, P.; Desteghe, L.; Haeusler, K.G.; Oldgren, J.; Reinecke, H.; Roldan-Schilling, V.; Rowell, N.; et al. 2021 European Heart Rhythm Association Practical Guide on the Use of Non-Vitamin K Antagonist Oral Anticoagulants in Patients with Atrial Fibrillation. *EP Eur.* **2021**, *23*, 1612–1676. [CrossRef] [PubMed]
25. Bolek, T.; Samoš, M.; Škorňová, I.; Stančiaková, L.; Staško, J.; Galajda, P.; Kubisz, P.; Mokáň, M. Dabigatran Levels in Elderly Patients with Atrial Fibrillation: First Post-Marketing Experiences. *Drugs Aging* **2018**, *35*, 539–544. [CrossRef] [PubMed]
26. Samoš, M.; Bolek, T.; Škorňová, I.; Stančiaková, L.; Urban, L.; Staško, J.; Galajda, P.; Kubisz, P.; Mokáň, M. Anti-Xa Activity in Elderly Xabans-Treated Patients With Atrial Fibrillation. *Am. J. Ther.* **2020**, *27*, e507–e509. [CrossRef]
27. Gommans, E.; Grouls, R.J.E.; Kerkhof, D.; Houterman, S.; Simmers, T.; Van der Linden, C. Dabigatran trough concentrations in very elderly patients. *Eur. J. Hosp. Pharm.* **2021**, *28*, 231–233. [CrossRef]
28. Stöllberger, C.; Finsterer, J. Update on drug interactions with non-vitamin-K-antagonist oral anticoagulants for stroke prevention in elderly patients. *Expert Rev. Clin. Pharmacol.* **2021**, *14*, 569–581. [CrossRef]
29. Bolek, T.; Samoš, M.; Škorňová, I.; Galajda, P.; Staško, J.; Kubisz, P.; Mokáň, M. Proton Pump Inhibitors and Dabigatran Therapy: Impact on Gastric Bleeding and Dabigatran Plasma Levels. *Semin. Thromb. Hemost.* **2019**, *45*, 846–850. [CrossRef] [PubMed]
30. Piran, S.; Traquair, H.; Chan, N.; Bhagirath, V.; Schulman, S. Peak plasma concentration of direct oral anticoagulants in obese patients weighing over 120 kilograms: A retrospective study. *Res. Pract. Thromb. Haemost.* **2018**, *2*, 684–688. [CrossRef]
31. Russo, V.; Cattaneo, D.; Giannetti, L.; Bottino, R.; Laezza, N.; Atripaldi, U.; Clementi, E. Pharmacokinetics of Direct Oral Anticoagulants in Patients With Atrial Fibrillation and Extreme Obesity. *Clin. Ther.* **2021**, *43*, e255–e263. [CrossRef] [PubMed]
32. Ballerie, A.; Nguyen Van, R.; Lacut, K.; Galinat, H.; Rousseau, C.; Pontis, A.; Nédelec-Gac, F.; Lescoat, A.; Belhomme, N.; Guéret, P.; et al. Apixaban and rivaroxaban in obese patients treated for venous thromboembolism: Drug levels and clinical outcomes. *Thromb. Res.* **2021**, *208*, 39–44. [CrossRef] [PubMed]
33. Russo, V.; Paccone, A.; Rago, A.; Maddaloni, V.; Iafusco, D.; Proietti, R.; Atripaldi, U.; D'Onofrio, A.; Golino, P.; Nigro, G. Apixaban in a Morbid Obese Patient with Atrial Fibrillation: A Clinical Experience Using the Plasmatic Drug Evaluation. *J. Blood Med.* **2020**, *11*, 77–81. [CrossRef] [PubMed]
34. Ji, Q.; Zhang, C.; Xu, Q.; Wang, Z.; Li, X.; Lv, Q. The impact of ABCB1 and CES1 polymorphisms on dabigatran pharmacokinetics and pharmacodynamics in patients with atrial fibrillation. *Br. J. Clin. Pharmacol.* **2021**, *87*, 2247–2255. [CrossRef]
35. Gouin-Thibault, I.; Delavenne, X.; Blanchard, A.; Siguret, V.; Salem, J.E.; Narjoz, C.; Gaussem, P.; Beaune, P.; Funck-Brentano, C.; Azizi, M.; et al. Interindividual variability in dabigatran and rivaroxaban exposure: Contribution of ABCB1 genetic polymorphisms and interaction with clarithromycin. *J. Thromb. Haemost.* **2017**, *15*, 273–283. [CrossRef]
36. Roșian, A.N.; Roșian, Ș.H.; Kiss, B.; Ștefan, M.G.; Trifa, A.P.; Ober, C.D.; Anchidin, O.; Buzoianu, A.D. Interindividual Variability of Apixaban Plasma Concentrations: Influence of Clinical and Genetic Factors in a Real-Life Cohort of Atrial Fibrillation Patients. *Genes* **2020**, *11*, 438. [CrossRef]
37. Sychev, D.; Ostroumova, O.; Cherniaeva, M.; Shakhgildian, N.; Mirzaev, K.; Abdullaev, S.; Denisenko, N.; Sozaeva, Z.; Kachanova, A.; Gorbatenkova, S.; et al. The Influence of ABCB1 (rs1045642 and rs4148738) Gene Polymorphisms on Rivaroxaban Pharmacokinetics in Patients Aged 80 Years and Older with Nonvalvular Atrial Fibrillation. *High Blood Press. Cardiovasc. Prev.* **2022**, *29*, 469–480. [CrossRef]
38. Vandell, A.G.; Lee, J.; Shi, M.; Rubets, I.; Brown, K.S.; Walker, J.R. An integrated pharmacokinetic/pharmacogenomic analysis of ABCB1 and SLCO1B1 polymorphisms on edoxaban exposure. *Pharm. J.* **2018**, *18*, 153–159. [CrossRef]
39. Suwa, M.; Morii, I.; Kino, M. Rivaroxaban or Apixaban for Non-Valvular Atrial Fibrillation—Efficacy and Safety of Off-Label Under-Dosing According to Plasma Concentration. *Circ. J.* **2019**, *83*, 991–999. [CrossRef]
40. Akpan, I.J.; Cuker, A. Laboratory assessment of the direct oral anticoagulants: Who can benefit? *Kardiol. Pol.* **2021**, *79*, 622–630. [CrossRef]

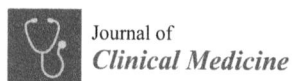

Article

# DNA Polymorphisms in Pregnant Women with Sticky Platelet Syndrome

Lucia Stančiaková [1,*], Jana Žolková [1], Ľubica Vadelová [1,2], Andrea Hornáková [3], Zuzana Kolková [3], Martin Vážan [4], Miroslava Dobrotová [1], Pavol Hollý [1], Zuzana Jedináková [1,5], Marián Grendár [6,7], Tomáš Bolek [8], Matej Samoš [8], Kamil Biringer [9], Ján Danko [9], Tatiana Burjanivová [3], Zora Lasabová [3], Peter Kubisz [1] and Ján Staško [1]

[1] National Centre of Haemostasis and Thrombosis, Department of Haematology and Transfusion Medicine, Jessenius Faculty of Medicine in Martin, Comenius University in Bratislava, Martin University Hospital, 036 59 Martin, Slovakia
[2] Centre of Immunology in Martin, s.r.o., 036 01 Martin, Slovakia
[3] Biomedical Centre Martin, Jessenius Faculty of Medicine in Martin, Comenius University in Bratislava, 036 01 Martin, Slovakia
[4] Department of Medical Genetics, Martin University Hospital, 036 59 Martin, Slovakia
[5] Centre of Haemostasis and Thrombosis, Unilabs Slovakia, s.r.o., 036 01 Martin, Slovakia
[6] Laboratory of Bioinformatics and Biostatistics, Biomedical Centre Martin, Jessenius Faculty of Medicine in Martin, Comenius University in Bratislava, 036 01 Martin, Slovakia
[7] Laboratory of Theoretical Methods, Institute of Measurement Science, Slovak Academy of Sciences, 841 04 Karlova Ves, Slovakia
[8] Department of Internal Medicine I., Jessenius Faculty of Medicine in Martin, Comenius University in Bratislava, Martin University Hospital, 036 59 Martin, Slovakia
[9] Department of Gynaecology and Obstetrics, Jessenius Faculty of Medicine in Martin, Comenius University in Bratislava, Martin University Hospital, 036 59 Martin, Slovakia
* Correspondence: stanciakova2@uniba.sk

**Abstract:** Sticky platelet syndrome (SPS) is a thrombophilia caused by the increased aggregability of platelets in response to the addition of low concentrations of epinephrine (EPI) and/or adenosine diphosphate (ADP). Some of the single nucleotide polymorphisms (SNP), alleles and haplotypes of platelet glycoprotein receptors were proved to have a role in the etiology of thrombotic episodes When comparing SPS and the control group, in VEGFA rs3025039, the $p$ value for both CC vs. TT and CT vs. TT analyses was <0.001. Interestingly, no minor TT genotype was present in the SPS group, suggesting the thrombotic pathogenesis of recurrent spontaneous abortions (RSA) in these patients. Moreover, we found a significant difference in the presence of AT containing a risky A allele and TT genotype of ALPP rs13026692 ($p$ = 0.034) in SPS patients when compared with the controls. Additionally, we detected a decreased frequency of the GG (CC) genotype of FOXP3 rs3761548 in patients with SPS and RSA when compared with the control group ($p$ value for the CC (GG) vs. AA (TT) 0.021). This might indicate an evolutionary protective mechanism of the A (T) allele in the SPS group against thrombotic complications in pregnancy. These results can be used for antithrombotic management in such pregnant patients.

**Keywords:** sticky platelet syndrome; DNA analysis; polymorphisms; antithrombotic treatment

## 1. Introduction

Sticky platelet syndrome (SPS) represents an autosomal dominant platelet function disorder associated with platelet hyperaggregability in platelet-rich plasma (PRP) with adenosine diphosphate (ADP) and/or epinephrine (EPI). Increased aggregability after the addition of both of these substances is defined as SPS type I, hyperaggregability after EPI alone as type II and increased aggregability only after the addition of ADP is SPS type III [1].

SPS can manifest as arterial thrombosis, such as acute myocardial infarction, angina pectoris, transient cerebral ischemic attack, stroke, peripheral arterial thrombosis, retinal thrombosis, or venous thromboembolism—frequently recurrent despite anticoagulant therapy or pregnancy complications (e.g., fetal growth retardation and fetal loss) [1–5]. Moreover, it has been reported that women with SPS have significantly more spontaneous abortions than patients in the general population [6].

Several mutations of genes encoding platelet glycoprotein receptors and further proteins associated with platelet function have been studied as potential etiopathogenetic factors of recurrent pregnancy loss (RPL) in women with SPS.

Single nucleotide polymorphisms (SNPs) rs9550270 and rs7400002 of the *GAS6* gene responsible for the function of alpha2-adrenergic and ADP receptors and activating endothelial and vascular smooth muscle cells are more common in women with SPS and pregnancy loss [7,8].

Moreover, SNPs 1,671,153, 1,613,662 and 1,654,419 of *GP6* as the gene encoding the receptor for collagen are more frequent in women with SPS and pregnancy loss. A significantly increased occurrence of CTGAG in haplotype 5 and CGATAG in haplotype 6, an increased presence of SNPs rs1671152, rs1654433, rs1654416, rs2304167 and rs1671215 in patients with platelet hyperaggregability and previous pregnancy loss and a significantly higher frequency of ccgt in *GP6_3reg* haplotype, acgg and aagg in *GP6_5reg* haplotype, SKTH and PEAN in *GP6_PEAN* haplotype and gg and ta in *GP6_REG* haplotype in this population have been confirmed [7,9–13].

Patients with SPS and spontaneous abortion had an increased prevalence of SNPs rs12566888 and rs12041331 of the *PEAR1* gene responsible for platelet contact [8].

Increased expression of platelet microRNA (miR-96) is expressed in patients with SPS and pregnancy complications [14]. Conclusively, different mutations of one or more genes might lead to a similar SPS phenotype. Additionally, platelets of individuals with atherosclerosis, renal and autoimmune diseases have hyperaggregability after EPI or other agonists, highlighting the possible existence of acquired forms of SPS [2,7].

In spite of several studies investigating the role of platelet glycoproteins in the activation and aggregation of platelets, the exact underlying defect causing the syndrome has not been fully elucidated [15].

In most patients, low doses of antiplatelet agents (usually 80–100 mg of acetylsalicylic acid (ASA) per day) lead to normalization of platelet hyperaggregability [15] and improvement of pregnancy outcome in comparison with SPS patients without such treatment [16]. However, in risky situations, such as a history of thromboembolic episodes or the presence of prothrombotic changes in hemostasis associated with RPL, both low-molecular-weight heparin (LMWH) and ASA are recommended, as also indicated by Bick and Hoppenstedt [17]. Therefore, pregnant patients in our study used a combination of ASA and LMWH to prevent further complications.

The term 'recurrent pregnancy loss' (RPL) is recommended for the description of repeated pregnancy demise and recurrent miscarriage (recurrent spontaneous abortion, RSA) when all pregnancy losses are confirmed as intrauterine miscarriages by histology or ultrasound [18,19]. A pregnancy loss is a spontaneous pregnancy demise before the fetus reaches viability—i.e., until 24 gestational weeks [20].

There is also a variation in the quantity defining recurrent miscarriage. It ranges from two miscarriages reported by the European Society of Human Reproduction and Embryology and the American Society for Reproductive Medicine to three subsequent pregnancy losses, as defined by the Royal College of Obstetricians and Gynaecologists [21].

In general, RPL affects approximately 2–5% of couples. Frequent causes are uterine anomalies, hormonal and metabolic disorders, antiphospholipid syndrome and genetic abnormalities. Further etiological factors that have been investigated include inherited thrombophilia, luteal phase deficiency, chronic endometritis and high sperm DNA fragmentation level [22]. However, it has been proved that approximately 55% of recurrent miscarriages are due to prothrombotic defects inducing infarction and thrombosis of placental vessels [23].

The *vascular endothelial growth factor A (VEGF-A)* gene encompasses 14 kb and is localized on the human chromosome 6, consisting of eight exons [24]. It is a member of the platelet-derived growth factor (PDGF)/vascular endothelial growth factor (VEGF) family. *VEGFA* encodes a heparin-binding protein inducing proliferation and migration of vascular endothelial cells. It is thus critical for physiological and pathological angiogenesis [25]. Additionally, *VEGFA* is essential for embryonic vasculature development, stimulation of trophoblast proliferation and both fetal and maternal blood cell growth in the course of early pregnancy. *VEGF* in general is also important for the implantation of the embryo into the placental wall, so its genetic defects have been studied in association with RPL [24]. A decrease in *VEGF* expression in first-trimester tissues can even indicate its involvement in RPL [26].

The *alkaline phosphatase, placental (ALPP)* gene encodes an alkaline phosphatase, a metalloenzyme catalyzing the hydrolysis of phosphoric acid monoesters. One of its main sources is the liver. However, in pregnant women, it is primarily expressed in placental and endometrial tissue. Strong ectopic expression of *ALPP* has been confirmed in ovarian adenocarcinoma, serous cystadenocarcinoma and further ovarian cancer cells [27].

*Fork head box protein 3 (FOXP3)* is an X-linked gene that codes a master transcription regulatory protein controlling the development and function of immunosuppressive T regulatory cells. These cells are key mediators of maternal fetal tolerance [28]. A decrease in T regulatory cells in peripheral blood and decidua leads to a decrease in *FOXP3* gene expression, which affects the development and function of CD4+ CD25+ T regulatory cells [29,30]. The protein encoded by the *FOXP3* gene represents a member of the fork head/winged-helix family of transcriptional regulators. Diseases associated with *FOXP3* include polyendocrinopathy, immunodysregulation, X-linked enteropathy and nonimmune and X-linked hydrops fetalis [31].

Based on this knowledge, the authors aimed to investigate the relationship between SPS, recurrent spontaneous abortions (RSA) and further thromboembolic complications and selected polymorphisms rs3025039 in *VEGFA*, rs2010963 in *VEGF*, rs13026692 in *ALPP* and rs3761548 in *FOXP3* genes.

## 2. Materials and Methods

### 2.1. Patients and the Control Group

A total of 53 pregnant women of Caucasian origin with a sticky platelet syndrome, 21 pregnant patients with a history of unprovoked or estrogen-related thromboembolic complications and 53 pregnant women with a history of RSA receiving antithrombotic thromboprophylaxis were included in the study.

SPS was diagnosed in patients before their inclusion in the study via light transmission aggregometry with the analysis of responsiveness of platelet-rich plasma to three different concentrations of adenosine diphosphate (ADP) and epinephrine (EPI) according to the criteria of Mammen and Bick [7] (Table 1). We suspect this diagnosis when the patient has a history of thromboembolic episodes and proved platelet hyperaggregability after mixing of the sample with 1 concentration of 1 of these reagents. The diagnosis of SPS is confirmed when the patient has one of the combinations of these situations:

- A history of thromboembolic episodes and hyperaggregability after the use of 2 concentrations of 1 reagent;
- A history of thromboembolic episodes and hyperaggregability after the use of 1 concentration of both reagents (ADP and EPI);
- A history of thromboembolic episodes and hyperaggregability after the use of 1 concentration of 1 reagent, but repeatedly tested [7].

**Table 1.** Diagnostic criteria of SPS.

| | Platelet Aggregation after the Addition of | | | | | |
|---|---|---|---|---|---|---|
| | ADP | | | EPI | | |
| Concentration (µM) | 0.58 | 1.17 | 2.34 | 0.55 | 1.1 | 11 |
| Reference range of aggregation (%) | 0–12 | 2–36 | 7.5–55 | 9–20 | 15–27 | 39–80 |

Legend: ADP—adenosine diphosphate, EPI—epinephrine, SPS—sticky platelet syndrome.

As mentioned above, the form of primary thromboprophylaxis in SPS is the use of ASA; however, in the case of the development of prothrombotic changes in hemostasis during pregnancy (e.g., significantly increased FVIII activity or decrease in free PS), combined antithrombotic prophylaxis composed of ASA and LMWH had to be used.

Due to the increased risk of bleeding during the use of such prophylaxis, pregnant patients with the following clinical conditions predisposing to bleeding were excluded from the study: a history of hemorrhagic stroke, disorder of blood coagulation or other diseases contributing to bleeding (severe thrombocytopenia, history of thrombocytopenia developed after the use of anticoagulant drugs, active gastroduodenal ulcerations, severe renal insufficiency (creatinine clearance <30 mL/min.), acute infective endocarditis and a history of severe allergic reaction to antithrombotics).

RSA was confirmed by a gynecologist with the exclusion of further causes of this complication, such as anatomic, hormonal or genetic changes or infections. Mean age was 31.93 years (age range 19–46 years), and the number of RSA varied from 2 to 8. Inclusion of patients was carried out from January 2014 to March 2019.

During clinical examination, data about family and personal history, drugs, allergies and gynecological history (previous abortions, interruptions, deliveries or thromboembolic complications) were collected.

The control group comprised 58 healthy non-pregnant women without any personal or family history of thromboembolism and no history of pregnancy complications, such as placental abruption, RPL in general, fetal demise, intrauterine growth restriction (IUGR) or VTE during pregnancy. These subjects did not take any agents that could have an impact on hemostasis—anticoagulant drugs, antiplatelet agents or oral contraceptives. The mean age was 29.05 years (age range 18–45 years).

We compared the frequency of genotypes of particular SNPs between four groups—the results of pregnant women with SPS (designated S in the figures and tables), of those with a history of RSA (group A in the figures and tables), of those with a history of thromboembolism (T) and of the control group (C).

### 2.2. Processing of Blood Samples for Genotyping

For genotyping, 10 mL of antecubital venous blood was obtained from each fasting pregnant woman included in the study and each fasting woman from the control group.

Blood was collected in Vacutainer® blood collection tubes with ethylenediaminetetraacetic acid (EDTA) as an anticoagulant, then immediately stored at 4 °C and further processed within 6 h. Centrifuging of the blood samples was carried out at 3000 rpm at 4 °C for 10 min to separate the serum plasma and buffy coat containing white blood cells, and then frozen at −20 °C for DNA extraction and genotyping.

Genomic DNA was isolated from buffy coat using a DNeasy Blood and Tissue Kit (Qiagen, Germany). All DNA samples were diluted to 20 ng per µL and were used as a template for genotyping.

The AB 7500 Fast Real-Time PCR system (Applied Biosystems, USA) was used to analyze polymorphisms rs3025039 in *VEGFA* (assay ID: C__16198794_10), rs2010963 in *VEGF* (assay ID: C__8311614_10), rs13026692 in *ALPP* (assay ID: C__11531497_10) and rs3761548 in *FOXP3* (assay ID: C__27476877_10). Each TaqMan genotyping assay mix contained a forward and reverse primer, one probe with perfect matching to the wild-type sequence variant labeled with VIC and the other probe labeled with FAM with perfect matching to the mutant sequence variant. TaqMan allelic discrimination real-time PCR was performed in a 20 µL volume, containing 0.5 µL TaqMan genotyping assay mix, 10 µL TaqMan Genotyping Master Mix (Applied Biosystems, Waltham, MA, USA), 7.5 µL DNase-free water and 2 µL of diluted genomic DNA. The real-time PCR conditions were as follows: an initial step at 95 °C for 10 min, followed by 50 cycles of denaturation at 92 °C for 15 s and annealing/extending at 60 °C for 1 min and 30 s. The genotypes were detected according to the strength of the fluorescent signals from VIC/FAM labeled probes.

### 2.3. Statistical Analysis

The role of this study was to explore how exactly the selected SNPs can predict the probability of the tested person belonging to one of the following groups: SPS/RSA/control group/thromboembolism. Therefore, we used multinomial logistic regression analysis, and the result was expressed as the significance of particular alleles of all SNPs and odds ratio (OR). The response was the group, and the predictors were all four SNPs.

For each of the SNPs, we made a contingency table showing the relationship genotype vs. study group. To obtain a summary contingency table, we performed a Chi-squared test and G-test of independence between genotype and study group. Cramér V was used for an effect size measurement in the contingency table. In cases where H0 was refused for any of the SNPs, we carried out pair post hoc tests (pair comparisons of particular levels of factor in the groups). A $p$ value $< 0.05$ was considered statistically significant. We also adjusted the $p$ value based on Holm's method and the Bonferroni correction.

Moreover, we calculated the estimated marginal means of frequencies of the alleles for each SNP and each group.

The control group was taken as the reference level in the group analysis. In each SNP, the minor allele was taken as the reference.

Not all pregnant women included in the study were treated with ASA or LMWH uniformly, so we performed a multivariate analysis to exclude the effect of antiplatelet drugs/anticoagulants on pregnancy outcomes or the occurrence of thromboembolism as potential confounding factors. For the same reason, we also analyzed the effect of the presence of concomitant thrombophilia in our pregnant patients as another confounding factor.

Statistical analysis was performed using the jamovi project, version 2.3, and the data were explored and analyzed in R (R), version 4.1 [32–35].

## 3. Results

### 3.1. Clinical Data

Family history in the form of thromboembolic and pregnancy complications (preeclampsia, RPL in general or intrauterine fetal death) was positive in 15 cases. SPS type I was detected in 16 patients and type II in 37 women; we did not include any pregnant woman with SPS type III. The most common dose of ASA used on patients was 100 mg taken daily (60%), while the minimal dosage confirmed as effective before the initiation of the study and used by patients was 50 mg (taken by 16.67%). The maximal dose of ASA was 150 mg daily for one woman.

Two patients with SPS were directly allergic to ASA and thus used only LMWH, while 29.13% of all included patients reported allergic reactions in the form of redness, resistances and local irritation of the skin at the site of administration of LMWH. For this reason, they switched between LMWH products, usually from nadroparin to enoxaparin.

In addition to SPS detected in the 53 mentioned patients, further thrombophilic states diagnosed in at-risk pregnant women were: antithrombin deficiency ($n = 5$), hyperhomocysteinemia ($n = 8$), factor V Leiden mutation present in the homozygous form ($n = 2$), heterozygous form ($n = 17$), prothrombin variant G20210A in the heterozygous form ($n = 7$), heterozygous form of mutation of $\beta$Fbgc.$-$39–424 G > A ($n = 24$), homozygous form ($n = 2$), PAI 4G/5G homozygous ($n = 7$) and heterozygous form ($n = 7$), mutation FXI c.1481-188 C > T ($n = 4$), SNP FXI rs2289252 ($n = 2$), variant FXII C46T in the homozygous form present in 2 patients and in heterozygous women (*n* = 1), CYP4V2 homozygous form of mutation (*n* = 3), homozygous form of mutation FXIII Val34Leu (*n* = 1) and the presence of antiphospholipid antibodies (*n* = 6).

No renal or liver function impairment developed. None of the included pregnant patients developed HELLP syndrome or heparin-induced thrombocytopenia. During the study, we did not detect any thromboembolic episode in the included patients.

The control group was composed of healthy non-pregnant women (mean age 29.42 years, age range 18–45 years). Based on the anamnestic data, none of them were pregnant or in menopause during the study.

### 3.2. Results of Genotyping

In the case of *VEGFA* rs2010963, the possible genotypes are GG, GC and CC. For *VEGFA* rs2010963 in our studied population, the global frequency of the GG genotype was 53%, while that of GC was 40% and that of CC 7% (Figure 1, Table 2).

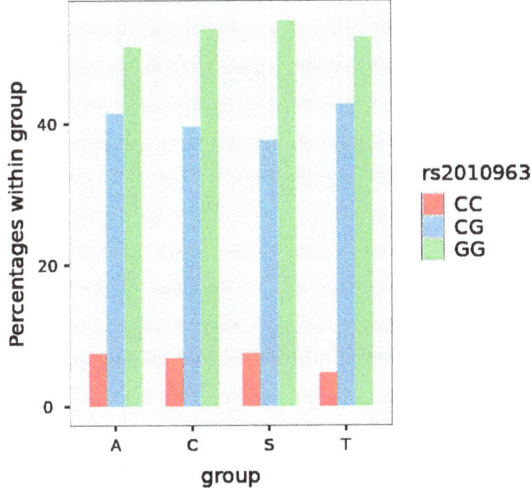

**Figure 1.** Plot with the frequency of the particular genotypes of *VEGFA* rs2010963 in the studied groups. Legend: group A—recurrent spontaneous abortions, group C—controls, group S—sticky platelet syndrome, group T—thromboembolism, VEGFA—vascular endothelial growth factor A.

**Table 2.** Contingency table showing the frequency of genotypes of VEGFA rs2010963 in the studied population.

| Group | | Rs2010963 | | | Total |
|---|---|---|---|---|---|
| | | CC | CG | GG | |
| A | Observed | 4 | 22 | 27 | 53 |
| | % within row | 7.5% | 41.5% | 50.9% | 100.0% |
| C | Observed | 4 | 23 | 31 | 58 |
| | % within row | 6.9% | 39.7% | 53.4% | 100.0% |
| S | Observed | 4 | 20 | 29 | 53 |
| | % within row | 7.5% | 37.7% | 54.7% | 100.0% |
| T | Observed | 1 | 9 | 11 | 21 |
| | % within row | 4.8% | 42.9% | 52.4% | 100.0% |
| Total | Observed | 13 | 74 | 98 | 185 |
| | % within row | 7.0% | 40.0% | 53.0% | 100.0% |

Legend: group A—recurrent spontaneous abortions, group C—controls, group S—sticky platelet syndrome, group T—thromboembolism, VEGFA—vascular endothelial growth factor A.

VEGFA rs3025039 has the possible genotypes CC, CT and TT. The general frequency of the CC genotype in SNP VEGFA rs3025039 was 70.8%, the CT genotype was present in 27% of the women included in the study and the TT genotype was detected only in 2.2% (Figure 2, Table 3).

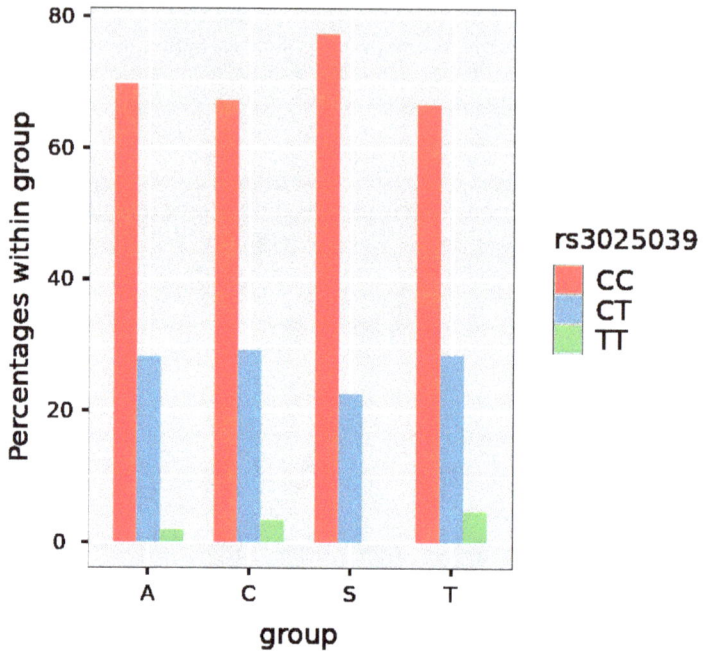

**Figure 2.** Plot with the frequency of the particular genotypes of VEGFA rs3025039 in the studied groups. Legend: group A—recurrent spontaneous abortions, group C—controls, group S—sticky platelet syndrome, group T—thromboembolism, VEGFA—vascular endothelial growth factor A.

**Table 3.** Contingency table showing the frequency of genotypes of VEGFA rs3025039 in the studied population.

| Group | | rs3025039 | | | |
|---|---|---|---|---|---|
| | | CC | CT | TT | Total |
| A | Observed | 37 | 15 | 1 | 53 |
| | % within row | 69.8% | 28.3% | 1.9% | 100.0% |
| C | Observed | 39 | 17 | 2 | 58 |
| | % within row | 67.2% | 29.3% | 3.4% | 100.0% |
| S | Observed | 41 | 12 | 0 | 53 |
| | % within row | 77.4% | 22.6% | 0.0% | 100.0% |
| T | Observed | 14 | 6 | 1 | 21 |
| | % within row | 66.7% | 28.6% | 4.8% | 100.0% |
| Total | Observed | 131 | 50 | 4 | 185 |
| | % within row | 70.8% | 27.0% | 2.2% | 100.0% |

Legend: group A—recurrent spontaneous abortions, group C—controls, group S—sticky platelet syndrome, group T—thromboembolism, VEGFA—vascular endothelial growth factor A.

ALPP rs13026692 has the possible genotypes AA, AT and TT. In the case of this polymorphism in our study, the frequency of the AA genotype was 44.9%, AT was present in 46.5% and TT only in 8.6% (Figure 3, Table 4).

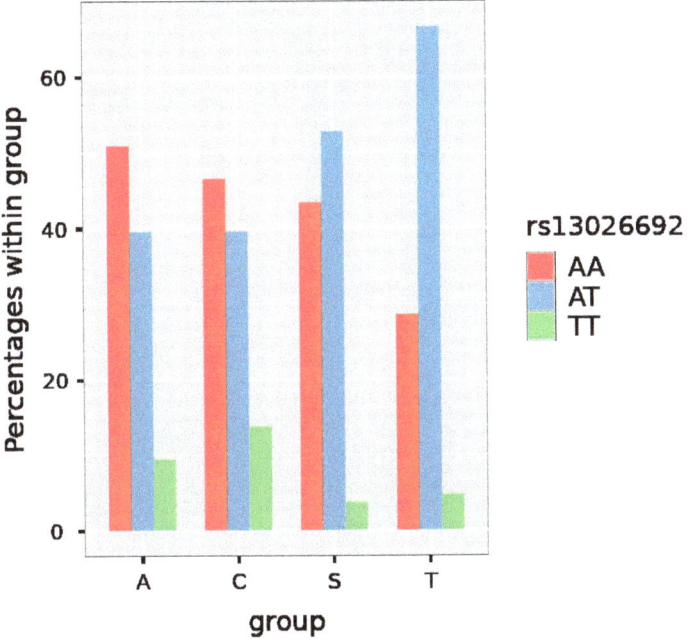

**Figure 3.** Plot with the frequency of the particular genotypes of *ALPP* rs13026692 in the studied groups. Legend: *ALPP*—alkaline phosphatase, placental, group A—recurrent spontaneous abortions, group C—controls, group S—sticky platelet syndrome, group T—thromboembolism.

**Table 4.** Contingency table showing the frequency of genotypes of *ALPP* rs13026692 in the studied population.

| Group | | rs13026692 | | | |
|---|---|---|---|---|---|
| | | AA | AT | TT | Total |
| A | Observed | 27 | 21 | 5 | 53 |
| | % within row | 50.9% | 39.6% | 9.4% | 100.0% |
| C | Observed | 27 | 23 | 8 | 58 |
| | % within row | 46.6% | 39.7% | 13.8% | 100.0% |
| S | Observed | 23 | 28 | 2 | 53 |
| | % within row | 43.4% | 52.8% | 3.8% | 100.0% |
| T | Observed | 6 | 14 | 1 | 21 |
| | % within row | 28.6% | 66.7% | 4.8% | 100.0% |
| Total | Observed | 83 | 86 | 16 | 185 |
| | % within row | 44.9% | 46.5% | 8.6% | 100.0% |

Legend: *ALPP*—alkaline phosphatase, placental, group A—recurrent spontaneous abortions, group C—controls, group S—sticky platelet syndrome, group T—thromboembolism.

SNP *FOX3* rs3761548 has the possible genotypes CC, CA and AA. For SNP *FOXP3* rs3761548 in our included women, the GG genotype was detected in 34.6% of the women, GT in 47% and TT in 18.4% (Figure 4, Table 5).

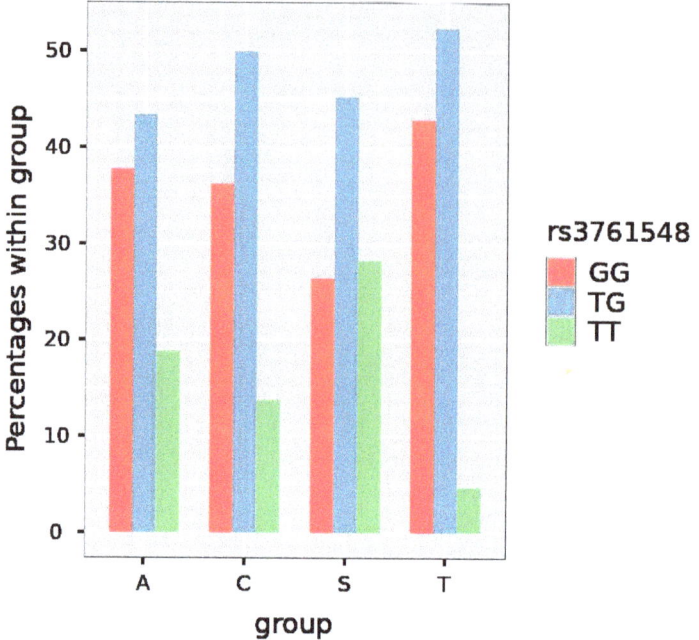

**Figure 4.** Plot with the frequency of the particular genotypes of *FOX3* rs3761548 in the studied groups. Legend: FOX 3—fork head box protein 3, group A—recurrent spontaneous abortions, group C—controls, group S—sticky platelet syndrome, group T—thromboembolism.

**Table 5.** Contingency table showing the frequency of genotypes of *FOX3* rs3761548 in the studied population.

| Group | | rs3761548 | | | |
|---|---|---|---|---|---|
| | | GG | TG | TT | Total |
| A | Observed | 20 | 23 | 10 | 53 |
| | % within row | 37.7% | 43.4% | 18.9% | 100.0% |
| C | Observed | 21 | 29 | 8 | 58 |
| | % within row | 36.2% | 50.0% | 13.8% | 100.0% |
| S | Observed | 14 | 24 | 15 | 53 |
| | % within row | 26.4% | 45.3% | 28.3% | 100.0% |
| T | Observed | 9 | 11 | 1 | 21 |
| | % within row | 42.9% | 52.4% | 4.8% | 100.0% |
| Total | Observed | 64 | 87 | 34 | 185 |
| | % within row | 34.6% | 47.0% | 18.4% | 100.0% |

Legend: FOX 3—fork head box protein 3, group A—recurrent spontaneous abortions, group C—controls, group S—sticky platelet syndrome, group T—thromboembolism.

Using multinomial logistic regression—group vs. SNPs—when taking into consideration the comparison of the SPS and the control group, in *VEGFA* rs3025039, both CC vs. TT and CT vs. TT analyses showed significant results ($p$ value for both of them was < 0.001) (Table 6).

Table 6. Multinomial logistic regression—group vs. SNPs.

| Group | Predictor | Estimate | SE | Z | p | Odds Ratio | 95% Confidence Interval Lower | 95% Confidence Interval Upper |
|---|---|---|---|---|---|---|---|---|
| A-C | Intercept | −0.593 | 1.575 | −0.377 | 0.707 | 0.5527 | 0.0252 | 12.11 |
| | rs2010963: | | | | | | | |
| | CG–CC | −0.159 | 0.785 | −0.202 | 0.84 | 0.8531 | 0.1832 | 3.972 |
| | GG–CC | −0.271 | 0.774 | −0.350 | 0.727 | 0.7629 | 0.1673 | 3.479 |
| | rs3025039: | | | | | | | |
| | CC–TT | 0.657 | 1.287 | 0.51 | 0.61 | 1.929 | 0.1548 | 24.039 |
| | CT–TT | 0.557 | 1.306 | 0.427 | 0.669 | 1.7459 | 0.1351 | 22.556 |
| | rs13026692: | | | | | | | |
| | AA–TT | 0.464 | 0.642 | 0.722 | 0.47 | 1.5903 | 0.4517 | 5.599 |
| | AT–TT | 0.405 | 0.655 | 0.618 | 0.536 | 1.4993 | 0.4154 | 5.411 |
| | rs3761548: | | | | | | | |
| | GG–TT | −0.272 | 0.587 | −0.464 | 0.643 | 0.7617 | 0.2413 | 2.405 |
| | TG–TT | −0.404 | 0.563 | −0.718 | 0.473 | 0.6675 | 0.2215 | 2.011 |
| S-C | Intercept | −14.105 | 0.765 | −18.446 | <0.001 | $7.49 \times 10^{-7}$ | $1.67 \times 10^{-7}$ | $3.35 \times 10^{-6}$ |
| | rs2010963: | | | | | | | |
| | CG–CC | −0.347 | 0.82 | −0.424 | 0.672 | 0.7065 | 0.1417 | 3.522 |
| | GG–CC | −0.382 | 0.803 | −0.475 | 0.635 | 0.6827 | 0.1414 | 3.296 |
| | rs3025039: | | | | | | | |
| | CC–TT | 13.961 | 0.422 | 33.1 | <0.001 | $1.16 \times 10^{6}$ | 506,157.2 | $2.64 \times 10^{6}$ |
| | CT–TT | 13.383 | 0.469 | 28.544 | <0.001 | 648,812 | 258,843.3 | $1.63 \times 10^{6}$ |
| | rs13026692: | | | | | | | |
| | AA–TT | 1.224 | 0.859 | 1.424 | 0.155 | 3.3993 | 0.6306 | 18.323 |
| | AT–TT | 1.819 | 0.86 | 2.116 | 0.034 | 6.1658 | 1.1435 | 33.246 |
| | rs3761548: | | | | | | | |
| | GG–TT | −1.320 | 0.594 | −2.223 | 0.026 | 0.2671 | 0.0834 | 0.856 |
| | TG–TT | −0.847 | 0.54 | −1.568 | 0.117 | 0.4286 | 0.1486 | 1.236 |
| T-C | Intercept | −3.057 | 2.239 | −1.365 | 0.172 | 0.047 | $5.84 \times 10^{-4}$ | 3.79 |
| | rs2010963: | | | | | | | |
| | CG–CC | 0.31 | 1.208 | 0.257 | 0.798 | 1.3633 | 0.1277 | 14.555 |
| | GG–CC | 0.293 | 1.197 | 0.244 | 0.807 | 1.34 | 0.1282 | 14.005 |
| | rs3025039: | | | | | | | |
| | CC–TT | −0.205 | 1.338 | −0.154 | 0.878 | 0.8143 | 0.0591 | 11.211 |
| | CT–TT | −0.169 | 1.372 | −0.123 | 0.902 | 0.8448 | 0.0574 | 12.434 |
| | rs13026692: | | | | | | | |
| | AA–TT | 0.611 | 1.163 | 0.525 | 0.599 | 1.8418 | 0.1886 | 17.988 |
| | AT–TT | 1.536 | 1.123 | 1.367 | 0.172 | 4.6452 | 0.5139 | 41.99 |
| | rs3761548: | | | | | | | |
| | GG–TT | 0.979 | 1.16 | 0.844 | 0.399 | 2.6613 | 0.2738 | 25.869 |
| | TG–TT | 0.973 | 1.138 | 0.855 | 0.393 | 2.6457 | 0.2841 | 24.634 |

Legend: group A—recurrent spontaneous abortions, group C—controls, group S—sticky platelet syndrome, group T—thromboembolism, p—p value, SE—standard error, SNP—single nucleotide polymorphism, Z—Z-score.

For SNP *ALPP* rs13026692, the comparison between genotypes AT and TT was significant ($p = 0.034$) as well. For SNP *FOXP3* rs3761548, GG vs. TT analysis also showed a significant value ($p = 0.026$). Thus, subjects with the GG genotype are at a four times lower risk of having SPS than subjects with the TT genotype (OR = 0.27). However, the decrease in risk is estimated with a low precision—the 95% confidence interval (95%CI) for odds ratio (OR) was (0.08, 0.86).

In the other group comparisons, we did not obtain significant data.

According to the results of estimated marginal means (estimates of the probability of the particular allele), for SNP *FOXP3* rs3761548, the TT (AA) genotype in the group of the patients with thromboembolism has a significant probability of presence ($p$ value = 0.0439).

Using post hoc tests, when analyzing *VEGFA* rs3025039 in the SPS group, the comparisons of the occurrence of genotypes CC vs. TT and CT vs. TT were statistically significant ($p$ values < 0.001 and 0.002, respectively) (Table 7).

Table 7. Post hoc comparisons—rs3025039.

| Response Groups | Comparison rs3025039 | rs3025039 | Difference | SE | z | p | pBonferroni | pholm |
|---|---|---|---|---|---|---|---|---|
| A | CC | CT | −0.02288 | 0.0794 | −0.2881 | 0.775 | 1 | 1 |
|   | CC | TT | 0.00906 | 0.246 | 0.0368 | 0.971 | 1 | 1 |
|   | CT | TT | 0.03195 | 0.2503 | 0.1277 | 0.899 | 1 | 1 |
| C | CC | CT | −0.05383 | 0.0793 | −0.6788 | 0.503 | 1 | 1 |
|   | CC | TT | −0.23849 | 0.2587 | −0.9219 | 0.365 | 1 | 1 |
|   | CT | TT | −0.18466 | 0.2625 | −0.7035 | 0.488 | 1 | 1 |
| S | CC | CT | 0.09291 | 0.0655 | 1.4191 | 0.167 | 0.502 | 0.167 |
|   | CC | TT | 0.31276 | 0.0585 | 5.3437 | <0.001 | <0.001 | <0.001 |
|   | CT | TT | 0.21986 | 0.0654 | 3.3641 | 0.002 | 0.007 | 0.005 |
| T | CC | CT | −0.01620 | 0.0392 | −0.4135 | 0.683 | 1 | 1 |
|   | CC | TT | −0.08334 | 0.1501 | −0.5552 | 0.583 | 1 | 1 |
|   | CT | TT | −0.06715 | 0.1517 | −0.4427 | 0.661 | 1 | 1 |

Legend: group A—recurrent spontaneous abortions, group C—controls, group S—sticky platelet syndrome, group T—thromboembolism, $p$—$p$ value, SE—standard error, SNP—single nucleotide polymorphism, Z—Z-score.

In the case of *ALPP* rs13026692, the comparison between AT and TT genotype in the SPS group was also significant ($p = 0.022$) (Table 8).

Table 8. Post hoc comparisons—rs13026692.

| Response Groups | rs13026692 | rs13026692 | Difference | SE | z | p | pBonferroni | pholm |
|---|---|---|---|---|---|---|---|---|
| A | AA | AT | 0.0824 | 0.075 | 1.099 | 0.282 | 0.845 | 0.845 |
|   | AA | TT | 0.0313 | 0.1276 | 0.245 | 0.808 | 1 | 1 |
|   | AT | TT | −0.0511 | 0.1271 | −0.402 | 0.691 | 1 | 1 |
| C | AA | AT | 0.0728 | 0.0789 | 0.923 | 0.364 | 1 | 0.54 |
|   | AA | TT | −0.1507 | 0.1338 | −1.126 | 0.27 | 0.81 | 0.54 |
|   | AT | TT | −0.2235 | 0.1348 | −1.658 | 0.109 | 0.327 | 0.327 |
| S | AA | AT | −0.0695 | 0.0488 | −1.424 | 0.166 | 0.497 | 0.309 |
|   | AA | TT | 0.0976 | 0.0666 | 1.465 | 0.155 | 0.464 | 0.309 |
|   | AT | TT | 0.1671 | 0.0688 | 2.43 | 0.022 | 0.066 | 0.066 |
| T | AA | AT | −0.0857 | 0.0618 | −1.385 | 0.177 | 0.532 | 0.532 |
|   | AA | TT | 0.0218 | 0.0675 | 0.323 | 0.749 | 1 | 0.749 |
|   | AT | TT | 0.1075 | 0.0835 | 1.287 | 0.209 | 0.627 | 0.532 |

Legend: group A—recurrent spontaneous abortions, group C—controls, group S—sticky platelet syndrome, group T—thromboembolism, $p$—$p$ value, SE—standard error, SNP—single nucleotide polymorphism, Z—Z-score.

Similarly, for SNP *FOXP3* rs3761548, in the SPS study group, the comparison between GG and TT genotype was evaluated as statistically significant ($p = 0.021$) (Table 9).

Table 9. Post hoc comparisons—rs3761548.

| Response Groups | rs3761548 | rs3761548 | Difference | SE | z | p | pBonferroni | pholm |
|---|---|---|---|---|---|---|---|---|
| A | GG | TG | 0.0457 | 0.0793 | 0.5765 | 0.569 | 1 | 1 |
| | GG | TT | −0.00977 | 0.1095 | −0.0892 | 0.93 | 1 | 1 |
| | TG | TT | −0.05547 | 0.1055 | −0.5259 | 0.603 | 1 | 1 |
| C | GG | TG | 0.004 | 0.086 | 0.0466 | 0.963 | 1 | 1 |
| | GG | TT | 0.06965 | 0.1155 | 0.6032 | 0.551 | 1 | 1 |
| | TG | TT | 0.06565 | 0.1097 | 0.5986 | 0.554 | 1 | 1 |
| S | GG | TG | −0.05293 | 0.0395 | −1.3417 | 0.191 | 0.573 | 0.229 |
| | GG | TT | −0.15178 | 0.0618 | −2.4573 | 0.021 | 0.062 | 0.062 |
| | TG | TT | −0.09885 | 0.0606 | −1.6315 | 0.114 | 0.343 | 0.229 |
| T | GG | TG | 0.00322 | 0.0559 | 0.0577 | 0.954 | 1 | 0.954 |
| | GG | TT | 0.09189 | 0.0714 | 1.2866 | 0.209 | 0.628 | 0.503 |
| | TG | TT | 0.08867 | 0.0625 | 1.4181 | 0.168 | 0.503 | 0.503 |

Legend: group A—recurrent spontaneous abortions, group C—controls, group S—sticky platelet syndrome, group T—thromboembolism, p—p value, SE—standard error, SNP—single nucleotide polymorphism, Z—Z-score.

In the case of *VEGFA* rs2010963, there were not any significant results between the probability of the presence of two studied genotypes. Moreover, the $p$ value in the Chi-squared test for this SNP was 0.999.

However, $R^2$McF was 0.0469—this generally indicates a poor prediction ability of the studied SNPs.

When investigating the association between thromboembolism/recurrent spontaneous abortions and SNP, the $p$ value for *VEGFA* rs2010963 polymorphism was 0.7486, and Pearson's Chi-squared test (X-squared) was 0.57917. For *VEGFA* rs3025039, the $p$ value was 0.69, and Pearson's Chi-squared test with Yates' continuity correction (X-squared) was 0.15906. Regarding SNP *ALPP* rs13026692, the $p$ value reached 0.47, and Pearson's Chi-squared test (X-squared) was 1.51. For SNP *FOXP3* rs3761548, $p$ was 0.233, and Pearson's Chi-squared test (X-squared) was 2.9136.

A multivariate analysis to evaluate the effect of ASA and LMWH on pregnancy outcome in terms of RSA or on the presence of thromboembolism is outlined in Table 10. The effect of concomitant thrombophilic state on the data obtained in the study is assessed in Table 10. In Table 10, we also tested the influence of the age of the patients on the results. Last but not least, post hoc comparisons for particular genotypes of selected SNPs in our study are provided in Tables 11–14.

Table 10. Model results of log likelihood ratio tests.

| | $X^2$ | df | p |
|---|---|---|---|
| rs2010963 | 1.22835 | 2 | 0.541 |
| rs3025039 | 0.39821 | 1 | 0.528 |
| rs13026692 | 1.50814 | 2 | 0.47 |
| rs3761548 | 3.13461 | 2 | 0.209 |
| age | 0.12124 | 1 | 0.728 |
| ASA and LMWH | 29.34294 | 4 | <0.001 |
| other thrombophilia | 0.00841 | 1 | 0.927 |

Legend: ASA—acetylsalicylic acid, df—degrees of freedom, LMWH—low molecular weight heparin, $p$—$p$ value, $X^2$—Chi-squared test.

Table 11. Post hoc comparisons—rs2010963.

| Comparison | | | | | | | |
|---|---|---|---|---|---|---|---|
| rs2010963 | rs2010963 | exp (B) | SE | z | p | pBonferroni | pholm |
| CC | CG | 0.217 | 0.482 | −0.689 | 0.491 | 1.000 | 0.982 |
| CC | GG | 0.652 | 1.296 | −0.215 | 0.830 | 1.000 | 0.982 |
| CG | GG | 3.001 | 3.134 | 1.053 | 0.293 | 0.878 | 0.878 |

Legend: exp(B)—exponential value of B, $p$—$p$ value, SE—standard error, z—Z-score.

Table 12. Post hoc comparisons—rs3025039.

| Comparison | | | | | | | |
|---|---|---|---|---|---|---|---|
| rs3025039 | rs3025039 | exp (B) | SE | z | p | pBonferroni | pholm |
| CC | CT | 2.02 | 2.32 | 0.613 | 0.540 | 0.540 | 0.540 |

Legend: exp(B)—exponential value of B, $p$—$p$ value, SE—standard error, z—Z-score.

Table 13. Post hoc comparisons—rs13026692.

| Comparison | | | | | | | |
|---|---|---|---|---|---|---|---|
| rs13026692 | rs13026692 | exp (B) | SE | z | p | pBonferroni | pholm |
| AA | AT | 1.19 | 1.17 | 0.17855 | 0.858 | 1.000 | 1.000 |
| AA | TT | $5.84 \times 10^8$ | $7.25 \times 10^{12}$ | 0.00163 | 0.999 | 1.000 | 1.000 |
| AT | TT | $4.90 \times 10^8$ | $6.08 \times 10^{12}$ | 0.00161 | 0.999 | 1.000 | 1.000 |

Legend: exp(B)—exponential value of B, $p$—$p$ value, SE—standard error, z—Z-score.

Table 14. Post hoc comparisons—rs3761548.

| Comparison | | | | | | | |
|---|---|---|---|---|---|---|---|
| rs3761548 | rs3761548 | exp (B) | SE | z | p | pBonferroni | pholm |
| GG | TG | 6.96 | 9.17 | 1.473 | 0.141 | 0.422 | 0.341 |
| GG | TT | 10.66 | 15.95 | 1.582 | 0.114 | 0.341 | 0.341 |
| TG | TT | 1.53 | 1.94 | 0.337 | 0.736 | 1.000 | 0.736 |

Legend: exp(B)—exponential value of B, $p$—$p$ value, SE—standard error, z—Z-score.

Post hoc comparisons of ASA vs. LMWH and those taking into account the influence of other thrombophilia are outlined in Tables 15 and 16.

Table 15. Post hoc comparisons—ASA_LMWH.

| Comparison | | | | | | | | |
|---|---|---|---|---|---|---|---|---|
| ASA_LMWH | ASA_LMWH | exp(B) | SE | z | p | pBonferroni | pholm |
| ASA | ASA | $3.14 \times 10^{8}$ | $3.07 \times 10^{12}$ | 0.00200 | 0.998 | 1.000 | 1.000 |
| ASA | ASA, LMWH | $1.01 \times 10^{9}$ | $4.30 \times 10^{12}$ | 0.00487 | 0.996 | 1.000 | 1.000 |
| ASA | LMWH | 0.344 | 0.334 | −1.10018 | 0.271 | 1.000 | 1.000 |
| ASA | LMWH a ASA | $5.04 \times 10^{-10}$ | $3.16 \times 10^{-6}$ | −0.00341 | 0.997 | 1.000 | 1.000 |
| ASA | ASA, LMWH | 3.223 | 34367.226 | $1.10 \times 10^{-4}$ | 1.000 | 1.000 | 1.000 |
| ASA | LMWH | $1.10 \times 10^{-9}$ | $1.07 \times 10^{-5}$ | −0.00211 | 0.998 | 1.000 | 1.000 |
| ASA | LMWH a ASA | $2.22 \times 10^{-16}$ | $2.58 \times 10^{-12}$ | −0.00353 | 0.997 | 1.000 | 1.000 |
| ASA, LMWH | LMWH | $3.40 \times 10^{-10}$ | $1.45 \times 10^{-6}$ | −0.00512 | 0.996 | 1.000 | 1.000 |
| ASA, LMWH | LMWH a ASA | $2.22 \times 10^{-16}$ | $1.68 \times 10^{-12}$ | −0.00555 | 0.996 | 1.000 | 1.000 |
| LMWH | LMWH a ASA | $1.46 \times 10^{9}$ | $9.20 \times 10^{-6}$ | −0.00324 | 0.997 | 1.000 | 1.000 |

Table 16. Post hoc comparisons—other thrombophilia.

| Comparison | | | | | | | |
|---|---|---|---|---|---|---|---|
| Other_Thrombophilia | Other_Thrombophilia | exp(B) | SE | z | p | pBonferroni | pholm |
| no | yes | 0.898 | 1.06 | −0.0915 | 0.927 | 0.927 | 0.927 |

Legend: exp(B)—exponential value of B, p—p value, SE—standard error, z—Z-score.

## 4. Discussion

It was confirmed that particularly rs1570360 (−1154G/A) (OR 1.51 (95%CI 1.13–2.03)), rs3025020 (−583C > T), rs833061 (460T/C), rs2010963 (−634G/C) and rs3025039 (+ 936C/T) *VEGF* genetic polymorphisms increase the probability of RSA or RPL [36–41]. The last two mentioned SNPs are even associated with an increased risk of preeclampsia in various ethnic groups [42].

In the case of SNP *VEGF* rs1570360 (−1154G > A), the variant allele A was significantly more common in patients with RPL (0.41) than in controls (0.19) ($p < 0.0001$). In *VEGF*-583 C > T, the CT genotype was significantly associated with this pathological state ($p = 0.003$) [43].

RPL is frequent in the population with *VEGF*-1154G/A (70.04%) and p53 Arg72Pro polymorphism (66.46%). The homozygous recessive genotype of *VEGF* and p53 thus exhibits significant association between these polymorphisms and RPL [44].

In *VEGF* 634 G > C, the allele C and CC genotype are significantly more frequent in individuals with RPL than in the control group ($p < 0.0001$) [43]. Thus, the frequency of idiopathic RSA can be dependent on the GC and CC genotype of rs2010963 *VEGF* polymorphism [45].

Moreover, placental −634 GC and CC genotypes might be involved in the development of preeclampsia and also in its severe form [46], with OR 1.85 (95%CI 1.25–2.75) and OR 1.90 (95%CI 1.28–2.83) in the maternal and fetal dominant model [47].

The C allele of SNP rs3025039 is associated with an increased risk of preeclampsia, and the T allele seems to have the opposite effect [48]. Interestingly, based on the results of the meta-analysis of 24 studies, rs2010963 polymorphism significantly contributes to the development of hypertensive disorders of pregnancy in the Caucasian and African population and rs3025039 in Asian women [49].

In our studied population, the GG genotype of *VEGFA* rs2010963 was most commonly found in the SPS group (54.7%). The less risky - minor CC genotype was more frequent in the group of pregnant patients with SPS and in the women with a history of RSA (7.5% in both of them) than in the group with a history of thromboembolism and the control group

(4.8% and 6.9%, respectively). However, the $p$ value in the Chi-squared test for this SNP was 0.999. This means the absence of a significant relationship between *VEGFA* rs2010963 and the study group and, thus, a poor predictive value.

The CC genotype of the SNP *VEGFA* rs3025039 was detected most commonly in the SPS group (77.4%). When compared with the controls, this was proved to be statistically significant ($p$ value for the comparison of CC vs. TT genotype < 0.001), as outlined in Tables 6 and 7. By contrast, interestingly, the minor TT genotype was not present in the SPS group. This finding confirms an increased frequency of the major (risky) genotype in the SPS population and suggests the thrombotic pathogenesis of RSA in this group of patients.

The T/T (Leu/leu) genotype of *ALPP* showed a protective effect for in vitro fertilization (IVF) failure and primary RSA (RR 0.438 (0.232–0.828, $p$ 0.002) and RR 0.532 (0.291–0.974, $p$ 0.016)). In the case of secondary RSA, the heterozygous genotype may be a risk factor with an RR of 2.226 (1.383–3.583, $p$ = 0.0031) [50].

Our study confirmed an increased frequency of the protective TT genotype in the control group (13.8%) and its lower incidence in the group of patients with SPS and a history of RSA (3.8%). These results were proven to be statistically significant ($p$ value for the comparison of AT vs. TT genotype in the SPS group was 0.022) (Table 8). Moreover, for the SPS vs. control group in the multinomial logistic regression analysis, when comparing AT and TT genotype, the $p$ value was 0.034 (Table 6). Such findings also correlate with an increased frequency of the risky AA genotype in the group of recurrent spontaneous abortions (50.9%) when compared with the controls (46.6%).

*FOXP3* rs3761548 polymorphism (−3279 C > A) is associated with a reduced expression of full-length FOXP3 protein in patients with unexplained RSA [28], and rs3761548 A/C polymorphism might be a significant risk factor for RPL [51,52]. Additionally, a potential relationship between further variants of *FOXP3* rs5902434, rs2232365 and rs2294021 and idiopathic recurrent miscarriage was confirmed [52,53].

Wu et al. suppose that functional polymorphisms of the *Foxp3* gene can represent an important factor of unexplained RSA in Chinese Han women, probably by altering Foxp3 expression and/or its function [52].

In addition to this relationship, *FOXP3* rs3761548 polymorphism was also tested for its association with preeclampsia. However, this causal link was not confirmed by Varshini et al. [54]. On the other hand, it was suggested that the A allele of this polymorphism might be protective against preeclampsia, and the C allele predisposes to this clinical condition in a dose-dependent manner [55].

We detected a decreased frequency of the GG (CC) genotype of *FOXP3* rs3761548 polymorphism in our study group of patients with SPS and RSA when compared with the control group ($p$ value for the CC (GG) vs. AA (TT) genotype in these two study groups = 0.021) (Table 9). This may indicate an evolutionary protective mechanism of the occurrence of the A (T) allele in the SPS group providing protection against thrombotic complications associated with pregnancy (preeclampsia or RSA).

Using a generalized linear model for logistic regression for the assessment of age as a potential factor, the $p$ value of the likelihood ratio test was 0.728, whereas in the case of consideration of treatment as a potential confounding factor, it was <0.001. When taking into consideration the presence of other thrombophilia, the $p$ value was 0.927, so the addition of this predictor to logistic regression does not improve the prediction regardless of whether the particular patient might be included in the group of thromboembolism or RSA (Table 10).

Thus, age does not have a significant influence on the results of our study. Moreover, after performance of post hoc tests, we did not find any significant difference between the genotypes of particular SNPs analyzed in our study (Tables 11–14). Regarding the influence of treatment with ASA or LMWH and the impact of the presence of concomitant thrombophilia on our results, we did not obtain any significant data, either (Tables 15 and 16).

However, when looking at the data of rs3761548, the comparison of the GG and TT genotype is close to statistical significance before the correction for multiple testing

($p$ value = 0.114). Therefore, patients with the GG (CC) genotype are approximately 11 times more at risk of thromboembolism than those with the TT (AA) genotype. This correlates with the above-described increased risk of RSA and RPL in carriers of A/C polymorphism and the increased risk of preeclampsia in the carriers of the C allele, as all these clinical states (RSA, RPL and preeclampsia) might be developed on the basis of thrombosis or vascular impairment in uteroplacental circulation. These results need to be confirmed using data from a higher number of patients, so we will continue to include further at-risk pregnant women to confirm our presumptions.

## 5. Conclusions

Our study confirmed the most frequent occurrence of the risky CC genotype of *VEGFA* polymorphism rs3025039, particularly in SPS patients ($p$ value < 0.001), in comparison with the TT genotype and the control group. Moreover, we found a significant difference in the presence of AT containing the risky A allele and TT genotype of *ALPP* rs13026692 polymorphism ($p$ = 0.034) in SPS patients when compared with the control group.

This might indicate that a diagnostic approach using genetic analysis of the presence of particular SNPs can predict clinically manifesting pregnancy complications developed on the basis of thrombotic events in uteroplacental circulation.

We are self-critically aware of the several limitations of our study—the fact that non-pregnant women were used as the control group, and the limited number of pregnant patients included because of health or personal issues. However, we will continue including patients to our study to contribute to improved knowledge in this field of research. Nevertheless, our study might be regarded as unique because, to the best of our knowledge, only our work has performed a genetic analysis of these selected polymorphisms associated with pregnancy complications in the specific population of at-risk pregnant women with SPS.

To conclude, we sincerely hope that our study might be useful and enrich the general knowledge around sticky platelet syndrome, helping in the management of at-risk pregnant women with SPS.

**Author Contributions:** Conceptualization, L.S., J.Ž., Ľ.V., A.H., Z.K., M.V., M.D., P.H., Z.J., J.S. and M.G.; methodology, L.S., J.Ž., Ľ.V., A.H., Z.K., M.V., J.S. and M.G.; software, L.S., M.G.; validation, T.B. (Tatiana Burjanivová), Z.L.; formal analysis, L.S., M.S., T.B. (Tomáš Bolek) and J.S.; investigation, L.S., J.Ž., Ľ.V., A.H., Z.K., M.V.; resources, L.S., J.S. and P.K.; data curation, L.S.; writing—original draft preparation, L.S.; writing—review and editing, L.S. and J.S.; visualization, L.S.; supervision, J.S., P.K., K.B. and J.D.; project administration, L.S. and J.S.; funding acquisition, L.S. and J.S. All authors have read and agreed to the published version of the manuscript.

**Funding:** It was supported by the project of the Scientific Grant Agency (Vega) 1/0549/19, Vega 1/0168/16, Vega 1/0479/21 and Agency for the Support of Research and Development (APVV) APVV-16-0020 received by our faculty.

**Institutional Review Board Statement:** All subjects gave their informed consent for inclusion before they participated in the study. The study was conducted in accordance with the Declaration of Helsinki, and the protocol was approved on 11 December 2013 by the Ethics Committee of the Jessenius Faculty of Medicine in Martin, Comenius University in Bratislava (Project identification code EK 1422/2013).

**Informed Consent Statement:** Informed consent was obtained from all subjects involved in the study.

**Data Availability Statement:** Not applicable.

**Conflicts of Interest:** The authors declare no conflict of interest. The funders in the form of the abovementioned projects in the section Funding had no role in the design, execution, interpretation or writing of the study.

## References

1. Mammen, E.F. Sticky platelet syndrome. *Semin. Thromb. Hemost.* **1999**, *25*, 361–365. [CrossRef] [PubMed]
2. Kubisz, P.; Ruiz-Argüelles, G.J.; Stasko, J.; Holly, P.; Ruiz-Delgado, G.J. Sticky platelet syndrome: History and future perspectives. *Semin. Thromb. Hemost.* **2014**, *40*, 526–534. [CrossRef]
3. Rac, M.W.F.; Minns Crawford, N.; Worley, K.C. Extensive thrombosis and first-trimester pregnancy loss caused by sticky platelet syndrome. *Obstet. Gynecol.* **2011**, *117 Pt 2*, 501–503. [CrossRef] [PubMed]
4. Azamar-Solis, B.; Cantero-Fortiz, Y.; Olivares-Gazca, J.C.; Olivares-Gazca, J.M.; Gómez-Cruz, G.B.; Murrieta-Álvarez, I.; Ruiz-Delgado, G.J.; Ruiz-Argüelles, G.J. Primary Thrombophilia in Mexico XIII: Localization of the Thrombotic Events in Mexican Mestizos with the Sticky Platelet Syndrome. *Clin. Appl. Thromb. Hemost.* **2019**, *25*, 1076029619841700. [CrossRef] [PubMed]
5. Kubisz, P.; Holly, P.; Stasko, J. Sticky Platelet Syndrome: 35 Years of Growing Evidence. *Semin. Thromb. Hemost.* **2019**, *45*, 61–68. [CrossRef]
6. Ruiz-Delgado, G.J.; Cantero-Fortiz, Y.; Mendez-Huerta, M.A.; Leon-Gonzalez, M.; Nuñez-Cortes, A.K.; Leon-Peña, A.A.; Olivares-Gazca, J.C.; Ruiz-Argüelles, G.J. Primary Thrombophilia in Mexico XII: Miscarriages Are More Frequent in People with Sticky Platelet Syndrome. *Turk. J. Haematol.* **2017**, *34*, 239–243. [CrossRef]
7. Kubisz, P.; Stanciakova, L.; Stasko, J.; Dobrotova, M.; Skerenova, M.; Ivankova, J.; Holly, P. Sticky platelet syndrome: An important cause of life-threatening thrombotic complications. *Expert Rev. Hematol.* **2016**, *9*, 21–35. [CrossRef]
8. Sokol, J.; Biringer, K.; Skerenova, M.; Stasko, J.; Kubisz, P.; Danko, J. Different models of inheritance in selected genes in patients with sticky platelet syndrome and fetal loss. *Semin. Thromb. Hemost.* **2015**, *41*, 330–335. [CrossRef]
9. Jung, S.M.; Moroi, M. Platelet glycoprotein VI. *Adv. Exp. Med. Biol.* **2008**, *640*, 53–63. [CrossRef]
10. Sokol, J.; Biringer, K.; Skerenova, M.; Hasko, M.; Bartosova, L.; Stasko, J.; Danko, J.; Kubisz, P. Platelet aggregation abnormalities in patients with fetal losses: The GP6 gene polymorphism. *Fertil. Steril.* **2012**, *98*, 1170–1174. [CrossRef]
11. Sokol, J.; Skerenova, M.; Biringer, K.; Lasabova, Z.; Stasko, J.; Kubisz, P. Genetic variations of the GP6 regulatory region in patients with sticky platelet syndrome and miscarriage. *Expert Rev. Hematol.* **2015**, *8*, 863–868. [CrossRef] [PubMed]
12. Sokol, J.; Skerenova, M.; Biringer, K.; Simurda, T.; Kubisz, P.; Stasko, J. Glycoprotein VI Gene Variants Affect Pregnancy Loss in Patients with Platelet Hyperaggregability. *Clin. Appl. Thromb. Hemost.* **2018**, *24* (Suppl. S9), 202S–208S. [CrossRef] [PubMed]
13. Stanciakova, L.; Skerenova, M.; Holly, P.; Dobrotova, M.; Ivankova, J.; Stasko, J.; Kubisz, P. Genetic origin of the sticky platelet syndrome. *Rev. Hematol. Mex.* **2016**, *17*, 139–143.
14. Vadelova, L.; Skerenova, M.; Ivankova, J.; Vazanova, A.; Sokol, J.; Zolkova, J.; Stanciakova, L.; Skornova, I.; Stasko, J. MicroRNA and hyperaggregability of platelets in women with sticky platelet syndrome and pregnancy complications. *Bratisl. Lek. Listy.* **2020**, *121*, 700–704. [CrossRef] [PubMed]
15. Kubisz, P.; Stasko, J.; Holly, P. Sticky platelet syndrome. *Semin. Thromb. Hemost.* **2013**, *39*, 674–683. [CrossRef]
16. Yagmur, E.; Bast, E.; Mühlfeld, A.S.; Koch, A.; Weiskirchen, R.; Tacke, F.; Neulen, J. High Prevalence of Sticky Platelet Syndrome in Patients with Infertility and Pregnancy Loss. *J. Clin. Med.* **2019**, *8*, 1328. [CrossRef]
17. Bick, R.L.; Hoppensteadt, D. Recurrent miscarriage syndrome and infertility due to blood coagulation protein/platelet defects: A review and update. *Clin. Appl. Thromb. Hemost.* **2005**, *11*, 1–13. [CrossRef]
18. Kolte, A.M.; Bernardi, L.A.; Christiansen, O.B.; Quenby, S.; Farquharson, R.G.; Goddijn, M.; Stephenson, M.D.; ESHRE Special Interest Group, Early Pregnancy. Terminology for pregnancy loss prior to viability: A consensus statement from the ESHRE early pregnancy special interest group. *Hum. Reprod.* **2015**, *30*, 495–498. [CrossRef]
19. Ford, H.B.; Schust, D.J. Recurrent Pregnancy Loss: Etiology, Diagnosis, and Therapy. *Rev. Obstet. Gynecol.* **2009**, *2*, 76–83.
20. Guideline on the Management of Recurrent Pregnancy Loss. Available online: https://www.eshre.eu/Guidelines-and-Legal/Guidelines/Recurrent-pregnancy-loss (accessed on 14 September 2022).
21. Green, D.M.; O'Donoghue, K. A review of reproductive outcomes of women with two consecutive miscarriages and no living child. *Obstet. Gynaecol.* **2019**, *39*, 816–821. [CrossRef]
22. Hachem, H.E.; Crepaux, V.; May-Panloup, P.; Descamps, P.; Legendre, G.; Bouet, P.-E. Recurrent pregnancy loss: Current perspectives. *Int. J. Womens Health* **2017**, *9*, 331–345. [CrossRef] [PubMed]
23. Bick, R.L. Recurrent miscarriage syndrome due to blood coagulation protein/platelet defects: Prevalence, treatment and outcome results. DRW Metroplex Recurrent Miscarriage Syndrome Cooperative Group. *Clin. Appl. Thromb. Hemost.* **2000**, *6*, 115–125. [CrossRef] [PubMed]
24. An, H.J.; Kim, J.H.; Ahn, E.H.; Kim, Y.R.; Kim, J.O.; Park, H.S.; Ryu, C.S.; Kim, E.-G.; Cho, S.H.; Lee, W.S.; et al. 3′-UTR Polymorphisms in the Vascular Endothelial Growth Factor Gene (VEGF) Contribute to Susceptibility to Recurrent Pregnancy Loss (RPL). *Int. J. Mol. Sci.* **2019**, *20*, 3319. [CrossRef] [PubMed]
25. VEGFA. Gene—Vascular Endothelial Growth Factor A. Available online: https://www.genecards.org/cgi-bin/carddisp.pl?gene=VEGFA&keywords=rs3025039,VEGF (accessed on 27 September 2022).
26. He, X.; Chen, Q. Reduced expressions of connexin 43 and VEGF in the first-trimester tissues from women with recurrent pregnancy loss. *Reprod. Biol. Endocrinol.* **2016**, *14*, 46. [CrossRef] [PubMed]
27. ALPP Gene—Alkaline Phosphatase, Placental. Available online: https://www.genecards.org/cgi-bin/carddisp.pl?gene=ALPP&keywords=alpp (accessed on 14 September 2022).

8. Dirsipam, K.; Ponnala, D.; Madduru, D.; Bonu, R.; Jahan, P. Association of FOXP3 rs3761548 polymorphism and its reduced expression with unexplained recurrent spontaneous abortions: A South Indian study. *Am. J. Reprod. Immunol.* **2021**, *86*, e13431. [CrossRef] [PubMed]
9. Effect of Forkhead Box Protein 3 Gene Polymorphisms in Recurrent Pregnancy Loss: A Meta-Analysis. Postgraduate Institute of Medical Education and Research (PGIMER), Department of Science and Technology (DST), New Delhi, India, 2022, a Preprint That Has Not Been Peer Reviewed by a Journal. Available online: https://www.researchsquare.com/article/rs-1532145/v1 (accessed on 16 September 2022).
10. Mishra, S.; Srivastava, A.; Mandal, K.; Phadke, S.R. Study of the association of forkhead box P3 (FOXP3) gene polymorphisms with unexplained recurrent spontaneous abortions in Indian population. *J. Genet.* **2018**, *97*, 405–410. [CrossRef] [PubMed]
11. FOXP3 Gene—Forkhead Box P3. Available online: https://www.genecards.org/cgi-bin/carddisp.pl?gene=FOXP3&keywords=rs3761548,FOXP3 (accessed on 24 September 2022).
12. The Jamovi Project. Jamovi. (Version 2.3) [Computer Software]. Available online: https://www.jamovi.org (accessed on 18 July 2022).
13. R Core Team. R: A Language and Environment for Statistical Computing. (Version 4.1) [Computer Software]. Available online: https://cran.r-project.org (accessed on 18 July 2022).
14. Meyer, D.; Zeileis, A.; Hornik, K.; Gerber, F.; Friendly, M. VCD: Visualizing Categorical Data. [R Package]. Available online: https://cran.r-project.org/package=vcd (accessed on 18 July 2022).
15. Gallucci, M. GAMLj: General Analyses for Linear Models. [Jamovi Module]. Available online: https://gamlj.github.io/ (accessed on 13 October 2022).
16. Xu, X.; Du, C.; Li, H.; Du, J.; Yan, X.; Peng, L.; Li, G.; Chen, Z.-J. Association of VEGF Genetic Polymorphisms with Recurrent Spontaneous Abortion Risk: A Systematic Review and Meta-Analysis. *PLoS ONE* **2015**, *10*, e0123696. [CrossRef]
17. El-Deeb, S.M.S.; ELSaeed, G.K.; Khodeer, S.A.; Dawood, A.A.; Omar, T.A.; Ibrahem, R.A.; ELShemy, A.M.; Montaser, B.A. Vascular endothelial growth factor and recurrent spontaneous abortion: A meta-analysis. *Menoufia Med. J.* **2022**, *35*, 26–33. [CrossRef]
18. Li, L.; Donghong, L.; Shuguang, W.; Hongbo, Z.; Jing, Z.; Shengbin, L. Polymorphisms in the vascular endothelial growth factor gene associated with recurrent spontaneous miscarriage. *J. Matern-Fetal Neonatal Med.* **2013**, *26*, 686–690. [CrossRef]
19. Su, M.-T.; Lin, S.-H.; Chen, Y.-C. Genetic association studies of angiogenesis- and vasoconstriction-related genes in women with recurrent pregnancy loss: A systematic review and meta-analysis. *Hum. Reprod. Update* **2011**, *17*, 803–812. [CrossRef]
40. Zhang, B.; Dai, B.; Zhang, X.; Wang, Z. Vascular endothelial growth factor and recurrent spontaneous abortion: A meta-analysis. *Gene* **2012**, *507*, 1–8. [CrossRef] [PubMed]
41. Yalcintepe, S.A.; Silan, F.; Hacivelioglu, S.O.; Uludag, A.; Cosar, E.; Ozdemir, O. Fetal Vegf Genotype is More Important for Abortion Risk than Mother Genotype. *Int. J. Mol. Cell Med.* **2014**, *3*, 88–94.
42. Duan, W.; Xia, C.; Wang, K.; Duan, Y.; Cheng, P.; Xiong, B. A meta-analysis of the vascular endothelial growth factor polymorphisms associated with the risk of pre-eclampsia. *Biosci. Rep.* **2020**, *40*, BSR20190209. [CrossRef] [PubMed]
43. Amin, I.; Pandith, A.A.; Manzoor, U.; Mir, S.H.; Afroze, D.; Koul, A.M.; Wani, S.; Ahmad, A.; Qasim, I.; Rashid, M.; et al. Implications of VEGF gene sequence variations and its expression in recurrent pregnancy loss. *Reprod. Biomed. Online* **2021**, *43*, 1035–1044. [CrossRef] [PubMed]
44. Subi, T.M.; Krishnakumar, V.; Kataru, C.R.; Panigrahi, I.; Kannan, M. Association of VEGF and p53 Polymorphisms and Spiral Artery Remodeling in Recurrent Pregnancy Loss: A Systematic Review and Meta-Analysis. *Thromb. Haemost.* **2022**, *122*, 363–376. [CrossRef]
45. Sajjadi, M.S.; Ghandil, P.; Shahbazian, N.; Saberi, A. Association of vascular endothelial growth factor A polymorphisms and aberrant expression of connexin 43 and VEGFA with idiopathic recurrent spontaneous miscarriage. *J. Obstet. Gynaecol. Res.* **2020**, *46*, 369–375. [CrossRef]
46. Keshavarzi, F.; Mohammadpour-Gharehbagh, A.; Shahrakipour, M.; Teimoori, B.; Yazdi, A.; Yaghmaei, M.; Naroeei-Nejad, M.; Salimi, S. The placental vascular endothelial growth factor polymorphisms and preeclampsia/preeclampsia severity. *Clin. Exp. Hypertens.* **2017**, *39*, 606–611. [CrossRef]
47. Chen, X.Z.; Yu, S.J.; Wei, M.H.; Li, C.Y.; Yan, W.R. Effects of maternal and fetal vascular endothelial growth factor a single nucleotide polymorphisms on pre-eclampsia: A hybrid design study. *Cytokine* **2020**, *127*, 154995. [CrossRef]
48. Amosco, M.D.; Villar, V.A.; Naniong, J.M.; David-Bustamante, L.M.; Jose, P.A.; Palmes-Saloma, C.P. VEGF-A and VEGFR1 SNPs associate with preeclampsia in a Philippine population. *Clin. Exp. Hypertens.* **2016**, *38*, 578–585.
49. Su, M.; Hu, Z.; Dong, C.; Xu, X. Vascular endothelial growth factor gene polymorphisms and hypertensive disorder of pregnancy: A meta-analysis. *Pregnancy Hypertens* **2019**, *17*, 191–196. [CrossRef]
50. Vatin, M.; Bouvier, S.; Bellazi, L.; Montagutelli, X.; Laissue, P.; Ziyyat, A.; Serres, C.; De Mazancourt, P.; Dieudonné, M.-N.; Mornet, E.; et al. Polymorphisms of human placental alkaline phosphatase are associated with in vitro fertilization success and recurrent pregnancy loss. *Am. J. Pathol.* **2014**, *184*, 362–368. [CrossRef] [PubMed]
51. Jaber, M.O.; Sharif, F.A. Association between functional polymorphisms of Foxp3 and Interleukin-21 genes with the occurrence of recurrent pregnancy loss in Gaza strip-Palestine. *Int. J. Res. Med. Sci.* **2014**, *2*, 1687–1693. [CrossRef]
52. Wu, Z.; You, Z.; Zhang, C.; Li, Z.; Su, X.; Zhang, X.; Li, Y. Association between functional polymorphisms of Foxp3 gene and the occurrence of unexplained recurrent spontaneous abortion in a Chinese Han population. *Clin. Dev. Immunol.* **2012**, *2012*, 896458. [CrossRef] [PubMed]

53. Saxena, D.; Misra, M.K.; Parveen, F.; Phadke, S.R.; Agrawal, S. The transcription factor Forkhead Box P3 gene variants affect idiopathic recurrent pregnancy loss. *Placenta* **2015**, *36*, 226–231. [CrossRef] [PubMed]
54. Sri Varshini, G.; Harshini, S.; Siham, M.A.; Tejaswini, G.K.; Santhosh Kumar, Y.; Kulanthaivel, L.; Subbaraj, G.K. Investigation of FOXP3 (rs3761548) polymorphism with the risk of preeclampsia and recurrent spontaneous abortion: A systemic review and meta-analysis. *Asian Pac. J. Reprod.* **2022**, *11*, 117–124. [CrossRef]
55. Jahan, P.; Sreenivasagari, R.; Goudi, D.; Komaravalli, P.L.; Ishaq, M. Role of Foxp3 gene in maternal susceptibility to pre-eclampsia—A study from South India. *Scand J. Immunol.* **2013**, *77*, 104–108. [CrossRef]

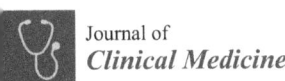 

*Review*

# Resistance on the Latest Oral and Intravenous P2Y12 ADP Receptor Blockers in Patients with Acute Coronary Syndromes: Fact or Myth?

Peter Blaško [1,2], Matej Samoš [1,*], Tomáš Bolek [1], Lucia Stančiaková [3], Ingrid Škorňová [3], Martin Jozef Péč [1], Jakub Jurica [1], Ján Staško [3] and Marián Mokáň [1]

1. Department of Internal Medicine I, Jessenius Faculty of Medicine in Martin, Comenius University in Bratislava, 036 59 Martin, Slovakia
2. Out-Patient Clinic of Cardiology, 957 01 Banovce nad Bebravou, Slovakia
3. Department of Hematology and Blood Transfusion, National Centre of Hemostasis and Thrombosis, Jessenius Faculty of Medicine in Martin, Comenius University in Bratislava, 036 59 Martin, Slovakia
* Correspondence: matej.samos@gmail.com; Tel.: +421-907-612-943 or +421-434-203-820

**Abstract:** Novel P2Y12 ADP receptor blockers (ADPRB) should be preferred in dual-antiplatelet therapy in patients with acute coronary syndrome. Nevertheless, there are still patients who do not respond optimally to novel ADP receptor blocker therapy, and this nonoptimal response (so-called "high on-treatment platelet reactivity" or "resistance") could be connected with increased risk of adverse ischemic events, such as myocardial re-infarction, target lesion failure and stent thrombosis. In addition, several risk factors have been proposed as factors associated with the phenomenon of inadequate response on novel ADPRB. These include obesity, multivessel coronary artery disease, high pre-treatment platelet reactivity and impaired metabolic status for prasugrel, as well as elderly, concomitant therapy with beta-blockers, morphine and platelet count for ticagrelor. There is no literature report describing nonoptimal therapeutic response on cangrelor, and cangrelor therapy seems to be a possible approach for overcoming HTPR on prasugrel and ticagrelor. However, the optimal therapeutic management of "resistance" on novel ADPRB is not clear and this issue requires further research. This narrative review article discusses the phenomenon of high on-treatment platelet reactivity on novel ADPRB, its importance in clinical practice and approaches for its therapeutic overcoming.

**Keywords:** prasugrel; ticagrelor; cangrelor; high on-treatment platelet reactivity; stent thrombosis; acute coronary syndrome

## 1. Introduction

Novel P2Y12 ADP receptor blockers (ADPRB), namely prasugrel, ticagrelor and cangrelor, have emerged as a potent therapeutic approach for ADP signaling pathway inhibition in patients with acute coronary syndromes (ACSs), with [1–3] or without planned percutaneous coronary intervention (PCI) [3], or patients who undergo PCI without oral ADPRB pre-treatment [4]. This therapy should be considered, especially in those patients who do not respond optimally to clopidogrel (patients with clopidogrel high on-treatment platelet reactivity = "clopidogrel resistance") [5]. Nevertheless, there are still patients who do not respond optimally to novel ADPRB therapy, and this nonoptimal response could be connected with increased risk of adverse ischemic events, such as myocardial re-infarction, target lesion failure and stent thrombosis [6,7]. This article discusses the phenomenon of "resistance" (high on-treatment platelet reactivity) on novel-generation ADPRB (the latest ADPRB available in clinical practice), its importance in clinical practice and approaches for its therapeutic overcoming.

## 2. Methods

The aim of this article is to provide a brief traditional (narrative) review, which summarizes current data regarding the prevalence and clinical significance of HTPR on novel-generation ADPRB, namely prasugrel, ticagrelor and cangrelor, in patients with acute coronary syndrome. To achieve this aim, the most relevant medical scientific literature databases—Web of Science, PubMed and Scopus—were searched, using selected keywords: "high on treatment platelet reactivity" or "resistance" or "insufficient response" and "prasugrel" or "ticagrelor" or "cangrelor" and "acute coronary syndrome" or "myocardial infarction" or "STEMI" or "NSTEMI" or "unstable angina". If needed, additional keywords, such as "major adverse cardiac event" or "stent thrombosis" or "stent failure" or "target lesion failure" were added, and the literature was researched. The authors non-systematically identified relevant articles matching their aim. Subsequently, a review of findings from these articles was provided, together with a discussion of the clinical implications of published observations.

## 3. Insufficient Response to ADPRB and the Risk of Future Events in Patients with ACS

ADPRB treatment failure is a major risk factor for stent thrombosis and early PCI failure [8]. Patients with high on-treatment platelet reactivity (HTPR) have an approximately 2–3-fold higher risk of adverse ischemic events and stent thrombosis than those without HTPR. Moreover, ADPRB HTPR has been observed in patients with ACS previously independently associated with unfavorable in-hospital clinical outcome [9], with increased risk of long-term thrombotic events in patients with implanted drug-eluting stents [10,11], connected with frequent recurrent angina and left ventricular failure [12] and predicted future cardiovascular events after PCI for ACS [13]. A previous observational study [14] showed that clopidogrel resistance was present in 72.5% of patients admitted for repeated ACS, which suggests that HTPR likely plays an important role in recurrent ACS. Additionally, the phenomenon was reported as a leading cause of stent thrombosis (including left main-chain and multi-vessel stent thrombosis) in several clinical cases [15–19].

Despite the abovementioned evidence, there is still an ongoing discussion about the association between antiplatelet drugs HTPR and major adverse cardiovascular events (MACE), and the clinical implication of antiplatelet therapy HTPR is not fully determined. Several factors could be responsible for this ambiguity. First, the results of so-far published studies are controversial (especially for aspirin HTPR), and there are studies that did not confirm the relation between HTPR and the risk of future ischemic adverse events [20–23]. Second, a MACE in a patient after previous coronary intervention is a complex phenomenon, which could be associated with stent failure itself (due to either stent thrombosis or stent restenosis) or due to "de novo" atherothrombotic events, which could develop due to progression of plaque instability or due to platelet activation or both mechanisms can be involved. Additionally, stent thrombosis, for example, could be connected with HTPR, stent malposition, inadequate stent expansion, stent undersizing, small stent diameter, stent fracture, edge dissection or drug non-compliance [24,25]. Therefore, one needs to understand that HTPR on ADPRB therapy is just one risk factor in a complex clinical problem. Third, there is still no definite answer for how to deal with HTPR, as multiple previously tested approaches failed to improve clinical outcomes [26–28]. Considering the fact that failure to reduce platelet reactivity in the settings of HTPR seems to be an independent predictor of future MACE [29], the issue of not having an optimal algorithm for HTPR-guided intensification of platelet inhibition could definitely play an important role in these uncertainties.

Fourth, there is an issue in laboratory testing for HTPR detection. In fact, various platelet function tests (PFTs) with different test principles have been tested (and validated) for the detection of HTPR [30]. Some of them are designed as point-of-care tests, others require complex laboratory equipment and skilled staff to perform the examination. Light transmission aggregometry (LTA) with a specific inducer (adenosine diphosphate—ADP) is still recognized as a standard laboratory test for PFT, which also includes the detection of HTPR, while the Vasodilator-Stimulated Phosphoprotein phosphorylation (VASP-P) by flow cytometric analysis is probably the most specific test for assessing the rate of P2Y12 ADP signaling pathway inhibition [31]. Both tests have important limitations (especially in the settings of daily clinical practice, including the need for measuring the antiplatelet drug response in a 24/7 ACS program), such as the need for special equipment, skilled staff, time demand and, in the case of LTA, the need to process the sample immediately (within first hour from blood sampling). Therefore, several point-of-care assays, namely Multiplate®, VerifyNow®, PFA-100® and platelet mapping thromboelastography® (TEG®), have been designed. Multiplate® (Roche Diagnostics, Indianapolis, IN, USA) is a point-of-care assay, which tests citrated whole blood samples using the electrical impedance aggregometry principle. The assay uses platelet stimulation with specific inducers (ADP) to activate platelet aggregation. Once the aggregated platelets attach the sensor wires in the Multiplate® device, electrical resistance (impedance) is detected and displayed as aggregation units (AUs) against time (area under the curve = AUC) [32]. VerifyNow® (Werfen, Barcelona, Spain) assay is performed as a point-of-care test using a citrated whole blood sample. In this turbidimetry-based assay, ADP induction is used to initiate platelet aggregation on fibrinogen-coated beads. Platelet aggregation is determined by the percentage of the light transmission and expressed in P2Y12 reaction units (PRUs). Low PRU indicates the high P2Y12 receptor inhibition and better response to P2Y12 ADPRB. VerifyNow® assay is a rapid test, which can be performed even at the bedside within 5 min, which is an advantage when compared with LTA and VASP-P assays. Moreover, the examination itself (due to a simple technique) and the interpretation of results can be carried out easily (there is no need for skilled staff to perform and/or evaluate the results). Both assays have been used for PFT in post-marketing studies, including randomized ones [26,30,32]. Platelet function assay-100 = PFA-100® (Siemens Medical Solutions, Malvern, PA, USA) is another point-of-care assay, which can be used to monitor the effect of P2Y12 ADPRB. The assay uses citrated whole blood sample and measures the platelet aggregation and effect of antiplatelet agents under higher shear stress. This test can be performed rapidly (in less time) and, similarly to VerifyNow® assay, has a simple test technique, which is an added advantage when compared with conventional PFT. PFA-100® has collagen-coated, epinephrine-coated and ADP-coated cartridges. If ADPRB is present in a sample, the blood will flow under higher shear rate through the capillary and through a small aperture of the PFA-100® analyzer. Subsequently, platelets will aggregate and form the ADP-induced platelet plug by blocking the aperture. The time taken for complete occlusion of the aperture is recorded as closure time (CT). Prolonged CT indicates a better response to ADPRB [32]. PFA-100® assay has been used in clinical studies mostly for the detection of aspirin resistance [33,34]; however, there are data to show that the test can be used also for the determination of response to ADPRB [35]. On the other side, it is questionable whether the use of point-of-care assays (compared to traditional PFT) has an impact (negative) on the clinical utility of PFT studies, as these assays are criticized for their limited sensitivity and/or specificity [36,37]. Additionally, it is possible that a single PFT will not reliably detect HTPR, and that confirmation of suspected HTPR with another PFT might be needed for establishment of final diagnosis (confirmation of results obtained from a point-of-care test by a laboratory-based test). Finally, there is an issue of inconsistent cut-off values for the detection of HTPR, especially when point-of-care assays are used for its determination. For example, for the VerifyNow® assay, cut-off values of >280 PRU, >272 PRU, >235 PRU and >230 PRU have been used to define HTPR in previously published studies [26,30]; for Multiplate®, at least two cut-off values (468 AUC, 450 AUC) have been reported. All these unclosed issues could explain the ongoing discussion regarding the clinical implication of HTPR.

Nonetheless, considering the fact that, with clopidogrel, ADP-induced platelet aggregation remains significantly high in ACS patients, even after 48 h from standard loading [38], it is unsurprising that a novel generation of ADPRB (Table 1) with more rapid and more potent platelet inhibitory effects has been developed and introduced to clinical practice, especially for the treatment of patients with ACS.

Table 1. Novel-generation ADP receptor blockers in current clinical practice.

| Drug | Route of Administration Dosing | Bioavailability | Receptor Inhibition | Time to Peak Platelet Inhibition | Clinical Application | HTPR (Prevalence) |
|---|---|---|---|---|---|---|
| Prasugrel | Oral Loading dose of 60 mg followed by 10 mg once daily (5 mg in elderly and low body weight) | Prodrug | Irreversible | 0.5–2 h | ACS with PCI | Described (1.6–25%; higher if time from drug administration to blood sampling is too short) |
| Ticagrelor | Oral Loading dose of 180 mg followed by 90 mg twice daily (60 mg twice daily in CAD) | Direct-acting | Reversible | 1.5–2 h | ACS High ischemic risk CAD | Described (8.6–13.7% if tested 30 to 90 days post drug loading; 0.0–1.9% on long-term therapy) |
| Cangrelor | Intravenous Bolus injection of 30 ug/kg followed by continuous intravenous infusion of 4 ug/kg/min. | Direct-acting | Reversible | 2 min | PCI (if not pretreated with oral agent) | Not described |

ACS—acute coronary syndromes; CAD—coronary artery disease; HTPR—high on-treatment platelet reactivity; PCI—percutaneous coronary intervention.

## 4. Novel-Generation ADPRB

### 4.1. Prasugrel

Prasugrel is an irreversible, 3$^{rd}$-generation thienopyridine P2Y12 ADPRB, which is indicated for combined (with aspirin) antiplatelet therapy in PCI-treated patients with ACS [1,2,39]. Prasugrel [39] provides more consistent inhibition of the P2Y12 ADP receptor and has lower intraindividual variability in efficacy compared with clopidogrel. It is hydrolyzed by plasma esterases, then metabolized by cytochrome P450 (CYP) 3A4 and 2B6 enzymes to form an active metabolite and has a plasma half-life of 7.4 h. The inactivation of the active metabolite is mediated trough drug S-methylation and drug conjugation. The inactive metabolites are excreted by urine (68%) and stool. The response to prasugrel is not affected by CYP 2C19 inhibition, loss of CYP 2C19 gene function or decreased function of P-glycoprotein (P-gp). Loading doses of 60 mg of prasugrel reach, in theory, full antiplatelet effects 15–30 min after administration. The benefit of prasugrel therapy seems to be the highest in patients with diabetes mellitus [1]. Prasugrel therapy was repeatedly used to overcome clopidogrel resistance [15,19].

### 4.2. Ticagrelor

Ticagrelor is a reversible, 3$^{rd}$-generation non-thienopyridine P2Y12 ADPRB, approved for combined antiplatelet therapy in patients with ACS (with or without PCI) and for long-term combined antiplatelet therapy in coronary artery disease (CAD) patients with high ischemic and low bleeding risk [3,40]. Ticagrelor offers rapid and consistent inhibition of the P2Y12 ADP signaling pathway, which is independent of previous metabolic activation and P-gp function. Ticagrelor reaches its maximal plasma activity approximately 1.5 h after ingestion and has a plasma half-life of 8.5 h. However, it undergoes metabolism, which is mediated by CYP 3A4 and, therefore, strong inducers/inhibitors of this enzyme complex could affect the concentrations of ticagrelor and lead to unexpected drug activity. Ticagrelor is, after metabolic transformation, eliminated by hepatic and renal excretion. A loading dose of 180 mg followed by a maintenance dose of 90 mg twice daily are recommended for patients with ACS, while a dose of 60 mg twice daily is recommended for long-term antiplatelet prophylaxis in high-ischemic-risk CAD patients [5,39,40]. Although a recent randomized study suggested better efficacy (with similar safety profile) of prasugrel compared to ticagrelor in ACS patients undergoing PCI [2], ticagrelor therapy had been repeatedly described as an effective approach for overcoming clopidogrel resistance [5,41,42] and is still preferred in those ACS patients who could not receive prasugrel.

*4.3. Cangrelor*

Cangrelor is a reversible, parenteral, 3rd-generation non-thienopyridine P2Y12 ADPRB, which is indicated for combined antiplatelet therapy in patients undergoing PCI (both for ACS and stable CAD) who are not pre-treated with oral ADPRB [4]. Cangrelor reaches the maximal antiplatelet effect within 2 min after bolus injection (30 ug per kg of body weight) and has a very short plasma half-life (2.6–3.3 min) requiring continuous intravenous infusion (4 ug per kg of body weight per minute) to maintain adequate ADP receptor inhibition. Cangrelor does not require metabolic transformation to form an active metabolite and is independent of CYP and P-gp activity. Cangrelor is deactivated by plasmatic de-phosphorylation; the inactive metabolite is eliminated by urine (58%) and stool (35%). Normal platelet function is restored within 1 h after stopping the cangrelor infusion [43]. Cangrelor administration could be, in theory, used as a bailout option for overcoming clopidogrel resistance in patients presenting with stent thrombosis [44].

## 5. Prasugrel Resistance in Patients with ACS

In one of the first studies examining the prevalence of insufficient response on prasugrel, Bonello et al. [45] reported that a significant portion of patients undergoing PCI for ACS did not achieve optimal platelet inhibition. In this study, with 301 patients receiving a prasugrel loading dose of 60 mg, 25.2% of patients had HTPR. Patients who experienced a thrombotic event after PCI had significantly higher residual platelet activity measured with VASP-P compared with those free of adverse thrombotic events. In our previous prospective study, which aimed to map the platelet reactivity in novel ADP receptor-blocker-treated patients with acute ST elevation myocardial infarction (STEMI), 60.9% of prasugrel-treated patients did not achieve sufficient platelet inhibition after a loading dose of 60 mg (measured $1.6 \pm 0.7$ h after loading dose administration) and 8.7% of prasugrel-treated patients remained non-responders in second blood sampling performed after $20.4 \pm 2.6$ h from loading dose administration [46]. In addition, Aradi et al. [47] tested platelet reactivity with LTA and whole blood impedance aggregometry (Multiplate®) in 103 consecutive, high-risk ACS patients 12 to 24 h after administration of loading dose (60 mg) of prasugrel. The authors of this study reported significant inter-patient variability in platelet reactivity after all doses of prasugrel, and the prevalence of HTPR was significantly higher during the maintenance dose administration. On the other side, another study enrolling PCI-treated ACS patients receiving prasugrel reported HTPR (defined as VASP-P index > 50%) 2 to 4 weeks after hospital discharge only in 6.8% of patients [48]. Similarly, only 9.1% of acute STEMI patients was identified as a non-responders on prasugrel (defined as VASP-P index > 50% 6 to 12 h after prasugrel loading dose administration) in a previous prospective study performed by Laine et al. [49]. A previous meta-analysis of 14 studies with 1822 patients reported the HTPR in 9.8% of prasugrel-treated patients [50]; Siller-Matula et al. [51] reported that only 3% of prasugrel-treated patients had HTPR in the maintenance phase of treatment. In another single-center retrospective analysis of 809 PCI-treated ACS patients, the prevalence of prasugrel HTPR was even lower and only 1.6% of prasugrel-treated patients fulfilled the criteria for HTPR [52]. However, this study measured platelet reactivity with whole blood impedance aggregometry. In a more recent analysis, Verdoia et al. [53,54], in their prospective studies, reported that HTPR on prasugrel was observed in 10% and 12.3% of patients, respectively. In these studies, whole blood impedance aggregometry was used for determination of HTPR.

Based on these data (Table 2), one could conclude that, although with significantly lower prevalence (compared to clopidogrel), HTPR on prasugrel exists, and its prevalence varies from 1.6 to approximately 25% of treated patients (depending on platelet function test used and chosen time from loading dose to blood sampling). In addition, if the time interval from drug administration to blood sampling is too short, the number of patients with inadequate response can be even higher [46]. Nevertheless, it seems that the phenomenon of prasugrel HTPR is connected with adverse ischemic events. This observation was repeatedly reported in previous prospective studies, including sub-analyses of randomized studies [45,55,56]. Aradi et al. [56], for example, reported, in a pre specified exploratory analysis of the TROPICAL-ACS trial, that, although infrequent, prasugrel HTPR was connected with increased risk of thrombotic events. The association between prasugrel HTPR and the higher risk of adverse ischemic events post PCI is also supported by multiple reported clinical cases of prasugrel "resistance", which consistently reported serious adverse thrombotic events, including repeated cases of stent thrombosis [6,57,58]. Hence, the HTPR on prasugrel could probably be considered as a risk factor for adverse ischemia/thrombosis, similarly to clopidogrel HTPR.

Table 2. Summary of studies reporting prasugrel HTPR.

| Study | Type of Study | Studied Population | Number of Patients | Test for HTPR | Cut Off | Main Results |
|---|---|---|---|---|---|---|
| Bonello et al. [45] | Prospective multicenter (non-randomized) | PCI for ACS | 301 | VASP-P | VASP-P: PRI > 50% | HTPR in 25.2% of patients; significantly higher PRI in those with thrombotic events |
| Škorňová et al. [46] | Prospective single-center (non-randomized) | STEMI with primary PCI | 44 | LTA with ADP induction, VASP-P | LTA: >50%, VASP-P: PRI > 50% | HTPR in 8.7% of patients |
| Aradi et al. [47] | Prospective multicenter (non-randomized) | high risk ACS | 104 | LTA, Multiplate® | LTA: >46%, Multiplate®: >47 AU | inter-patient variability after prasugrel loading dosing; no effect of PPI on prasugrel activity |
| Cayla et al. [48] | Prospective two high-volume centers (non-randomized) | ACS with PCI | 444 | VASP-P, VerifyNow®, LTA | VASP-P: PRI ≥ 50%, VerifyNow®: ≥235 PRU, LTA: ≥46.2% | HTPR in 3.2–6.8% of patients according to method used for detection |
| Laine et al. [49] | Prospective single-center (randomized) | STEMI with primary PCI | 44 | VASP-P | VASP-P: PRI ≥ 50% | HTPR in 9.1% of patients |
| Lemesle et al. [50] | Meta-analysis (14 studies included) | CAD | 1822 | VASP-P, VerifyNow® | VASP-P: PRI ≥ 50%, different cut off for VerifyNow in included studies (208–235 PRU) | HTPR in 9.8% of patients |
| Siller-Matula et al. [51] | Prospective single-center (non-randomized) | ACS | 200 | Multiplate® | Multiplate®: >46 AU | HTPR in 3% of patients |
| Selhorst et al. [52] | Retrospective single-center | ACS with primary PCI | 809 | Multiplate® | Multiplate®: >468 AUC | HTPR in 1.6% of patients |
| Verdoia et al. [53] | Prospective single-center (non-randomized) | ACS with PCI | 190 | Multiplate® | Multiplate®: >417 AUC | HTPR in 10% of patients |
| Verdoia et al. [54] | Prospective single-center (non-randomized) | ACS with PCI | 105 | Multiplate® | Multiplate®: >417 AUC | HTPR in 12.3% of patients |

ACS—acute coronary syndrome; ADP—adenosine diphosphate; AU—aggregation units; AUC—area under the curve; CAD—coronary artery disease; HTPR—high on treatment platelet reactivity; LTA—light transmission aggregometry; PCI—percutaneous coronary intervention; PRI—platelet reactivity index; PRU—P2Y12 reactivity units; VASP-P—Vasodilator-Stimulated Phosphoprotein phosphorylation.

A question regarding the mechanism of prasugrel HTPR could be posed. In fact, right now, no satisfactory answer to this question exists, as there is no study examining this problem. Theoretically, several factors could be responsible for this insufficient drug response (Figure 1). Prasugrel HTPR can be caused by decreased bioavailability—either due to decreased absorption or increased drug elimination, by impaired drug metabolism (either due to genetic polymorphism or drug interactions), leading to decreased formation of an active metabolite, due to ineffective inhibition of the platelet P2Y12 ADP receptor via an active metabolite or due to impaired response on ADP receptor inhibition on the level of the post-receptor signaling pathway [59].

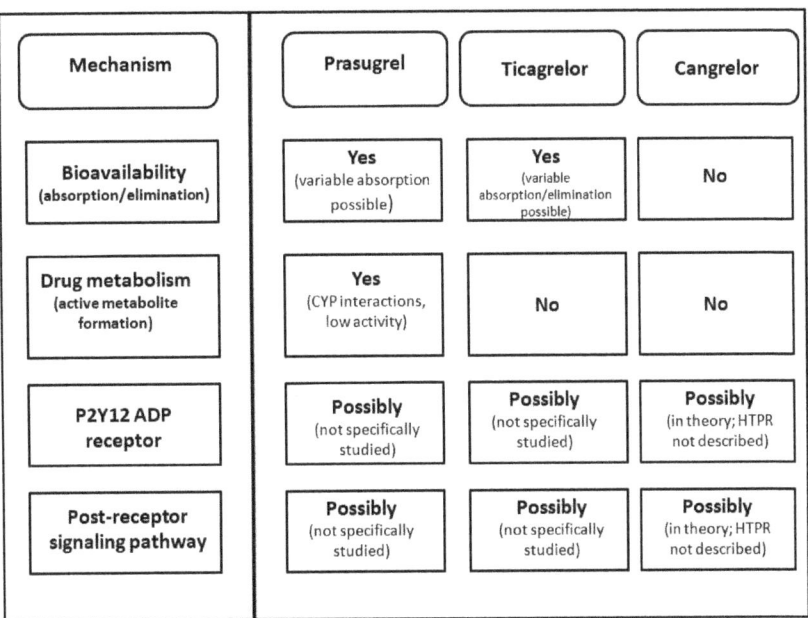

**Figure 1.** Possible mechanism of HTPR on novel-generation ADPRB [59]. ADP—adenosine diphosphate; ADPRB—P2Y12 ADP receptor blockers; CYP—cytochrome P450 enzyme; HTPR—high on-treatment platelet reactivity.

## 6. Ticagrelor Resistance in Patients with ACS

Although first observations reported no risk of HTPR on ticagrelor [60,61], Laine et al. [62] subsequently reported, in their multicenter prospective observational study enrolling 115 ticagrelor-treated patients, that platelet inhibition post 180 mg of ticagrelor loading dose is not uniform and that 3.5% of patients had HTPR (defined as VASP-P index > 50%, blood sampling was performed 6 to 24 h post drug loading). In our previously mentioned analysis of STEMI patients planned for primary PCI [46], platelet inhibition after 180 mg of ticagrelor loading dose was not sufficient in 42.9% of patients in a sample taken $1.4 \pm 0.6$ h and in 14.3% of patients in a sample taken $21.0 \pm 2.0$ h post drug loading, respectively. In other studies, the range of ticagrelor HTPR after loading dose administration ranged from 1.5 to 60.2%, depending on studied patient population, method used for HTPR detection and timing of blood sampling [50,51,63–67]. Although Verdoia et al. reported in their studies [54,68,69] 8.6 to 13.7% prevalence of ticagrelor HTPR on maintenance dosing (tested 30 to 90 days post drug loading), it seems that a longer duration of ticagrelor therapy probably achieves sufficient platelet inhibition in the majority of patients, as the majority of so-far published studies, including meta-analyses, reported very low rates (0.0–1.9%) of ticagrelor HTPR (Table 3) on long-term therapy [49,52,70–76]. This prevalence practically limits the occurrence of ticagrelor HTPR to occasional clinical cases. However, although the evidence is still limited and the phenomenon of ticagrelor resistance is relatively rare, ticagrelor HTPR seems to be connected with a higher risk of adverse ischemic events [67], very similarly to clopidogrel HTPR and prasugrel HTPR. Additionally, Musallam et al. reported a case of a patient with subacute stent thrombosis in whom ticagrelor HTPR was verified [7], and Malik [77] described a case of stent thrombosis 22 days after successful drug eluting coronary stent implantation in a 62-year-old man with diabetes who did not respond adequately to ticagrelor therapy. In this particular case, intravascular imaging with optical coherence tomography was performed, and stent underexpansion, stent strunt mal-apposition and edge dissection were excluded. Finally, Jariwala et al. [78] described a case of subacute stent thrombosis after uncomplicated implantation of sirolimus-eluting coronary stent, which developed despite ticagrelor therapy (in this case, authors were unable to verify HTPR with laboratory testing). In summary, current evidence suggests that ticagrelor HTPR exists, but its prevalence is lower compared to clopidogrel and prasugrel HTPR. Nevertheless, this phenomenon seems to be connected with a higher risk of ischemic adverse events, including stent throcccmbosis.

Table 3. Summary of studies reporting ticagrelor HTPR.

| Study | Type of Study | Studied Population | Number of Patients | Test for HTPR | Cut Off | Main Results |
|---|---|---|---|---|---|---|
| Alexopoulos et al. [60] | Prospective single-center (randomized) | ACS with PCI and HTPR on clopidogrel | 44 | VerifyNow® | VerifyNow®: ≥235 PRU | HTPR in 0% of patients |
| Alexopoulos et al. [61] | Prospective single-center (randomized) | ACS with PCI and T2D | 30 | VerifyNow® | VerifyNow®: ≥230 PRU | HTPR in 0% of patients |
| Laine et al. [62] | Prospective multicenter (non-randomized) | ACS with PCI | 115 | VASP-P | VASP-P: PRI ≥ 50% | HTPR in 3.5% of patients |
| Škorňová et al. [46] | Prospective single-center (non-randomized) | STEMI with primary PCI | 44 | LTA with ADP induction, VASP-P | LTA: >50%, VASP-P: PRI ≥ 50% | HTPR in 14.3% of patients |
| Lemesle et al. [50] | Meta-analysis (14 studies included) | CAD | 1822 | VASP-P, VerifyNow® | VASP-P: PRI ≥ 50%, different cut off for VerifyNow in included studies (208–235 PRU) | HTPR in 1.5% of patients |
| Siller-Matula et al. [51] | Prospective single-center (non-randomized) | ACS | 200 | Multiplate® | Multiplate®: >46 AU | HTPR in 2% of patients |
| Laine et al. [63] | Prospective single-center (randomized) | ACS with PCI and T2D | 100 | VASP-P | VASP-P: PRI ≥ 50% | HTPR in 6% of patients |
| Verdoia et al. [64] | Prospective single-center (non-randomized) | ACS | 190 | Multiplate® | Multiplate®: >417 AUC | HTPR in 11% of patients |
| Barbieri et al. [65] | Prospective single-center (non-randomized) | PCI | 537 | Multiplate® | Multiplate®: >417 AUC | HTPR in 12.7% of patients |
| Li et al. [66] | Prospective single-center (non-randomized) | ACS | 176 | TEG® | TEG®: MA > 47 mm | HTPR in 3.98% of patients |
| Laine et al. [67] | Prospective multicenter (non-randomized) | ACS with PCI | 530 | VASP-P | VASP-P: PRI ≥ 50% | HTPR in 5.3% of patients |
| Verdoia et al. [54] | Prospective single-center (non-randomized) | ACS with PCI | 105 | Multiplate® | Multiplate®: >417 AUC | HTPR in 8.6% of patients |
| Verdoia et al. [68] | Prospective single-center (non-randomized) | ACS with PCI | 195 | Multiplate® | Multiplate®: >417 AUC | HTPR in 13.3% of patients |
| Verdoia et al. [69] | Prospective single-center (non-randomized) | ACS with PCI | 432 | Multiplate® | Multiplate®: >417 AUC | HTPR in 11.4% of patients |
| Laine et al. [49] | Prospective single-center (randomized) | STEMI with primary PCI | 44 | VASP-P | VASP-P: PRI ≥ 50% | HTPR in 0% of patients |
| Selhorst et al. [52] | Retrospective single-center | ACS with primary PCI | 809 | Multiplate® | Multiplate®: >468 AUC | HTPR in 1.9% of patients |
| Alexopoulos et al. [70] | Prospective single-center (non-randomized) | ACS with PCI | 512 | VerifyNow® | VerifyNow®: >208 PRU | HTPR in 0% of patients |
| Alexopoulos et al. [71] | Meta-analysis (8 studies included) | CAD or ACS (with or without PCI) | 445 | VerifyNow® | VerifyNow®: >230 PRU | HTPR in 0% of patients |

Table 3. Cont.

| Study | Type of Study | Studied Population | Number of Patients | Test for HTPR | Cut Off | Main Results |
|---|---|---|---|---|---|---|
| Gaglia et al. [72] | Prospective single-center (non-randomized) | ACS and black rase | 29 | LTA, VASP-P, VerifyNow® | LTA: >60%, VASP-P: PRI > 50%, VerifyNow®: >208 PRU | HTPR in 0% of patients |
| Sweeny et al. [73] | post-hoc analysis of prospective multicenter study (randomized) | ACS (troponin negative) with PCI | 100 | VerifyNow® | VerifyNow®: >208 PRU | HTPR in 5.9% of patients |
| Liu et al. [74] | Prospective multicenter (randomized) | NSTE ACS | 278 | VASP-P | VASP-P: PRI ≥ 50% | HTPR in 3.1–5.3% of patients (according to ticagrelor loading dose) |
| Wen et al. [75] | Meta-analysis (14 studies included) | ACS | 2629 | VASP-P, VerifyNow® | VASP-P: PRI ≥ 50%, VerifyNow®: ≥208 PRU or ≥230 PRU | HTPR in 0.66–2.67% of patients (according to method used for detection) |
| Dai et al. [76] | Meta-analysis (25 studies included) | ACS | 5098 | VASP-P, VerifyNow®, Multiplate® | Not reported | low incidence of HTPR on ticagrelor maintenance dosing (exact rate was not reported) |
| Musallam et al. [7] | Case report | stent thrombosis on ticagrelor therapy | 1 | VerifyNow® | - | HTPR (339 PRU) at the time of stent thrombosis |
| Malik [77] | Case report | stent thrombosis on ticagrelor therapy | 1 | TEG® | TEG®: MA > 47 mm | HTPR (MA of 66 mm) at the time of stent thrombosis |
| Jariwala et al. [78] | Case report | stent thrombosis on ticagrelor therapy | 1 | Not tested | - | stent thrombosis on ticagrelor—stent-related complication excluded by intravascular coronary imaging |

ACS—acute coronary syndrome; ADP—adenosine diphosphate; AU—aggregation units; AUC—area under the curve; CAD—coronary artery disease; HTPR—high on treatment platelet reactivity; LTA—light transmission aggregometry; MA—maximum amplitude; NSTE—non-ST segment elevation; PCI—percutaneous coronary intervention; PRI—platelet reactivity index; PRU—P2Y12 reactivity units; T2D—type 2 diabetes; TEG®—thromboelastography; VASP-P—Vasodilator-Stimulated Phosphoprotein phosphorylation.

Looking at the mechanism of ticagrelor HTPR, it is obvious that impaired (pro)drug conversion (metabolism) does not play a role, as ticagrelor is an active metabolite, which does not require metabolic transformation to achieve its drug activity. In theory, all the other possible mechanisms discussed in connection with prasugrel HTPR (Figure 1) could be responsible [59]. Nevertheless, similarly to prasugrel HTPR, there is no study specifically examining the mechanism of this HTPR; therefore, clarification of this matter is still open for future research.

## 7. Cangrelor Resistance in Patients with ACS

Looking at the currently available data, there is no study examining the prevalence of cangrelor HTPR in patients with acute coronary syndrome, no study describing this phenomenon or clinical case report describing a case of ischemic adverse post-PCI event related to failure of cangrelor therapy. Moreover, cangrelor seems to be a promising agent for treatment (overcoming) prasugrel HTPR [79,80] or to bridge the gap until optimal platelet inhibition with ticagrelor is achieved [81]. Nevertheless, cangrelor has been approved for clinical use in patients undergoing PCI relatively recently; thus, it might be possible that the phenomenon of cangrelor HTPR just awaits its description.

## 8. Risk Factors of Novel ADPRB Resistance

The next question should be what are the risk factors for HTPR on novel-generation ADPRB? Searching the literature, several factors have been proposed as factors associated with this phenomenon. For prasugrel, obesity (BMI > 30 kg/m$^2$) [48,82–84], multivessel coronary artery disease [48], carrying a CYP 2C19*2 or 2C19*17 loss-of-function allele [85,86], high pre-treatment platelet reactivity and smoking status [87] and impaired metabolic status (with higher levels of glycosylated hemoglobin and low-density lipoprotein cholesterol) [53] have been reported as factors independently predicting HTPR. Several other clinical factors, namely chronic kidney disease [53], type 2 diabetes [88], elderly and proton pump inhibition co-therapy [47], were studied, but an association was not found. For ticagrelor, in a previous study, age and BMI positively and smoking negatively affected on-treatment platelet reactivity [71]. Verdoia et al. [68] reported that, using multivariable analysis, age (≥70 years), concomitant therapy with beta-blockers and platelet count independently predicted HRPR on ticagrelor. In another prospective study in ticagrelor-treated ACS patients, Adamski et al. reported that the presence of ST-segment elevation and morphine co-administration were the strongest predictors of ticagrelor HTPR [89]. Other clinical factors, such as chronic kidney disease, diabetes or proton pump inhibitor co-administration, probably do not affect the efficacy of ticagrelor therapy [88,90,91].

## 9. How to Manage Insufficient Response to Novel ADPRB?

In theory, novel-generation ADPRB HTPR can be managed by modification of drug dosing (either with re-loading or increasing the maintenance dosage) [92], by adding other antithrombotic agents, to bridge the time until the drug achieves its full activity (glycoprotein IIb/IIIa inhibitor or parenteral ADPRB—cangrelor) [93] or to achieve more potent platelet inhibition in long-term therapy (cilostazol or low-dose rivaroxaban) [94], or by switching the novel-generation ADPRB (prasugrel to ticagrelor in prasugrel HTPR and ticagrelor to prasugrel in ticagrelor HTPR) [54,95]. One must say that each of the strategies has its disadvantages and that none of them was tested in a randomized trial. For example, adding the third antithrombotic agent to long-term therapy can increase the risk of bleeding, while the effect on a reduction in adverse thrombotic events remains unclear. In addition, increasing the drug dose leads to long-term drug dosing, for which efficacy and safety were not previously tested in clinical trials. Furthermore, cangrelor has been approved only in ADPRB-naïve patients who are planned for PCI, and the safety of its administration in those who already received ADPRB loading (although with insufficient platelet response) remains unclear. In the majority of so-far published cases [6,7,57,58,77,78], the authors used a switch strategy, either alone or with bridging the ineffective antiplatelet response with adding glycoprotein IIb/IIIa inhibition. This strategy appears to be safe and effective, as there were no reports of repeated ischemic or serious bleeding adverse events in these cases. However, the evidence for any approach is still limited to a small number of clinical cases, and further research on the issue of optimal management of HTPR on novel-generation ADPRB is definitely needed.

## 10. Conclusions

Based on the limited evidence discussed in this review article, we can conclude that the phenomenon of HTPR or resistance on novel-generation ADPRB therapy might exist. The prevalence of novel-generation ADPRB HTPR is lower compared to clopidogrel HTPR. Additionally, several studies suggested that this phenomenon could be connected with a high risk of adverse ischemic events; however, the evidence for this association is still limited. Therefore, there is a need for future research dedicated to clinical impact and optimal management of this phenomenon.

**Author Contributions:** P.B., M.S., T.B. and L.S. designed the study; P.B., M.S. and T.B. drafted the manuscript; I.Š., M.J.P. and J.J. performed the search of the literature, analyzed and interpreted the data; L.S., J.J., J.S. and M.M. revised the manuscript critically. All authors have read and agreed to the published version of the manuscript.

**Funding:** This study was supported by project APVV (Slovak Research and Development Agency) 16-0020, by projects of Research Agency of Slovak Ministry of Education, Science and Sports (VEGA) 1/0090/20 and 1/0549/19.

**Institutional Review Board Statement:** This research was conducted according to ethical standards. There is no need for formal consent for this type of study (a narrative review article).

**Informed Consent Statement:** Not applicable.

**Data Availability Statement:** All the source data are available from the corresponding author upon reasonable request.

**Acknowledgments:** This study was supported by project APVV (Slovak Research and Development Agency) 16-0020, by projects of Research Agency of Slovak Ministry of Education, Science and Sports (VEGA) 1/0090/20 and 1/0549/19.

**Conflicts of Interest:** The authors declare no conflict of interest.

## References

1. Wiviott, S.D.; Braunwald, E.; McCabe, C.H.; Montalescot, G.; Ruzyllo, W.; Gottlieb, S.; Neumann, F.-J.; Ardissino, D.; De Servi, S.; Murphy, S.A.; et al. Prasugrel versus Clopidogrel in Patients with Acute Coronary Syndromes. *N. Engl. J. Med.* **2007**, *357*, 2001–2015. [CrossRef] [PubMed]
2. Schüpke, S.; Neumann, F.J.; Menichelli, M.; Mayer, K.; Bernlochner, I.; Wöhrle, J.; Richardt, G.; Liebetrau, C.; Witzenbichler, B.; Antoniucci, D.; et al. Ticagrelor or Prasugrel in Patients with Acute Coronary Syndromes. *N. Engl. J. Med.* **2019**, *381*, 1524–1534. [CrossRef] [PubMed]
3. Wallentin, L.; Becker, R.C.; Budaj, A.; Cannon, C.P.; Emanuelsson, H.; Held, C.; Horrow, J.; Husted, S.; James, S.; Katus, H.; et al. Ticagrelor versus Clopidogrel in Patients with Acute Coronary Syndromes. *N. Engl. J. Med.* **2009**, *361*, 1045–1057. [CrossRef]
4. Bhatt, D.L.; Stone, G.W.; Mahaffey, K.W.; Gibson, C.M.; Steg, P.G.; Hamm, C.W.; Price, M.J.; Leonardi, S.; Gallup, D.; Bramucci, E.; et al. Effect of platelet inhibition with cangrelor during PCI on ischemic events. *N. Engl. J. Med.* **2013**, *368*, 1303–1313. [CrossRef] [PubMed]
5. Samoš, M.; Fedor, M.; Kovář, F.; Duraj, L.; Stančiaková, L.; Galajda, P.; Staško, J.; Kubisz, P.; Mokáň, M. Ticagrelor: A safe and effective approach for overcoming clopidogrel resistance in patients with stent thrombosis? *Blood Coagul. Fibrinolysis* **2016**, *27*, 117–120. [CrossRef] [PubMed]
6. Fiore, M.; Horovitz, A.; Pons, A.-C.; Leroux, L.; Casassus, F. First report of a subacute stent thrombosis in a prasugrel resistant patient successfully managed with ticagrelor. *Platelets* **2013**, *25*, 636–638. [CrossRef] [PubMed]
7. Musallam, A.; Lev, E.I.; Roguin, A. Stent thrombosis in a patient with high on-treatment platelet reactivity despite ticagrelor treatment. *Eur. Heart J. Acute Cardiovasc. Care* **2014**, *4*, 85–87. [CrossRef]
8. Thomas, M.R.; Storey, R.F. Clinical significance of residual platelet reactivity in patients treated with platelet P2Y12 inhibitors. *Vasc. Pharmacol.* **2016**, *84*, 25–27. [CrossRef]
9. Małek, Ł.A.; Spiewak, M.; Filipiak, K.J.; Grabowski, M.; Szpotańska, M.; Rosiak, M.; Główczyńska, R.; Imiela, T.; Huczek, Z.; Opolski, G. Persistent platelet activation is related to very early cardiovascular events in patients with acute coronary syndromes. *Kardiol. Pol.* **2007**, *65*, 40–45.
10. Wang, L.; Wang, X.; Chen, F. Clopidogrel resistance is associated with long-term thrombotic events in patients implanted with drug-eluting stents. *Drugs R D* **2010**, *10*, 219–224. [CrossRef]
11. Liang, Z.-Y.; Han, Y.-L.; Zhang, X.-L.; Li, Y.; Yan, C.-H.; Kang, J. The impact of gene polymorphism and high on-treatment platelet reactivity on clinical follow-up: Outcomes in patients with acute coronary syndrome after drug-eluting stent implantation. *EuroIntervention* **2013**, *9*, 316–327. [CrossRef]
12. Costache, I.I.; Rusu, C.; Ivanov, I.; Popescu, R.; Petriş, A. Impact of clopidogrel response on the clinical evolution in patients with acute coronary syndromes. *Rev. Med. Chir. Soc. Med. Nat. IASI* **2012**, *116*, 962–967. [PubMed]
13. Li, M.; Wang, H.; Xuan, L.; Shi, X.; Zhou, T.; Zhang, N.; Huang, Y. Associations between P2RY12 gene polymorphisms and risks of clopidogrel resistance and adverse cardiovascular events after PCI in patients with acute coronary syndrome. *Medicine* **2017**, *96*, e6553. [CrossRef] [PubMed]
14. Guha, S.; Mookerjee, S.; Guha, P.; Sardar, P.; Deb, S.; Das Roy, P.; Karmakar, R.; Mani, S.; Hema, M.B.; Pyne, S.; et al. Antiplatelet drug resistance in patients with recurrent acute coronary syndrome undergoing conservative management. *Indian Heart J.* **2010**, *61*, 348–352.
15. Samoš, M.; Šimonová, R.; Kovář, F.; Duraj, L.; Fedorová, J.; Galajda, P.; Staško, J.; Fedor, M.; Kubisz, P.; Mokáň, M. Clopidogrel resistance in diabetic patient with acute myocardial infarction due to stent thrombosis. *Am. J. Emerg. Med.* **2014**, *32*, 461–465. [CrossRef] [PubMed]
16. Lee, J.S.; Dunn, S.P.; Marshall, H.M.; Cohen, M.G.; Smyth, S.S. A case report of simultaneous thrombosis of two coronary artery stents in association with clopidogrel resistance. *Clin. Cardiol.* **2007**, *30*, 200–203. [CrossRef]
17. Schäfer, A.; Bonz, A.W.; Eigenthaler, M.; Bauersachs, J. Late thrombosis of a drug-eluting stent during combined anti-platelet therapy in a clopidogrel nonresponsive diabetic patient: Shall we routinely test platelet function? *Thromb Haemost* **2007**, *97*, 862–865.

18. Jung, H.-J.; Sir, J.-J. Recurrent myocardial infarction due to one subacute and two very late thrombotic events of drug-eluting stent associated with clopidogrel resistance. *J. Invasive Cardiol.* **2011**, *23*, E13–E18.
19. Kim, Y.-S.; Lee, S.-R. Successful Prasugrel Therapy for Recurrent Left Main Stent Thrombosis in a Clopidogrel Hyporesponder. *Tex. Heart Inst. J.* **2015**, *42*, 483–486. [CrossRef]
20. Redfors, B.; Ben-Yehuda, O.; Lin, S.-H.; Furer, A.; Kirtane, A.J.; Witzenbichler, B.; Weisz, G.; Stuckey, T.D.; Maehara, A.; Généreux, P.; et al. Quantifying Ischemic Risk After Percutaneous Coronary Intervention Attributable to High Platelet Reactivity on Clopidogrel (From the Assessment of Dual Antiplatelet Therapy with Drug-Eluting Stents Study). *Am. J. Cardiol.* **2017**, *120*, 917–923. [CrossRef]
21. Olędzki, S.; Kornacewicz-Jach, Z.; Safranow, K.; Kiedrowicz, R.; Gawrońska-Szklarz, B.; Jastrzębska, M.; Gorący, J. Variability of platelet response to clopidogrel is not related to adverse cardiovascular events in patients with stable coronary artery disease undergoing percutaneous coronary intervention. *Eur. J. Clin. Pharmacol.* **2017**, *73*, 1085–1094. [CrossRef] [PubMed]
22. Bolliger, D.; Filipovic, M.; Matt, P.; Tanaka, K.A.; Gregor, M.; Zenklusen, U.; Seeberger, M.D.; Buse, G.L. Reduced aspirin responsiveness as assessed by impedance aggregometry is not associated with adverse outcome after cardiac surgery in a small low-risk cohort. *Platelets* **2015**, *27*, 254–261. [CrossRef] [PubMed]
23. Chung, C.J.; Kirtane, A.J.; Zhang, Y.; Witzenbichler, B.; Weisz, G.; Stuckey, T.D.; Brodie, B.R.; Rinaldi, M.J.; Neumann, F.-J.; Metzger, D.C.; et al. Impact of high on-aspirin platelet reactivity on outcomes following successful percutaneous coronary intervention with drug-eluting stents. *Am. Heart J.* **2018**, *205*, 77–86. [CrossRef] [PubMed]
24. Redfors, B.; Chen, S.; Généreux, P.; Witzenbichler, B.; Weisz, G.; Stuckey, T.D.; Maehara, A.; McAndrew, T.; Mehran, R.; Ben-Yehuda, O.; et al. Relationship Between Stent Diameter, Platelet Reactivity, and Thrombotic Events After Percutaneous Coronary Artery Revascularization. *Am. J. Cardiol.* **2019**, *124*, 1363–1371. [CrossRef]
25. Gori, T.; Polimeni, A.; Indolfi, C.; Räber, L.; Adriaenssens, T.; Münzel, T. Predictors of stent thrombosis and their implications for clinical practice. *Nat. Rev. Cardiol.* **2018**, *16*, 243–256. [CrossRef]
26. Price, M.J.; Berger, P.B.; Teirstein, P.S.; Tanguay, J.F.; Angiolillo, D.J.; Spriggs, D.; Puri, S.; Robbins, M.; Garratt, K.N.; Bertrand, O.F.; et al. Standard- vs. high-dose clopidogrel based on platelet function testing after percutaneous coronary intervention: The GRAVITAS randomized trial. *JAMA* **2011**, *305*, 1097–1105. [CrossRef]
27. Chandrasekhar, J.; Baber, U.; Mehran, R.; Aquino, M.; Sartori, S.; Yu, J.; Kini, A.; Sharma, S.; Skurk, C.; Shlofmitz, R.A.; et al. Impact of an integrated treatment algorithm based on platelet function testing and clinical risk assessment: Results of the TRIAGE Patients Undergoing Percutaneous Coronary Interventions to Improve Clinical Outcomes Through Optimal Platelet Inhibition study. *J. Thromb. Thrombolysis* **2016**, *42*, 186–196. [CrossRef]
28. Xing, Z.; Tang, L.; Zhu, Z.; Huang, J.; Peng, X.; Hu, X. Platelet reactivity-adjusted antiplatelet therapy in patients with percutaneous coronary intervention: A meta-analysis of randomized controlled trials. *Platelets* **2017**, *29*, 589–595. [CrossRef]
29. Robledo-Nolasco, R.; Godínez-Montes de Oca, A.; Zaballa-Contreras, J.F.; Suárez-Cuenca, J.A.; Mondragón-Terán, P.; Rubio-Guerra, A.F.; Meléndez-Alcántara, M.A. Efficacy of Change to New P2Y12 Receptor Antagonists in Patients High on Treatment Platelet Reactivity Undergoing Percutaneous Coronary Intervention. *Clin. Appl. Thromb. Hemost.* **2015**, *21*, 619–625. [CrossRef]
30. Tantry, U.S.; Bonello, L.; Aradi, D.; Price, M.J.; Jeong, Y.-H.; Angiolillo, D.J.; Stone, G.W.; Curzen, N.; Geisler, T.; ten Berg, J.; et al. Consensus and Update on the Definition of On-Treatment Platelet Reactivity to Adenosine Diphosphate Associated with Ischemia and Bleeding. *J. Am. Coll. Cardiol.* **2013**, *62*, 2261–2273. [CrossRef]
31. Fedor, M.; Samoš, M.; Šimonová, R.; Fedorová, J.; Škorňová, I.; Duraj, L.; Staško, J.; Kovář, F.; Mokáň, M.; Kubisz, P. Monitoring the efficacy of ADP inhibitor treatment in patients with acute STEMI post-PCI by VASP-P flow cytometry assay. *Clin. Appl. Thromb. Hemost.* **2015**, *21*, 334–338. [CrossRef] [PubMed]
32. Alvitigala, B.Y.; Gooneratne, L.V.; Constantine, G.R.; Wijesinghe, R.A.N.K.; Arawwawala, L.D.A.M. Pharmacokinetic, pharmacodynamic, and pharmacogenetic assays to monitor clopidogrel therapy. *Pharmacol. Res. Perspect.* **2020**, *8*, e00686. [CrossRef] [PubMed]
33. Kinsella, J.A.; Tobin, W.O.; Cox, D.; Coughlan, T.; Collins, R.; O'Neill, D.; Murphy, R.P.; McCabe, D.J. Prevalence of Ex Vivo High On-treatment Platelet Reactivity on Antiplatelet Therapy after Transient Ischemic Attack or Ischemic Stroke on the PFA-100® and VerifyNow®. *J. Stroke Cerebrovasc. Dis.* **2013**, *22*, e84–e92. [CrossRef] [PubMed]
34. Crescente, M.; Mezzasoma, A.M.; Del Pinto, M.; Palmerini, F.; Di Castelnuovo, A.; Cerletti, C.; De Gaetano, G.; Gresele, P. Incomplete inhibition of platelet function as assessed by the platelet function analyzer (PFA-100) identifies a subset of cardiovascular patients with high residual platelet response while on aspirin. *Platelets* **2011**, *22*, 179–187. [CrossRef] [PubMed]
35. Koessler, J.; Kobsar, A.L.; Rajkovic, M.S.; Schafer, A.; Flierl, U.; Pfoertsch, S.; Bauersachs, J.; Steigerwald, U.; Rechner, A.R.; Walter, U. The new INNOVANCE® PFA P2Y cartridge is sensitive to the detection of the $P2Y_{12}$ receptor inhibition. *Platelets* **2011**, *22*, 20–27. [CrossRef] [PubMed]
36. Paniccia, R.; Antonucci, E.; Gori, A.M.; Marcucci, R.; Poli, S.; Romano, E.; Valente, S.; Giglioli, C.; Fedi, S.; Gensini, G.F.; et al. Comparison of Different Methods to Evaluate the Effect of Aspirin on Platelet Function in High-Risk Patients with Ischemic Heart Disease Receiving Dual Antiplatelet Treatment. *Am. J. Clin. Pathol.* **2007**, *128*, 143–149. [CrossRef]
37. Kweon, O.J.; Lim, Y.K.; Kim, B.; Lee, M.-K.; Kim, A.H.R. Effectiveness of Platelet Function Analyzer-100 for Laboratory Detection of Anti-Platelet Drug-Induced Platelet Dysfunction. *Ann. Lab. Med.* **2019**, *39*, 23–30. [CrossRef]

38. Guha, S.; Mookerjee, S.; Lahiri, P.; Mani, S.; Saha, J.; Guha, S.; Majumdar, D.; Mandal, M.; Bhattacharya, R. A study of platelet aggregation in patients with acute myocardial infarction at presentation and after 48 hrs of initiating standard anti platelet therapy. *Indian Heart J.* **2013**, *63*, 409–413.
39. Dobesh, P.P.; Varnado, S.; Doyle, M. Antiplatelet Agents in Cardiology: A Report on Aspirin, Clopidogrel, Prasugrel, and Ticagrelor. *Curr. Pharm. Des.* **2016**, *22*, 1918–1932. [CrossRef]
40. Bonaca, M.P.; Bhatt, D.L.; Cohen, M.; Steg, P.G.; Storey, R.F.; Jensen, E.C.; Magnani, G.; Bansilal, S.; Fish, M.P.; Im, K.; et al. Long-Term Use of Ticagrelor in Patients with Prior Myocardial Infarction. *N. Engl. J. Med.* **2015**, *372*, 1791–1800. [CrossRef]
41. Wang, W.; Wang, B.; Chen, Y.; Wei, S. Late Stent Thrombosis After Drug-Coated Balloon Coronary Angioplasty for In-Stent Restenosis. *Int. Heart J.* **2021**, *62*, 171–174. [CrossRef] [PubMed]
42. Lee, S.-Y.; Cho, J.Y.; Yun, K.H.; Oh, S.K. Successful Therapy with Ticagrelor in Three-Vessel Stent Thrombosis Related to Clopidogrel Resistance. *Can. J. Cardiol.* **2021**, *37*, 1278–1280. [CrossRef] [PubMed]
43. Keating, G.M. Cangrelor: A Review in Percutaneous Coronary Intervention. *Drugs* **2015**, *75*, 1425–1434. [CrossRef] [PubMed]
44. Chen, Y.; Bernardo, N.L.; Waksman, R. Cangrelor for the Rescue of Intra-Procedural Stent Thrombosis in Percutaneous Coronary Intervention. *Cardiovasc. Revascularization Med.* **2019**, *20*, 624–625. [CrossRef]
45. Bonello, L.; Pansieri, M.; Mancini, J.; Bonello, R.; Maillard, L.; Barnay, P.; Rossi, P.; Ait-Mokhtar, O.; Jouve, B.; Collet, F.; et al. High On-Treatment Platelet Reactivity after Prasugrel Loading Dose and Cardiovascular Events after Percutaneous Coronary Intervention in Acute Coronary Syndromes. *J. Am. Coll. Cardiol.* **2011**, *58*, 467–473. [CrossRef]
46. Skorňová, I.; Samoš, M.; Šimonová, R.; Žolková, J.; Stančiaková, L.; Vádelová, L.; Bolek, T.; Urban, L.; Kovář, F.; Staško, J.; et al. On-treatment platelet reactivity in the era of new ADP receptor blockers: Data from a real-world clinical practice. *Acta Med. Martiniana* **2018**, *18*, 34–39. [CrossRef]
47. Kuliczkowski, W.; Atar, D.; Serebruany, V.L.; Aradi, D. Inter-patient variability and impact of proton pump inhibitors on platelet reactivity after prasugrel. *Thromb. Haemost.* **2012**, *107*, 338–345. [CrossRef]
48. Cayla, G.; Cuisset, T.; Silvain, J.; O'Connor, S.A.; Kerneis, M.; Castelli, C.; Quilici, J.; Bonnet, J.-L.; Alessi, M.-C.; Morange, P.-E.; et al. Prasugrel Monitoring and Bleeding in Real World Patients. *Am. J. Cardiol.* **2013**, *111*, 38–44. [CrossRef]
49. Laine, M.; Gaubert, M.; Frère, C.; Peyrol, M.; Thuny, F.; Yvorra, S.; Chelini, V.; Bultez, B.; Luigi, S.; Mokrani, Z.; et al. Comparison of Platelet reactivity following prAsugrel and ticagrelor loading dose in ST-Segment elevation myocardial infarction patients: The COMPASSION study. *Platelets* **2015**, *26*, 570–572. [CrossRef]
50. Lemesle, G.; Schurtz, G.; Bauters, C.; Hamon, M. High on-treatment platelet reactivity with ticagrelor versus prasugrel: A systematic review and meta-analysis. *J. Thromb. Haemost.* **2015**, *13*, 931–942. [CrossRef]
51. Siller-Matula, J.M.; Akca, B.; Neunteufl, T.; Maurer, G.; Lang, I.M.; Kreiner, G.; Berger, R.; Delle-Karth, G. Inter-patient variability of platelet reactivity in patients treated with prasugrel and ticagrelor. *Platelets* **2015**, *27*, 373–377. [CrossRef] [PubMed]
52. Selhorst, G.; Schmidtler, F.; Ott, A.; Hitzke, E.; Tomelden, J.; Antoni, D.; Hoffmann, E.; Rieber, J. Platelet reactivity in patients with acute coronary syndrome treated with prasugrel or ticagrelor in comparison to clopidogrel: A retrospective pharmacodynamic analysis. *Platelets* **2018**, *30*, 341–347. [CrossRef] [PubMed]
53. Verdoia, M.; Pergolini, P.; Nardin, M.; Rolla, R.; Barbieri, L.; Marino, P.; Carriero, A.; Suryapranata, H.; De Luca, G. Prevalence and predictors of high-on treatment platelet reactivity during prasugrel treatment in patients with acute coronary syndrome undergoing stent implantation. *J. Cardiol.* **2018**, *73*, 198–203. [CrossRef] [PubMed]
54. Verdoia, M.; Pergolini, P.; Nardin, M.; Rolla, R.; Suryapranata, H.; Kedhi, E.; De Luca, G. Ticagrelor and prasugrel in acute coronary syndrome: A single-arm crossover platelet reactivity study. *J. Cardiovasc. Med.* **2021**, *22*, 686–692. [CrossRef]
55. Bonello, L.; Mancini, J.; Pansieri, M.; Maillard, L.; Rossi, P.; Collet, F.; Jouve, B.; Wittenberg, O.; Laine, M.; Michelet, P.; et al. Relationship between post-treatment platelet reactivity and ischemic and bleeding events at 1-year follow-up in patients receiving prasugrel. *J. Thromb. Haemost.* **2012**, *10*, 1999–2005. [CrossRef]
56. Aradi, D.; Gross, L.; Trenk, D.; Geisler, T.; Merkely, B.; Kiss, R.G.; Komócsi, A.; Dézsi, C.A.; Ruzsa, Z.; Ungi, I.; et al. Platelet reactivity and clinical outcomes in acute coronary syndrome patients treated with prasugrel and clopidogrel: A pre-specified exploratory analysis from the TROPICAL-ACS trial. *Eur. Heart J.* **2019**, *40*, 1942–1951. [CrossRef]
57. Silvano, M.; Zambon, C.-F.; De Rosa, G.; Plebani, M.; Pengo, V.; Napodano, M.; Padrini, R. A case of resistance to clopidogrel and prasugrel after percutaneous coronary angioplasty. *J. Thromb. Thrombolysis* **2010**, *31*, 233–234. [CrossRef]
58. Ohno, Y.; Okada, S.; Kitahara, H.; Nishi, T.; Nakayama, T.; Fujimoto, Y.; Kobayashi, Y. Repetitive stent thrombosis in a patient who had resistance to both clopidogrel and prasugrel. *J. Cardiol. Cases* **2016**, *13*, 139–142. [CrossRef]
59. Warlo, E.M.K.; Arnesen, H.; Seljeflot, I. A brief review on resistance to P2Y12 receptor antagonism in coronary artery disease. *Thromb. J.* **2019**, *17*, 1–9. [CrossRef]
60. Alexopoulos, D.; Galati, A.; Xanthopoulou, I.; Mavronasiou, E.; Kassimis, G.; Theodoropoulos, K.C.; Makris, G.; Damelou, A.; Tsigkas, G.; Hahalis, G.; et al. Ticagrelor versus prasugrel in acute coronary syndrome patients with high on-clopidogrel platelet reactivity following percutaneous coronary intervention: A pharmacodynamic study. *J. Am. Coll. Cardiol.* **2012**, *60*, 193–199. [CrossRef]
61. Alexopoulos, D.; Xanthopoulou, I.; Mavronasiou, E.; Stavrou, K.; Siapika, A.; Tsoni, E.; Davlouros, P. Randomized Assessment of Ticagrelor Versus Prasugrel Antiplatelet Effects in Patients with Diabetes. *Diabetes Care* **2013**, *36*, 2211–2216. [CrossRef] [PubMed]

62. Laine, M.; Toesca, R.; Berbis, J.; Frere, C.; Barnay, P.; Pansieri, M.; Peyre, J.-P.; Michelet, P.; Bessereau, J.; Camilleri, E.; et al. Platelet reactivity evaluated with the VASP assay following ticagrelor loading dose in acute coronary syndrome patients undergoing percutaneous coronary intervention. *Thromb. Res.* **2013**, *132*, e15–e18. [CrossRef] [PubMed]
63. Laine, M.; Frere, C.; Toesca, R.; Berbis, J.; Barnay, P.; Pansieri, M.; Michelet, P.; Bessereau, J.; Camilleri, E.; Ronsin, O.; et al. Ticagrelor versus prasugrel in diabetic patients with an acute coronary syndrome. *Thromb. Haemost.* **2014**, *111*, 273–278. [CrossRef]
64. Verdoia, M.; Sartori, C.; Pergolini, P.; Nardin, M.; Rolla, R.; Barbieri, L.; Schaffer, A.; Marino, P.; Bellomo, G.; Suryapranata, H.; et al. Immature platelet fraction and high-on treatment platelet reactivity with ticagrelor in patients with acute coronary syndromes. *J. Thromb. Thrombolysis* **2015**, *41*, 663–670. [CrossRef]
65. Barbieri, L.; Pergolini, P.; Verdoia, M.; Rolla, R.; Nardin, M.; Marino, P.; Bellomo, G.; Suryapranata, H.; De Luca, G. Platelet reactivity in patients with impaired renal function receiving dual antiplatelet therapy with clopidogrel or ticagrelor. *Vasc. Pharmacol.* **2016**, *79*, 11–15. [CrossRef] [PubMed]
66. Li, D.-D.; Wang, X.-Y.; Xi, S.-Z.; Liu, J.; Qin, L.-A.; Jing, J.; Yin, T.; Chen, Y.-D. Relationship between ADP-induced platelet-fibrin clot strength and anti-platelet responsiveness in ticagrelor treated ACS patients. *J. Geriatr. Cardiol.* **2016**, *13*, 282–289. [CrossRef] [PubMed]
67. Laine, M.; Panagides, V.; Frère, C.; Cuisset, T.; Gouarne, C.; Jouve, B.; Thuny, F.; Paganelli, F.; Alessi, M.; Mancini, J.; et al. Platelet reactivity inhibition following ticagrelor loading dose in patients undergoing percutaneous coronary intervention for acute coronary syndrome. *J. Thromb. Haemost.* **2019**, *17*, 2188–2195. [CrossRef]
68. Verdoia, M.; Sartori, C.; Pergolini, P.; Nardin, M.; Rolla, R.; Barbieri, L.; Schaffer, A.; Marino, P.; Bellomo, G.; Suryapranata, H.; et al. Prevalence and predictors of high-on treatment platelet reactivity with ticagrelor in ACS patients undergoing stent implantation. *Vasc. Pharmacol.* **2015**, *77*, 48–53. [CrossRef]
69. Verdoia, M.; Rolla, R.; Negro, F.; Tonon, F.; Pergolini, P.; Nardin, M.; Marcolongo, M.; De Luca, G. Homocysteine levels and platelet reactivity in coronary artery disease patients treated with ticagrelor. *Nutr. Metab. Cardiovasc. Dis.* **2019**, *30*, 292–299. [CrossRef]
70. Stavrou, K.; Koniari, I.; Gkizas, V.; Perperis, A.; Kontoprias, K.; Vogiatzi, C.; Bampouri, T.; Xanthopoulou, I.; Alexopoulos, D. Ticagrelor vs. prasugrel one-month maintenance therapy: Impact on platelet reactivity and bleeding events. *Thromb. Haemost.* **2014**, *112*, 551–557. [CrossRef]
71. Alexopoulos, D.; Xanthopoulou, I.; Storey, R.F.; Bliden, K.P.; Tantry, U.S.; Angiolillo, D.J.; Gurbel, P.A. Platelet reactivity during ticagrelor maintenance therapy: A patient-level data meta-analysis. *Am. Heart J.* **2014**, *168*, 530–536. [CrossRef] [PubMed]
72. Gaglia, M.A., Jr.; Lipinski, M.J.; Lhermusier, T.; Steinvil, A.; Kiramijyan, S.; Pokharel, S.; Torguson, R.; Angiolillo, D.J.; Wallentin, L.; Storey, R.F.; et al. Comparison of Platelet Reactivity in Black Versus White Patients with Acute Coronary Syndromes After Treatment with Ticagrelor. *Am. J. Cardiol.* **2017**, *119*, 1135–1140. [CrossRef]
73. Sweeny, J.M.; Angiolillo, D.J.; Franchi, F.; Rollini, F.; Waksman, R.; Raveendran, G.; Dangas, G.; Khan, N.D.; Carlson, G.F.; Zhao, Y.; et al. Impact of Diabetes Mellitus on the Pharmacodynamic Effects of Ticagrelor Versus Clopidogrel in Troponin-Negative Acute Coronary Syndrome Patients Undergoing Ad Hoc Percutaneous Coronary Intervention. *J. Am. Heart Assoc.* **2017**, *6*, e005650. [CrossRef] [PubMed]
74. Liu, H.L.; Wei, Y.J.; Ding, P.; Zhang, J.; Li, T.C.; Wang, B.; Wang, M.S.; Li, Y.T.; Zhang, J.J.; Ren, Y.H.; et al. Antiplatelet Effect of Different Loading Doses of Ticagrelor in Patients with Non-ST-Elevation Acute Coronary Syndrome Undergoing. *Can. J. Cardiol.* **2017**, *33*, 1675–1682. [CrossRef] [PubMed]
75. Wen, M.; Li, Y.; Qu, X.; Zhu, Y.; Tian, L.; Shen, Z.; Yang, X.; Shi, X. Comparison of platelet reactivity between prasugrel and ticagrelor in patients with acute coronary syndrome: A meta-analysis. *BMC Cardiovasc. Disord.* **2020**, *20*, 430. [CrossRef]
76. Dai, L.; Xu, J.; Jiang, Y.; Chen, K. Impact of Prasugrel and Ticagrelor on Platelet Reactivity in Patients with Acute Coronary Syndrome: A Meta-Analysis. *Front. Cardiovasc. Med.* **2022**, *9*, 905607. [CrossRef]
77. Malik, J. A Case of Ticagrelor Resistance. *Eur. J. Case Rep. Intern. Med.* **2021**, *8*, 002719. [CrossRef]
78. Jariwala, P.; Bhatia, H.; Kumar, E.A.P. Sub-acute stent thrombosis secondary to ticagrelor resistance-Myth or reality! *Indian Heart J.* **2017**, *69*, 804–806. [CrossRef]
79. Rollini, F.; Franchi, F.; Tello-Montoliu, A.; Patel, R.; Darlington, A.; Ferreiro, J.L.; Cho, J.R.; Muñiz-Lozano, A.; Desai, B.; Zenni, M.M.; et al. Pharmacodynamic effects of cangrelor on platelet P2Y12 receptor-mediated signaling in prasugrel-treated patients. *JACC Cardiovasc. Interv.* **2014**, *7*, 426–434. [CrossRef]
80. Valenti, R.; Muraca, I.; Marcucci, R.; Ciatti, F.; Berteotti, M.; Gori, A.M.; Carrabba, N.; Migliorini, A.; Marchionni, N.; Valgimigli, M. "Tailored" antiplatelet bridging therapy with cangrelor: Moving toward personalized medicine. *Platelets* **2021**, *33*, 687–691. [CrossRef]
81. Franchi, F.; Rollini, F.; Rivas, A.; Wali, M.; Briceno, M.; Agarwal, M.; Shaikh, Z.; Nawaz, A.; Silva, G.; Been, L.; et al. Platelet Inhibition with Cangrelor and Crushed Ticagrelor in Patients with ST-Segment–Elevation Myocardial Infarction Undergoing Primary Percutaneous Coronary Intervention. *Circulation* **2019**, *139*, 1661–1670. [CrossRef]
82. Cuisset, T.; Gaborit, B.; Dubois, N.; Quilici, J.; Loosveld, M.; Beguin, S.; Loundou, A.D.; Moro, P.J.; Morange, P.E.; Alessi, M.-C.; et al. Platelet reactivity in diabetic patients undergoing coronary stenting for acute coronary syndrome treated with clopidogrel loading dose followed by prasugrel maintenance therapy. *Int. J. Cardiol.* **2013**, *168*, 523–528. [CrossRef]

3. Pankert, M.; Quilici, J.; Loundou, A.D.; Verdier, V.; Lambert, M.; Deharo, P.; Bonnet, G.; Gaborit, B.; Morange, P.E.; Valéro, R.; et al. Impact of Obesity and the Metabolic Syndrome on Response to Clopidogrel or Prasugrel and Bleeding Risk in Patients Treated After Coronary Stenting. *Am. J. Cardiol.* **2014**, *113*, 54–59. [CrossRef]
4. Silvain, J.; Cayla, G.; Hulot, J.-S.; Finzi, J.; Kerneis, M.; O'Connor, S.A.; Bellemain-Appaix, A.; Barthélémy, O.; Beygui, F.; Collet, J.-P.; et al. High on-thienopyridine platelet reactivity in elderly coronary patients: The SENIOR-PLATELET study. *Eur. Heart J.* **2011**, *33*, 1241–1249. [CrossRef]
5. Cuisset, T.; Loosveld, M.; Morange, P.E.; Quilici, J.; Moro, P.J.; Saut, N.; Gaborit, B.; Castelli, C.; Beguin, S.; Grosdidier, C.; et al. CYP2C19*2 and *17 Alleles Have a Significant Impact on Platelet Response and Bleeding Risk in Patients Treated with Prasugrel After Acute Coronary Syndrome. *JACC Cardiovasc. Interv.* **2012**, *5*, 1280–1287. [CrossRef]
6. Grosdidier, C.; Quilici, J.; Loosveld, M.; Camoin, L.; Moro, P.J.; Saut, N.; Gaborit, B.; Pankert, M.; Cohen, W.; Lambert, M.; et al. Effect of CYP2C19*2 and *17 Genetic Variants on Platelet Response to Clopidogrel and Prasugrel Maintenance Dose and Relation to Bleeding Complications. *Am. J. Cardiol.* **2013**, *111*, 985–990. [CrossRef]
7. Alexopoulos, D.; Xanthopoulou, I.; Perperis, A.; Siapika, A.; Stavrou, K.; Tsoni, E.; Davlouros, P.; Hahalis, G. Factors Affecting Residual Platelet Aggregation in Prasugrel Treated Patients. *Curr. Pharm. Des.* **2013**, *19*, 5121–5126. [CrossRef]
8. Samoš, M.; Fedor, M.; Kovář, F.; Galajda, P.; Bolek, T.; Stančiaková, L.; Fedorová, J.; Staško, J.; Kubisz, P.; Mokáň, M. The Impact of Type 2 Diabetes on the Efficacy of ADP Receptor Blockers in Patients with Acute ST Elevation Myocardial Infarction: A Pilot Prospective Study. *J. Diabetes Res.* **2016**, *2016*, 2909436. [CrossRef]
9. Adamski, P.; Buszko, K.; Sikora, J.; Niezgoda, P.; Fabiszak, T.; Ostrowska, M.; Barańska, M.; Karczmarska-Wódzka, A.; Navarese, E.P.; Kubica, J. Determinants of high platelet reactivity in patients with acute coronary syndromes treated with ticagrelor. *Sci. Rep.* **2019**, *9*, 3924. [CrossRef]
90. Ilardi, F.; Gargiulo, G.; Paolillo, R.; Ferrone, M.; Cimino, S.; Giugliano, G.; Schiattarella, G.G.; Verde, N.; Stabile, E.; Perrino, C.; et al. Impact of chronic kidney disease on platelet aggregation in patients with acute coronary syndrome. *J. Cardiovasc. Med.* **2020**, *21*, 660–666. [CrossRef]
91. Bolek, T.; Samoš, M.; Šimonová, R.; Kovář, F.; Fedor, M.; Galajda, P.; Staško, J.; Kubisz, P.; Mokáň, M. Does Pantoprazole Affect the On-Treatment Platelet Reactivity in Patients With Acute STEMI Treated With ADP Receptor Blockers?—A Pilot Prospective Study. *Am. J. Ther.* **2017**, *24*, e162–e166. [CrossRef] [PubMed]
92. Ferreiro, J.L.; Ueno, M.; Tello-Montoliu, A.; Tomasello, S.D.; Seecheran, N.; Desai, B.; Rollini, F.; Guzman, L.A.; Bass, T.A.; Angiolillo, D.J. Impact of Prasugrel Reload Dosing Regimens on High On-Treatment Platelet Reactivity Rates in Patients on Maintenance Prasugrel Therapy. *JACC Cardiovasc. Interv.* **2013**, *6*, 182–184. [CrossRef] [PubMed]
93. Christ, G.; Hafner, T.; Siller-Matula, J.M.; Francesconi, M.; Grohs, K.; Wilhelm, E.; Podczeck-Schweighofer, A. Platelet Inhibition by Abciximab Bolus-Only Administration and Oral ADP Receptor Antagonist Loading in Acute Coronary Syndrome Patients: The Blocking and Bridging Strategy. *Thromb. Res.* **2013**, *132*, e36–e41. [CrossRef] [PubMed]
94. Niazi, A.K.; Dinicolantonio, J.J.; Lavie, C.J.; O'Keefe, J.H.; Meier, P.; Bangalore, S. Triple versus dual antiplatelet therapy in acute coronary syndromes: Adding cilostazol to aspirin and clopidogrel? *Cardiology* **2013**, *126*, 233–243. [CrossRef]
95. Bassez, C.; Deharo, P.; Pankert, M.; Bonnet, G.; Quilici, J.; Lambert, M.; Verdier, V.; Morange, P.; Alessi, M.-C.; Bonnet, J.-L.; et al. Effectiveness of switching 'low responders' to prasugrel to ticagrelor after acute coronary syndrome. *Int. J. Cardiol.* **2014**, *176*, 1184–1185. [CrossRef]

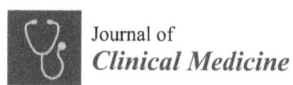 

*Review*

# COVID-19 and the Response to Antiplatelet Therapy

Tomáš Bolek [1], Matej Samoš [1,*], Jakub Jurica [1], Lucia Stančiaková [2], Martin Jozef Péč [1], Ingrid Škorňová [2], Peter Galajda [1], Ján Staško [2], Marián Mokáň [1] and Peter Kubisz [2,†]

[1] Department of Internal Medicine I, Jessenius Faculty of Medicine in Martin, Comenius University in Bratislava, 036 59 Martin, Slovakia
[2] National Centre of Hemostasis and Thrombosis, Department of Hematology and Blood, Transfusion, Jessenius Faculty of Medicine in Martin, Comenius University in Bratislava, 036 59 Martin, Slovakia
* Correspondence: matej.samos@gmail.com; Tel.: +421-907-612-943 or +421-43-4203-820
† In memoriam.

**Abstract:** The coronavirus SARS-CoV2 disease (COVID-19) is connected with significant morbidity and mortality (3.4%), disorders in hemostasis, including coagulopathy, activation of platelets, vascular injury, and changes in fibrinolysis, which may be responsible for an increased risk of thromboembolism. Many studies demonstrated relatively high rates of venous and arterial thrombosis related to COVID-19. The incidence of arterial thrombosis in severe/critically ill intensive care unit–admitted COVID-19 patients appears to be around 1%. There are several ways for the activation of platelets and coagulation that may lead to the formation of thrombi, so it is challenging to make a decision about optimal antithrombotic strategy in patients with COVID-19. This article reviews the current knowledge about the role of antiplatelet therapy in patients with COVID-19.

**Keywords:** antiplatelet therapy; aspirin; arterial thrombosis; COVID-19

## 1. Introduction

The coronavirus SARS-CoV2 disease (COVID-19) is known to be associated with significant morbidity and mortality. Globally, there are approximately 616 million COVID-19 cases reported to date, with a mortality of 3.4%. Studies have highlighted an astonishing rate of venous thromboembolism (VTE) and pulmonary embolism (PE) in patients with a severe form of COVID-19 reaching 42% and 17%, respectively [1]. However, arterial thrombotic events have also been described at various sites, such as coronary arteries, cerebral arteries, and peripheral arteries [2,3]. A pharmacologic thromboprophylaxis is recommended in all hospitalized patients with COVID-19 unless the risk of bleeding on prophylactic anticoagulation is higher than the risk of thrombosis. In non-hospitalized patients with COVID-19, pharmacological prevention of VTE is not recommended, unless the patient has other indications for the therapy or participates in a clinical trial [4,5]. Nevertheless, the incidence of arterial thrombosis (AT) in severe/critically ill COVID-19 patients admitted to intensive care units (ICU) across the five cohort studies was 4.4% (95% confidence interval [CI] 2.8–6.4) [6]. Thus, this raises a question about the need for antiplatelet therapy (APT) in these patients. In this article, we review the current knowledge about the use of APT and its efficacy and safety in COVID-19 patients.

## 2. COVID-19 and Arterial Thrombosis

The clinical manifestations of COVID-19 disease are variable, and the risk of AT seems to be dependent on the severity of the disease [7,8].

### 2.1. COVID-19 and the Incidence of Arterial Thrombosis

The incidence of VTE in COVID-19 patients ranged from 1.7 to 16.5% in 35 observational studies reported worldwide [9]. In a multicenter, cohort, retrospective database

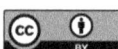

Citation: Bolek, T.; Samoš, M.; Jurica, J.; Stančiaková, L.; Péč, M.J.; Škorňová, I.; Galajda, P.; Staško, J.; Mokáň, M.; Kubisz, P. COVID-19 and the Response to Antiplatelet Therapy. *J. Clin. Med.* 2023, 12, 2038. https://doi.org/10.3390/jcm12052038

Academic Editor: Ferdinando Mannello

Received: 28 November 2022
Revised: 1 March 2023
Accepted: 3 March 2023
Published: 4 March 2023

Copyright: © 2023 by the authors. Licensee MDPI, Basel, Switzerland. This article is an open access article distributed under the terms and conditions of the Creative Commons Attribution (CC BY) license (https://creativecommons.org/licenses/by/4.0/).

analysis of COVID-19 patients (with 3531 patients), the reported incidence of VTE was 6.68% [10]. However, reports describing the incidence of AT are inconsistent [11,12]. In a retrospective analysis of the RECOVER database, which enrolled 26,974 patients, the incidence of AT was 0.13% in COVID-19-positive patients. These patients experienced a greater proportion of AT in peripheral arteries [13]. In a retrospective U.S. cohort study, a comparison between a hospital stay due to COVID-19 and a hospital stay due to influenza showed a higher risk for venous, but not arterial, thrombotic events in the former [14]. On the other hand, in a recently published study analyzing 909,473 COVID-19 cases, AT ranged from 0.1% to 0.8% and increased to 3.1% among those who needed in-hospital admission. The occurrence of VTE and AT in patients with COVID-19 carried an increased risk of death (adjusted hazard ratios [HR] for VTE 4.42 [3.07–6.36] for those not hospitalized and 1.63 [1.39–1.90] for those hospitalized; and adjusted HR for AT 3.16 [2.65–3.75] and 1.93 [1.57–2.37], respectively) [15]. In summary, based on the latest available data, the incidence of AT in patients with COVID-19 is thought to be around 1% [13–15].

*2.2. Pathophysiology of Arterial Thrombosis in COVID-19 Patients*

COVID-19 is known to be associated with several abnormalities in hemostasis, including coagulopathy, activation of platelets, vessel injury, and alterations in fibrinolysis, which may be responsible for thrombosis related to this disease [1,16]. Such pathophysiological changes may cause AT or VTE, especially in patients with a severe course of the disease. These events occur more frequently in the lung, where both macro- and microthrombi have been reported [17]. In a post-mortem study, fibrin- and platelet-rich thrombi in pulmonary arterioles were reported together with congestion in capillaries and alveolar bleeding [18,19]. Subsequently, there is a greater chance of platelet aggregation and activation of the coagulation system due to COVID-19-related endothelial dysfunction. Furthermore, COVID-19 is related to platelet activation which has been repeatedly described in patients suffering from this disease [20–22]. Yatim et al. [20] reported that elevated soluble P-selectin (a marker of platelet activation) was associated with disease severity and in-hospital mortality and predicted the need for intubation and mechanical ventilatory support. Another observational, prospective study performed by Jakobs et al. on a sample of hospitalized patients with COVID-19 showed that adenosine diphosphate- (ADP), thrombin receptor activator peptide 6- (TRAP), and arachidonic acid- (AA) induced platelet reactivity was significantly higher in those with COVID-19 [22]. In addition, there is a dysregulation of the renin-angiotensin system due to SARS-CoV-2-induced consumption of the angiotensin-converting enzyme 2 (ACE-2) resulting in an intensive immune response that might lead to further endothelial damage [23], and aggravate the risk of AT development. There are several pathways of platelet-coagulation system activation with subsequent thrombus formation; therefore, it is challenging to make an optimal decision regarding the antithrombotic strategy in COVID-19 patients.

Additionally, the pro-thrombotic state in COVID-19 patients has been linked to the increased formation of neutrophil extracellular traps (NETs) [24]. Although the exact mechanisms and signaling pathways involved in neurophil/platelet interaction which leads to increased NETs formation are not fully understood, it is known that platelets can activate neutrophils to form NETs and that NETs themselves can be detected in thrombi, which points to a possible interaction between inflammatory cells (neutrophils), platelets, and thrombosis [25]. This interaction had also been described in COVID-19-related arterial thrombosis [26]. Interestingly, Petito et al. [27] observed in their prospective study on COVID-19-related thrombosis that NETs, but not platelet activation, correlated with disease activity and predicted thrombosis. However, it is not currently known whether the formation of NETs can be modified (reduced) by the administration of antiplatelet (or anticoagulant) therapy as there is no study dealing with this issue.

## 3. COVID-19 and the Response to Aspirin

Aspirin (Acetylsalicylic acid) is one of the most commonly used drugs worldwide [28] for its anti-platelet, analgesic, anti-inflammatory, and anti-pyretic effect. Aspirin exerts its major activity by inhibiting the cyclooxygenase enzyme (COX), which exists in two forms: COX-1 and COX-2 [29]. As a result, it inhibits the conversion of arachidonic acid into prostaglandins and thromboxane. Its activity expands to several other target structures leading to a number of anti-inflammatory and anti-thrombotic effects [28,29].

Endothelial inflammation and the exposure of von-Willebrand factor to sub-endothelial collagen in COVID-19 patients, in turn, precipitate thrombus formation manifesting as AT or VT [30].

A previous study suggested that aspirin could, in theory, offer protection against the severe form of COVID-19 infection [30]. This theory was examined in a retrospective study, which included 35,370 patients with and also without active aspirin prescriptions prior to becoming infected with SARS-CoV-2. Aspirin significantly reduced the risk of mortality in this study by 32%. After propensity score matching and confounding covariate adjustments, mortality decreased from 6.3 to 2.5% at 14 days and from 10.5 to 4.3% at 30 days in the propensity-matched cohorts [31]. Confounding covariate adjustments included age, gender, comorbidities, and the Care Assessment Needs [CAN] 1-year mortality score. In the RECOVERY trial [32], 14,892 patients were eligible for randomization to aspirin (7351 patients) or usual care alone (7541 patients). In this trial, 150 mg of aspirin did not reduce 28-day mortality, and among patients who were not receiving invasive mechanical ventilation at randomization, aspirin therapy did not reduce the probability of progression to the composite outcome of invasive mechanical ventilation or death. Aspirin therapy was associated with an increase in the rate of being discharged alive within 28 days, but the magnitude of the effect was small (1% absolute difference). Afterwards, Chow et al. published the results of a retrospective cohort study assessing COVID-19 patients, who received aspirin within the period of one week before admission involving the first day of hospital stay as well. After adjustment to sex, ethnicity, age, body mass index (BMI), comorbidities, and beta-blocker use, patients taking aspirin showed a reduced risk of intensive care unit (ICU) admission, mechanical ventilation, and in-hospital mortality [33]. Furthermore, a study carried out by Meizlish et al. analyzed the efficacy of aspirin in patients with SARS-CoV-2 infection. In this study, using multivariate analysis, patients taking aspirin had a lower cumulative incidence of in-hospital death [34]. A meta-analysis evaluating 12 retrospective studies in SARS-CoV-2 positive patients demonstrated a clear benefit of aspirin therapy in preventing a fatal course of COVID-19 disease [35].

Despite the fact that many studies have demonstrated the benefit of aspirin in SARS-CoV-2 patients, there is also a certain degree of evidence in the literature arguing against its use. In a recently released single-center, open-label, randomized controlled trial, 900 COVID-19 patients (with positive PCR), who needed in-hospital treatment were randomized to receive either atorvastatin 40 mg, aspirin 75 mg, or both (N = 225) added to standard care for 10 days or until discharge, whichever came first, or only standard therapy (N = 226). The primary endpoint was clinical deterioration to the level $\geq 6$ of the WHO Ordinal Scale for Clinical Improvement. There was no difference in the primary endpoint across the study groups ($p = 0.463$); hence, aspirin treatment in this study did not prevent clinical deterioration [36]. Another randomized, double-blind, placebo-controlled phase two clinical trial in adult patients with adult respiratory distress syndrome assigned patients randomly at a 1:1 ratio to aspirin (75 mg) or placebo, for a maximum of 14 days. The primary endpoint was defined as the value of the oxygenation index (OI) on day seven. In this study, no significant difference in day 7 OI was found (aspirin group: $54.4 \pm 26.8$; vs. placebo group: $42.4 \pm 25$; mean difference, 12.0; 95% CI, -6.1 to 30.1; $p = 0.19$) [37]. Finally, in a meta-analysis of 34 studies, including randomized controlled trials (3 trials), prospective cohort studies (4 studies), or retrospective studies (27 studies) on associations between aspirin or other antiplatelet therapy administration and all-cause mortality in COVID-19 patients performed by Su et al. [38], aspirin showed no significant effect on all-cause mortality in randomized controlled trials, decreased all-cause mortality by 15% in prospective studies, and reduced all-cause mortality by 20% in retrospective studies.

In summary, the anti-platelet, anti-inflammatory, anti-pyretic, and analgesic effects of aspirin seem to be promising in COVID-19 patients; however, the results of available studies are still controversial (Table 1). More studies are needed to better define recommendations for aspirin treatment in COVID-19 patients.

**Table 1.** Aspirin therapy in patients with COVID-19 [31–38].

| Author | Study Design | ICU Care | Number of Patients | Conclusion |
|---|---|---|---|---|
| Osborne T.F et al., 2021 [31] | Retrospective, cohort | Not reported | 32,836 | Aspirin was strongly associated with decreased mortality rates for Veterans with COVID-19. |
| RECOVERY Collaborative Group 2022, [32] | Randomised, open-label, platform trial | Not reported (non-invasive or invasive respiratory support in 33% of patients) | 14,892 | Aspirin did not reduce 28-day mortality, and in patients who were not on invasive ventilation at randomisation, aspirin did not reduce the probability of the composite outcome of mechanical ventilation or death |
| Chow J.H. et al. 2022, [33] | Observational, cohort | No (patients with moderate disease severity included) | 112,269 | Early aspirin use was associated with lower odds of 28-day in-hospital mortality. |
| Meizlish M.L. et al., 2021 [34] | Retrospective study | Not reported | 2785 | Aspirin therapy was associated with a lower incidence of in-hospital death |
| Kow C.S. et al., 2021 [35] | Meta-analysis of retrospective studies | Not reported | 14,377 | Significantly reduced risk of a fatal course of COVID-19 with the use of aspirin in patients with COVID-19. |
| Ghati N. et al., 2022 [36] | Randomized, open-label, controlled | Not reported | 900 | Aspirin treatment among patients admitted with mild to moderate COVID-19 infection did not prevent clinical deterioration |
| Toner P. et al., 2022 [37] | Randomized, placebo-controlled | Yes | 49 | Aspirin did not improve oxygen index or other physiological outcomes. |
| Su W. et al., 2022 [38] | Meta-analysis of randomized controlled, prospective cohort, and retrospective studies | Not reported | 233,796 | Aspirin reduced all-cause mortality in prospective and retrospective studies; no impact in randomized controlled studies |

## 4. COVID-19 and the Response on P2Y12 ADP Receptor Blockers

As previously mentioned, the increased risk of AT and VT observed during moderate-to-severe COVID-19 disease is associated with the increased morbidity and mortality of these patients [8,9]. In addition, patients with COVID-19 were demonstrated to require lower amounts of thrombin for the aggregation of platelets compared to healthy controls [39,40]. Furthermore, as mentioned, there is a study demonstrating ADP-, TRAP-, and AA-induced platelet hyper-reactivity in COVID-19 [22]. This (ADP-induced) platelet hyperreactivity could be, in theory, affected by treatment with P2Y12 ADP receptor blockers (ADPRB). However, there is limited information about the efficacy of P2Y12 ADPRB in patients with COVID-19 (Table 2). A small case-control study was performed enrolling five patients with severe respiratory failure as a result of SARS-CoV-2 infection. These patients required helmet continuous positive airway pressure (CPAP) and received a dose of 25 µg/kg/body weight of tirofiban as bolus infusion, followed by a continuous infusion of 0.15 µg/kg/body weight per minute for 48 h. Prior to the tirofiban infusion, patients received 250 mg of aspirin and 300 mg of clopidogrel. Both antiplatelet drugs continued at a dose of 75 mg daily for 30 days. All controls received a prophylactic or therapeutic dose of heparin, according to local standard operating procedures. Patients consistently experienced a mean (SD) reduction in A-a O2 gradient of $-32.6$ mmHg (61.9, $p = 0.154$), $-52.4$ mmHg (59.4, $p = 0.016$), and $-151.1$ mmHg (56.6, $p = 0.011$; $p = 0.047$ vs. controls) at 24, 48 h, and 7 days after treatment [41]. This study included a very limited number of patients (only five patients were enrolled), and this should definitely be taken into consideration when interpreting these results. An open-label, bayesian, adaptive randomized clinical trial was designed to evaluate the benefits and risks of adding a P2Y12 ADPRB (ticagrelor/clopidogrel) to anticoagulant treatment among non-critically ill patients hospitalized for COVID-19. In this trial, patients were randomized to a therapeutic dose of heparin and a P2Y12 ADPRB (N = 293 [ticagrelor = 63.2%/clopidogrel = 36.8%]) or a therapeutic dose of heparin only (usual care, N = 269) in a 1:1 ratio for 14 days or until hospital discharge. The composite primary outcome was organ support-free days evaluated on an ordinal scale that combined in-hospital death and the primary safety outcome was a major bleeding event within the first 28 days. The median number of organ support-free days was 21 days (interquartile range [IQR], 20–21 days) among patients in the P2Y12 ADPRB group and 21 days (IQR, 21–21 days) in the standard treatment group (adjusted OR, 0.83 [95% credible interval (CrI), 0.55–1.25]), and a major bleeding event occurred in six patients (2.0%) in the P2Y12 ADPRB group and in two patients (0.7%) in the control group; so no benefit of P2Y12 ADPRB was found in a group of non-critically ill COVID-19 patients with a higher risk of bleeding [42]. Likewise, in the REMAP-CAP trial (Randomized, Embedded, Multifactorial Adaptive Platform Trial), 1557 critically ill adult COVID-19 patients were enrolled and randomized to receive either open-label aspirin (N = 565), a P2Y12 ADPRB (N = 455), or no antiplatelet therapy (control group; N = 529). The median for organ support-free days was 7 (IQR, $-1$ to 16) in both antiplatelet and control groups (median-adjusted OR, 1.02 [95% CrI, 0.86–1.23]; 95.7% posterior probability of futility) and among survivors, the median for organ support-free days was 14 in both P2Y12 ADPRB group and control group [43]. Thus, no benefit of the addition of P2Y12 ADPRB (clopidogrel or ticagrelor) was found in non-critically ill and critically ill SARS-CoV-2 patients. Furthermore, in the COVD-PACT (Prevention of Arteriovenous Thrombotic Events in Critically-ill COVID-19 Patients Trial) trial [44], a multi-center randomized trial, 290 patients who required intensive care unit level of care for COVID-19 were randomly assigned to clopidogrel (300 mg orally once on the day of randomization, followed by 75 mg orally once daily on subsequent days of in-hospital stay) or no antiplatelet therapy in addition to the standard or full-dose anticoagulation. The primary efficacy end-point of the study was a composite of venous and arterial thrombosis and the primary safety end-point was a composite of fatal or life-threatening bleeding. In this randomized trial, there were no differences in the primary efficacy or safety end-points with clopidogrel versus no antiplatelet therapy. On the other hand, in a recently published international multicenter prospective registry, COVID-19 patients were treated with aspirin (oral or venous), clopidogrel, ticlopidine, prasugrel, and ticagrelor, either with single or dual antiplatelet therapy and were compared with patients without antiplatelet therapy. Patients who received antiplatelet therapy had a shorter duration of mechanical ventilation ($8 \pm 5$ days vs. $11 \pm 7$ days, $p = 0.01$); and lower mortality (log-rank $p < 0.01$, RR 0.79, 95% CI 0.70 to 0.94) compared to patients who did not receive antiplatelet agents [45]. There are no available data about the use of cangrelor in COVID-19 patients. In summary, a limited number of published studies on the role of P2Y12 ADPRB in SARS-CoV-2 infection have shown controversial results. Therefore, further studies will be needed in future.

Table 2. P2Y12 ADPRB therapy in patients with COVID-19 [41–45].

| Author | Study Design | ICU Care | Number of Patients | Conclusion |
|---|---|---|---|---|
| Veicca M. et al., 2020 [41] | Prospective, case series | Yes | 5 | Improvement in blood oxygenation with combined antiplatelet therapy (including P2Y12 ADPRB) |
| Berger J.S. et al., 2022 [42] | Open-label, bayesian, adaptive randomized clinical trial | No | 562 | P2Y12 ADPRB therapy did not result in an increased odds of improvement in organ support–free days during hospitalization |
| Bradbury C.A. et al., 2022 [43] | Prospective, adaptive platform trial | Yes | 1824 | P2Y12 ADPRB therapy did not result in an increased odds of improvement in organ support–free days during hospitalization |
| Bohula E. A. et al., 2022 [44] | Open-label, randomized, controlled trial | Yes | 292 | No effect of P2Y12 ADPRB on thrombotic complications |
| Santoro F. et al., 2022 [45] | Multicentre international prospective registry | No (only 9% of enrolled patients were admitted to ICU) | 7824 | Antiplatelet therapy (including P2Y12 ADPRB) was associated with lower mortality and shorter duration of mechanical ventilation |

## 5. COVID-19 and the Response to Glycoprotein (GP) IIb/IIIa Inhibitors

Glycoprotein (GP) IIb/IIIa inhibitors (GPIIb/IIIaI) are potent, rapid, and selective blockers of platelet aggregation. These agents might, in theory, facilitate the dissolution of blood clots and prevent the formation of new clots in COVID-19 patients [46,47]. Additionally, patients with COVID-19 and acute ST-segment elevation myocardial infarction (STEMI) were shown to have higher rates of multivessel thrombosis, stent thrombosis, and higher modified thrombus grade post-first-device implantation with consequently a higher use of glycoprotein IIb/IIIa inhibitors and thrombus aspiration compared to COVID-19 negative patients [46]. There is little evidence about the benefit of the use of GPIIb/IIIaI in patients with COVID-19 (Table 3), which comes from a case describing a successful outcome of GPIIb/IIIaI administration in a patient with a severe form of COVID-19 viral pneumonia and non-ST-elevation myocardial infarction (NSTEMI) [47]; and from the above-mentioned study including five patients with a laboratory-confirmed SARS-CoV-2 infection, severe respiratory failure, who received tirofiban infusion (together with dual antiplatelet therapy) and who consistently experienced a reduction in blood gas oxygen gradient [41]. Although several cases showed a possible benefit of GPIIb/IIIaI in patients with COVID-19, right now there is no study examining the specificity of GPIIb/IIIaI use in COVID-19 versus non-COVID-19 cardiac patients. Furthermore, to date, there is no prospective, randomized trial to confirm this benefit, and further studies will be needed to adopt any final recommendations.

Table 3. GPIIb/IIIaI therapy in patients with COVID-19.

| Author | Study Design | ICU Care | Number of Patients | Conclusion |
|---|---|---|---|---|
| Veicca M. et al., 2020 [41] | Prospective, case series | Yes | 5 | Improvement in blood oxygenation with combined antiplatelet therapy (including GPIIb/IIIaI) |
| Merrill P.J. and Bradburne R.M., 2021 [47] | Case report | Yes | 1 | Successful use of GPIIb/IIIaI for NSTEMI |

## 6. The Effect of Time of Antiplatelet Agent Admission on COVID-19-Related Outcomes

Another possible question is whether there is a difference between patients already on antiplatelet therapy before admission and those randomly assigned to antiplatelet drugs or placebo on top of anticoagulation after admission.

Looking at the studies in which antiplatelet therapy was started at the time of patient admission (patients who used antiplatelet therapy prior to admission were excluded) [32,34,36,37,43,44], only a single observational study performed by Meizlish et al. [34] showed a reduced risk of in-hospital death in patients receiving aspirin. In the rest of the studies, no overall benefit of antiplatelet therapy (either with aspirin or with a P2Y12 ADPRB) was shown.

In contrast, in studies which included patients with pre-event antiplatelet therapy [31,35,45], antiplatelet therapy reduced mortality [31], the risk of a fatal course of COVID-19 [35] and the risk of mortality or the duration of mechanical ventilation [45]. This observation could suggest that previous antiplatelet therapy could be more beneficial than starting the therapy after the estimation of the diagnosis of COVID-19, or that pre-existing antiplatelet therapy should not be stopped after the diagnosis of COVID-19. However, due to different study designs, it is difficult to compare their results, and these differences should be interpreted with caution until a study directly comparing pre-event antiplatelet therapy with an on-admission one is performed and published.

Summarizing, although the results of trials published so far indicate that antiplatelet agents might protect against the development of AT complications of severe COVID-19 disease, current recommendations [4,5] state that in non-hospitalized patients with symptomatic COVID-19, the initiation of antiplatelet therapy is not effective (does not reduce risk of hospitalization, arterial or venous thrombosis, or mortality) [48]. Among non-critically ill patients hospitalized for COVID-19, there is a strong recommendation against the addition of an antiplatelet agent. Adding an antiplatelet agent to prophylactic anticoagulation might be considered in selected critically ill patients (although the selection of patients is not well established). Nevertheless, only randomized studies with a minimum sample size of 100 patients and observational studies with a minimum sample size of 400 patients were included in the preparation of these recommendations [5]. As repeatedly discussed within the article, the majority of studies on antiplatelet agents had limited patient samples and therefore were not included in current recommendations. In addition, there is a report showing that the addition of an antiplatelet agent (aspirin) might be beneficial in frail cardiovascular patients, as was shown, for example, in the HOPE COVID-19 registry [49]. Going further, right now there is no satisfactory explanation for the differences between the results observed in the randomized and non-randomized clinical studies. One should consider the usual disadvantages of non-randomized and retrospective studies, such as selection bias or missing data; however, non-randomized studies might better copy the settings of real-world clinical practice and so far, available randomized trials also have their limitations (mostly relatively low sample sizes, exclusion criteria limiting the ability to enroll the patients in the highest risk, etc.). Therefore, the role of antiplatelet therapy in patients with COVID-19 disease should be probably re-questioned in future treatment recommendations.

## 7. Conclusions

The results of trials published so far indicate that antiplatelet agents (especially if administered prior to the development of the disease) might protect against AT complications of COVID-19; however, this evidence comes mostly from non-randomized studies and is not in line with current recommendations. Randomized controlled trials (with sufficient patient samples) are highly required to investigate whether pre-existing or newly added antiplatelet therapy might be beneficial in SARS-CoV-2 infection.

**Author Contributions:** M.S., T.B. and L.S. designed the study; T.B. and M.S. drafted the manuscript; M.J.P., J.J. and I.Š. performed the search of the literature, analyzed and interpreted the data; L.S., I.Š., P.G., J.S., M.M. and P.K. revised the manuscript critically. P.K., unfortunately, died before the submission of the final version of the manuscript. All the remaining authors have read and agreed to the published version of the manuscript.

**Funding:** This study was funded by project APVV (Slovak Research and Development Agency) 16-0020, and by Projects of Research Agency of Slovak Ministry of Education, Science and Sports (VEGA) 1/0549/19 and 1/0090/20.

**Institutional Review Board Statement:** The study was conducted in accordance with the Declaration of Helsinki. Formal Ethical review and approval were waived for this study as there is no need for a formal approval for this type of study.

**Informed Consent Statement:** Not applicable.

**Data Availability Statement:** The source data are available at the Corresponding Author upon request.

**Acknowledgments:** This study was supported by project APVV (Slovak Research and Development Agency) 16-0020, and by Projects of Research Agency of Slovak Ministry of Education, Science and Sports (VEGA) 1/0549/19 and 1/0090/20.

**Conflicts of Interest:** The authors have no conflicts of interest to declare.

## References

1. Wu, C.; Liu, Y.; Cai, X.; Zhang, W.; Li, Y.; Fu, C. Prevalence of Venous Thromboembolism in Critically Ill Patients with Coronavirus Disease 2019: A Meta-Analysis. *Front. Med.* **2021**, *8*, 603558. [CrossRef] [PubMed]
2. De Roquetaillade, C.; Chousterman, B.G.; Tomasoni, D.; Zeitouni, M.; Houdart, E.; Guedon, A.; Reiner, P.; Bordier, R.; Gayat, E.; Montalescot, G.; et al. Unusual arterial thrombotic events in Covid-19 patients. *Int. J. Cardiol.* **2021**, *323*, 281–284. [CrossRef] [PubMed]
3. Guillan, M.; Villacieros-Alvarez, J.; Bellido, S.; Perez-Jorge Peremarch, C.; Suarez-Vega, V.M.; Aragones-Garcia, M.; Cabrera-Rojo, C.; Fernandez-Ferro, J. Unusual simultaneous cerebral infarcts in multiple arterial territories in a COVID-19 patient. *Thromb. Res.* **2020**, *193*, 107–109. [CrossRef]
4. Cuker, A.; Tseng, E.K.; Nieuwlaat, R.; Angchaisuksiri, P.; Blair, C.; Dane, K.; Davila, J.; DeSancho, M.T.; Diuguid, D.; Griffin, D.O.; et al. American Society of Hematology 2021 guidelines on the use of anticoagulation for thromboprophylaxis in patients with COVID-19. Blood Adv. *Blood. Adv.* **2021**, *5*, 872–888. [CrossRef] [PubMed]
5. Schulman, S.; Sholzberg, M.; Spyropoulos, A.C.; Zarychanski, R.; Resnick, H.E.; Bradbury, C.A.; Broxmeyer, L.; Connors, J.M.; Falanga, A.; Iba, T.; et al. International Society on Thrombosis and Haemostasis. ISTH guidelines for antithrombotic treatment in COVID-19. *J. Thromb. Haemost.* **2022**, *20*, 2214–2225. [CrossRef] [PubMed]
6. Cheruiyot, I.; Kipkorir, V.; Ngure, B.; Misiani, M.; Munguti, J.; Ogeng'o, J. Arterial Thrombosis in Coronavirus Disease 2019 Patients: A Rapid Systematic Review. *Ann. Vasc. Surg.* **2021**, *70*, 273–281. [CrossRef]
7. Azouz, E.; Yang, S.; Monnier-Cholley, L.; Arrivé, L. Systemic arterial thrombosis and acute mesenteric ischemia in a patient with COVID-19. *Intensive. Care. Med.* **2020**, *46*, 1464–1465. [CrossRef]
8. Gallo Marin, B.; Aghagoli, G.; Lavine, K.; Yang, L.; Siff, E.J.; Chiang, S.S.; Salazar-Mather, T.P.; Dumenco, L.; Savaria, M.C.; Aung, S.N.; et al. Share. Predictors of COVID-19 severity: A literature review. *Rev. Med. Virol.* **2021**, *31*, 1–10. [CrossRef]
9. Kunutsor, K.S.; Laukkanen, A.J. Incidence of venous and arterial thromboembolic complications in COVID-19: A systematic review and meta-analysis. *Thromb. Res.* **2020**, *196*, 27–30. [CrossRef]
10. Lee, Y.; Jehangir, Q.; Li, P.; Gudimella, D.; Mahale, P.; Lin, C.H.; Apala, D.R.; Krishnamoorthy, G.; Halabi, A.; Patel, K.; et al. Venous thromboembolism in COVID-19 patients and prediction model: A multicenter cohort study. *BMC Infect. Dis.* **2022**, *22*, 462. [CrossRef]
11. Indes, J.E.; Koleilat, I.; Hatch, A.N.; Choinski, K.; Jones, D.B.; Aldailami, H.; Billett, H.; Denesopolis, J.M.; Lipsitz, E. Early experience with arterial thromboembolic complications in patents with COVID-19. *J. Vasc. Surg.* **2021**, *73*, 381–389. [CrossRef] [PubMed]
12. Bellosta, R.; Luzzani, L.; Natalini, G.; Pegorer, M.A.; Attisani, L.; Cossu, L.G.; Ferrandina, C.; Fossati, A.; Conti, E.; Bush, R.L.; et al. Acute limb ischemia in patients with COVID-19 pneumonia. *J. Vasc. Surg.* **2020**, *72*, 1864–1872. [CrossRef]
13. Glober, N.; Stewart, L.; Seo, J.; Kabrhel, C.; Nordenholz, K.; Camargo, C.; Kline, J. Incidence and characteristics of arterial thromboemboli in patients with COVID-19. *Thromb. J.* **2021**, *19*, 104. [CrossRef] [PubMed]
14. Hana, M.; El Sahly, M.D. Association of COVID-19 vs influenza with risk of arterial and venous thrombotic events among hospitalized patients. *JAMA* **2022**, *328*, 637.

15. Burn, E.; Duarte-Salles, T.; Fernandez-Bertolin, S.; Reyes, C.; Kostka, K.; Delmestri, A.; Rijnbeek, P.; Verhamme, K.; Prieto-Alhambra, D. Venous or arterial thrombosis and deaths among COVID-19 cases: A European network cohort study. *Lancet Infect. Dis.* **2022**, *22*, 1142–1152. [CrossRef]
16. Leentjens, J.; Van Haaps, T.F.; Wessels, F.P.; Schutgens, R.E.; Middeldorp, S. COVID-19-associated coagulopathy and antithrombotic agents-lessons after 1 year. *Lancet Haematol.* **2021**, *8*, e524–e533. [CrossRef] [PubMed]
17. Asakura, H.; Ogawa, H. COVID-19-associated coagulopathy and disseminated intravascular coagulation. *Int. J. Hematol.* **2021**, *113*, 45–57. [CrossRef] [PubMed]
18. Carsana, L.; Sonzogni, A.; Nasr, A.; Rossi, R.S.; Pellegrinelli, A.; Zerbi, P.; Rech, R.; Colombo, R.; Antinori, S.; Corbellino, M.; et al. Pulmonary post-mortem findings in a series of COVID-19 cases from northern Italy: A two-centre descriptive study. *Lancet Infect. Dis.* **2020**, *20*, 1135–1140. [CrossRef]
19. Varga, Z.; Flammer, A.J.; Steiger, P.; Haberecker, M.; Andermatt, R.; Zinkernagel, A.S.; Mehra, M.R.; Schuepbach, R.A.; Ruschitzka, F.; Moch, H. Endothelial cell infection and endotheliitis in COVID-19. *Lancet* **2020**, *395*, 1417–1418. [CrossRef]
20. Yatim, N.; Boussier, J.; Chocron, R.; Hadjadj, J.; Philippe, A.; Gendron, N.; Barnabei, L.; Charbit, B.; Szwebel, T.A.; Carlier, N.; et al. Platelet activation in critically ill COVID-19 patients. *Ann. Intensive. Care.* **2021**, *11*, 113. [CrossRef]
21. Smęda, M.; Hosseinzadeh Maleki, E.; Pełesz, A.; Chłopicki, S. Platelets in COVID-19 disease: Friend, foe, or both? *Pharmacol Rep.* **2022**, *74*, 1182–1197. [CrossRef]
22. Jakobs, K.; Reinshagen, L.; Puccini, M.; Friebel, J.; Wilde, A.B.; Alsheik, A.; Rroku, A.; Landmesser, U.; Haghikia, A.; Kränkel, N.; et al. Disease Severity in Moderate-to-Severe COVID-19 Is Associated With Platelet Hyperreactivity and Innate Immune Activation. *Front. Immunol.* **2022**, *13*, 844701. [CrossRef] [PubMed]
23. Amraei, R.; Rahimi, N. COVID-19, Renin-Angiotensin System and Endothelial Dysfunction. *Cells* **2020**, *9*, 1652. [CrossRef]
24. Zebardast, A.; Latifi, T.; Shabani, M.; Hasanzadeh, A.; Danesh, M.; Babazadeh, S.; Sadeghi, F. Thrombotic storm in coronavirus disease 2019: From underlying mechanisms to its management. *J. Med. Microbiol.* **2022**, *71*, 001591. [CrossRef]
25. Wienkamp, A.K.; Erpenbeck, L.; Rossaint, J. Platelets in the NETworks interweaving inflammation and thrombosis. *Front. Immunol.* **2022**, *13*, 953129. [CrossRef] [PubMed]
26. Nappi, F.; Giacinto, O.; Ellouze, O.; Nenna, A.; Avtaar Singh, S.S.; Chello, M.; Bouzguenda, A.; Copie, X. Association between COVID-19 Diagnosis and Coronary Artery Thrombosis: A Narrative Review. *Biomedicines* **2022**, *10*, 702. [CrossRef] [PubMed]
27. Petito, E.; Falcinelli, E.; Paliani, U.; Cesari, E.; Vaudo, G.; Sebastiano, M.; Cerotto, V.; Guglielmini, G.; Gori, F.; Malvestiti, M.; et al. COVIR study investigators. Association of Neutrophil Activation, More Than Platelet Activation, With Thrombotic Complications in Coronavirus Disease 2019. *J. Infect. Dis.* **2021**, *223*, 933–944. [CrossRef]
28. Vane, J.R.; Botting, R.M. The mechanism of action of aspirin. *Thromb. Res.* **2003**, *110*, 255–258. [CrossRef]
29. Patrono, C.; Coller, B.; Dalen, J.E.; FitzGerald, G.A.; Fuster, V.; Gent, M.; Hirsh, J.; Roth, G. Platelet-active drugs: The relationships among dose, effectiveness, and side effects. *Chest* **2001**, *119*, 39S–63S. [CrossRef]
30. Choudhary, S.; Sharma, K.; Singhb, P.K. Von Willebrand factor: A key glycoprotein involved in thrombo-inflammatory complications of COVID-19. *Chem. Biol. Interact.* **2021**, *348*, 109657. [CrossRef]
31. Osborne, T.F.; Veigulis, Z.P.; Arreola, D.M.; Mahajan, S.M.; Röösli, E.; Curtin, M.C. Association of mortality and aspirin prescription for COVID-19 patients at the Veterans Health Administration. *PLoS ONE* **2021**, *16*, e0246825. [CrossRef]
32. RECOVERY Collaborative Group. Aspirin in patients admitted to hospital with COVID-19 (RECOVERY): A randomised, controlled, open-label, platform trial. *Lancet* **2022**, *399*, 143–151. [CrossRef]
33. Chow, J.H.; Rahnavard, A.; Gomberg-Maitland, M.; Chatterjee, R.; Patodi, P.; Yamane, D.P.; Levine, A.R.; Davison, D.; Hawkins, K.; Jackson, A.M.; et al. N3C Consortium and ANCHOR Investigator. Association of Early Aspirin Use With In-Hospital Mortality in Patients With Moderate COVID-19. *JAMA. Netw. Open* **2022**, *5*, e223890. [CrossRef]
34. Meizlish, M.L.; Goshua, G.; Liu, Y.; Fine, R.; Amin, K.; Chang, E.; DeFilippo, N.; Keating, C.; Liu, Y.; Mankbadi, M.; et al. Intermediate-dose anticoagulation, aspirin, and in-hospital mortality in COVID-19: A propensity score-matched analysis. *Am. J. Hematol.* **2021**, *96*, 471–479. [CrossRef] [PubMed]
35. Kow, C.S.; Hasan, S.S. Use of Antiplatelet Drugs and the Risk of Mortality in Patients with COVID-19: A Meta-Analysis. *J. Thromb. Thrombolysis.* **2021**, *52*, 124–129. [CrossRef] [PubMed]
36. Ghati, N.; Bhatnagar, S.; Mahendran, M.; Thakur, A.; Prasad, K.; Kumar, D.; Dwivedi, T.; Mani, K.; Tiwari, P.; Gupta, R.; et al. Statin and aspirin as adjuvant therapy in hospitalised patients with SARS-CoV-2 infection: A randomised clinical trial (RESIST trial). *BMC Infect. Dis.* **2022**, *22*, 606. [CrossRef]
37. Toner, P.; Boyle, A.J.; McNamee, J.J.; Callaghan, K.; Nutt, C.; Johnston, P.; Trinder, J.; McFarland, M.; Verghis, R.; McAuley, D.F.; et al. Aspirin as a Treatment for ARDS: A Randomized, Placebo-Controlled Clin Trial. *Chest* **2022**, *161*, 1275–1284. [CrossRef] [PubMed]
38. Su, W.; Miao, H.; Guo, Z.; Chen, Q.; Huang, T.; Ding, R. Associations between the use of aspirin or other antiplatelet drugs and all-cause mortality among patients with COVID-19: A meta-analysis. *Front. Pharmacol.* **2022**, *13*, 989903. [CrossRef] [PubMed]
39. Guo, T.; Fan, Y.; Chen, M.; Wu, X.; Zhang, L.; He, T.; Wang, H.; Wan, J.; Wang, X.; Lu, Z. CardiovascularImplications of Fatal Outcomes of Patients With Coronavirus Disease 2019(COVID-19). *JAMA. Cardiol.* **2020**, *5*, 811–818. [CrossRef]
40. Canzano, P.; Brambilla, M.; Porro, B.; Cosentino, N.; Tortorici, E.; Vicini, S.; Poggio, P.; Cascella, A.; Pengo, M.F.; Veglia, F.; et al. Platelet and Endothelial Activation as Potential Mechanisms Behind theThrombotic Complications of COVID-19 Patients. *JACC Basic Transl Sci.* **2021**, *6*, 202–218. [CrossRef] [PubMed]

41. Viecca, M.; Radovanovic, D.; Forleo, B.G.; Santus, P. Enhanced platelet inhibition treatment improves hypoxemia in patients with severe Covid-19 and hypercoagulability. A case control, proof of concept study. *Pharmacol. Res.* **2020**, *158*, 104950. [CrossRef]
42. Berger, J.S.; Kornblith, L.Z.; Gong, M.N.; Reynolds, H.R.; Cushman, M.; Cheng, Y.; McVerry, B.J.; Kim, K.S.; Lopes, R.D.; Atassi, B.; et al. ACTIV-4a Investigators Effect of P2Y12 Inhibitors on Survival Free of Organ Support Among Non-Critically Ill Hospitalized Patients With COVID-19: A Randomized Clinical Trial. *JAMA* **2022**, *327*, 227–236. [CrossRef] [PubMed]
43. REMAP-CAP Writing Committee for the REMAP-CAP Investigators; Bradbury, C.A.; Lawler, P.R.; Stanworth, S.J.; McVerry, B.J.; McQuilten, Z.; Higgins, A.M.; Mouncey, P.R.; Al-Beidh, F.; Rowan, K.M.; et al. Effect of Antiplatelet Therapy on Survival and Organ Support-Free Days in Critically Ill Patients With COVID-19: A Randomized Clinical Trial. *JAMA* **2022**, *327*, 1247–1259. [CrossRef]
44. Bohula, E.A.; Berg, D.D.; Lopes, M.S.; Connors, J.M.; Babar, I.; Barnett, C.F.; Chaudhry, S.P.; Chopra, A.; Ginete, W.; Ieong, M.H.; et al. COVID-PACT Investigators. Anticoagulation and Antiplatelet Therapy for Prevention of Venous and Arterial Thrombotic Events in Critically Ill Patients With COVID-19: COVID-PACT. *Circulation* **2022**, *146*, 1344–1356. [CrossRef] [PubMed]
45. Santoro, F.; Nuñez-Gil, I.J.; Vitale, E.; Viana-Llamas, M.C.; Reche-Martinez, B.; Romero-Pareja, R.; Feltez Guzman, G.; Fernandez Rozas, I.; Uribarri, A.; Becerra-Muñoz, V.M.; et al. Antiplatelet therapy and outcome in COVID-19: The Health Outcome Predictive Evaluation Registry. *Heart* **2022**, *108*, 130–136. [CrossRef] [PubMed]
46. Choudry, F.A.; Hamshere, S.M.; Rathod, K.S.; Akhtar, M.M.; Archbold, R.A.; Guttmann, O.P.; Woldman, S.; Jain, A.K.; Knight, C.J.; Baumbach, A.; et al. High Thrombus Burden in Patients With COVID-19 Presenting With ST-Segment Elevation Myocardial Infarction. *Am. Coll. Cardiol.* **2020**, *76*, 1168–1176. [CrossRef] [PubMed]
47. Merrill, P.J.; Bradburne, R.M. Successful Use of Glycoprotein IIb/IIIa Inhibitor Involving Severely Ill COVID-19 Patient. *Perm. J.* **2021**, *25*, 21.125. [CrossRef]
48. Connors, J.M.; Brooks, M.M.; Sciurba, F.C.; Krishnan, J.A.; Bledsoe, J.R.; Kindzelski, A.; Baucom, A.L.; Kirwan, B.A.; Eng, H.; Martin, D.; et al. ACTIV-4B Investigators. Effect of Antithrombotic Therapy on Clinical Outcomes in Outpatients With Clinically Stable Symptomatic COVID-19: The ACTIV-4B Randomized Clinical Trial. *JAMA* **2021**, *326*, 1703–1712. [CrossRef]
49. Santoro, F.; Núñez-Gil, I.J.; Vitale, E.; Viana-Llamas, M.C.; Romero, R.; Maroun Eid, C.; Feltes Guzman, G.; Becerra-Muñoz, V.M.; Fernández Rozas, I.; Uribarri, A.; et al. Aspirin Therapy on Prophylactic Anticoagulation for Patients Hospitalized With COVID-19: A Propensity Score-Matched Cohort Analysis of the HOPE-COVID-19 Registry. *J. Am. Heart Assoc.* **2022**, *11*, e024530. [CrossRef]

**Disclaimer/Publisher's Note:** The statements, opinions and data contained in all publications are solely those of the individual author(s) and contributor(s) and not of MDPI and/or the editor(s). MDPI and/or the editor(s) disclaim responsibility for any injury to people or property resulting from any ideas, methods, instructions or products referred to in the content.

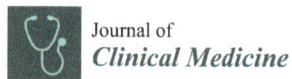 

Article

# The Influence of Hyperthyroidism on the Coagulation and on the Risk of Thrombosis

Nebojsa Antonijevic [1,2,*,†], Dragan Matic [1,2,†], Biljana Beleslin [2,3], Danijela Mikovic [4], Zaklina Lekovic [1], Marija Marjanovic [1], Ana Uscumlic [1,2], Ljubica Birovljev [1] and Branko Jakovljevic [2,5]

1. Clinic for Cardiology, University Clinical Center of Serbia, 11 000 Belgrade, Serbia; dragan4m@gmail.com (D.M.); lekoviczaklina@gmail.com (Z.L.); marija4m@yahoo.co.uk (M.M.); anauscumlic@gmail.com (A.U.); drljubicabirovljev@gmali.com (L.B.)
2. Faculty of Medicine, University of Belgrade, 11 000 Belgrade, Serbia; biljana_beleslin@yahoo.com (B.B.); jakovljevic@dr.com (B.J.)
3. Clinic for Endocrinology, University Clinical Center of Serbia, 11 000 Belgrade, Serbia
4. Blood Transfusion Institute of Serbia, 11 000 Belgrade, Serbia
5. Institute for Hygiene and Medical Ecology, 11 000 Belgrade, Serbia
* Correspondence: drantoni@gmail.com
† These authors contributed equally to this work.

**Abstract: Introduction**: Apart from the well-known fact that hyperthyroidism induces multiple prothrombotic disorders, there is no consensus in clinical practice as to the impact of hyperthyroidism on the risk of thrombosis. The aim of this study was to examine the various hemostatic and immunologic parameters in patients with hyperthyroidism. **Methods**: Our study consists of a total of 200 patients comprised of 64 hyperthyroid patients, 68 hypothyroid patients, and 68 euthyroid controls. Patient thyroid status was determined with standard tests. Detailed hemostatic parameters and cardiolipin antibodies of each patient were determined. **Results**: The values of factor VIII (FVIII), the Von Willebrand factor (vWF), fibrinogen, plasminogen activator inhibitor-1 (PAI-1), and anticardiolipin antibodies of the IgM class were significantly higher in the hyperthyroid patients than in the hypothyroid patients and euthyroid controls. The rate of thromboembolic manifestations was much higher in hyperthyroid patients (6.25%) than in hypo-thyroid patients (2.9%) and euthyroid controls (1.4%). Among hyperthyroid patients with an FVIII value of ≥1.50 U/mL, thrombosis was recorded in 8.3%, while in hyperthyroid patients with FVIII value ≤ 1.50 U/mL the occurrence of thrombosis was not recorded. The incidence of atrial fibrillation (AF) was significantly higher (8.3%) in the hyperthyroid patients compared to the hypothyroid patients (1.5%) and euthyroid controls (0%). **Conclusions**: High levels of FVIII, vWF, fibrinogen, PAI-1, and anticardiolipin antibodies along with other hemostatic factors contribute to the presence of a hypercoaguable state in patients with hyperthyroidism. The risk of occurrence of thrombotic complications is especially pronounced in patients with a level of FVIII exceeding 150% and positive anticardiolipin antibodies of the IgM class. Patients with AF are at particularly high risk of thrombotic complications due to a hyperthyroid prothrombotic milieu.

**Keywords**: hyperthyroidism; prothrombotic; risk of thrombosis

**Citation**: Antonijevic, N.; Matic, D.; Beleslin, B.; Mikovic, D.; Lekovic, Z.; Marjanovic, M.; Uscumlic, A.; Birovljev, L.; Jakovljevic, B. The Influence of Hyperthyroidism on the Coagulation and on the Risk of Thrombosis. *J. Clin. Med.* **2024**, *13*, 1756. https://doi.org/10.3390/jcm13061756

Academic Editor: Boyoung Joung

Received: 12 January 2024
Revised: 24 February 2024
Accepted: 12 March 2024
Published: 19 March 2024

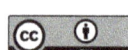

**Copyright**: © 2024 by the authors. Licensee MDPI, Basel, Switzerland. This article is an open access article distributed under the terms and conditions of the Creative Commons Attribution (CC BY) license (https://creativecommons.org/licenses/by/4.0/).

## 1. Introduction

The significance of the data on hyperthyroidism as a probable prothrombotic condition has not been sufficiently implemented in clinical practice, nor are large studies consistent in asserting the association between elevated thyroid hormone values and thrombotic events [1,2]. The results of a new meta-analysis and the findings of other authors indicate that the prothrombotic milieu induced by hyperthyroidism contributes to the increased risk of venous thromboembolism (OR 1.322, 95% CI: 1.278–1.368) [1]. It is believed that the emergence of a prothrombotic (hypercoagulable and hypofibrinolytic) state in hyperthyroidism is significantly contributed to by an elevated level of factor VIII (FVIII), von Willebrand factor (vWF), fibrinogen, and plasminogen activator inhibitor-1 (PAI-1), the level of which increases gradually with the level of thyroid hormones [2–5]. Atrial fibrillation (AF)—as a special risk factor for cerebral and peripheral thromboembolism—is registered in 5–15% of patients with hyperthyroidism. Besides the unquestionable position that AF itself is a risk for thromboembolism even in non-thyroid patients, the existence of a prothrombotic state in hyperthyroidism and its correlation with thromboembolic complications is not mentioned in the most important recommendations or marked as controversial (American College of Cardiology/American Heart Association 2014 (ACC/AHA 2014), European Society of Cardiology 2020 (ESC 2020)).

The most important and most frequently applied risk scores for the occurrence of cerebral infarction (stroke) and peripheral thromboembolism (CHADS2-VASc, GARFIELD-AF, ATRIA, ABC-stroke) do not include the existence of hyperthyroidism as a risk factor for the occurrence of thromboembolic events [6–9].

Considering hemostatic prothrombotic factors in patients with thyroid dysfunction, some authors emphasize the possibility of the influence of elevated levels of anticardiolipin antibodies (aCLA) on the occurrence of a prothrombotic state in hyperthyroid patients [10].

The aim of this study was to examine the various hemostatic and immunologic parameters in patients with hyperthyroidism and compare them with the parameters of the patients with hypothyroidism as well as with the euthyroid controls.

## 2. Materials and Methods

### 2.1. The Studied Population

The study is prospective and included 200 participants. The study was conducted in the University Clinical Center of Serbia, Belgrade, between March 2022 and April 2023.

The diagnosis of hyperthyroidism was established in those patients with decreased TSH levels below the reference range and elevated levels of fT4 [11]. The diagnosis of overt (clinically manifested) hypothyroidism was established in those with elevated TSH levels above the reference range and decreased levels of fT4.

A standard clinical and electrocardiographic examination was performed on all subjects.

The exclusion criteria included the presence of infection, malignancy, moderate to severe renal insufficiency, other significant comorbidities, oral contraceptive therapy, and other medications that could potentially affect the analyses.

### 2.2. Laboratory Analysis

Laboratory analyses were conducted in the morning before meals. Tests for detecting thrombophilia, including antithrombin (AT), protein C (PC), protein S (PS), and lupus anticoagulants (LA), were performed outside the acute thrombotic phase of the disease.

The value of T4 was determined using the radioimmunoassay (RIA) method. Detection of thyroid hormone levels (fT4, TSH) was performed on a gamma counter from LKB 1272 CLINIGAMA. CIS tests were used. The reference range for T4 is 55–160 nmol/L. The fT4 value was determined using the CIS RIA method, with reference values of 7–18 ng/L. The TSH value was determined using the immunoradiometric (IRMA) method, with reference values of 0.15–5.9 mU/L.

The assessment of hemostasis was conducted using standard laboratory tests that included the analysis of prothrombin time (PT), activated partial thromboplastin time (APTT), PC, PS, antithrombin, fibrinogen, and PAI-1. These analyses were performed on a "Dade Behring BCS XP System; Siemens Healthtineers; 91301 Forchheim; Germany" apparatus.

For the determination of coagulation activity of FVIII and vWF activity, a coagulometric method was employed using IL tests on an "Instrumentation Laboratory ACL 6000; Beckman; Brea-California; USA" apparatus.

To detect the presence of lupus anticoagulants, the following tests were used:

1. Activated partial thromboplastin time using IL cephaloplastin reagent, with reference values of 24–36 s. The test was performed on the ACL 6000 apparatus.

2. Dilute Russell's Viper Venom Time (DRVVT) using IL Test LAC Screen and IL Test LAC Confirm. The test result is calculated as the ratio of LAC Screen to LAC Confirm. Reference value: 0.8 to 1.2; a value higher than 1.2 indicates the presence of lupus anticoagulants [12,13].

Anticardiolipin antibodies were determined using a commercial ELISA test (Binding Site UK) on a spectrophotometer. Reference values for the aCLA IgG class are less than 10 GPL U/mL, and for the aCLA IgM class, values are less than 10 MPL U/mL.

The semiquantitative negativity of anticardiolipin antibodies (0) is defined as a value below the upper limit of the reference range. Semiquantitative weak positivity of anticardiolipin antibodies is defined as a value one to two times higher than the upper reference limit. Semiquantitative strong positivity is defined as a value two times higher than the defined upper limit of normal values. The same methodology was applied for the semiquantitative description of aCLA IgG and IgM classes.

*2.3. Statistical Analysis*

In the first phase of data processing, a database was formed, followed by sorting, grouping, and tabulating the results based on the examined characteristics of both the study and control groups. Categorical variables were presented as absolute values and percentages, and comparisons were made using the $\chi^2$ test and Fisher's exact test for probabilities. Continuous variables were presented as mean values with standard deviation (SD). Continuous variables with a normal distribution were compared using the Student's t-test, while those without a normal distribution were compared using the Mann–Whitney U test. To assess the significance of differences among three continuous variables, analysis of variance (ANOVA) was used for variables with a normal distribution, and the Kruskal–Wallis test was used for variables without a normal distribution. A $p$-value less than 0.05 was considered statistically significant. All statistical analyses were conducted using an IBM SPSS Statistics V.20.0 software package.

## 3. Results

The prospective study included 200 participants overall. Of these, 68 were patients with hypothyroidism, 64 patients with hyperthyroidism, and 68 healthy euthyroid participants of equivalent age.

The average age of the entire group (including hypothyroid, hyperthyroid, and euthyroid individuals) was 45.17 years ± 14.86 years. The youngest patient was 16, and the oldest was 83 years old. Although the average age was highest in the hypothyroid group, no statistically significant difference in age was found among the examined groups ($p = 0.129$), Table 1.

The mean body-mass index (BMI) in hypothyroid patients was significantly higher than that in euthyroid participants and hyperthyroid patients. There was no statistically significant difference in mean BMI between hyperthyroid and euthyroid participants—Table 1.

In the total study population, there were 51 males (25.5%) and 149 females (74.5%). In each of the three groups, the female gender was more represented. The difference in gender distribution among the examined groups was statistically highly significant ($p < 0.001$)—Table 1.

The analysis of patients with hypothyroidism, hyperthyroidism, and euthyroid controls in relation to the presence or absence of absolute arrhythmia, and their mutual comparison, is shown in Table 1.

Atrial fibrillation was significantly more common in patients with hyperthyroidism than in patients with hypothyroidism and euthyroid controls ($p = 0.022$). Patients with hyperthyroidism and electrocardiographically documented AF were significantly older (average age 62.2 ± 17.4 years) than patients with hyperthyroidism without absolute arrhythmia (average age 41.63 ± 12.3 years) ($p = 0.012$).

Table 1. Clinical characteristics and immunologic parameters of patients in relation to thyroid status.

| Variable | Hyperthyroidism n = 64 | Hypothyroidism n = 68 | Euthyreosis n = 68 | p |
|---|---|---|---|---|
| Age, years ± SD | 43.23 ± 13.77 | 48.09 ± 13.63 | 44.06 ± 14.86 | 0.129 |
| BMI, kg/m² ± SD | 23.16 ± 3.74 | 27.21 ± 6.08 | 24.37 ± 3.84 | >0.05 |
| Female, % | 82.8 | 85.3 | 55.9 | 0.000 |
| Atrial fibrillation, % | 8.3 | 1.5 | 0.0 | 0.022 |
| Thrombotic events, % | 6.3 | 2.6 | 1.5 | 0.313 |
| aCLA IgG p.o., % | 5.9 | 10.6 | 0.0 | 0.113 |
| aCLA IgG p.s., % | 0.0 | 5.3 | 0.0 | 0.113 |
| aCLA IgG p.m., % | 5.9 | 5.3 | 0.0 | 0.113 |
| aLCA IgM p.o., % | 37.6 | 5.6 | 0.0 | 0.000 |
| aLCA IgM p.s., % | 18.8 | 5.6 | 0.0 | 0.000 |
| aCLA IgM p.m., % | 18.8 | 0.0 | 0.0 | 0.000 |

BMI—body-mass index, aCLA—anticardiolipin antibodies, p.o.—positive overall, p.s.—positive strong, p.m.—positive mildly.

During the follow-up, through the active phase of the disease, thrombotic manifestations occurred in the group of hyperthyroid patients with the highest frequency (6.3%) (one with myocardial infarction, two with cerebrovascular infarction, one with pulmonary embolism) compared to 2.9% of patients with hypothyroidism (two patients with myocardial infarction) and 1.5% of euthyroid patients (one patient with myocardial infarction). Despite the evident differences between the groups, due to the small number of patients with thromboses, a statistically higher frequency of thrombosis in hyperthyroid and hypothyroid patients compared to euthyroid control subjects was not proven.

Among five patients with AF and hyperthyroidism, two had thrombotic episodes (one had a cerebrovascular infarction, and the other had a pulmonary embolism). Three patients with AF and hyperthyroidism did not have thrombotic manifestations. Out of 59 patients with hyperthyroidism without AF, 2 patients had thrombotic episodes.

Semiquantitative analysis of aCLA of the IgG class found that in the group of hypothyroid patients, 89.5% were negative, 5.3% were weakly positive, and 5.3% were strongly positive. In the hyperthyroid patient group, 94.1% of participants were negative, while 5.9% were weakly positive. There were no patients with strong positivity for the aCLA IgG class in the hyperthyroid patient group (0%). In the euthyroid group, all participants were negative for the presence of aCLA IgG (100%). Statistical analysis did not find a significant difference in the examined groups regarding semiquantitative analysis of anticardiolipin antibodies of the IgG class ($p = 0.113$).

Semiquantitative analysis of anticardiolipin antibodies of the IgM class revealed that in the group of hypothyroid patients, 94.4% were negative, 5.6% were strongly positive, and there were no patients with weak positivity (0%). In the hyperthyroid patient group, 62.2% were negative, 18.8% were weakly positive, and 18.8% were strongly positive. In the euthyroid group, all participants were negative for the presence of the aCLA IgM class. Statistical analysis found a significant difference among the examined groups in a semiquantitative analysis of anticardiolipin antibodies of the IgM class ($p = 0.000$).

The values of fibrinogen and natural anticoagulants (antithrombin III, PC, PS) in relation to thyroid status are presented in Table 2 and Figure 1. By comparing fibrinogen values between defined groups, it was found that patients with hyperthyroidism had a significantly higher mean fibrinogen value compared to patients with hypothyroidism and control euthyroid subjects ($p = 0.000$). Additionally, it was established that patients with hyperthyroidism more frequently had a fibrinogen value above 4.1 g/L compared to the euthyroid participant group.

Patients with hyperthyroidism had significantly higher levels of FVIII and vWF compared to those patients with hypothyroidism and euthyroid individuals. The rate of FVIII values over 1.5 U/mL was significantly higher in patients with hyperthyroidism (79.4%) than in patients with hypothyroidism (17.6%) and in euthyroid individuals (2.9%).

In the group of hyperthyroid patients, the mean value of PC was significantly lower compared to the group of hypothyroid patients and the control euthyroid group ($p = 0.000$)—Table 2,

Figure 1. The representation of PC values below the lower limit of normal (<69%) was similar among the examined groups.

**Table 2.** Hemostatic parameter characteristics in relation to thyroid status.

| Variable | Hyperthyroidism n = 64 | Hypothyroidism n = 68 | Euthyreosis n = 68 | p |
|---|---|---|---|---|
| Fibrinogen (g/L), mean ± SD | 3.74 ± 0.79 | 3.41 ± 1.06 | 2.96 ± 0.74 | 0.000 |
| Antithrombin III (%), mean ± SD | 110.60 ± 14.50 | 91.65 ± 16.68 | 105.41 ± 10.67 | 0.000 |
| FVIII (U/mL), mean ± SD | 1.67 ± 0.78 | 0.93 ± 0.40 | 0.95 ± 0.24 | 0.000 |
| FVIII (U/mL) ≥ 1.5 U/mL, % | 79.4 | 17.6 | 2.9 | 0.000 |
| vWF (%), mean ± SD | 115.8 ± 20.3 | 81.6 ± 19.6 | 91.0 ± 12.8 | 0.000 |
| Protein C (%), mean ± SD | 104.84 ± 24.10 | 123.91 ± 22.90 | 121.30 ± 21.45 | 0.000 |
| Protein S (%), mean ± SD | 99.33 ± 20.88 | 114.52 ± 21.65 | 98.48 ± 26.26 | 0.001 |
| Plasminogen (%), mean ± SD | 97.67 ± 20.39 | 119.28 ± 19.28 | 107.23 ± 18.51 | 0.000 |
| PAI-1 (U/mL), mean ± SD | 5.08 ± 1.94 | 3.62 ± 2.13 | 4.81 ± 1.56 | 0.001 |
| Fibrinogen > 4 g/L, % | 30.4 | 18.3 | 10.6 | 0.022 |
| Antithrombin > 75%, % | 98.1 | 86.5 | 100.0 | 0.001 |
| Protein C < 69%, % | 2.0 | 0.0 | 0.0 | 0.326 |
| Protein S < 65%, % | 4.8 | 2.3 | 9.7 | 0.266 |
| Plasminogen > 75%, % | 90.4 | 100.0 | 97.0 | 0.068 |
| PAI-1 > 3.5 U/mL, % | 73.0 | 53.6 | 73.8 | 0.133 |

FVIII—factor VIII, vWF—Von Willebrand factor, PAI-1—plasminogen activator inhibitor-1.

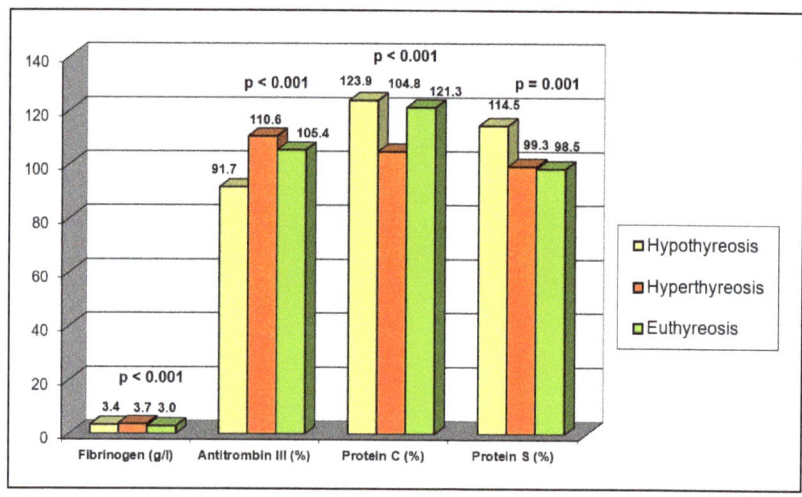

**Figure 1.** Fibrinogen and Natural Anticoagulant Values in Relation to Thyroid Status.

A significantly lower mean value of PS was found in the group of hyperthyroid patients and the group of euthyroid participants compared to the group with hypothyroidism ($p = 0.001$)—Table 2, Figure 1. The representation of PS values below the lower limit of normal (<65%) was similar among the examined groups.

The mean value of antithrombin III was significantly higher in the group of hyperthyroid patients in comparison to the euthyroid control and group of hypothyroid patients ($p = 0.001$)—Table 2 and Figure 1. Furthermore, patients with hypothyroidism had antithrombin III values below the lower limit of normal (<75%) significantly more frequently than patients with hyperthyroidism and participants from the euthyroid control group.

The values of plasminogen and PAI-1 in relation to thyroid status are presented in Table 2 and Figure 2. Although a higher percentage of patients with hyperthyroidism had plasminogen values below the reference limit (<75%) compared to euthyroid patients and patients with hypothyroidism, this difference was not statistically significant. However, by comparing the mean values of plasminogen, a significantly lower value was found in the group of patients with hyperthyroidism compared to the value in the group of hypothyroid patients and the value in the group of euthyroid participants ($p = 0.000$).

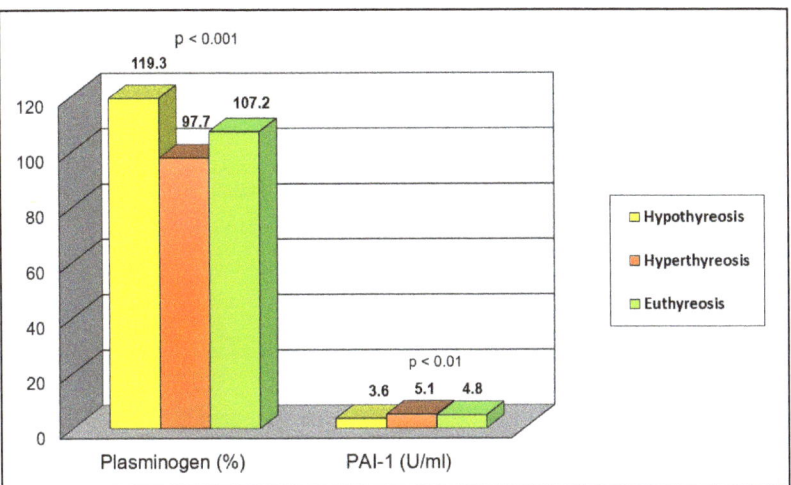

**Figure 2.** Fibrinolytic System Parameter Values in Relation to Thyroid Status.

The PAI-1 value above the lower limit of normal (>3.5 U/mL) did not significantly differ among the examined groups. However, by comparing the mean values of PAI-1 in the defined groups, a significantly higher value of this parameter was found in the group of hyperthyroid patients compared to the mean value in the group of hypothyroid patients ($p < 0.001$) and a not-significantly higher mean value compared to euthyroid participants.

## 4. Discussion

### 4.1. Changes in FVIII Values in Hyperthyroid Patients

Patients with hyperthyroidism had significantly higher levels of FVIII and vWF compared to those patients with hypothyroidism and euthyroid individuals. When interpreting the significance of the increase in FVIII values, it should be kept in mind that FVIII, together with FV, is a key procoagulant factor capable of dramatically increasing FIXa activity and catalyzing FX activation in a dose-dependent manner, noting that small changes in FVIII concentration can have a critical impact [14]. Elevated levels of the mentioned coagulation factors become normalized after appropriate thyroid-suppressive therapy [15]. Several studies indicate that patients with hyperthyroidism in comparison to euthyroid controls show a significant increase in the levels of fibrinogen, FVIII, FIX, and vWF [5,15].

In our study, among hyperthyroid patients with an FVIII value of ≥1.50 U/mL, thrombosis was recorded in 8.3%, while in hyperthyroid patients with an FVIII value ≤1.50 U/mL the occurrence of thrombosis was not recorded. The existence of data indicating a 3–6 times higher relative risk of venous thrombosis and the impact on the occurrence of recurrent venous thrombosis in individuals with FVIII values above 1.5 U/mL (over 150%), as well as the role of FVIII in the pathogenesis of atherothrombosis, highlights the significance of these findings in inducing a prothrombotic state, atherothrombotic complications, and venous thromboembolism in patients with hyperthyroidism [16,17]. Several authors observe a positive correlation between the concentration of FVIII and serum T4 [18,19], while others argue that, among all examined coagulation factors (FV, FVII, FVIII, FIX, FXI, FXII), FVIII is the most sensitive to changes in thyroid hormone concentration and plays a crucial role in thrombus formation during the hyperthyroid stage of the disease [19].

*4.2. Changes in vWF Values in Hyperthyroid Patients*

In our study, values of vWF were significantly higher in hyperthyroid patients than in patients with hypothyroidism and euthyroid controls. It is considered that elevated levels of vWF, FVIII, and fibrinogen, along with reduced fibrinolytic activity and decreased levels of plasminogen, contribute to the presence of a hypercoagulable state and a predisposition to thromboembolism and vascular diseases in patients with hyperthyroidis [20].

*4.3. Changes in the Concentration of Fibrinogen*

In our study, patients with hyperthyroidism had significantly higher levels of fibrinogen compared to both the hypothyroid group and the euthyroid subjects. In studies by other authors, the level of fibrinogen, a well-known acute-phase reactant, is higher in patients with hyperthyroidism compared to euthyroid control subjects [21].

Many studies have confirmed the connection between plasma fibrinogen concentration and coronary heart disease, indicating that elevated fibrinogen is an independent predictor of both initial and recurrent coronary events [22–24]. Fibrinogen is a risk factor not only for cardiovascular diseases but also for stroke, transient ischemic attack, and mortality in middle-aged men and men older than 65 years (with little evidence suggesting it as a risk factor in older women) [15].

*4.4. Hyperthyroidism and Dysfunction of the Fibrinolytic System*

In our study, hyperthyroid patients had significantly lower levels of plasminogen than hypothyroid patients and euthyroid subjects. Despite the well-known physiological role of plasminogen in the fibrinolysis system and the expectation that defects in plasminogen synthesis reduce clot lysis and contribute to a prothrombotic tendency [25], only a small number of authors find clinical expression of thrombosis in patients with severe hypoplasminogenemia [25–27]. Plasminogen deficiency is considered a rare cause of thrombophilia, and as an individual defect, it does not represent a strong thrombotic risk factor [28].

In our study, even though the mean values of PAI-1 in hyperthyroid patients were higher than those of the euthyroid group ($4.81 \pm 1.56$ U/mL), statistical analysis did not reveal a significant difference between these two groups. The activity of the endogenous fibrinolytic system depends on the balance between plasminogen activators and inhibitors, with PAI-1 being the most significant. It is considered that elevated plasma PAI-1 concentrations alongside fibrinolysis suppression and findings of increased plasma levels of FVIII, vWF, fibrinogen, t-PA, and D-dimer lead to an additional risk of the occurrence of myocardial infarction [5,29]. Dysfunction of the fibrinolytic system may also play a role in the pathogenesis of venous thromboembolism. Increased concentrations of PAI-1 are observed in over 40% of patients with venous thromboembolism [30].

*4.5. Anticardiolipin Antibodies and Thrombosis*

Considering hemostatic prothrombotic factors in patients with thyroid dysfunction, some authors emphasize the possibility of the influence of elevated levels of anticardiolipin antibodies on the occurrence of a prothrombotic state in hyperthyroid patients [15]. In our study, patients with hyperthyroidism had a significantly higher rate of positive titer of aCLA in the IgM class compared to hypothyroid patients and euthyroid controls. Some authors consider aCLA of the IgM class, especially when present in low titers, to be nonpathogenic, unlike the findings of IgG or IgA class aCLA, which are persistently found at higher titers in patients with thromboembolic diseases. However, there are studies that also link IgM aCLA to the occurrence of thrombotic events [31]. Despite the possible explanation that elevated levels of IgM class anticardiolipin antibodies represent an epiphenomenon reflecting the immune background of hyperthyroidism, it is also possible that this factor may contribute to the development of a prothrombotic tendency in patients with hyperthyroidism. Elevated levels of anticardiolipin antibodies, whether in high or low titers, are associated with the occurrence of myocardial infarction and cerebrovascular insult, while only high positive titers of anticardiolipin antibodies are associated with the development of deep vein thrombosis [32]. In our study, among patients with hyperthyroidism there was a low rate of positive IgG anticardiolipin antibodies, and no significant differences were found compared to the hypothyroid patients.

*4.6. Atrial Fibrillation in Patients with Hyperthyroidism*

In our study, AF was significantly more common in patients with hyperthyroidism than in patients with hypothyroidism and euthyroid controls. In a Danish registry with over 40,000 patients with hyperthyroidism, as in our study, AF or Afl was registered in 8.3% of patients within 30 days of the hyperthyroidism diagnosis (11). In studies by other authors, AF is recorded in 10–30% of patients with thyrotoxicosis of all age groups [33,34]. The data indicating that our patients with hyperthyroidism and electrocardiographically registered AF were significantly ($p = 0.012$) older (average age $62.2 \pm 17.4$ years) than patients with hyperthyroidism without AF (average age $41.63 \pm 12.3$ years) are consistent with well-established facts that the incidence of AF in hyperthyroid individuals increases with age. In certain studies, the incidence of AF in hyperthyroid patients older than 60 years has been estimated to be between 25–45% in these individuals [33–35]. Highlighting the data on the danger of thyrotoxic AF in older individuals should not overshadow the risk of complications in younger patients with the same disease. Results from a study involving 3176 adults with hyperthyroidism and 25,408 euthyroid young adults (18–44 years old), monitored over 5 years, indicate a 1.44 times higher risk of ischemic stroke among the thyrotoxic population. Hyperthyroidism is associated with a prothrombotic state and ischemic stroke independently of AF or flutter findings. Undocumented paroxysmal AF may also contribute to embolic phenomena [8,34].

Various studies estimate the incidence of thrombosis in hyperthyroid states ranging from 8% to 40%, with cerebral embolization being the most commonly registered event [8]. Findings from other authors indicate that thyrotoxic AF is associated with an increased risk of embolization compared to non-thyrotoxic AF [33,34,36–38]. The rate of thromboembolic episodes in patients with hyperthyroidism varies from 8.5% to 18.1% in the Hurley et al. study [33,35]. Of the overall of thromboembolic episodes, 53% are cerebral embolism [33]. In our study group, two patients (3.1%) experienced cerebral infarctions—one hyperthyroid patient with AF and one patient with hyperthyroidism in a sinus rhythm. Results from certain studies indicate the association between hyperthyroid prothrombotic conditions and ischemic stroke independently of registered atrial tachycardia, despite the possibility that certain episodes of paroxysmal AF remain undiagnosed [8].

Although AF is a known risk factor for cardio-embolism, the presence of the hypercoagulability parameters in hyperthyroidism further contributes to the occurrence of thrombotic complications [39]. In other words, the thromboembolic potential of patients depends not only on their predisposition to thromboembolic complications with AF, but is significantly enhanced by the endogenous prothrombotic biochemical milieu resulting from high levels of thyroid hormones [39]. In addition to the mentioned data on cerebral and peripheral arterial thromboembolism in patients with hyperthyroidism, certain studies also indicate the risk of venous thromboembolism in patients with hyperthyroidism. A large population study of 53,418 patients registers that in patients with hyperthyroidism, the risk of pulmonary embolism is 2.31 times higher than the control group during a 5-year follow-up after adjusting for confounding factors [40]. A meta-analysis that included 15 studies up until October 2022 found an increased risk of venous thromboembolism (VTE) even in patients with subclinical hyperthyroidism (OR 1.33, 95% CI: 1.29–1.38) [1].

## 5. Study Limitations

Our study was conducted on a relatively small number of patients, so it would be advisable to perform the investigation on a larger sample. The presence of AF was detected through clinical examination and routine electrocardiographic findings, so the number of patients with AF might be higher if continuous ECG monitoring were used for detection. Correlations of other coagulation and hemostasis parameters not investigated in this study might reveal additional risks of thromboembolism. The use of more sensitive techniques for the diagnosis of ischemic stroke, such as NMR, and high-quality CT diagnostics could further establish the association between fibrinogen levels, other coagulation factors, and ischemic stroke or other thromboembolic events.

## 6. Conclusions

The results of our study indicate the presence of a prothrombotic milieu, in patients with hyperthyroidism, that could potentially lead to an increased incidence of thrombotic complications. The risk of thromboembolism is not only higher in older individuals but also in younger people with hyperthyroidism. High levels of hemostatic factors can lead to multiple clinical forms of thromboembolism, especially in the active phase of the disease. The risk of occurrence of a thrombotic complication is especially pronounced in patients with levels of FVIII exceeding 150%, as well as in patients with positive anticardiolipin antibodies of the IgM class.

Given the lack of clear evidence, despite the fact that ACC/AHA from 2006 classified hyperthyroidism as a moderate risk factor, and considering the omission of this classification in later recommendations, due to a larger number of studies and congruent data indicating a prothrombotic tendency induced by hyperthyroidism, it seems reasonable to recommend starting anticoagulant therapy along with adequate thyrostatic therapy when there are no contraindications. New evidence-based studies would be needed to clarify this clinically important issue.

**Author Contributions:** Conceptualization, N.A. and D.M. (Dagan Matic); Investigation N.A., D.M. (Dragan Matic), Z.L., B.B., D.M. (Danijela Mikovic), M.M., B.J. and L.B.; Data curation, A.U., M.M. and Z.L.; Writing—original draft preparation, N.A. and D.M. (Dragan Matic); Writing—review and editing, N.A., D.M. (Dragan Matic), B.B., D.M. (Danijela Mikovic) and B.J.; Visualization N.A. and D.M. (Dragan Matic); Supervision, N.A. and D.M. (Dragan Matic); Project administration, N.A. and D.M. (Dragan Matic). All authors have read and agreed to the published version of the manuscript.

**Funding:** This research received no external funding.

**Institutional Review Board Statement:** The ethics committee of the University Clinical Center of Serbia approved this study. The number of the approval: 837/9-1. Date of the approval: 25 January 2024.

**Informed Consent Statement:** Not applicable.

**Data Availability Statement:** The data presented in this study are available on request from the corresponding author.

**Conflicts of Interest:** The authors declare no conflicts of interest.

## References

1. Wang, Y.; Ding, C.; Guo, C.; Wang, J.; Liu, S. Association between thyroid dysfunction and venous thromboembolism: A systematic review and meta-analysis. *Medicine* **2023**, *102*, e33301. [CrossRef]
2. Elbers, L.P.B.; Fliers, E.; Cannegieter, S.C. The influence of thyroid function on the coagulation system and its clinical consequences. *J. Thromb. Haemost.* **2018**, *16*, 634–645. [CrossRef] [PubMed]
3. Stuijver, D.J.; van Zaane, B.; Romualdi, E.; Brandjes, D.P.; Gerdes, V.E.; Squizzato, A. The effect of hyperthyroidism on procoagulant, anticoagulant and fibrinolytic factors: A systematic review and meta-analysis. *Thromb. Haemost.* **2012**, *108*, 1077–1088. [PubMed]
4. Debeij, J.; van Zaane, B.; Dekkers, O.M.; Doggen, C.J.; Smit, J.W.; van Zanten, A.P.; Brandjes, D.P.; Büller, H.R.; Gerdes, V.E.; Rosendaal, F.R.; et al. High levels of procoagulant factors mediate the association between free thyroxine and the risk of venous thrombosis: The MEGA study. *J. Thromb. Haemost.* **2014**, *12*, 839–846. [CrossRef]
5. Davis, P.J.; Mousa, S.A.; Schechter, G.P. New Interfaces of Thyroid Hormone Actions with Blood Coagulation and Thrombosis. *Clin. Appl. Thromb. Hemost.* **2018**, *24*, 1014–1019. [CrossRef] [PubMed]
6. Fuster, V.; Rydén, L.E.; Cannom, D.S.; Crijns, H.J.; Curtis, A.B.; Ellenbogen, K.A.; Halperin, J.L.; Le Heuzey, J.Y.; Kay, G.N.; Lowe, J.E.; et al. ACC/AHA/ESC 2006 guidelines for the management of patients with atrial fibrillation: Full Text: A report of the American College of Cardiology/American Heart Association Task Force on practice guidelines and the European Society of Cardiology Committee for Practice Guidelines (Writing Committee to Revise the 2001 guidelines for the management of patients

7. with atrial fibrillation) developed in collaboration with the European Heart Rhythm Association and the Heart Rhythm Society. *Europace* **2006**, *8*, 651–745. [PubMed]
8. Klein, I.; Danzi, S. Thyroid disease and the heart. *Circulation* **2007**, *116*, 725–735. [CrossRef]
9. Traube, E.; Coplan, N.L. Embolic risk in atrial fibrillation that arises from hyperthyroidism: Review of the medical literature. *Tex. Heart Inst. J.* **2011**, *38*, 225–228. [PubMed]
10. Petersen, P. Thromboembolic complications in atrial fibrillation. *Stroke* **1990**, *21*, 4–13. [CrossRef]
11. Versini, M. Thyroid Autoimmunity and Antiphospholipid Syndrome: Not Such a Trivial Association. *Front. Endocrinol.* **2017**, *8*, 175. [CrossRef]
12. Bithell, T.C. The diagnostic approach to the bleeding disorders. In *Wintrobe's Clinical Hematology*; Lee R.G. Lea & Febiger: Philadelphia, PA, USA; London, UK, 1993; pp. 1301–1328.
13. Bithell, T.C. Blood coagulation; fibrinolysis. In *Wintrobe's Clinical Hematology*; Lee R.G. Lea & Febiger: Philadelphia, PA, USA; London, UK, 1993; pp. 592–615.
14. Kellett, H.A.; Sawars, J.S.; Boulton, E.F.; Cholerton, S.; Park, B.K.; Toft, A.D. Problems of anticoagulation with warfarin in hyperthyroidism. *Q. J. Med.* **1986**, *225*, 43–51.
15. Horne, K.M.; Singh, K.K.; Rosenfeld, G.K.; Wesley, R.; Skarulis, C.M.; Merryman, K.P.; Cullinane, A.; Costelo, R.; Patterson, A.; Eggerman, T.; et al. Is thyroid hormone suppression therapy prothrombotic? *J. Clin. Endocrinol. Metab.* **2004**, *89*, 4469–4473. [CrossRef]
16. Tracy, P.R.; Arnold, M.A.; Ettinger, W.; Fried, L.; Meilahn, E.; Savage, P. The relationship of fibrinogen and factor VII and VIII to incident cardiovascular disease and death in the elderly: Result from the cardiovascular health study. *Arterioscler. Thromb. Vasc. Biol.* **1999**, *19*, 1776–1783. [CrossRef]
17. Klein, I.; Levey, G.S. Unusual Manifestation of hypothyroidism. *Arch. Intern. Med.* **1984**, *144*, 123–128. [CrossRef]
18. Li, Y.; Chen, H.; Tan, J.; Wang, X.; Liang, S.; Sun, H. Impaired release of tissue plasminogen activator from the endothelium in Graves' disease-indicator of endothelial dysfunction and reduced fibrinolytic capacity. *Eur. J. Clin. Investig.* **1998**, *28*, 1050–1054. [CrossRef]
19. Homoncik, M.; Alois, G.; Bernd, J.; Heinrich, V. Altered platelet plug formation in hyperthyroidism and hypothyroidism. *J. Clin. Endocrinol. Metab.* **2007**, *92*, 3006–3012. [CrossRef]
20. Thögersen, M.A.; Jansson, J.H.; Boman, K.; Nilsson, K.T.; Weinehall, L.; Huhtasaari, F.; Hallmans, G. High plasminogen activator inhibitor and tissue plasminogen activator levels in plasma precede a first acute myocardial infarction in both men and women. Evidence for the fibrinolytic system as an independent primary risk factor. *Circulation* **1998**, *98*, 2241–2247. [CrossRef]
21. Thompson, S.G.; Kienast, J.; Pyke, S.D.; Haverkate, F.; van den Loo, W.C. Hemostatic factors and the risk of myocardial infarction or sudden death in patients with angina pectoris. *N. Engl. J. Med.* **1995**, *332*, 635–641. [CrossRef] [PubMed]
22. Desforges, J.F. Hematologic manifestations of endocrine disorders. In *Hematology; Basic Principles and Practice*, 2nd ed.; Hoffman, A., Benz, E.J., Shattil, S.J., Furie, B., Cohen, J.H., Silberstein, L.E., Eds.; Churchill Livingstone: New York, NY, USA, 1995; pp. 2155–2156.
23. Ma, J.; Hannekens, H.C.; Ridkrer, P.M.; Stamfer, J.M. A prospective study of fibrinogen and risk of myocardial infarction in the physicians Health study. *J. Am. Coll. Cardiol.* **1999**, *33*, 1347–1352. [CrossRef] [PubMed]
24. Dörr, M.; Wolf, B.; Robinson, M.D.; John, U.; Lüdeman, J.; Meg, W.; Felix, B.S.; Wölzke, H. The association of thyroid function with cardiac mass and left ventricular hypertrophy. *J. Clin. Endocrinol. Metab.* **2005**, *90*, 673–677. [CrossRef] [PubMed]
25. Triplett, D.A. Protein S deficiency. In *Disorders of Haemostasis and Thrombosis*; Goodnight, S.H., Hathaway, W.E., Eds.; The McGraw-Hill Companies: New York, NY, USA, 2001; pp. 374–380.
26. Squizzato, A.; Romualdi, E.; Büller, H.R.; Gerdes, V.E. Clinical review: Thyroid dysfunction and effects on coagulation and fibrinolysis: A systematic review. *J. Clin. Endocrinol. Metab.* **2007**, *92*, 2415–2420. [CrossRef]
27. Bovill, E.G. Fibrinolytic defects and thrombosis. In *Disorders of Haemostasis and Thrombosis*; Goodnight, S.H., Hathaway, W.E., Eds.; The McGraw-Hill Companies: New York, NY, USA, 2001; pp. 389–396.
28. Kohler, P.H.; Grant, J.P. Plasminogen-activator inhibitor type 1 and coronary artery disease. *N. Engl. J. Med.* **2000**, *342*, 1792–1801. [CrossRef]
29. Tofler, G.H.; D'Agostino, R.B.; Jacques, P.F.; Bostom, A.G.; Wilson, P.W.; Lipinska, I.; Mittleman, M.A.; Selhub, J. Association between increases homocysteine levels and impaired fibrinolytic potential: Potential mechanism for cardiovascular risk. *Thromb. Haemost.* **2002**, *88*, 799–804.
30. Hamsten, A.; Walldius, G.; Szamosi, A.; Blombäck, M.; de Faire, U.; Dahlén, G.; Landou, C.; Wiman, B. Plasminogen activator inhibitors in plasma: Risk factor for recurrent myocardial infarction. *Lancet* **1987**, *8549*, 3–9. [CrossRef]
31. Bauer, K.A. Hypercoagulable states. In *Hematology: Basic Principles and Practice*; Hoffman, R., Benz, E.J., Shattil, S.J., Furie, B., Cohen, H.J., Silberstein, L.E., McGlave, P., Eds.; Elsevier Churchill Livingstone: Philadelphia, PA, USA, 2005; pp. 2197–2224.
32. Rand, J.H.; Senzel, L. Antiphospholipid antiboidies and the antiphospholipid syndrome. In *Haemostasis and Thrombosis: Basic Principles and Clinical Practice*; Colman, R.W., Clowes, A.W., Goldhaber, S.Z., Marder, V.J., George, J.N., Eds.; Lippincott Williams&Wilkins: Philadelphia, PA, USA, 2006; pp. 1621–1636.
33. McCrae, K.R.; Feinstein, D.I.; Cines, D.B. Antiphospholipid antibodies and the antiphospholipid syndrome. In *Haemostasis and Thrombosis: Basic Principles and Clinical Practice*; Colman, R.W., Hirsh, J., Marder, V.J., Clowes, A.W., George, J.N., Eds.; Lippincott Williams&Wilkins: Philadelphia, PA, USA, 2001; pp. 1339–1356.

33. Petersen, P.; Hansen, M.J. Stroke in thyrotoxicosis with atrial fibrilation. *Stroke* **1989**, *19*, 15–18. [CrossRef]
34. Sheu, J.J.; Kang, J.H.; Lin, H.C.; Lin, H.C. Hyperthyroidism and risk of ischemic stroke in young adults: A 5-year follow-up study. *Stroke* **2010**, *5*, 961–966. [CrossRef] [PubMed]
35. Staffurth, J.S.; Gibberd, M.C.; Fui, S.N. Arterial embolism in thyrotoxicosis with atrial fibrillation. *Br. Med. J.* **1977**, *2*, 688–690. [CrossRef] [PubMed]
36. Parker, L.J.; Lawson, D.H. Death from thyrotoxicosis. *Lancet* **1973**, *2*, 894–895. [CrossRef]
37. Parle, V.J.; Maisonneuve, P.; Sheppard, C.M.; Boyle, P.; Franklyn, A.J. Prediction of all-cause and cardiovascular mortality in elderly people from one low serum thyrothropin result: A 10-year cohort study. *Lancet* **2001**, *358*, 861–865. [CrossRef]
38. Siu, C.W.; Pong, V.; Zhang, X.; Siu, C.W.; Pong, V.; Zhang, X.; Chan, Y.H.; Jim, M.H.; Liu, S.; Yiu, K.H.; et al. Risk of ischemic stroke after new-onset atrial fibrillation in patients with hyperthyroidism. *Heart Rhythm* **2009**, *6*, 169–173. [CrossRef] [PubMed]
39. Rietveld, I.M.; Lijfering, W.M.; le Cessie, S.; Bos, M.H.A.; Rosendaal, F.R.; Reitsma, P.H.; Cannegieter, S.C. High levels of coagulation factors and venous thrombosis risk: Strongest association for factor VIII and von Willebrand factor. *J. Thromb. Haemost.* **2019**, *17*, 99–109. [CrossRef] [PubMed]
40. Lin, H.C.; Yang, Y.; Kan, H. Increased risk of pulmonary embolism among patients with hyperthyroidism: A 5-year follow-up study. *J. Thromb. Haemost.* **2010**, *8*, 2176–2181. [CrossRef] [PubMed]

**Disclaimer/Publisher's Note:** The statements, opinions and data contained in all publications are solely those of the individual author(s) and contributor(s) and not of MDPI and/or the editor(s). MDPI and/or the editor(s) disclaim responsibility for any injury to people or property resulting from any ideas, methods, instructions or products referred to in the content.

MDPI
St. Alban-Anlage 66
4052 Basel
Switzerland
www.mdpi.com

*Journal of Clinical Medicine* Editorial Office
E-mail: jcm@mdpi.com
www.mdpi.com/journal/jcm

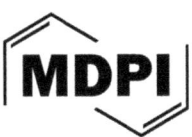

Disclaimer/Publisher's Note: The statements, opinions and data contained in all publications are solely those of the individual author(s) and contributor(s) and not of MDPI and/or the editor(s). MDPI and/or the editor(s) disclaim responsibility for any injury to people or property resulting from any ideas, methods, instructions or products referred to in the content.